PRINCIPLES OF INTERNAL MEDICINE

TWELFTH EDITION

COMPANION HANDBOOK

Editors

JEAN D. WILSON

EUGENE BRAUNWALD

KURT J. ISSELBACHER

ROBERT G. PETERSDORF

JOSEPH B. MARTIN

ANTHONY S. FAUCI

RICHARD K. ROOT

McGRAW-HILL BOOK COMPANY
Health Professions Division

New York St. Louis San Francisco Auckland Bogotá Caracas
Colorado Springs Hamburg Lisbon London Madrid Mexico
Milan Montreal New Delhi Paris San Juan São Paulo
Singapore Sydney Tokyo Toronto

NOTICE
Medicine is an ever-changing science. As new research and clinical experience broaden our knowledge, changes in treatment and drug therapy are required. The editors and the publisher of this work have made every effort to ensure that the drug dosage schedules herein are accurate and in accord with the standards accepted at the time of the publication. Readers are advised, however, to check the product information sheet included in the package of each drug they plan to administer to be certain that changes have not been made in the recommended dose or in the contraindications for administration. This recommendation is of particular importance in regard to new or infrequently used drugs.

Harrison's
Principles of Internal Medicine
Twelfth Edition
Companion Handbook

1234567890   DOCDOC   9654321

ISBN 0-07-081208-X

This book was set in Times Roman by Monotype Composition Company. The editors were J. Dereck Jeffers and Stuart D. Boynton; the production supervisor was Clare Stanley; the designer was Marsha Cohen. The index was prepared by Irving Conde Tullar.
R. R. Donnelley & Sons Company was printer and binder.

Library of Congress Cataloging-in-Publication Data

Harrison's principles of internal medicine, twelfth
  edition. Companion handbook / editors, Jean D. Wilson . . . [et al.].
     p.   cm.
  An extension of: Harrison's principles of internal medicine, 12th ed. © 1991.
  Includes bibliographical references and index.
  ISBN 0-07-081208-X
  1. Internal medicine—Handbooks, manuals, etc. I. Harrison, Tinsley Randolph, date   . II. Wilson, Jean D., date   . III. Principles of internal medicine.
  [DNLM: 1. Internal Medicine—handbooks. WB 115 P957 Suppl.]
RC46.H333   1991 Suppl. 2
616—dc20
DNLM/DLC
for Library of Congress   90-13683
                                                              CIP

ABBREVIATED CONTENTS

CONTENTS

SECTION 3

INFECTIOUS DISEASES

SECTION 4

CARDIOVASCULAR DISEASES

SECTION 5

RESPIRATORY DISEASES

SECTION 6

RENAL DISEASE

SECTION 10

ENDOCRINOLOGY AND METABOLISM

SECTION 11

NEUROLOGY

SECTION 12

PSYCHIATRIC AND DEPENDENCY DISORDERS

SECTION 13

DERMATOLOGY

SECTION 14

NUTRITION

SECTION 15

SECTION 16

LIST OF CONTRIBUTORS

Numbers in parentheses indicate the chapters for which each contributor is responsible.

EUGENE BRAUNWALD, A.B., M.D., M.A. (Hon.), M.D. (Hon.) (2, 10–13, 23–25, 66–72, 74–83, 85–91, 129, 130, 189)
Hersey Professor of the Theory and Practice of Medicine, Harvard Medical School; Chairman, Department of Medicine, Brigham and Women's Hospital, Boston

STEVEN I. CHUCK, M.D. (6, 30, 32, 33, 35–65, 84, 98, 160, 161)
Fellow in Infectious Disease, Department of Medicine; School of Medicine, University of California at San Francisco, San Francisco

ANTHONY S. FAUCI, M.D. (22, 31, 115–128, 136–139, 181–183)
Director, National Institute of Allergy and Infectious Disease; Chief, Laboratory of Immunoregulation; Director, Office of AIDS Research, National Institutes of Health, Bethesda

LAWRENCE S. FRIEDMAN, M.D. (17, 19, 103, 104, 106, 108, 111–114)
Associate Professor of Medicine and Vice Chairman of the Department, Jefferson Medical College, Thomas Jefferson University, Philadelphia

KURT J. ISSELBACHER, M.D. (3, 14, 16–19, 103–114, 131–135)
Mallinckrodt Professor of Medicine, Harvard Medical School; Director, Cancer Center, Massachusetts General Hospital, Boston

ELIZABETH P. JENKINS, M.D. (15, 20, 21, 28, 34, 92–97, 99–102, 140–153, 184–188)
Fellow in Endocrinology and Metabolism, Department of Internal Medicine, University of Texas Southwestern Medical Center, Dallas

LEE M. KAPLAN, M.D., Ph.D. (3, 16, 18, 107, 110)
Assistant Professor of Medicine, Harvard Medical School, Boston

WALTER KOROSHETZ, M.D. (8, 9, 26, 29, 159, 174–177, 180)
Instructor in Neurology, Harvard Medical School, Boston

LEONARD S. LILLY, M.D. (2, 13, 23–25, 66–72, 74–79)
Assistant Professor of Medicine, Harvard Medical School, Boston

JOSEPH B. MARTIN, M.D., Ph.D., F.R.C.P.(C), M.A. (Hon) (1, 4, 5, 27, 164, 169, 172, 179)
Professor of Neurology and Dean, School of Medicine, University of California at San Francisco, San Francisco

NORMAN S. NISHIOKA, M.D. (14, 105, 109)
Assistant Professor of Medicine, Harvard Medical School; Assistant in Medicine, Massachusetts General Hospital, Boston

RICHARD K. ROOT, M.D. (6, 30, 32, 33, 35–65, 73, 84, 98, 160, 161)
Associate Dean for Clinical Education, School of Medicine, University of California at San Francisco, San Francisco

M. ELIZABETH ROSS, M.D., Ph.D. (7, 155, 156, 158, 166, 167, 169)
Assistant Professor of Neurology, University of Minnesota School of Medicine, Minneapolis

ROBERT I. TEPPER, M.D. (131–135)
Assistant Professor of Medicine, Harvard Medical School, Boston

KENNETH TYLER, M.D. (154, 157, 162, 163, 165, 170, 173, 179)
Assistant Professor of Neurology, Harvard Medical School, Boston

J. WOODROW WEISS, M.D. (10–12, 80–83, 85–91)
Assistant Professor of Medicine, Harvard Medical School, Boston

JEAN D. WILSON, M.D. (15, 20, 21, 28, 34, 92–97, 99–102, 140–153, 184–188)
Charles C. Sprague Professor of Internal Medicine, The University of Texas Southwestern Medical Center, Dallas

K. RANDALL YOUNG, M.D. (22, 31, 115–128, 136–139, 181–183)
Assistant Professor of Medicine, Uiversity of Alabama–Birmingham Medical Center, Birmingham

PREFACE

Most students of medicine are overwhelmed by the sheer quantity of medical information potentially applicable to the diagnosis and treatment of patients. The editors and authors summarize this vast amount of information in *Harrison's Principles of Internal Medicine,* which is revised and updated every three to four years. Although *HPIM* represents a distillate of the broad field of internal medicine, along with its deep roots in the basic sciences, the total information presented in the book grows steadily, as does the base of useful medical knowledge.

While it would be ideal to have a copy of *HPIM* available at all times, the sheer bulk and weight of the book make this impractical. The editors, with the aid of selected contributors, have condensed the clinical portions of *HPIM* into this pocket-sized *Companion Handbook* which residents and students can carry through the inpatient, outpatient, and emergency services of a teaching hospital. The *Companion Handbook* contains brief summaries of the key features of the diagnosis and treatment of the principal diseases that are likely to be encountered on a medical service. The inside cover (front and back) contain a glossary listing the abbreviations used throughout the book.

It is important to emphasize that the *Companion Handbook* should not and cannot be a replacement for a textbook of internal medicine. Rather it is an extension of the Twelfth Edition of *HPIM*. The *Companion Handbook* is meant to be used when the house officer or student requires a brief introduction to or reminder of some aspect of clinical medicine but does not have immediate access to or the time to consult *HPIM*. Since the amount of material presented is too brief to stand on its own, it is recommended that the relevant subjects in a standard text book be consulted as soon as time permits. Thus, we consider the two books, *HPIM* and the *Companion Handbook*, a single educational package.

THE EDITORS

SECTION 1 IMPORTANT SYMPTOMS AND SIGNS

1 PAIN AND ITS MANAGEMENT

Pain is the most common symptom of disease. Its management depends on determining its cause and alleviating triggering and potentiating factors.

ORGANIZATION OF PAIN PATHWAYS (See HPIM-12, Fig. 15-1.) Pain-producing (nociceptive) sensory stimuli in skin and viscera activate nerve endings of bipolar neurons of spinal dorsal root or cranial nerve ganglia. After synapse in cord or medulla, crossed ascending pathways reach thalamus and are projected to cortex. An indirect multisynaptic afferent system connects with brainstem reticular formation and projects to intralaminar and medial thalamic nuclei and limbic system. Pain transmission is regulated at the dorsal horn level by descending bulbospinal pathways that contain serotonin, norepinephrine, and several neuropeptides.

Agents that modify pain perception may act to reduce tissue inflammation (glucocorticoids, NSAIDs, prostaglandin synthesis inhibitors), to interfere with pain transmission (narcotics), or to enhance descending modulation (tricyclic antidepressants). Anticonvulsants (phenytoin, carbamazepine) may alter aberrant pain sensations arising from neurogenic sources, e.g., demyelination of peripheral nerves.

EVALUATION Pain may be of *somatic* (skin, deep tissues, joints, muscles) or *neuropathic* (injury to nerves, spinal cord pathways, or thalamus) origin. Characteristics of each are summarized in Table 1-1.

Sensory symptoms and signs in neuropathic pain are described by the following definitions: *neuralgia:* pain in distribution of a single nerve, as in trigeminal neuralgia; *dysesthesia:* spontaneous background pain of aching, burning quality; *hyperalgesia* and *hyperesthesia:* exaggerated responses to nociceptive or touch stimulus, respectively; *allodynia:* perception of nonnociceptive stimulus as painful, as when vibration evokes painful sensation. Reduced pain

TABLE 1-1 Characteristics of somatic and neuropathic pain

Somatic pain:
   Nociceptive stimulus usually evident.
   Usually well localized; visceral pain may be referred.
   Similar to other somatic pains in pt's experience.
   Relieved by anti-inflammatory or narcotic analgesics.

Neuropathic pain:
   No obvious nociceptive stimulus.
   Often poorly localized.
   Unusual, dissimilar from somatic pain.
   Only partially relieved by narcotic analgesics.

Modified from Maciewicz R, Martin JB: HPIM-12, p. 94.

perception is called *hypalgesia* or, when absent, *analgesia*. *Causalgia* is continuous severe burning pain with indistinct boundaries and accompanying sympathetic nervous system dysfunction (sweating, vascular, skin, and hair changes—sympathetic dystrophy) that occurs after injury to a peripheral nerve.

MANAGEMENT Acute somatic pain Usually effectively treated with nonnarcotic analgesic agents (Table 1-2). Narcotic analgesics are usually required for relief of severe pain.

Neuropathic pain Often chronic; management is particularly difficult. The following drugs, in combination with careful assessment of underlying factors that contribute to pain (depression, "compensation neurosis"), may be beneficial:

1. Anticonvulsants: In pts with neuropathic pain and little or no evidence of sympathetic dysfunction; diabetic neuropathy, trigeminal neuralgia (tic douloureux).

2. Antisympathetic agents: In pts with causalgia and sympathetic dystrophy, surgical or chemical sympathectomy may be tried (see HPIM-12, Chap. 15).

3. Tricyclic antidepressants: Pharmacologic effects include facilitation of monoamine neurotransmitters by inhibition of transmitter reuptake. Are useful in management of pts with chronic pain, postherpetic neuralgia, atypical facial pain (see Chap. 4), chronic low back pain (see Chap. 5).

For a more detailed discussion, see Maciewicz R, Martin JM: Pain: Pathophysiology and Management, Chap. 15 in HPIM-12, p. 93

TABLE 1-2 Drugs used to relieve pain

Nonnarcotic analgesics		
Generic name	PO dose, mg	Interval
Aspirin	650	q 4 h
Acetaminophen	650	q 4 h
Ibuprofen	400	q 4–6 h
Naproxen	250–500	q 12 h
Indomethacin	25–50	q 8 h

Narcotic analgesics		
Generic name	Parenteral dose, mg	PO dose, mg
Codeine	30–60 q 4 h	30–60 q 4 h
Oxycodone	—	5–10 q 4–6 h
Morphine	10 q 4 h	60 q 4 h
Hydromorphone	1–2 q 4 h	2–4 q 4 h
Levorphanol	2 q 6–8 h	4 q 6–8 h
Methadone	10 q 6–8 h	20 q 6–8 h
Meperidine	75–100 q 3–4 h	300 q 4 h

Anticonvulsants		
Generic name	PO dose, mg	Interval
Phenytoin	100	q 6–8 h
Carbamazepine	200–300	q 6 h
Clonazepam	1	q 6 h

Antidepressants		
Generic name	PO dose, mg/d	Range, mg/d
Doxepin	200	75–400
Amitriptyline	150	75–300
Imipramine	200	75–400
Nortriptyline	100	40–150
Desipramine	150	75–300

2 CHEST PAIN

There is little correlation between the severity of chest pain and the seriousness of its cause.

POTENTIALLY SERIOUS CAUSES

MYOCARDIAL ISCHEMIA Angina pectoris (Chap. 75) Substernal pressure, squeezing, constriction, with radiation typically to left arm; usually on exertion, especially after meals or with emotional arousal. Characteristically relieved by rest and nitroglycerin.

Acute myocardial infarction (Chap. 74) Similar to angina but more severe, of longer duration (≥ 30 min), and not immediately relieved by rest or nitroglycerin. S_3 and S_4 common.

PULMONARY EMBOLISM (Chap. 85) May be substernal or lateral, pleuritic in nature, and associated with hemoptysis, tachycardia, hypoxemia.

AORTIC DISSECTION (Chap. 78) Very severe, in center of chest, a "ripping quality," radiates to back, not affected by changes in position. May be associated with weak or absent peripheral pulses.

MEDIASTINAL EMPHYSEMA Sharp, intense, localized to substernal region; often associated with audible crepitus.

ACUTE PERICARDITIS (Chap. 76) Usually steady, crushing, substernal; often has pleuritic component aggravated by cough, deep inspiration, supine position, and relieved by sitting upright; one-, two-, or three-component pericardial friction rub often audible.

PLEURISY Due to inflammation; less commonly tumor and pneumothorax. Usually unilateral, knifelike, superficial, aggravated by cough and respiration.

LESS SERIOUS CAUSES

COSTOCHONDRAL PAIN In anterior chest, usually sharply localized, may be brief and darting or a persistent dull ache. Can be reproduced by pressure on costochondral and/or chondrosternal junctions. In Tietze's syndrome (costochondritis), joints are swollen, red, and tender.

CHEST WALL PAIN Due to strain of muscles or ligaments from excessive exercise or rib fracture from trauma; accompanied by local tenderness.

ESOPHAGEAL PAIN Deep thoracic discomfort; may be accompanied by dysphagia and regurgitation.

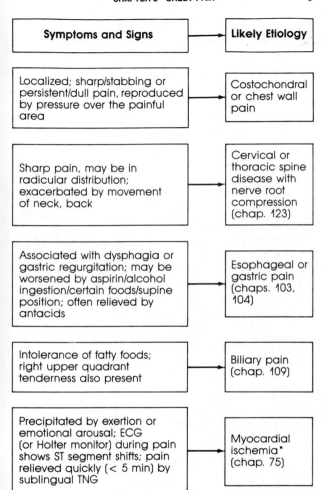

Symptoms and Signs	Likely Etiology
Localized; sharp/stabbing or persistent/dull pain, reproduced by pressure over the painful area	Costochondral or chest wall pain
Sharp pain, may be in radicular distribution; exacerbated by movement of neck, back	Cervical or thoracic spine disease with nerve root compression (chap. 123)
Associated with dysphagia or gastric regurgitation; may be worsened by aspirin/alcohol ingestion/certain foods/supine position; often relieved by antacids	Esophageal or gastric pain (chaps. 103, 104)
Intolerance of fatty foods; right upper quadrant tenderness also present	Biliary pain (chap. 109)
Precipitated by exertion or emotional arousal; ECG (or Holter monitor) during pain shows ST segment shifts; pain relieved quickly (< 5 min) by sublingual TNG	Myocardial ischemia* (chap. 75)

* If myocardial ischemia suspected, also consider aortic valve disease (chap. 71) and hypertrophic obstructive cardiomyopathy (chap. 77) if systolic murmur present.

FIGURE 2-1 Differential diagnosis of recurrent chest pain.

	Acute myocardial infarction (chap. 74)	Aortic dissection (chap. 78)	Acute pericarditis (chap. 76)	Pulmonary embolism (chap. 85)	Acute pneumothorax (chap. 88)	Rupture of esophagus
Description of Pain	Oppressive, constrictive, or squeezing; may radiate to arm(s), neck, back	"Tearing" or "ripping"; may travel from anterior chest to mid-back	Crushing, sharp, pleuritic; relieved by sitting forward	Pleuritic, sharp; possibly accompanied by cough/hemoptysis	Very sharp, pleuritic	Intense substernal and epigastric; accompanied by vomiting ± hematemesis
Background history	Less severe, similar pain on exertion; + coronary risk factors (chap. 75)	Hypertension or Marfan's syndrome (chap. 118)	Recent upper respiratory tract infection, or other conditions which predispose to pericarditis (chap. 76)	Recent surgery or other immobilization	Recent chest trauma, or history of chronic obstructive lung disease	Recent recurrent vomiting/retching
Key Physical findings	Diaphoresis, pallor; S4 common; S3 less common	Weak, asymmetric peripheral pulses; possible diastolic murmur of aortic insufficiency (chap. 71)	Pericardial friction rub (usually 3 components, best heard by sitting patient forward)	Tachypnea; possible pleural friction rub	Tachypnea; breath sounds & hyperresonance over affected lung field	Subcutaneous emphysema; audible crepitus adjacent to the sternum
Consider	Acute myocardial infarction (chap. 74)	Aortic dissection (chap. 78)	Acute pericarditis (chap. 76)	Pulmonary embolism (chap. 85)	Acute pneumothorax (chap. 88)	Rupture of esophagus
Confirmatory Tests	• Serial ECGs • Serial cardiac enzymes (esp. CK, LDH)	• CXR—widened mediastinal silhouette • MRI, CT, or echogram: intimal flap visualized • Aortic angiogram: definitive diagnosis	• ECG: diffuse ST elevation and PR segment depression • Echogram: pericardial effusion often visualized	• Arterial blood gas: hypoxemia & respiratory alkalosis • Lung scan: V/Q mismatch • Pulmonary angiogram: arterial luminal filling defects	• CXR: radiolucency within pleural space; poss. collapse of adjacent lung segment; if tension pneumothorax, mediastinum is shifted to opp. side	• CXR: pneumomediastinum • Esophageal endoscopy is diagnostic

EMOTIONAL DISORDERS   Prolonged ache or dartlike, brief, flashing pain; associated with fatigue, emotional strain.

OTHER CAUSES

(1) Cervical disk; (2) osteoarthritis of cervical or thoracic spine; (3) abdominal disorders: peptic ulcer, hiatus hernia, pancreatitis, biliary colic; (4) tracheobronchitis, pneumonia; (5) diseases of the breast (inflammation, tumor); (6) intercostal neuritis (herpes zoster)

APPROACH TO THE PATIENT

A meticulous history of the behavior of pain, what precipitates it and what relieves it, aids diagnosis of recurrent chest pain (Fig. 2–1). Figure 2–2 presents clues to diagnosis and workup of acute, life-threatening chest pain.

For a more detailed discussion, see Goldman L, Braunwald E: Chest Discomfort and Palpitation, Chap. 16, in HPIM-12, p. 98

---

3 ABDOMINAL PAIN

Numerous causes, ranging from acute, life-threatening emergencies to chronic functional disease and disorders of several organ systems can generate abdominal pain. Evaluation of acute pain requires rapid assessment of likely causes and early initiation of appropriate therapy. A more detailed and leisurely approach to diagnosis may be followed in less acute situations. Table 3-1 lists the common causes of abdominal pain.

APPROACH TO THE PATIENT WITH ABDOMINAL PAIN

History Extremely important. Physical examination may be unrevealing or misleading and laboratory and radiologic exams delayed or unhelpful.

Characteristic features of abdominal pain *Duration and pattern* Provide clues to nature and severity, although acute abdominal crisis may occasionally present insidiously or on background of chronic pain.

Type and location provide rough guide to nature of disease. *Visceral pain* (due to distention of a hollow viscus) localizes poorly and is often perceived in the midline. Intestinal pain tends to be crampy; when originating proximal to the ileocecal valve, it usually localizes above and around the umbilicus. Pain of colonic origin is perceived in the hypogastrium and lower quadrants. Pain from biliary or ureteral obstruction often causes patients to writhe in discomfort. *Somatic pain* (due to peritoneal inflammation) is usually sharper and more precisely localized to the diseased region (e.g., acute appendicitis, capsular distention of liver, kidney, or spleen), exacerbated by movement, causing patients to remain still. Pattern of radiation may be helpful: right shoulder (hepatobiliary origin), left shoulder (splenic), midback (pancreatic), flank (proximal urinary tract), groin (genital or distal urinary tract).

Factors that precipitate or relieve pain Relationship to eating (e.g., upper gastrointestinal, biliary, pancreatic, ischemic bowel disease), defecation (colorectal), urination (genitourinary or colorectal), respiratory (pleuropulmonary, hepatobiliary), position (pancreatic, gastroesophageal reflux, musculoskeletal), menstrual cycle/menarche (tuboovarian, endometrial, including endometriosis), exertion (coronary/intestinal ischemia, musculoskeletal), medication/specific foods

TABLE 3-1 Common etiologies of abdominal pain

Mucosal or muscle inflammation in hollow viscera: Acid-peptic disease (ulcers, erosions, inflammation), hemorrhagic gastritis, gastroesophageal reflux, appendicitis, diverticulitis, cholecystitis, cholangitis, inflammatory bowel diseases (Crohn's, ulcerative colitis, Behçet's), infectious gastroenteritis, mesenteric lymphadenitis, colitis, cystitis, or pyelonephritis

Visceral spasm or distention: Intestinal obstruction (adhesions, tumor, intussusception), appendiceal obstruction with appendicitis, strangulation of hernia, irritable bowel syndrome (muscle hypertrophy and spasm), acute biliary obstruction, pancreatic ductal obstruction (chronic pancreatitis, stone), ureteral obstruction (kidney stone, blood clot), fallopian tubes (tubal pregnancy)

Vascular disorder: Mesenteric thromboembolic disease (arterial or venous), arterial dissection or rupture (e.g., aortic aneurysm), occlusion from external pressure or torsion (e.g., volvulus, hernia, tumor, intussusception), hemoglobinopathy (esp. sickle cell disease)

Distention or inflammation of visceral surfaces: Hepatic capsule (hepatitis, hemorrhage, tumor, Budd-Chiari syndrome, Fitz-Hugh–Curtis syndrome), renal capsular distention (tumor, infection, infarction, venous occlusion), splenic capsular distention (hemorrhage, abscess, infarction), pancreas (pancreatitis, pseudocyst, abscess), ovary (hemorrhage into cyst, ectopic pregnancy, abscess)

Peritoneal inflammation: Bacterial infection (perforated viscus, pelvic inflammatory disease, infected ascites), intestinal infarction, chemical irritation, pancreatitis, perforated viscus (esp. stomach and duodenum, mittelschmerz), reactive inflammation (neighboring abscess, incl. diverticulitis, pleuropulmonary infection or inflammation), serositis (collagen-vascular diseases, familial Mediterranean fever)

Abdominal wall disorders: Trauma, hernias, muscle inflammation or infection, hematoma (trauma, anticoagulant therapy), traction from mesentery (e.g., adhesions)

Toxins: Lead poisoning, black widow spider bite

Metabolic disorders: Uremia, ketoacidosis (diabetic, alcoholic), Addisonian crisis, porphyria, angioedema (C_1 esterase deficiency), narcotic withdrawal

Neurologic: Tabes dorsalis, herpes zoster, causalgia, compression or inflammation of spinal roots, (e.g., arthritis, herniated disk, tumor, abscess), psychogenic

Referred pain: From heart, lungs, esophagus, genitalia (e.g., cardiac ischemia, pneumonia, pneumothorax, pulmonary embolism, esophagitis, esophageal rupture)

(motility disorders, gastroesophageal reflux, porphyria, adrenal insufficiency, ketoacidosis, toxins), stress (motility disorders, acid-peptic disease).

Associated symptoms Fevers/chills (infection, inflammatory disease, infarction), weight loss (tumor, inflammatory diseases, malabsorption, ischemia), nausea/vomiting (obstruction, infection, inflammatory disease, metabolic disease), dysphagia/odynophagia (esophageal), early satiety (gastric), hematemesis (esophageal, gastric, duodenal), constipation (colorectal, perianal, genitourinary), jaundice (hepatobiliary, hemolytic), diarrhea (inflammatory disease, infection, malabsorption, secretory tumors, ischemia, genitourinary), dysuria/hematuria/vaginal or penile discharge (genitourinary), hematochezia (colorectal, urinary), skin/joint/eye disorders (inflammatory disease, infection).

Predisposing factors Family history (inflammatory disease, tumors, pancreatitis), hypertension (ischemia), diabetes mellitus (motility disorders, ketoacidosis), connective tissue disease (motility disorders, serositis), depression (motility disorders, tumors), smoking (ischemia), recent smoking cessation (inflammatory disease), ethanol (motility disorders, hepatobiliary, pancreatic, acid-peptic disease).

Physical examination Evaluate abdomen for prior trauma or surgery, current trauma; abdominal distention, fluid, or air; direct, rebound, and referred tenderness; liver and spleen size; masses, bruits, altered bowel sounds, hernias, arterial masses. Rectal examination for masses, tenderness, blood (gross or occult). Pelvic examination in women is essential. General examination: evaluate for evidence of hemodynamic instability, acid-base disturbances, nutritional deficiency, coagulopathy, arterial occlusive disease, stigmata of liver disease, cardiac dysfunction, lymphadenopathy, and skin lesions.

Routine laboratory and radiologic studies Choices depend on clinical setting. Generally include CBC, serum electrolytes, arterial blood gases, coagulation parameters, serum glucose, and biochemical tests of liver, kidney, and pancreatic function; chest radiographs to determine the presence of diseases involving heart, lung, mediastinum, and pleura; ECG is helpful to exclude referred pain from cardiac disease; plain abdominal radiographs to evaluate bowel displacement, intestinal distention, fluid and gas pattern, free peritoneal air, liver size, and abdominal calcifications (e.g., gallstones, renal stones, chronic pancreatitis).

Special studies May include abdominal ultrasonography (most helpful to visualize biliary ducts, gallbladder, liver, and kidneys); gastrointestinal barium contrast radiographs (barium swallow, upper GI series, small bowel follow-through, barium enema, enteroclysis); upper GI endoscopy, sigmoidoscopy, or colonoscopy; CT or MRI, cholangiography, angiography, and radionuclide scanning. In selected cases, biopsy of the liver, pancreas, or abdominal mass, laparoscopy, and sometimes exploratory laparotomy are required.

ACUTE, CATASTROPHIC ABDOMINAL PAIN

Intense abdominal pain of acute onset or pain associated with syncope, hypotension, or toxic appearance of patient, necessitates rapid yet orderly evaluation. Consider obstruction, perforation or rupture of hollow viscus, dissection or rupture of major blood vessels (esp. aortic aneurysm), ulceration, abdominal sepsis, ketoacidosis, and adrenal crisis.

Brief history and physical exam   Should focus on presence of hypothermia, hyperventilation, cyanosis, direct or rebound abdominal tenderness, pulsating abdominal mass, abdominal bruits, ascites, rectal blood, rectal or pelvic tenderness, evidence of coagulopathy. Useful laboratory studies include hematocrit (may be normal with acute hemorrhage or elevated with dehydration), WBC, arterial blood gases, serum electrolytes, BUN, creatinine, glucose, lipase or amylase, and urinalysis. Radiologic studies should include supine and upright abdominal films (left lateral decubitus view if upright unobtainable) to evaluate bowel caliber and presence of free peritoneal air, cross-table lateral film to assess aortic diameter. Abdominal paracentesis (or peritoneal lavage in cases of trauma) to detect evidence of bleeding or spontaneous peritonitis. Abdominal ultrasound (when readily available) to disclose evidence of abscess, cholecystitis, or hematoma and to determine aortic diameter.

Immediate therapy   Should include intravenous fluids, correction of life-threatening acid-base disturbances, and assessment of need for emergent surgery; careful follow-up with frequent reexamination (when possible, by the same examiner) is essential. Narcotic analgesics may best be withheld pending establishment of diagnosis and therapeutic plan, since masking of diagnostic signs may delay needed intervention.

For a more detailed discussion, see Silen W: Abdominal Pain, Chap. 17, in HPIM-12, p. 105

---

4 HEADACHE AND FACE PAIN

Headache is a common complaint, often chronic or recurrent, signifying either *vascular* (migraine) or *tension* (muscle contraction) origin in most pts. Recurrent headache of either type may be unilateral or generalized. Migraine is commonly stereotyped in presentation (classic, common, or cluster). A classification of causes of headache is given in Table 4-1.

Headaches can occur as a result of: (1) distention, traction, or dilatation of intracranial or extracranial arteries; (2) traction or displacement of intracranial veins or their dural envelope; (3) compression, traction, or inflammation of cranial or upper spinal nerves; (4) spasm, inflammation, and trauma of cranial or cervical muscles; (5) meningeal irritation (infection or subarachnoid hemorrhage); (6) infection or congestion of paranasal sinuses; (7) lesions that affect cranial bones (infections or tumors); or (8) secondary to raised or lowered intracranial pressure.

TABLE 4-1 Classification of headache

   I. Migraine
      A. Common migraine
      B. Classic migraine
      C. Cluster migraine
  II. Tension
 III. Cerebrovascular disease
      A. Hypertension
      B. Subarachnoid hemorrhage
      C. Arteriovenous malformation
      D. Arteritis (temporal artery)
  IV. Meningeal irritation
      A. Meningitis (bacterial or viral)
      B. Encephalitis
   V. Changes in intracranial pressure
      A. Decreased intracranial pressure (post-LP headache)
      B. Increased intracranial pressure
         1. Brain tumor
         2. Venous sinus thrombosis
         3. Benign intracranial hypertension (pseudotumor cerebri)
  VI. Posttraumatic
 VII. Miscellaneous
      A. Coital
      B. Hangover
      C. Diseases of the sinuses (sinusitis) and of the eyes (glaucoma)
      D. Cough
      E. "Ice-pick"
      F. "Ice-cream"

General considerations   The quality, location, duration, and time course of the headache and the conditions that produce, exacerbate, or relieve it should be reviewed. Except for the headache of temporal arteritis and of occipital neuralgia, physical exam of the head is rarely useful.

MIGRAINE

CLASSIC MIGRAINE   The onset is usually in childhood, adolescence, or early adulthood. First attacks occurring in adults after age 50 are described. There is often a positive family history, and migraine is more common in women. The classic triad is visual scotomata or scintillations, unilateral throbbing headache (occurring on either left or right), accompanied by nausea and vomiting. An attack lasting 2–6 h is common, with relief after sleep. Attacks may be triggered by wine, cheese, chocolate, contraceptives, stress, exercise, or travel.

COMMON MIGRAINE   Unilateral (alternating side-to-side) or bilateral headache with nausea, but rarely with vomiting or visual complaints. More common in women. The onset is usually more gradual than in classic migraine, and pain becomes more generalized and may persist for hours or days. Commonly combined with or fades into typical tension headache and differentiation may be difficult.

CLUSTER MIGRAINE   Characterized by recurrent, nocturnal, unilateral, retroorbital searing pain. Typically a young male (90%) awakens 2–4 h after sleep onset with severe pain, accompanied by unilateral lacrimation, and nasal and conjunctival congestion. Visual complaints or nausea and vomiting are rare. Pain lasts 20–60 min and subsides quickly but tends to recur at the same time of night or several times each 24 h over several weeks (a cluster). A pain-free period of months or years may be followed by another cluster of headaches. A cerebral artery berry aneurysm may mimic retroorbital pain.

MUSCLE CONTRACTION (TENSION) HEADACHES

The onset is often in adolescence or young adulthood; nonfamilial. Pain is bilateral, generalized, bitemporal, or suboccipital; usually felt as a pressure or a tight band, but may be throbbing. Nausea and vomiting are rare; no nasal congestion or lacrimation. Tends to occur late in day, related to stress. Headaches may persist for hours or days.

OTHER TYPES OF HEADACHES AND FACIAL PAIN

Headaches associated with *CNS infection* are usually accompanied by fever and stiff neck. *Temporal arteritis* is diagnosed by unilateral or bilateral headache in elderly (occasionally in younger) pts, accompanied by visual loss; tender, swollen temporal arteries; and an elevated ESR. Early diagnosis and treatment are important to preserve vision (compromised due to optic nerve ischemia). *Lumbar puncture* headaches are caused by reduced intracranial pressure and usually subside spontaneously after 5–7 d. Hypertension rarely causes headache. Increased intracranial pressure due to any cause can produce severe headaches, usually with nausea and vomiting. Coital headaches are usually benign but must be distinguished from subarachnoid hemorrhage.

Benign intracranial hypertension   Obese women under age 40; increased CSF pressure without focal neurologic signs, and normal CT or MRI. Treat with acetazolamide, repeat LPs, or in severe cases with optic nerve fenestration (see HPIM-12, p. 2014).

Headaches with onset after age 50   Should alert to possibility of (cranial) temporal arteritis (positive biopsy for giant cell arteritis), brain tumor (personality change, vomiting, papilledema, focal neurologic signs), subdural hematoma (recent fall, altered consciousness).

Trigeminal neuralgia   Stabbing, lancinating pain lasting 10–30 s, unilateral location, most commonly mandibular or (less often) maxillary division of the trigeminal nerve. Pain occurs after age 50. Trigger point in gum or cheek may limit eating. Neurologic exam is normal. Similar pain in younger person may indicate multiple sclerosis, aneurysm or vascular anomaly, or trigeminal neuroma. Treatment with carbamazepine is effective initially in about two-thirds of pts. Therapeutic dose ranges from 600–1400 mg daily. Recurrent or refractory pain is treated surgically with nerve section (see HPIM-12, p. 2077).

Postherpetic (zoster) neuralgia   Pain following herpetic eruptions of ophthalmic, maxillary, or (rarely) mandibular division of trigeminal nerve. May be accompanied by sensory loss (anesthesia dolorosa). Management is difficult but pain usually subsides in 4–8 weeks.

Atypical facial pain   Not restricted to a cranial nerve distribution; generalized; sometimes associated with temporomandibular joint (TMJ) dysfunction.

Occipital neuralgia   Entrapment of greater occipital nerve at exit from skull causing unilateral, lancinating pain in occipital region. Local pain and trigger point usually found over nerve at exit point. Treatment is surgical.

PRINCIPLES OF TREATMENT OF HEADACHE

1. Establish clinical diagnosis.
2. After diagnosis, initiate therapy based on frequency, severity, and incapacitation caused by headache. Therapy for migraine may be directed towards abating or ameliorating an attack or be prophylactic if attacks are severe or frequent.

MIGRAINE   Acute attack; manage with ergotamines, alone or in combination with caffeine or analgesics (aspirin, acetaminophen, or ibuprofen). Treat early with ergotamine tartrate 1–3 mg PO, repeated q 30 min up to 4–6 tablets (6 mg/d or 12 mg/week maximum). Treatment combinations include Cafergot or Wigraine, which contain 1 mg ergotamine tartrate and 100 mg caffeine. Two tablets are given at onset of headache or during aura, if present, followed by another each 30 min to maximum of 6. Rectal suppositories containing ergotamine 1–2 mg may also be beneficial. A second suppository given after 15–30 min may be required to abort an attack. If nausea and vomiting are severe, early administration of metaclopramide, 10 mg, or trimethobenzamide, 200 mg, may be beneficial, followed by ergotamine.

Prophylaxis (Table 4-2)   A number of options exist; frequently need to be given as successive trials to determine most effective drug. Treat pts who experience more than three or four severe attacks each month. Bellergal 1 or 2 tablets daily, propranolol 40 mg tid or qid, amitriptyline 150 mg qhs (start gradually), or calcium channel blockers (nife-

TABLE 4-2   Prophylaxis of migraine

Drug	Daily dose range	Side effects
Ergonovine	0.4–2.0 mg	Nausea, abdominal pain
Bellergal	1–4 tabs	Nausea, sedation
Propranolol	40–320 mg	Lethargy, insomnia, constipation
Amitriptyline	25–150 mg	Sedation, dry mouth
Cyproheptadine	12–24 mg	Sedation, weight gain
Phenelzine	15–75 mg	Insomnia, postural dizziness
Methysergide	2–8 mg	Nausea, abdominal cramps, insomnia, *retroperitoneal fibrosis*
Nifedipine	10–40 mg	Constipation, flushing of skin
Verapamil	320 mg	

dipine 10–40 mg qd or verapamil 80 mg tid). Methysergide may be used in otherwise refractory pts (2 mg q 8 h), but never for more than 4–6 months because of retroperitoneal fibrosis.

TENSION HEADACHES   Acetaminophen, aspirin, or Fiorinal.

TEMPORAL ARTERITIS   Prednisone in doses sufficient to lower ESR to normal (usually 60–120 mg qd × 2–4 weeks, then taper as ESR returns toward normal). Treatment may need to continue for months or years.

For a more detailed discussion, see Martin JB: Headache, Chap. 18, in HPIM-12, p. 108

---

5 LOW BACK PAIN

Pain in the lower back is a common complaint. It may be acute or chronic; it may arise from lesions of spinal column or nerve roots or be referred from deeper structures (kidney, pancreas, colon, pelvic organs, or retroperitoneal tumors).

ETIOLOGY

ACUTE LOW BACK PAIN Acute strain Clear evidence by history of acute trauma. Pain is localized with paraspinal muscular spasm, restriction of movements. There is no radiation of pain to groin or legs.

Vertebral fractures Usually result from flexion injury or fall onto legs; may occur with minimal or no trauma in patients with bone disease, osteoporosis, Cushing's disease, hyperparathyroidism, multiple myeloma, metastatic bone disease, Paget's disease.

Lumbar intervertebral disk protrusion Most common site is L5–S1, then L4–L5, rarely L3–L4 or higher. Clinical findings include backache, abnormal posture, and limitation of movement. Nerve root involvement is indicated by radiating radicular pain, usually unilateral, sensory disturbances (paresthesias, hyperesthesia, or hypalgesia), and impairment of ankle jerk (S1 or S2 root) or rarely of quadriceps reflex (L3–L4). Localizing signs are summarized in Table 5-1. Herniation of an intervertebral disk usually affects the root below the level of the disk; i.e., L4–L5 disk affects L5

TABLE 5-1 Symptoms and signs of disk protrusion

Symptoms and signs	L3–L4 (L4 root)	L4–L5 (L5 root)	L5–S1 (S1 root)
Radicular pain, paresthesias, and/or sensory loss	Medial leg + arch of foot	Dorsum of foot and great toe	Lateral leg, foot and sole, 4th and 5th toes
Weakness or muscle atrophy	Quadriceps	Peroneals and extensor hallucis longus	Gastrocnemius, extensor digitorum brevis
Reflex change	Decreased knee jerk	No change	Decreased ankle jerk
Straight leg raising	May be positive with extension in prone position (reversed)	Positive	Positive

root, L5–S1 disk affects S1 root. Bladder or bowel symptoms usually indicate lesion in conus medullaris of spinal cord or in cauda equina, but large central disc protrusion may also impair these functions.

Facet syndromes   Entrapment of nerve roots at sites of exit from spinal canal may cause radicular pain unrelated to disk disease. Unilateral facet syndrome, which most often affects L5 root, is caused by enlarged superior or inferior facet with narrowing of intervertebral canal or foramen.

Epidural abscess   Occurs most commonly in thoracic region; may cause acute back pain with tenderness to percussion or pressure on spinous process. Requires rapid diagnosis and surgical treatment if spinal cord compression is found (see HPIM-12, p. 2028).

Hip disease   Can cause pain that radiates to buttocks and leg as far as knee.

CHRONIC LOW BACK PAIN   Osteoarthritis   Also called lumbar spondylosis due to degenerative disease of lumbar vertebrae with bony spurs, narrowing of lumbar canal, and impingement on nerve roots. Lumbosacral pain with neurologic symptoms on walking (numbness, paresthesia, or weakness in both legs) suggests syndrome of *intermittent claudication of the spinal cord* due to spinal canal stenosis. Diagnosis is confirmed by CT or MRI or by metrizamide myelography (see HPIM-12, p. 1475).

Ankylosing spondylitis   Presents in young men with low back pain radiating to thighs; 90% are positive for HLA-B27 antigen. Limitation of movement and morning stiffness are followed by limitation of chest expansion, progressive kyphosis, and flexion of thoracic spine. Radiologic hallmarks are destruction and obliteration of the sacroiliac joints and formation of "bamboo" spine. Similar patterns of restricted movements of lower spine may occur in psoriatic arthritis, Reiter's syndrome, and chronic inflammatory bowel disease.

Neoplastic, metastatic, metabolic diseases   Metastatic carcinoma (breast, lung, prostate, thyroid, kidney, GI tract), multiple myeloma, and lymphoma should be excluded by radiologic studies, CT, MRI, or myelography.

Osteomyelitis   From pyogenic bacteria (usually staphylococcus) or tuberculosis; should be considered and excluded by ESR, bone x-rays, tuberculin skin tests.

Intradural tumors   Neurofibromas, meningiomas, and lipomas may cause chronic pain before neurologic findings appear.

REFERRED PAIN FROM VISCERAL DISEASE   Pelvic diseases refer pain to sacral region; lower abdominal diseases, to the lumbar region L3–L5; and upper abdominal diseases, to lower thoracic and upper lumbar region T10–L2. Characteristically, no local signs or stiffness of back; full range of movement of back does not augment pain.

1. Peptic ulcer and tumors of stomach, duodenum, or pancreas, particularly with retroperitoneal involvement, may cause T10–L2 back pain.
2. Ulcerative colitis, diverticulitis, and tumors of colon may cause low back pain.
3. Chronic pelvic inflammatory disease, endometriosis, or carcinoma of the ovary or uterus in women may cause low back pain. In men, chronic prostatitis and prostate carcinoma need to be excluded.
4. Renal disease can cause pain in costovertebral angle.
5. Aortic dissecting aneurysm can cause thoracic-lumbar pain.

MANAGEMENT

Careful attention should be given to onset, duration, location, and factors that exacerbate or alleviate. Examination should include abdomen and pelvic regions, movements of spine, and evidence of neurologic dysfunction. In acute pain, plain radiographs are rarely helpful except after trauma. CT, MRI, and lumbar myelography are used to assess spondylosis, acute herniated disk, and tumor. Chronic pain should be assessed by ESR, serum acid phosphatase, carcinoembryonic antigen, and x-ray studies.

For a more detailed discussion, see Mankin HJ: Back and Neck Pain, Chap. 19, in HPIM-12, p. 116

---

6 CHILLS AND FEVER

GENERAL CONSIDERATIONS

Causes of fever • All infections • Immune mechanisms (connective tissue disorders, drug reactions, AIDS, immune hemolytic anemia) • Vascular inflammation or thrombosis, infarction, or trauma (phlebitis, arteritis, myocardial, pulmonary, or cerebral infarction) • Granulomatous disorders (sarcoid) • Inflammatory bowel disease • Neoplasms (lymphoma, hypernephroma, hepatoma) • Acute metabolic disorders (gout, porphyria, Addisonian or thyroid crises)

Accompaniments of fever • Systemic symptoms (headache, back pain, myalgia) • Chills (differentiate true *shaking* chill from chilly sensations; chills may be evoked by antipyretics) • Herpes labialis (common in pneumococcal, streptococcal, and meningococcal infections) • Delirium (common in old age, alcoholism) • Convulsions (watch for in children)

Management of fever • Do not lower temperature unless very high (heat stroke, delirium, seizures, heart failure) • Cooling blankets; sponging with cool water • If antipyretics (aspirin 0.650 g or acetaminophen 0.5 g) are used, do so around clock (q 2–3 h) to mitigate sweats, abrupt fall in temperature, and compensatory chills with more fever • Glucocorticoids are potent antipyretics; use with caution to prevent abrupt fall in temperature • NSAIDs useful in fever due to neoplasia (see Chap. 33 for treatment of extreme hyperthermia)

Diagnostic considerations • Fever patterns rarely of diagnostic value • In U.S., fever usually due to common diseases • Most febrile illness of short duration

Clues to acute infections • High fever ± chills • Respiratory Sx • Severe malaise • Nausea, vomiting, diarrhea • Acute enlargement of lymph nodes or spleen • Meningeal signs • WBC ≥12,000 or ≤5000 • Dysuria, frequency, flank pain

Fever of unknown origin: prolonged, undiagnosed fever • Temperature ≥38.3°C (≥101°F) for ≥3 weeks • Undiagnosed after 1 week of extensive studies • Rigid criteria eliminate common infections, easily diagnosed diseases, and tandem diseases (e.g., myocardial infarction followed by thrombophlebitis followed by pulmonary emboli)

CAUSES OF PROLONGED FEVER

Infections • Abscesses • Mycobacterial infections (usually extrapulmonary; watch for *Mycobacterium avium-intracellulare* in AIDS) • Renal infections (usually complicated by stone or obstruction) • Other bacterial: sinusitis, vertebral osteomyelitis, infected IV catheters • Subacute bacterial endocarditis (rare cause of fever of unknown origin) • Iatrogenic (watch for IV lines, infected bandages or casts, wounds) • Viral, rickettsial, and chlamydial infections (rare in U.S. in immunocompetent individuals) • Parasitic (obtain travel history)

Neoplasms • Lymphomas of all types • Malignant histiocytosis • Leukemias (telltale cells usually absent at onset) • Solid tumors (usually metastatic to liver) • Atrial myxomas • Renal cell carcinoma

Connective tissue diseases • Systemic lupus erythematosus • Rheumatic fever (now rare) • Rheumatoid arthritis (usually juvenile without joint changes) • Granulomas (nonpulmonary sarcoid, regional enteritis, granulomatous hepatitis)

Miscellaneous • Drug fever (often multiple drugs) • Multiple pulmonary emboli • Cryptic hematomas • Nonspecific pericarditis • Familial Mediterranean fever (ethnic origin; peritonitis; pleuritis; pericarditis; well between episodes; renal failure secondary to amyloidosis now rare; responds to colchicine 0.6 mg 2–3 times per day) • Psychogenic fever [habitual hyperthermia 37.2–38.1°C (99–100.5°F); young women; psychoneurosis; do not do extensive workup] • Factitious fever (malingerers; young women with professional/medical background; prove by personally being in room with thermometer in place; note dissociation of pulse and temperature; refractory to psychotherapy)

Undiagnosed • Some patients' fever is steroid suppressible • Rarely life-threatening

DIAGNOSTIC PROCEDURES

Routine • Must individualize workup • Careful Hx and PE • Hematology, chemistry, and immunologic battery rarely diagnostic • Microbiology; avoid repeated (more than 6) blood cultures; look at Gram and acid-fast bacillus smears; culture for anaerobes (do not withold therapy if otherwise indicated) • Skin tests rarely helpful

Imaging • Chest x-rays most helpful; other films only if signs or symptoms warrant • Ultrasonography (best for kidneys and RUQ diseases) • CT scans (best for abscesses, nodes, tumors, hematomas) • MRI scan best for pelvis, bone/soft tissue and intracranial infections • Radionuclide scans (technetium liver and spleen scans may be helpful in RUQ and LUQ diseases; gallium: too many false positives or negatives; indium 111 helpful for abscesses)

Biopsies • Abnormal-appearing tissues better than blind biopsy • Bone marrow if patient is anemic • Lung if decreased $P_{A_{O_2}}$ or infiltrate and bronchoalveolar lavage unrevealing • Liver: low yield unless function tests abnormal • Lymph node useful except for inguinal nodes

Exploratory laparotomy   Only if there are clinical, laboratory, or imaging clues.

Therapeutic trials   Only useful if specific (isoniazid and rifampin for tuberculosis, but not multiple antibiotics).

Prognosis generally favorable   Repeated history, physical, and chart reviews (not lab tests) may lead to diagnosis that was missed originally.

For a more detailed discussion, see Root RK, Petersdorf RG: Chills and Fever, Chap. 20, in HPIM-12, p. 125

7 SYNCOPE AND SEIZURES

SYNCOPE Defined as generalized weakness, with loss of postural tone, inability to stand upright, and loss of consciousness. Begins with a sense of "feeling bad," with dimming vision, ringing in ears, or sweating. May occur so rapidly that there is no warning. Patient appears pale and ashen, with faint pulse. Complete loss of consciousness may be averted if subject can promptly lie down. Once horizontal, cerebral perfusion is no longer hindered by gravity. Pulse then becomes stronger, color returns to face, and consciousness is regained.

FAINTNESS A lack of strength with sensation of impending loss of consciousness (presyncope).

SEIZURE An abrupt alteration in cortical electrical activity manifested clinically by change in consciousness or by a motor, sensory, or behavioral symptom. See also Chap. 157, Epilepsy.

FEATURES DISTINGUISHING SYNCOPE FROM SEIZURE Seizures may occur day or night, regardless of patient's posture; syncope rarely occurs when recumbent (exception: Stokes-Adams attack). Pallor is invariable in syncope, whereas cyanosis or plethora may occur in seizure. Seizures are often heralded by an aura of localizing significance. Injury from falling is common in seizure, rare in syncope. Unconsciousness usually lasts longer in seizure than in syncope; return to alertness is usually slow after a seizure, prompt with syncope. Urinary incontinence is common in seizure, rare in syncope. Repeated spells of unconsciousness (several per day or per month) in a young person suggest seizure rather than syncope. These points, when taken as a group and supplemented by EEG findings characteristic of seizure, provide the basis on which to distinguish syncope from seizure.

ETIOLOGY OF SYNCOPE Most often due to processes resulting in reduced cerebral blood flow (see Table 7-1).

For a more detailed discussion, see Martin JB, Ruskin J: Faintness, Syncope, and Seizures, Chap. 21, HPIM-12, p. 134

TABLE 7-1 Causes of recurrent weakness, faintness, and disturbances of consciousness

I. Circulatory (reduced cerebral blood flow)
  A. Inadequate vasoconstrictor mechanisms
    1. Vasovagal (vasodepressor)
    2. Postural hypotension
    3. Primary autonomic insufficiency
    4. Sympathectomy (pharmacologic, due to antihypertensive medications such as methyldopa and hydralazine, or surgical)
    5. Diseases of central and peripheral nervous systems, including autonomic nerves
    6. Carotid sinus syncope (see also ''Bradyarrhythmias,'' below)
  B. Hypovolemia
    1. Blood loss—gastrointestinal hemorrhage
    2. Addison's disease
  C. Mechanical reduction of venous return
    1. Valsalva maneuver
    2. Cough
    3. Micturition
    4. Atrial myxoma, ball valve thrombus
  D. Reduced cardiac output
    1. Obstruction to left ventricular outflow: aortic stenosis, hypertrophic subaortic stenosis
    2. Obstruction to pulmonary flow: pulmonic stenosis, primary pulmonary hypertension, pulmonary embolism
    3. Myocardial: massive myocardial infarction with pump failure
    4. Pericardial: cardiac tamponade
  E. Arrhythmias
    1. Bradyarrhythmias
      a. Atrioventricular (AV) block (second- and third-degree), with Stokes-Adams attacks
      b. Ventricular asystole
      c. Sinus bradycardia, sinoatrial block, sinus arrest, sick-sinus syndrome
      d. Carotid sinus syncope (see also inadequate vasoconstrictor mechanisms, above)
      e. Glossopharyngeal neuralgia (and other painful states)
    2. Tachyarrhythmias
      a. Episodic ventricular tachycardia with or without associated bradyarrhythmias
      b. Supraventricular tachycardia without AV block
II. Other causes of weakness and episodic disturbances of consciousness
  A. Altered state of blood to the brain
    1. Hypoxia
    2. Anemia
    3. Hypoventilation—CO_2 is diminished (faintness common, syncope seldom occurs)
    4. Hypoglycemia (episodic weakness common, faintness occasional, syncope rare)

TABLE 7-1   Continued

 B. Cerebral
   1. Transient ischemic attack
      a. Extracranial vascular insufficiency (vertebral-basilar, carotid)
      b. Diffuse spasm of cerebral arterioles (hypertensive encephalopathy)
   2. Emotional disturbances, anxiety attacks, and hysterical seizures

---

Modified from Martin JB, Ruskin J: HPIM-12, p. 134.

8 DIZZINESS AND VERTIGO

Patients use the term *dizziness* to describe several unusual head sensations or gait unsteadiness. With a careful history, the patient's symptoms can be placed into more specific neurologic categories, of which faintness and vertigo are most important.

DEFINITIONS Faintness A symptom of insufficient blood, oxygen or, rarely, glucose supply to the brain. Usually described as light-headedness followed by visual blurring and postural swaying. Occurs with hyperventilation, hypoglycemia, and prior to a syncopal event (Chap. 7). Light-headedness also can occur as an aura before a seizure. Chronic light-headedness is a common somatic complaint in patients with depression.

Vertigo The illusion of self or environmental movement, most commonly a sensation of spinning. Physiologic vertigo is due to unfamiliar head movement or visual-proprioceptive-vestibular mismatch, i.e., seasickness, height vertigo, visual vertigo. True vertigo almost never occurs in the presyncopal state.

Pathologic vertigo Caused by abnormalities of visual, somatosensory, or vestibular inputs, most commonly the latter. Frequently accompanied by nausea, postural unsteadiness, and gait ataxia, vertigo is provoked or worsened by head movement. May be caused by peripheral (labyrinth or eighth nerve) or CNS lesions. The distinction is prognostically important.

PERIPHERAL VERTIGO Usually severe, accompanied by nausea and emesis. Tinnitus, a feeling of ear fullness, or hearing loss may occur. Patient may be pale and diaphoretic. A characteristic jerk nystagmus almost always present. The nystagmus is unidirectional, horizontal with a torsional component, and has its fast phase to side of normal ear. It is inhibited by visual fixation. Patient senses spinning motion in direction of slow phase and falls or mispoints to that side. Usually no other neurologic abnormalities.

Etiology Peripheral vertigo is common and usually episodic because central compensatory mechanisms ultimately diminish it. An attack of acute peripheral vestibulopathy may be followed by multiple recurrent episodes. Common causes of peripheral vertigo include recent head trauma, labyrinthine infection, toxins, Ménière's disease (recurrent vertigo accompanied by tinnitus and deafness), and acoustic neuroma. The latter also may cause facial weakness and facial sensory loss due to involvement of cranial nerves V and VII. Drug toxicity (streptomycin, gentamicin, neomycin) can cause peripheral vestibulopathy. Psychogenic vertigo should be suspected in patients with chronic incapacitating vertigo who also have agoraphobia, a normal neurologic exam, and no nystagmus.

CENTRAL VERTIGO   Identified by associated abnormal brainstem or cerebellar signs such as dysarthria, diplopia, paresthesia, headache, weakness, limb ataxia. The nystagmus can take almost any form, i.e., vertical, multidirectional, but is often purely horizontal without a torsional component. Central nystagmus is not inhibited by fixation. Central vertigo may be chronic or mild and is less likely to be accompanied by tinnitus or hearing loss. It usually is a sign of brainstem dysfunction and may be due to demyelinating, vascular, or neoplastic disease. Rarely it occurs as a manifestation of temporal lobe epilepsy.

EVALUATION   The "dizzy" patient usually requires provocative tests to reproduce the symptoms. Valsalva maneuver, hyperventilation, or postural changes may reproduce faintness. Rapid rotation of the patient in a swivel chair may reproduce vertigo. Benign positional vertigo is identified by positioning the turned head of a recumbent patient in extension over the edge of the bed to elicit vertigo and a characteristic type of nystagmus. If patient does not exhibit signs of peripheral vertigo or has other neurologic abnormalities, then prompt evaluation for central pathology is indicated, i.e., CT or MRI scan of the posterior fossa, electronystagmography, evoked potential tests, or vertebrobasilar angiography.

TREATMENT   For acute vertigo, bed rest and vestibular suppressant drugs such as antihistamines (meclizine, dimenhydrinate, promethazine), anticholinergics (scopolamine), or hypnotics. Ménière's may respond to a low-salt diet with a diuretic. A mild exercise program is prescribed for patients with a prolonged episode of peripheral vertigo to induce central compensatory mechanisms. Patients with central vertigo should be carefully evaluated for potentially life-threatening brainstem lesions.

For a more detailed discussion, see Daroff RB: Dizziness and Vertigo, Chap. 22, in HPIM-12, p. 140

9 ALTERATIONS IN CONSCIOUSNESS (CONFUSION, STUPOR, AND COMA)

Disorders of consciousness are common in medical practice. Assessment of consciousness abnormalities should determine whether there is a change in *level* of consciousness (drowsy, stuporous, comatose) and/or *content* of consciousness (confusion, perseveration, hallucinations). *Confusion* is a lack of clarity in thinking with inattentiveness; *stupor,* a state in which vigorous stimuli are needed to elicit a response; *coma,* a condition of unresponsiveness. Patients in such states are usually seriously ill and etiologic factors must be assessed.

APPROACH TO PATIENT

1. Support the patient's vital functions.
2. Administer glucose, thiamine, and naloxone if etiology is not clear.
3. Utilize history, examination, and laboratory and radiologic information to rapidly establish the cause of the disorder.
4. Provide the appropriate medical or surgical treatment.

HISTORY   Patient should be aroused, if possible, and questioned regarding use of insulin, narcotics, anticoagulants, other prescription drugs, suicidal intent, recent trauma, headache, epilepsy, significant medical problems, and preceding symptoms. Witnesses and family members should be interrogated, often by phone. History of sudden headache followed by loss of consciousness suggests intracranial hemorrhage; preceding vertigo, nausea, diplopia, ataxia, hemisensory disorder suggest basilar insufficiency; chest pain, palpitations, and faintness suggest cardiovascular cause.

IMMEDIATE ASSESSMENT   Vital signs should be evaluated, and appropriate support initiated. Blood should be drawn for glucose, Na, K, Ca, BUN, ammonia, alcohol, liver transaminase levels; also screen for presence of toxins. Fever, especially with petechial rash, should suggest meningitis. Fever with dry skin suggests heat shock or intoxication with anticholinergics. Hypothermia suggests myxedema, intoxication, or hypoglycemia. Marked hypertension occurs with increased intracranial pressure and hypertensive encephalopathy.

NEUROLOGIC EVALUATION   Focuses on establishing patient's best level of function and uncovering signs that enable a specific diagnosis. Although confused states may occur with unilateral cerebral lesions, stupor and coma are signs of bihemispheral dysfunction or damage to midbrain-tegmentum (reticular activating system).

Responsiveness Stimuli of increasing intensity are applied to body parts to gauge the degree of unresponsiveness and any asymmetry in sensory or motor function. Motor responses may be purposeful or reflexive. Spontaneous flexion of elbows with leg extension, termed *decortication,* accompanies severe damage to contralateral hemisphere above midbrain. Extension of elbows, wrists, and legs, termed *decerebration,* suggests damage to diencephalon or midbrain. Postural reflexes can occur in profound encephalopathic states.

Pupils In patients with coma, equal, round, reactive pupils exclude midbrain damage as cause and suggest a metabolic abnormality. Pinpoint pupils occur in narcotic overdose (except meperidine, which causes midsize pupils). Small pupils also occur with hydrocephalus and thalamic or pontine damage. A unilateral, enlarged, often oval, poorly reactive pupil is caused by midbrain lesions or compression of third cranial nerve, as occurs in transtentorial herniation. Bilaterally dilated, unreactive pupils indicate severe bilateral midbrain damage, anticholinergic overdose, or ocular trauma.

Eye movements Spontaneous and reflex eye movements should be examined for limitations of ocular movement, involuntary movements, and misalignment of ocular axes. Intermittent horizontal divergence is common in drowsiness. An *adducted* eye at rest with impaired ability to turn eye laterally indicates an abducens (VI) nerve palsy, common in raised intracranial pressure or pontine damage. The eye with a dilated, unreactive pupil often is *abducted* at rest and cannot adduct fully due to third nerve dysfunction, as occurs with transtentorial herniation. Vertical separation of ocular axes occurs in pontine or cerebellar lesions. *Doll's head maneuver* and *cold caloric*–induced eye movements allow accurate diagnosis of gaze or cranial nerve palsies in patients who do not move their eyes purposefully. Oculocephalic reflex is tested by observing eye movements in response to lateral rotation of head (significant neck injury is a contraindication). Loose movement of eyes with the doll's head maneuver occurs in bihemispheric dysfunction. In comatose patients with an intact brainstem, raising head to 60° above the horizontal and irrigating external auditory canal with cold water causes tonic deviation of gaze to irrigated ear. In conscious patients, it causes nystagmus, vertigo, and emesis.

Respiration Respiratory pattern may suggest site of neurologic damage. Cheyne-Stokes (periodic) breathing occurs in bihemispheral dysfunction and is common in metabolic encephalopathies. Respiratory patterns composed of gasps or apneustic breathing are indicative of lower brainstem damage; patients usually require intubation and ventilatory assistance.

Other   Comatose patient's best motor and sensory function should be assessed by testing reflex responses to noxious stimuli; carefully note any asymmetric responses, which suggest a focal lesion. If possible, patient with disordered consciousness should have gait examined. Ataxia may be the prominent neurologic finding in a stuporous patient with a cerebellar mass.

RADIOLOGIC EXAMINATION   Lesions causing raised intracranial pressure commonly cause impaired consciousness. CT or MRI scans of the brain are often abnormal in coma but are not usually diagnostic in patients with metabolic encephalopathy, meningitis, early infarction, early encephalitis, diffuse anoxic injury, or drug overdose. Postponing appropriate therapy in these patients while awaiting a CT or MRI scan may be deleterious. Patients with disordered consciousness due to high intracranial pressure can deteriorate rapidly; emergent CT study is necessary to confirm presence of mass effect and to guide surgical consideration. CT scan is normal in some patients with subarachnoid hemorrhage; the diagnosis then rests on clinical history combined with RBC in spinal fluid. Cerebral angiography is frequently necessary to establish basilar artery insufficiency as cause of coma in patients with brainstem signs.

Brain death   This results from total cessation of cerebral function and blood flow at a time when cardiopulmonary function continues but is dependent on ventilatory assistance. EEG is isoelectric at high gain, patient is unresponsive, brainstem reflexes are absent, drug toxicity and hypothermia are excluded. Diagnosis should be made only if the state persists for some agreed upon period, 6–24 h. Demonstration of apnea requires that the P_{CO_2} be high enough to stimulate respiration.

For a more detailed discussion, see Ropper AH, Martin JB: Coma and Other Disorders of Consciousness, Chap. 31, in HPIM-12, p. 617

10 DYSPNEA

DEFINITION An uncomfortable awareness of breathing; intensity can be quantified by establishing the amount of physical exertion necessary to produce the sensation.

CAUSES **Heart disease** Dyspnea is due to ↑ pulmonary capillary pressure, left atrial hypertension, and sometimes fatigue of respiratory muscles. Vital capacity and lung compliance are ↓ and airway resistance ↑. Begins as exertional breathlessness → orthopnea → paroxysmal nocturnal dyspnea and dyspnea at rest. Diagnosis depends on recognition of heart disease, e.g., Hx of MI, presence of S_3, S_4, murmurs, cardiomegaly, jugular vein distention, hepatomegaly, and peripheral edema (see Chap. 68).

Obstructive disease of the airways May occur with obstruction anywhere from extrathoracic airways to lung periphery. Acute dyspnea with difficulty *inhaling* suggests *upper* airway obstruction. Physical exam may reveal inspiratory stridor and retraction of supraclavicular fossae. Acute intermittent dyspnea with expiratory wheezing suggests reversible intrathoracic obstruction due to asthma. Chronic, slowly progressive exertional dyspnea characterizes emphysema and CHF.

Diffuse parenchymal lung diseases Many parenchymal lung diseases, ranging from sarcoidosis to the pneumoconioses, may cause dyspnea. Dyspnea is usually related to exertion early in the course of the illness. Physical exam typically reveals late tachypnea and inspiratory rales.

Pulmonary embolism (See Chap. 85) Repeated discrete episodes of dyspnea may occur with recurrent pulmonary emboli, but others describe slowly progressive dyspnea without abrupt worsening; tachypnea is frequent. Finding of deep venous thrombosis often absent in chronic pulmonary embolism.

Disease of the chest wall or respiratory muscles Severe kyphoscoliosis may produce chronic dyspnea, often with chronic cor pulmonale. The spinal deformity must be severe before respiratory function is compromised. Pts with bilateral diaphragmatic paralysis appear normal while standing, but complain of severe orthopnea and display paradoxical abnormal respiratory movement when supine.

APPROACH TO PATIENT Elicit a description of the amount of physical exertion necessary to produce the sensation and whether it varies under different conditions.

- If acute upper airway obstruction is suspected, lateral neck films or a fiberoptic exam of upper airway may be helpful. Patient should be accompanied by a physician adept in all aspects of airway management during the evaluation. With chronic upper airway obstruction the respiratory flow-volume curve may show inspiratory cutoff of flow, suggesting variable extrathoracic obstruction.
- Dyspnea due to emphysema is reflected in a reduction in expiratory flow rates (FEV_1).
- Patients with intermittent dyspnea due to asthma may have normal pulmonary function if tested when asymptomatic.
- Patients with dyspnea due to both cardiac and pulmonary diseases may report orthopnea. Paroxysmal nocturnal dyspnea occurring after awakening from sleep is characteristic of CHF.
- Dyspnea of chronic obstructive lung disease tends to develop more gradually than that of heart disease.
- PFTs should be performed in pts in whom the etiology is not clear.
- Management depends on elucidating etiology.

Differentiation between cardiac and pulmonary dyspnea is summarized in Table 10–1.

TABLE 10-1   Differentiation between cardiac and pulmonary dyspnea

1. Careful history: Dyspnea of lung disease usually more gradual in onset than that of heart disease; nocturnal exacerbations common with each.

2. Examination: Usually obvious evidence of cardiac or pulmonary disease. Findings may be absent at rest when symptoms are present only with exertion.

3. Pulmonary function tests: Pulmonary disease rarely causes dyspnea unless tests of obstructive disease (FEV_1, FEV_1/FVC) or restrictive disease (total lung capacity) are reduced (<80% predicted).

4. Ventricular performance: LV ejection fraction at rest and/or during exercise usually depressed in cardiac dyspnea.

For a more detailed discussion, see Ingram RH Jr, Braunwald E: Dyspnea and Pulmonary Edema, Chap. 36, in HPIM-12, p. 220

11 COUGH AND HEMOPTYSIS

COUGH

Produced by inflammatory, mechanical, chemical, and thermal stimulation of cough receptors.

ETIOLOGY **Inflammatory** Edema and hyperemia of airways and alveoli due to laryngitis, tracheitis, bronchitis, bronchiolitis, pneumonitis, lung abscess.

Mechanical Inhalation of particulates (dust) or compression of airways (pulmonary neoplasms, foreign bodies, granulomas, bronchospasm).

Chemical Inhalation of irritant fumes, including cigarette smoke.

Thermal Inhalation of cold or very hot air.

APPROACH TO THE PATIENT **Diagnosis** *History* should consider: (1) duration; (2) presence of fever or chills; (3) sputum quantity and character; (4) temporal or seasonal pattern; (5) risk factors for underlying disease; and (6) past medical history. Short duration with associated fever suggests acute viral or bacterial infection. Change in sputum character, color, or volume in a smoker with "smoker's cough" necessitates investigation. Seasonal cough may indicate "cough asthma." Environmental exposures may suggest occupational asthma or interstitial lung disease. Past history of recurrent pneumonias may indicate bronchiectasis.

Physical exam should assess upper and lower airways and lung parenchyma. Stridor suggests upper airway obstruction; wheezing suggests bronchospasm as the cause of cough. Midinspiratory crackles indicate airways disease (e.g., chronic bronchitis); fine end-inspiratory crackles occur in interstitial fibrosis and heart failure. *CXR* may show neoplasm, infection, interstitial disease. *Pulmonary function tests* may reveal obstruction or restriction. *Sputum exam* can indicate malignancy or infection.

COMPLICATIONS (1) Syncope, due to transient decrease in venous return; (2) rupture of an emphysematous bleb with pneumothorax; (3) rib fractures—may occur in otherwise normal individuals.

Treatment When possible, therapy of cough is that of underlying disease. If no etiology can be found, an irritative nonproductive cough may be suppressed with an antitussive agent such as codeine, 15–30 mg up to qid. Cough productive of significant volumes of sputum should generally not be suppressed.

HEMOPTYSIS

Includes both streaked sputum and coughing up of gross blood.

ETIOLOGY (Table 11-1) Bronchitis and bronchiectasis are most common causes. Neoplasm may be cause, particularly in smokers and when hemoptysis is persistent. Hemoptysis rare in metastatic neoplasm to lung. Pulmonary thromboembolism, infection, CHF are other causes. Five to 15% of cases with hemoptysis remain undiagnosed.

APPROACH TO THE PATIENT Diagnosis Essential to determine that blood is coming from respiratory tract. Often frothy, may be preceded by a desire to cough. History may suggest diagnosis: chronic hemoptysis in otherwise asymptomatic young woman suggests bronchial adenoma; recurrent hemoptysis in pts with chronic copious sputum production suggests bronchiectasis; hemoptysis, weight loss, and anorexia in a smoker suggest carcinoma; hemoptysis with acute pleuritic pain suggests infarction.

Physical exam may also suggest diagnosis: pleural friction rub raises possibility of pulmonary embolism or some other pleural-based lesion (lung abscess, coccidioidomycosis cavity, vasculitis); diastolic rumble suggests mitral stenosis; localized wheeze suggests bronchogenic carcinoma. Initial evaluation includes CXR. A normal CXR does not exclude tumor or bronchiectasis as a source of bleeding. The CXR

TABLE 11-1 Causes of hemoptysis

Inflammatory:
  Bronchitis
  Bronchiectasis
  Tuberculosis
  Lung abscess
  Pneumonia, particularly *Klebsiella*
Neoplastic:
  Lung cancer: squamous cell, adenocarcinoma, oat cell
  Bronchial adenoma
Other:
  Pulmonary thromboembolism
  Left ventricular failure
  Mitral stenosis
  Traumatic, including foreign body and lung contusion
  Primary pulmonary hypertension; AV malformation; Eisenmenger's syndrome; pulmonary vasculitis, including Wegener's granulomatosis and Goodpasture's syndrome; idiopathic pulmonary hemosiderosis; and amyloid
  Hemorrhagic diathesis, including anticoagulant therapy

Reproduced from Braunwald E: HPIM-12, p. 219.

may show an air-fluid level suggesting an abscess or atelectasis distal to an obstructing carcinoma.

Most pts should then have chest CT scan followed by bronchoscopy. While rigid bronchoscopy is particularly helpful when bleeding is massive or from proximal airway lesion and when endotracheal intubation is contemplated, most pts should be assessed by fiberoptic bronchoscopy.

Treatment   Mainstays of treatment are bed rest and cough suppression with an opiate (codeine, 15–30 mg, or hydrocodone, 5 mg q 4–6 h). Pts with massive hemoptysis (>600 mL/d) and pts with respiratory compromise due to aspiration of blood should have suction and intubation equipment close by so that intubation by balloon tube to isolate the bleeding lung can be accomplished. In massive hemoptysis, choice of medical or surgical therapy relates often to the anatomic site of hemorrhage and the pt's baseline pulmonary function.

For a more detailed discussion, see Braunwald E: Cough and Hemoptysis, Chap. 35, in HPIM-12, p. 217

12 CYANOSIS

The circulating quantity of reduced hemoglobin is elevated [>50 g/L (>5 g/dL)] resulting in bluish discoloration of the skin and/or mucous membranes.

CENTRAL CYANOSIS Results from arterial desaturation.

1. Impaired pulmonary function: Poorly ventilated alveoli or impaired oxygen diffusion; most frequent in pneumonia, pulmonary edema, and chronic obstructive pulmonary disease.

2. Anatomic vascular shunting: Shunting of desaturated venous blood into the arterial circulation may result from congenital heart disease or pulmonary AV fistula.

3. Decreased inspired O_2: Cyanosis may develop at ascents to altitudes >2400 m (>8000 ft).

4. Abnormal hemoglobins: Methemoglobinemia, sulfhemoglobinemia, and mutant hemoglobins with low oxygen affinity (see HPIM-12, Chap. 295).

PERIPHERAL CYANOSIS Occurs with normal arterial O_2 saturation with increased extraction of O_2 from capillary blood caused by decreased localized blood flow. Vasoconstriction due to cold exposure, decreased cardiac output (in shock, Chap. 24), and peripheral vascular disease (Chap. 79) with arterial obstruction or vasospasm (Table 12-1).

APPROACH TO THE PATIENT

- Inquire about congenital heart disease or exposure to chemicals that result in abnormal hemoglobins.
- Examine nailbeds, lips, and mucous membranes for cyanosis; clubbing of fingers and toes may be present; combination of clubbing and cyanosis is frequent in congenital heart disease and occasionally with pulmonary disease (lung abscess, pulmonary AV shunts).
- Examine chest for evidence of pulmonary disease, pulmonary edema, or murmurs associated with congenital heart disease.
- If cyanosis is localized to an extremity, evaluate for peripheral vascular obstruction.
- Obtain arterial blood gas to measure systemic O_2 saturation. Repeat while patient inhales 100% O_2; if saturation fails to increase to >95%, intravascular shunting of blood bypassing the lungs is likely (e.g., right-to-left intracardiac shunts).
- Evaluate abnormal hemoglobins by hemoglobin electrophoresis and measurement of methemoglobin level.

TABLE 12-1 Causes of cyanosis

I. Central cyanosis
  A. Decreased arterial oxygen saturation
    1. Decreased atmospheric pressure—high altitude
    2. Impaired pulmonary function
      a. Alveolar hypoventilation
      b. Uneven relationships between pulmonary ventilation and perfusion (perfusion of hypoventilated alveoli)
      c. Impaired oxygen diffusion
    3. Anatomic shunts
      a. Certain types of congenital heart disease
      b. Pulmonary arteriovenous fistulas
      c. Multiple small intrapulmonary shunts
    4. Hemoglobin with low affinity for oxygen
  B. Hemoglobin abnormalities
    1. Methemoglobinemia—hereditary, acquired
    2. Sulfhemoglobinema—acquired
    3. Carboxyhemoglobinemia (not true cyanosis)
II. Peripheral cyanosis
  A. Reduced cardiac output
  B. Cold exposure
  C. Redistribution of blood flow from extremities
  D. Arterial obstruction
  E. Venous obstruction

From E Braunwald: HPIM-12, p. 227.

For a more detailed discussion, see Braunwald E: Hypoxia, Polycythemia, and Cyanosis, Chap. 37, in HPIM-12, p. 224

13 **EDEMA**

DEFINITION   Soft-tissue swelling due to abnormal expansion of interstitial fluid volume. Edema fluid is a plasma transudate that accumulates when movement of fluid from vascular to interstitial space is favored. Since detectable diffuse edema in the adult reflects a gain of ≥ 3 L, renal retention of salt and water is necessary for edema to occur. Distribution of edema can be an important guide to cause.

Localized edema   Limited to a particular organ or vascular bed; easily distinguished from generalized edema. Unilateral extremity edema is usually due to venous or lymphatic obstruction (e.g., deep venous thrombosis, tumor obstruction, primary lymphedema). Stasis edema of a paralyzed lower extremity also may occur. Allergic reactions (''angioedema'') and superior vena caval obstruction are causes of localized facial edema. Bilateral lower extremity edema may have localized causes: e.g., inferior vena caval obstruction, compression due to ascites, abdominal mass. Ascites (fluid in peritoneal cavity) and hydrothorax (in pleural space) may also present as isolated localized edema, due to inflammation or neoplasm.

Generalized edema   (See Fig. 13-1)   Soft-tissue swelling of most or all regions of the body. Bilateral lower extremity swelling, more pronounced after standing for several hours, and pulmonary edema are usually cardiac in origin. Periorbital edema noted on awakening often results from renal disease and impaired Na excretion. Ascites and edema of lower extremities and scrotum are frequent in cirrhosis or CHF. In the latter, diminished cardiac output and effective arterial blood volume result in both decreased renal perfusion and increased venous pressure with resultant renal Na retention due to renal vasoconstriction, intrarenal blood flow redistribution, and secondary hyperaldosteronism.

In *cirrhosis,* arteriovenous shunts lower effective renal perfusion resulting in Na retention. Ascites accumulates when ↑ intrahepatic vascular resistance produces portal hypertension. Reduced serum albumin and increased abdominal pressure promote lower extremity edema.

In *nephrotic syndrome,* massive renal loss of albumin lowers plasma oncotic pressure, promoting fluid transudation into interstitium; lowering of effective blood volume stimulates renal Na retention.

In acute or chronic *renal failure,* edema occurs if Na intake exceeds kidney's ability to excrete Na secondary to marked

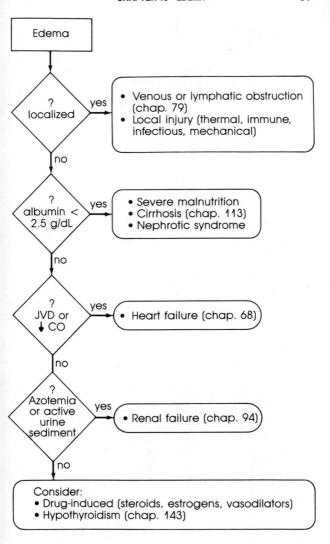

FIGURE 13-1 Diagnostic approach to edema. JVD = jugular venous distension. CO = cardiac output.

TABLE 13-1 Diuretics for edema (See also Table 13-2.)

Drug	Usual Dose	Comments
DISTAL, K-LOSING		
Hydrochlorothiazide	25–200 mg	First choice; causes hypokalemia; need GFR > 25 mL/min
Chlorthalidone	100 mg qd or qod	Long-acting (up to 72 h); hypokalemia; need GFR > 25 mL/min
Metolazone	1–10 mg qd	Long-acting; hypokalemia; effective with low GFR, especially when combined with a loop diuretic
LOOP (MAY BE ADMINISTERED PO OR IV)		
Furosemide	40–120 mg qd or bid	Short-acting; potent; effective with low GFR
Bumetanide	0.5–2 mg qd or bid	May be used if allergic to furosemide
Ethacrynic acid	50–200 mg qd	Longer-acting
DISTAL, K-SPARING		
Spironolactone	25–100 mg qid	Hyperkalemia; acidosis; blocks aldosterone; gynecomastia, impotence, amenorrhea; onset takes 2–3 days; avoid use in renal failure or in combination with ACE inhibitors or potassium supplements
Amiloride	5–10 mg qd or bid	Hyperkalemia; once daily; less potent than spironolactone
Triamterene	100 mg bid	Hyperkalemia; less potent than spironolactone; renal stones

TABLE 13-2 Complications of diuretics

Common	Uncommon
Volume depletion	Interstitial nephritis (thiazides, furosemide)
Prerenal azotemia	
Potassium depletion	Pancreatitis (thiazides)
Hyponatremia (thiazides)	Loss of hearing (loop diuretics)
Metabolic alkalosis	Anemia, leukopenia, thrombocytopenia (thiazides)
Hypercholesterolemia	
Hyperglycemia (thiazides)	
Hyperkalemia (K-sparing)	
Hypomagnesemia	
Hyperuricemia	
Hypercalcemia (thiazides)	
GI complaints	
Rash (thiazides)	

reductions in glomerular filtration. Severe *hypoalbuminemia* [<25 g/L (2.5 g/dL)] of any cause (e.g., nephrosis, nutritional deficiency states, chronic liver disease) may lower plasma oncotic pressure sufficiently to cause edema.

Less common causes of generalized edema: *idiopathic edema,* a syndrome of recurrent rapid weight gain and edema in women of reproductive age; *hypothyroidism,* in which myxedema is typically located in pretibial region; *drugs* such as steroids, estrogens, and vasodilators; *pregnancy; refeeding* after starvation.

TREATMENT Primary management is to identify and treat the underlying cause of edema (Fig. 13-1).

Dietary Na restriction (<500 mg/d) may prevent further edema formation. Bed rest enhances response to salt restriction in CHF and cirrhosis. Supportive stockings and elevation of edematous lower extremities will help mobilize interstitial fluid. If severe hyponatremia (<132 mmol/L) is present, water intake should also be reduced (<1500 mL/d). Diuretics (Table 13-1) are indicated for marked peripheral edema, pulmonary edema, CHF, inadequate dietary salt restriction. Side effects are listed in Table 13-2. Weight loss by diuretics should be limited to 1–1.5 kg/d. Metolazone may be added to loop diuretics for enhanced effect. Note that intestinal edema may impair absorption of oral diuretics and reduce effectiveness. When desired weight is achieved, diuretic doses should be reduced.

In CHF (Chap. 68), avoid overdiuresis as it may bring a fall in cardiac output and prerenal azotemia. Avoid diuretic-induced hypokalemia, which predisposes to digitalis toxicity.

In *cirrhosis,* spironolactone is the diuretic of choice, but may produce acidosis and hyperkalemia. Thiazides or small doses of loop diuretics also may be added. However, renal failure may result from volume depletion. Overdiuresis may result in hyponatremia and alkalosis, which may worsen hepatic encephalopathy (Chap. 113).

In *nephrotic syndrome,* albumin infusion should be limited to very severe cases (patients with associated hypotension) as rapid renal excretion prevents any sustained rise in serum albumin.

For a more detailed discussion, see Braunwald E: Edema, Chap. 38, in HPIM-12, p. 228

---

14 NAUSEA AND VOMITING

DEFINITION *Nausea* refers to the imminent desire to vomit and often precedes or accompanies vomiting. *Vomiting* refers to the forceful expulsion of gastric contents through the mouth. *Retching* refers to labored rhythmic respiratory activity that precedes emesis. *Regurgitation* refers to the expulsion of gastric contents in the absence of nausea and abdominal diaphragmatic muscular contraction. *Rumination* refers to the regurgitation, rechewing, and reswallowing of food from the stomach.

PATHOPHYSIOLOGY Gastric contents are propelled into the esophagus when there is relaxation of the gastric fundus and gastroesophageal sphincter followed by a rapid increase in intraabdominal pressure produced by contraction of the abdominal and diaphragmatic musculature. Increased intrathoracic pressure results in further movement of the material to the mouth. Reflex elevation of the soft palate and closure of the glottis protects the nasopharynx and trachea and completes the act of vomiting. Vomiting is controlled by two brainstem areas, the vomiting center and chemoreceptor trigger zone.

ETIOLOGY Nausea and vomiting are manifestations of a large number of disorders. Clinical classification:

- Acute abdominal emergency: appendicitis, acute cholecystitis, acute intestinal obstruction (adhesions, malignancy, hernia, volvulus), acute peritonitis.
- Chronic indigestion: peptic ulcer disease, aerophagia.
- Disordered GI motility: gastroparesis (postvagotomy, diabetic, idiopathic), abnormal gastric myoelectric activity ("dysrhythmia"), achalasia, intestinal pseudoobstruction.
- Infections: bacterial, viral, and parasitic infections of the GI tract. Systemic infection not involving the GI tract directly, especially in children.
- CNS disorders: increased intracranial pressure (neoplasms, encephalitis, hydrocephalus) may result in vomiting, often of a projectile nature.

  Labyrinthine disorders (acute labyrinthitis, Ménière's disease) that underlie vertigo are often associated with nausea and vomiting.

- Cardiac: acute myocardial infarction (especially inferior MI) and congestive heart failure.

43

- Metabolic and endocrine disorders: diabetic ketoacidosis, adrenal insufficiency, hyperthyroid crisis, pregnancy, uremia.
- Medicines/toxins: nausea is a common side effect of many medications and toxins. Enterotoxins produced by bacteria cause food poisoning.
- Psychogenic: emotional upset, anorexia, bulimia.
- GI hemorrhage: blood in the stomach from any cause can result in nausea and vomiting.

EVALUATION   The history, including a careful drug history, and the timing and character of the vomitus can be helpful. For example, vomiting that occurs predominantly in the morning is often seen in pregnancy, uremia, and alcoholic gastritis; feculent emesis implies distal intestinal obstruction or gastrocolic fistula; projectile vomiting suggests increased intracranial pressure. Associated symptoms may also be helpful: vertigo and tinnitus in Ménière's disease, relief of abdominal pain with vomiting in peptic ulcer, and early satiety in gastroparesis. Plain radiographs can suggest diagnoses such as intestinal obstruction. The upper GI series assesses motility of the proximal GI tract as well as the mucosa. Other studies may be indicated such as gastric emptying scans (diabetic gastroparesis) and CT scan of the brain.

COMPLICATIONS   Rupture of the esophagus (Boerhaave's syndrome), hematemesis from a mucosal tear (Mallory-Weiss syndrome), dehydration, malnutrition, dental caries, metabolic alkalosis, hypokalemia, and aspiration pneumonitis.

TREATMENT   This should be directed towards correcting the specific etiology. The effectiveness of antiemetic medications depends upon etiology of symptoms, patient responsiveness, and side effects. Antihistamines such as dimenhydrinate and promethazine hydrochloride are effective for nausea due to inner ear dysfunction. Anticholinergics such as scopolamine are effective for nausea associated with motion sickness. Haloperidol and phenothiazine derivatives such as prochlorperazine are often effective in controlling mild nausea and vomiting, but sedation, hypotension, and Parkinson-like symptoms are common side effects. Selective dopamine antagonists such as metoclopramide may be superior to the phenothiazines in treating severe nausea and vomiting and are particularly useful in treatment of gastroparesis. Intravenous metoclopramide may be effective as prophylaxis against nausea when given prior to chemotherapy.

For a more detailed discussion, see Friedman LS, Isselbacher KJ: Anorexia, Nausea, Vomiting, and Indigestion, Chap. 43, in HPIM-12, p. 251

15 WEIGHT LOSS AND WEIGHT GAIN

Changes in weight may involve body fluid or tissue mass. Rapid fluctuations of weight over days suggest loss or gain of fluid, whereas long-term changes usually involve body mass and reflect the balance of energy intake and expenditure.

WEIGHT GAIN Fluid accumulation can be due to congestive heart failure, cirrhosis of the liver, nephrosis, or renal disease. The most common cause of increased tissue mass is endogenous obesity, usually from overeating. The history may be misleading, and excess intake should be documented by calorie counts. Secondary causes of obesity include Cushing's syndrome, hypothyroidism, hypogonadism, and insulin-secreting tumors. Rarely, neoplasms of the CNS such as craniopharyngiomas cause a central drive to overeat. Congenital disorders such as Prader-Willi and Laurence-Moon-Biedl syndromes cause obesity early in life.

WEIGHT LOSS In the absence of dieting, weight loss has more import than weight gain. Weight loss in the setting of an increased appetite suggests accelerated metabolism or loss of calories in the urine or stool. Thyrotoxicosis causes enhanced energy expenditure from increase in metabolic rate and physical activity. Weight loss in pheochromocytoma is due to catecholamine-mediated hypermetabolism. Diabetes mellitus typically causes polyuria, polydipsia, polyphagia, and weight loss. Initial weight loss is secondary to osmotic diuresis, but subsequent loss of body mass reflects caloric wastage in the urine (glycosuria). Malabsorption with steatorrhea, as in sprue, chronic pancreatitis, or cystic fibrosis, and chronic diarrhea of diverse causes also may cause weight loss despite increased food intake. A variety of other GI tract disorders cause weight loss: inflammatory bowel disease, parasite infestations, esophageal strictures, obstruction secondary to chronic peptic ulcer, pernicious anemia, and cirrhosis.

Weight loss with a diminished appetite is due to the inadequacy of intake for metabolic needs and suggests occult malignancy. The search for malignancy should include GI tract, pancreas, liver, lymphoma, and leukemia. Weight loss and anorexia also can be due to tuberculosis, fungal disease, amebic abscess, bacterial endocarditis, and AIDS. The mechanism involves both anorexia and acceleration of cellular metabolic demands. Adrenal insufficiency rarely causes weight loss due to a diminished appetite, as may anorexia nervosa, depressive states, and schizophrenia. One of the earliest manifestations of uremia is anorexia.

For a more detailed discussion, see Foster DW: Gain and Loss in Weight, Chap. 45, in HPIM-12, p. 259

16 DIARRHEA, CONSTIPATION, AND MALABSORPTION SYNDROMES

NORMAL GASTROINTESTINAL FUNCTION

ABSORPTION OF FLUID AND ELECTROLYTES   Fluid delivery to GI tract is 8–10 L/d, including 2 L ingested; most is absorbed in small bowel. Colonic absorption is normally 500–2000 mL, with capacity for 6 L/d if required. Water absorption passively follows active transport of Na^+, Cl^-, and glucose. Additional transport mechanisms include Cl^-/HCO_3^- exchange, H^+, K^+, and HCO_3^- secretion, and Na^+-glucose cotransport.

NUTRIENT ABSORPTION   (1) Proximal small intestine: iron, calcium, folate, fats (after hydrolysis of triglycerides to fatty acids by pancreatic lipase and colipase), proteins (after hydrolysis by pancreatic and intestinal peptidases), carbohydrates (after hydrolysis by amylases and disaccharidases); triglycerides absorbed as micelles after solubilization by bile salts; amino acids and dipeptides absorbed via specific carriers; sugars absorbed by active transport; (2) distal small intestine: vitamin B_{12}, bile salts, water; (3) colon: water, electrolytes.

INTESTINAL MOTILITY   Allows propulsion of intestinal contents from stomach to anus and separation of components to facilitate nutrient absorption. Propulsion is controlled by neural, myogenic, and hormonal mechanisms; mediated by migrating motor complex, an organized wave of neuromuscular activity that originates in the distal stomach during fasting and migrates slowly down the small intestine. Colonic motility is mediated by local peristalsis to propel feces. Defecation is effected by relaxation of internal anal sphincter in response to rectal distention, with voluntary control by contraction of external anal sphincter.

DIARRHEA

PHYSIOLOGY   Formally defined as fecal output greater than 200 g/d on low-fiber (western) diet; *diarrhea* also frequently used to connote loose or watery stools. Mediated by one or more of the following mechanisms:

Osmotic diarrhea   Nonabsorbed solutes increase intraluminal oncotic pressure, causing outpouring of water; usually ceases with fasting; stool osmolal gap greater than 40 (see below). Causes include disaccharidase (e.g., lactase) deficiencies, lactulose ingestion, polyvalent laxative abuse.

Lactase deficiency either primary (more prevalent in blacks and Asians, usually presenting in early adulthood) or secondary (from viral, bacterial, or protozoal gastroenteritis, celiac or tropical sprue, or kwashiorkor).

Secretory diarrhea Active ion secretion causes obligatory water loss; diarrhea usually watery, often profuse, unaffected by fasting; stool Na^+ and K^+ elevated with osmolal gap less than 40. Causes include viral infections (e.g., rotavirus, Norwalk virus), bacterial infections (e.g., cholera, enterotoxigenic *E. coli, Staphylococcus aureus*), protozoa (e.g., *Giardia, Cryptosporidia*), AIDS-associated disorders (including mycobacterial and HIV-induced), Zollinger-Ellison syndrome (excess gastrin production), vasoactive intestinal peptide (VIP)-producing tumors, carcinoid tumors (histamine and serotonin), medullary thyroid carcinoma (prostaglandins and serotonin), systemic mastocytosis, basophilic leukemia, and distal colonic villous adenomas (direct secretion of electrolyte-rich fluid).

Exudative Inflammation, necrosis, and sloughing of colonic mucosa; may include component of secretory diarrhea due to prostaglandin release by inflammatory cells; stools usually contain PMNs as well as occult or gross blood. Causes include bacterial infections [e.g., *Campylobacter, Salmonella, Shigella, Yersinia,* invasive or enterotoxigenic *E. coli, Vibrio parahemolyticus, Clostridium difficile* colitis (frequently antibiotic-induced)], colonic parasites (e.g., *Entamoeba histolytica*), Crohn's disease, ulcerative proctocolitis, idiopathic inflammatory bowel disease, diverticulitis, radiation enterocolitis, cancer chemotherapeutic agents, and intestinal ischemia.

Altered intestinal motility Alteration of coordinated control of intestinal propulsion; diarrhea often intermittent or alternating with constipation. Causes include diabetes mellitus, adrenal insufficiency, hyperthyroidism, collagenvascular diseases, parasitic infestations, gastrin and VIP hypersecretory states, amyloidosis, laxatives (esp. magnesium-containing agents), antibiotics (esp. erythromycin), cholinergic agents, primary neurologic dysfunction (e.g., Parkinson's disease), and irritable bowel syndrome. Blood in intestinal lumen is cathartic, and major upper GI bleeding leads to diarrhea from increased motility.

Decreased absorptive surface Usually arises from surgical manipulation (e.g., extensive bowel resection or rearrangement) that leaves inadequate absorptive surface for fluid and electrolyte absorption; occurs spontaneously from enteroenteric fistulas (esp. gastrocolic).

EVALUATION History Diarrhea must be distinguished from fecal incontinence, change in stool caliber, rectal bleeding, and small, frequent, but otherwise normal stools. Alternating diarrhea and constipation suggests fixed colonic obstruction or irritable bowel disease. Sudden, acute course is typical of viral and bacterial diverticulitis infections, and drug-induced diarrhea and may represent the initial presentation of inflammatory bowel disease. A longer, more insidious course suggests malabsorption, inflammatory bowel disease, metabolic or endocrine disturbance, pancreatic insufficiency, laxative abuse, ischemia, neoplasm (hypersecretory state or partial obstruction), or irritable bowel syndrome. Parasitic and certain forms of bacterial enteritis also can produce chronic symptoms. Particularly foul-smelling or oily stool suggests fat malabsorption. Fecal impaction may cause apparent diarrhea because only liquids pass partial obstruction.

Physical exam   Signs of dehydration are often prominent in acute diarrhea. Fever and abdominal tenderness suggest infection or inflammatory disease but are often absent in viral enteritis. Evidence of malnutrition suggests chronic course. Certain signs are frequently associated with specific deficiency states secondary to malabsorption (e.g., cheilosis with riboflavin deficiency, glossitis with B_{12}, folate deficiency).

Stool examination   Culture for bacterial pathogens, examination for leukocytes, measurement of *Clostridium difficile* toxin, and examination for ova and parasites are important components of evaluation of pts with severe, protracted, or bloody diarrhea. Presence of blood (fecal occult blood test) or leukocytes (Wright's stain) suggests inflammation (e.g., Crohn's disease, ulcerative colitis, infection, or ischemia). Gram's stain of stool can be diagnostic of *Staphylococcus, Campylobacter,* or *Candida* infection. Steatorrhea (determined with Sudan III stain of stool sample or 72-h quantitative fecal fat analysis) suggests malabsorption or pancreatic insufficiency. Measurement of Na^+ and K^+ levels in fecal water helps to distinguish osmotic from other types of diarrhea [stool osmolal gap $\approx$ $(osmol)_{serum} - (Na^+ + K^+)_{stool}$].

Laboratory studies   CBC may indicate anemia (acute or chronic blood loss or malabsorption of iron, folate, or B_{12}), leukocytosis (inflammation), eosinophilia (parasitic, neoplastic, and inflammatory bowel diseases). Serum levels of calcium, albumin, iron, cholesterol, folate, and B_{12}, serum iron-binding capacity, and PT can provide evidence of intestinal malabsorption.

Other studies   Sigmoidoscopy or colonoscopy useful in the diagnosis of colitis (esp. pseudomembranous and ischemic); it may not allow distinction between infectious and noninfectious (esp. idiopathic ulcerative) colitis. Barium contrast x-ray studies may suggest malabsorption (thickened bowel folds), inflammatory bowel disease (ileitis or colitis), tuberculosis (ileocecal inflammation), diverticulitis, neo-plasm, intestinal fistula, or motility disorders. D-Xylose absorption test is a convenient screen for small bowel absorptive function. Small-bowel biopsy is especially useful for evaluating intestinal malabsorption. Specialized studies include Schilling test (B_{12} malabsorption), lactose H_2 breath test (carbohydrate malabsorption), [^{14}C]xylose and lactulose H_2 breath tests (bacterial overgrowth), glycocholic breath test (ileal malabsorption), triolein breath test (fat malabsorption), and bentiromide and secretin tests (pancreatic insufficiency).

TREATMENT Varies widely depending on etiology. Table 16-1 lists treatment options for common causes of diarrhea. In addition, symptomatic therapy includes vigorous rehydration (IV or with oral glucose-electrolyte solutions), electrolyte replacement, binders of osmotically active substances (e.g., kaolin-pectin), and opiates to decrease bowel motility (e.g., loperamide, diphenoxylate); opiates may be contraindicated in infectious or inflammatory causes of diarrhea.

MALABSORPTION SYNDROMES

Intestinal malabsorption of ingested nutrients may produce osmotic diarrhea, steatorrhea, or specific deficiencies (e.g., iron, folate, B_{12}, vitamins A, D, E, and K). Table 16-2 lists common causes of intestinal malabsorption. Protein-losing enteropathy may result from several causes of malabsorption; it is associated with hypoalbuminemia and can be detected by measuring stool α_1-antitrypsin or radiolabeled albumin levels. Therapy is directed at the underlying disease.

CONSTIPATION

Decrease in frequency of stools or difficulty in defecation; may result in abdominal pain, distention, and fecal impaction, with consequent obstruction or, rarely, perforation. A frequent and often subjective complaint. Contributory factors may include inactivity, low-roughage diet, and inadequate allotment of time for defecation.

SPECIFIC CAUSES Altered colonic motility due to neurologic dysfunction (diabetes mellitus, spinal cord injury, multiple sclerosis, Hirschsprung's disease, chronic idiopathic intestinal pseudoobstruction, idiopathic megacolon), scleroderma, drugs (esp. anticholinergic agents, opiates, aluminum-based antacids), hypothyroidism, Cushing's syndrome, hypokalemia, hypercalcemia, dehydration, mechanical causes (colorectal tumors, diverticulitis, volvulus, hernias, intussusception), and anorectal pain (from fissures, hemorrhoids,

TABLE 16-1   Treatment of common causes of diarrhea

I. Infectious: (uncomplicated enteritis or colitis)
  A. Viral
    1. Rotavirus, Norwalk virus, unclassified enteritis—symptomatic therapy only
    2. AIDS-associated—symptomatic therapy; octreotide possibly helpful
  B. Bacterial
    1. *Staphylococcus, Yersinia enterocolitica*, salmonellae, *Vibrio*—supportive therapy; avoid opiates
    2. Enterotoxigenic *E. coli*, traveler's diarrhea—bismuth subsalicylate; trimethoprim/sulfamethoxazole; doxycycline, ciprofloxacin
    3. *Shigella*—bismuth subsalicylate; ampicillin
    4. *Campylobacter*—symptomatic therapy; erythromycin
    5. *Clostridium difficile*—metronidazole; oral vancomycin
  C. Protozoal
    1. *Giardia*—metronidazole; quinacrine
    2. *Cryptosporidium*—symptomatic therapy; spiramycin
    3. *Entameba histolytica*—metronidazole; iodoquinone
II. Inflammatory
  A. Crohn's disease—glucocorticoids, aminosalicylates (esp. for colitis), metronidazole, azathioprine
  B. Ulcerative proctocolitis—glucocorticoids (oral or rectal), aminosalicylates
  C. Diverticulitis—tetracycline
III. Malabsorptive
  A. Pancreative insufficiency—low fat diet, pancreatic enzyme replacement
  B. Lactase deficiency—lactose-free diet; lactase preparations (e.g., Lactaid)
  C. Nontropical (celiac) sprue (gluten-sensitive enteropathy)—gluten-free diet; glucocorticoids for refractory disease
  D. Bacterial overgrowth, tropical sprue—tetracycline (with folic acid for sprue)
  E. Whipple's disease—penicillin
  F. Short-bowel syndrome—symptomatic therapy; opiates, elemental diet, medium chain triglycerides; octreotide possibly helpful
  G. Postgastrectomy—symptomatic therapy; frequent small meals; low carbohydrate diet; octreotide for dumping syndrome
  H. Postileal resection—symptomatic therapy; cholestyramine
  I. Lymphangiectasia—medium chain triglycerides; treat underlying disease if possible
IV. Endocrine
  A. Adrenal insufficiency, hyperkalemia, hypocalcemia, thyrotoxicosis, diabetes mellitus—treat underlying disorder
V. Neoplastic
  A. Gastrinoma (Zollinger-Ellison)—H_2 blockers, omeprazole, gastrectomy, tumor resection
  B. Carcinoid syndrome—symptomatic therapy; resection/tumor ablation, octreotide
  C. Secretory villous adenoma—resection

TABLE 16-1   **Treatment of common causes of diarrhea** (*Continued*)

VI. Ischemic
    A. Supportive therapy; avoid opiates; resection of nonviable bowel
VII. Radiation-induced
    A. Symptomatic therapy; opiates
VIII. Irritable bowel disease
    A. High-fiber diet (e.g., Metamucil), anticholinergic agents

---

abscesses, or proctitis) leading to retention, constipation, and fecal impaction.

TREATMENT   In absence of identifiable cause, constipation may improve with reassurance, exercise, increased dietary roughage, and increased fluid intake. Specific therapies include removal of bowel obstruction (fecolith, tumor), discontinuance of nonessential hypomotility agents (esp. aluminum-containing antacids, opiates). For symptomatic relief, magnesium-containing agents or other cathartics are occasionally needed. With severe hypo- or dysmotility or in presence of opiates, osmotically active agents (e.g., oral lactulose, intestinal polyethylene glycol–containing lavage solutions) and mineral oil (orally or rectally) are most effective.

TABLE 16-2   **Common causes of malabsorption**

Maldigestion: Chronic pancreatitis, cystic fibrosis, pancreatic carcinoma
Bile salt deficiency: Cirrhosis, cholestasis, bacterial overgrowth (blind loop syndromes, intestinal diverticula, hypomotility disorders), impaired ileal reabsorption (resection, Crohn's disease), bile salt binders (cholestyramine, calcium carbonate, neomycin)
Inadequate absorptive surface: Massive intestinal resection, gastrocolic fistula, jejunoileal bypass
Lymphatic obstruction: Lymphoma, Whipple's disease, intestinal lymphangiectasia
Vascular disease: Constrictive pericarditis, right-sided heart failure, mesenteric vascular disease
Mucosal disease: Inflammatory diseases (infectious enteridites, Crohn's disease), radiation enteritis, eosinophilic enteritis, ulcerative jejunitis, mastocytosis, tropical sprue, infiltrative disorders (amyloidosis, scleroderma, lymphoma, collagenous sprue), biochemical abnormalities (gluten-sensitive enteropathy, disaccharidase deficiency, hypogammaglobulinemia, abetalipoproteinemia), endocrine disorders (diabetes mellitus, hypoparathyroidism, adrenal insufficiency, hyperthyroidism, Zollinger-Ellison syndrome, carcinoid syndrome)

For a more detailed discussion, see Goldfinger SE: Constipation and Diarrhea, Chap. 44, p. 256; and Greenberger NJ, Isselbacher KJ: Disorders of Absorption, Chap. 240, p. 1252, in HPIM-12

17 GASTROINTESTINAL BLEEDING

PRESENTATION

1. Hematemesis: Vomiting of blood or altered blood ("coffee grounds"); indicates bleeding proximal to ligament of Treitz.

2. Melena: Altered (black) blood per rectum (≥100 mL blood required for one melenic stool); usually indicates bleeding proximal to ligament of Treitz, but may be as distal as ascending colon; pseudomelena may be caused by iron, bismuth, licorice, beets, blueberries, charcoal.

3. Hematochezia: Bright red or maroon rectal bleeding; usually implies bleeding beyond ligament of Treitz, but may be due to rapid upper GI bleeding (≥1000 mL).

4. Positive fecal occult blood test (see Chap. 131).

5. Iron deficiency anemia (see Chap. 129).

Hemodynamic changes Orthostatic hypotension >110 mmHg; usually indicates >20% reduction in blood volume ($\pm$ syncope, light-headedness, nausea, sweating, thirst).

Shock BP <100 mmHg systolic; usually indicates >30% reduction in blood volume ($\pm$ pallor, cool skin).

Laboratory changes Hematocrit may not reflect extent of blood loss because of delayed equilibration with extravascular fluid. Mild leukocytosis and thrombocytosis and elevated BUN are common in upper GI bleeding.

Adverse prognostic signs Age >60, presentation with shock, rebleeding, endoscopic stigmata of recent bleeding [e.g., "visible vessel" in ulcer base (see below)].

UPPER GI BLEEDING

CAUSES Common Peptic ulcer, gastritis (alcohol, aspirin, NSAIDs, stress), esophagitis, Mallory-Weiss tear (mucosal tear at gastroesophageal junction due to retching), gastroesophageal varices.

Less common Swallowed blood (nosebleed); esophageal, gastric, or intestinal neoplasm; anticoagulant and fibrinolytic therapy; hypertrophic gastropathy (Ménétrier's disease); aortic aneurysm; aortoenteric fistula (from aortic graft); AV malformation; telangiectases (Osler-Rendu-Weber syndrome); vasculitis; connective-tissue disease (pseudoxanthoma elasticum, Ehlers-Danlos syndrome); blood dyscrasias; neurofibroma; amyloidosis; hemobilia (biliary origin).

EVALUATION Only *after* hemodynamic resuscitation (see below).

- History and physical examination: Drugs, prior ulcer, bleeding history, family history, features of cirrhosis or vasculitis, etc.
- Nasogastric aspirate for blood if upper source not clear from history; may be falsely negative if bleeding has ceased.
- Upper endoscopy: Accuracy >90%; allows visualization of bleeding site and possibility of therapeutic intervention; mandatory for suspected varices, aortoenteric fistulas; preferable to radiography for suspected ulcer to identify "visible vessel" (protruding artery in ulcer crater), which connotes high (~50%) risk of rebleeding.
- Upper GI barium radiography: Accuracy ~80%; acceptable alternative to endoscopy in resolved or chronic low-grade bleeding.
- Selective mesenteric arteriography: When brisk bleeding precludes adequate endoscopic examination.
- Radioisotope scanning (e.g., ^{99m}Tc tagged to red blood cells or albumin): Used primarily as screening test to assess feasibility of arteriography in intermittent bleeding of unclear origin.

LOWER GI BLEEDING

CAUSES Anal lesions (hemorrhoids, fissures), rectal trauma, proctitis, colitis (ulcerative colitis, Crohn's disease, infectious colitis, ischemic colitis), colonic polyps, colonic carcinoma, angiodysplasia (vascular ectasia), diverticulosis, intussusception, solitary ulcer, blood dyscrasias, vasculitis, connective-tissue disease, neurofibroma, amyloidosis, anticoagulation.

EVALUATION

- History and physical examination.
- Anoscopy and sigmoidoscopy: Exclude hemorrhoids, fissure, ulcer, proctitis, neoplasm.
- Nasogastric aspirate (if any suspicion of upper GI source, best to do upper endoscopy).
- Barium enema: No role in active bleeding.
- Arteriography (requires bleeding rate >0.5 mL/min; may require prestudy radioisotope bleeding scan as above): Defines site of bleeding or abnormal vasculature.
- Colonoscopy: May be impossible if bleeding is massive.
- Surgical exploration (last resort).

BLEEDING OF OBSCURE ORIGIN Often small-bowel source. Consider small-bowel enteroclysis x-ray (careful barium radiography via peroral intubation of small bowel), Meckel's

scan, or exploratory laparotomy with intraoperative enter-
oscopy.

MANAGEMENT

- Venous access with large bore IV (14–18 gauge); central
  venous line for major bleed and pts with cardiac disease;
  monitor vital signs, urine output, hemoglobin (fall may
  lag). Gastric lavage of unproven benefit, but clears stomach
  before endoscopy; ice may lyse clots, room-temperature
  fluid may be preferable.
- Type and cross match blood (6 units for major bleed).
- Surgical standby.
- Support blood pressure with isotonic fluids (normal saline),
  albumin and fresh frozen plasma in cirrhotics, then packed
  red blood cells when available (whole blood if massive
  bleeding); maintain Hct ≥25–30.
- Fresh frozen plasma and vitamin K (10 mg SC or IV) in
  cirrhotics with coagulopathy.
- IV calcium (e.g., up to 10–20 mL 10% calcium gluconate
  IV over 10–15 min) if serum calcium falls (due to transfusion
  of citrated blood).
- Empiric drug therapy (antacids, H-2-receptor blockers) of
  unproven benefit; experimental—IV somatostatin, prostaglandins; ethinylestradiol/norethisterone (0.05/1.0 mg PO
  qd) may prevent recurrent bleeding from GI vascular
  malformations.
- Specific measures: *Varices:* IV vasopressin (0.4–0.9 U/
  min), Blakemore-Sengstaken tube tamponade, endoscopic
  sclerosis (see Chap. 114); *ulcer with visible vessel or active
  bleeding:* endoscopic electro-, heater-probe, or laser coagulation; *gastritis:* embolization or vasopressin infusion
  of left gastric artery; *diverticulosis:* mesenteric arteriography with intraarterial vasopressin; *angiodysplasia:* colonoscopic electro- or laser coagulation, may regress with
  replacement of stenotic aortic valve.
- Indications for emergency surgery: Uncontrolled or prolonged bleeding, severe rebleeding, aortoenteric fistula.

For a more detailed discussion, see Richter JM, Isselbacher
KJ, Gastrointestinal Bleeding, Chap. 46, in HPIM-12, p. 261

18 ASSESSMENT OF LIVER FUNCTION, JAUNDICE, AND HEPATOMEGALY

BLOOD TESTS OF LIVER FUNCTION

Used to evaluate functional status of liver and to discriminate among different types of liver disease (inflammatory, infiltrative, metabolic, vascular, hepatobiliary). (See Table 18-1.)

Bilirubin Provides indication of hepatic uptake, metabolic (conjugation), and excretory functions; conjugated fraction (direct-reacting) distinguished from unconjugated by chemical assay (see Table 18-2).

Aminotransferases (transaminases) Aspartate aminotransferase (AST; SGOT) and alanine aminotransferase (ALT; SGPT); sensitive indicators of liver cell integrity; greatest elevations seen in hepatocellular necrosis (e.g., viral hepatitis, toxic liver injury, circulatory collapse); levels correlate poorly with severity of disease; milder abnormalities in cholestatic, cirrhotic, and infiltrative disease; ALT more specific measure of liver injury, since AST also found in striated muscle; ethanol-induced liver injury usually produces

TABLE 18-1   Patterns of liver test abnormalities

| Test | Type of liver disease | | | |
	Hepato-cellular	Obstructive	Ischemic	Infiltrative
AST, ALT*	↑ ↑ ↑	↑	↑ – ↑ ↑ ↑	N– ↑
Alkaline phosphatase	↑ – ↑ ↑	↑ ↑ ↑	↑ – ↑ ↑	↑ – ↑ ↑ ↑
5'-Nucleotidase	↑ – ↑ ↑	↑ ↑ ↑	↑	↑ – ↑ ↑ ↑
Bilirubin	↑ – ↑ ↑ ↑	↑ – ↑ ↑ ↑	N– ↑	N
Prothrombin time	↑ – ↑ ↑ ↑	N†	N– ↑ ↑	N
Albumin	N– ↓ ↓ ↓	N‡	N– ↓	N

* In *acute complete obstruction,* serum transaminases may rise rapidly and dramatically, but return to near normal levels after 1–3 days even in the presence of continued obstruction.

† May increase with prolonged biliary obstruction and secondary biliary cirrhosis.

‡ May decrease with prolonged biliary obstruction and secondary biliary cirrhosis.

Note: N, normal; ↑, elevated; ↓, decreased. (Modified from Podolsky DK, Isselbacher KJ, HPIM-12, p. 1308.)

TABLE 18-2 Causes of hyperbilirubinemia

PREDOMINANTLY UNCONJUGATED (INDIRECT-REACTING) BILIRUBIN

Overproduction of bilirubin pigments: Intravascular hemolysis, hematoma resorption, ineffective erythropoiesis (bone marrow)

Decreased hepatic uptake: Sepsis, prolonged fasting, right-sided heart failure, drugs (e.g., rifampin, probenecid)

Decreased conjugation: Severe hepatocellular disease (e.g., hepatitis, cirrhosis), sepsis, drugs (e.g., chloramphenicol), inherited glucuronyl transferase deficiency (Gilbert's syndrome, Crigler-Najjar syndrome type II, or Crigler-Najjar syndrome type I)

PREDOMINANTLY CONJUGATED (DIRECT-REACTING) BILIRUBIN

Impaired hepatic excretion: Hepatocellular disease (e.g., drug-induced, viral, or ischemic hepatitis, cirrhosis), drug-induced cholestasis (e.g., oral contraceptives, methyltestosterone), sepsis, postoperative state, inherited disorders (Dubin-Johnson syndrome, Rotor syndrome, cholestasis of pregnancy, benign familial recurrent cholestasis)

Biliary obstruction: Biliary cirrhosis (primary or secondary), sclerosing cholangitis, mechanical obstruction (e.g., stone, tumor, stricture)

Modified from Isselbacher KJ, HPIM-12, p. 267.

---

modest increases with more prominent elevation of AST than ALT.

Lactate dehydrogenase (LDH) Less specific measure of hepatocellular integrity with little value in evaluation of liver disease.

Alkaline phosphatase Sensitive indicator of cholestasis (more sensitive than serum bilirubin) and liver infiltration; mild elevations in other forms of liver disease; limited specificity because of wide tissue distribution; elevations also seen in childhood, pregnancy, and bone diseases; tissue-specific isoenzymes can be distinguished by differences in heat stability (liver enzyme activity stable under conditions that destroy bone enzyme activity).

5′-Nucleotidase (5′-NT) Pattern of elevation in hepatobiliary disease similar to alkaline phosphatase; has greater specificity for liver disorders; used to determine whether liver is source of elevation in serum alkaline phosphatase, esp. in children, pregnant women, pts with possible concomitant bone disease.

γ-Glutamyltranspeptidase Correlates with serum alkaline phosphatase activity; greater sensitivity for hepatobiliary disease, but also elevated in pancreatic, renal, pulmonary, and cardiac disorders.

Prothrombin time (see also Chap. 133) Measure of clotting factor activity; prolongation results from clotting-factor deficiency or inactivity; all clotting factors except factor VIII are synthesized in the liver, and deficiency commonly results from widespread liver necrosis, as in hepatitis, toxic injury, or cirrhosis; clotting factors II, VII, IX, X function only in the presence of the fat-soluble vitamin K; PT prolongation from fat malabsorption distinguished from hepatic disease by rapid response to vitamin K replacement.

Albumin   Decreased serum levels result from decreased hepatic synthesis (chronic liver disease or prolonged malnutrition) or excessive losses in urine or stool; insensitive indicator of acute hepatic dysfunction, since serum half-life is 2 to 3 weeks; in pts with chronic liver disease, degree of hypoalbuminemia correlates with severity of dysfunction.

Globulin   Mild polyclonal hyperglobulinemia often seen in chronic liver diseases; marked elevation frequently seen in the autoimmune, idiopathic form of chronic active hepatitis.

Ammonia   Elevated blood levels result from deficiency of hepatic detoxification pathways and portal-systemic shunting, as in fulminant hepatitis, hepatotoxin exposure, and severe portal hypertension (e.g., from cirrhosis); for many (but not all) pts, blood ammonia level correlates with degree of portal-systemic encephalopathy; asterixis correlates with encephalopathy more accurately, but does not distinguish among several metabolic causes, including hepatic dysfunction, uremia, and hypercarbia.

HEPATOBILIARY IMAGING PROCEDURES

Used in evaluation of jaundice, hepatomegaly, and liver biochemical test abnormalities.

Ultrasonography   Rapid, noninvasive examination of abdominal structures; no radiation exposure; relatively low cost, equipment portable; images and interpretation strongly dependent on expertise of examiner; particularly valuable for detecting biliary duct dilatation and gallbladder stones (>95%); much less sensitive for intraductal stones (~40%); most sensitive means of detecting ascites; only moderately sensitive for detecting hepatic masses but excellent for discriminating solid from cystic structures; useful in directing percutaneous needle biopsies of suspicious lesions; Doppler ultrasonography useful to determine patency and flow in portal, hepatic veins and portal-systemic shunts; imaging improved by presence of ascites but severely hindered by bowel gas; endoscopic ultrasonography less affected by bowel gas and is sensitive for determination of depth of tumor invasion through bowel wall.

CT   Particularly useful for detecting, differentiating, and directing percutaneous needle biopsy of abdominal masses, cysts, and lymphadenopathy; imaging enhanced by intestinal or intravenous contrast dye and unaffected by intestinal gas; less sensitive than ultrasound for detecting stones in gallbladder but more sensitive for choledocholithiasis; may be useful in distinguishing certain forms of diffuse hepatic disease (e.g., fatty infiltration, iron overload).

MRI   Holds promise for most sensitive detection of hepatic masses and cysts; allows easy differentiation of hemangiomas from other hepatic tumors; most accurate *noninvasive* means of assessing hepatic and portal vein patency, vascular invasion by tumor; useful for monitoring iron, copper deposition in liver (e.g., hemochromatosis, Wilson's disease).

Radionuclide scanning   Using various radiolabeled compounds, different scanning methods allow sensitive assessment of biliary excretion (HIDA, PIPIDA, DISIDA scans), parenchymal changes (technetium sulfur colloid liver/spleen scan), and selected inflammatory and neoplastic processes (gallium scan); HIDA and related scans particularly useful for assessing biliary patency and excluding acute cholecystitis; colloid scans and CT have similar sensitivity for detecting liver tumors and metastases; colloid scans provide most accurate assessment of spleen size and can provide strong indirect evidence for cirrhosis and portal hypertension; combination of colloidal liver and lung scans sensitive for detecting right subphrenic (suprahepatic) abscesses.

Cholangiography   Most sensitive means of detecting biliary ductal calculi, biliary tumors, sclerosing cholangitis, choledochal cysts, fistulas, and bile duct leaks; may be performed via endoscopic (transampullary) or percutaneous (transhepatic) route; allows sampling of bile for cytologic analysis and culture, placement of biliary drainage catheter, stricture dilatation, and gallstone dissolution; endoscopic route (ERCP) permits manometric evaluation of sphincter of Oddi, sphincterotomy, and stone extraction.

Angiography   Most accurate means of determining portal pressures and assessing patency and direction of flow in portal and hepatic veins; highly sensitive for detecting small vascular lesions and hepatic tumors (esp. primary hepatocellular carcinoma); ''gold standard'' for differentiating hemangiomas from solid tumors; most accurate means of studying vascular anatomy in preparation for complicated hepatobiliary surgery (e.g., portal-systemic shunting, biliary reconstruction) and determining resectability of hepatobiliary and pancreatic tumors.

JAUNDICE

Definition Yellow skin pigmentation caused by elevation in serum bilirubin level. *Icterus* refers to similar pigmentation in sclerae, which is often more easily discernible. Jaundice and icterus become clinically evident at a serum bilirubin level of 34–43 μmol/L (2–2.5 mg/dL) (approximately twice normal); yellow skin discoloration also occurs with elevated serum carotene levels, but there is no pigmentation of the sclerae.

BILIRUBIN METABOLISM Bilirubin is the major breakdown product of hemoglobin released from senescent erythrocytes. Initially it is bound to albumin, transported into the liver, conjugated to a water-soluble form (glucuronide) by glucuronyl transferase, excreted into the bile, and converted to urobilinogen in colon. Urobilinogen is mostly excreted in the stool; a small portion is reabsorbed and excreted by the kidney. Bilirubin can only be filtered by the kidney in its conjugated form (measured as the "direct" fraction); thus increased *direct* serum bilirubin level is associated with bilirubinuria. Increased bilirubin production and excretion (even without hyperbilirubinemia, as in hemolysis) produce elevated urinary urobilinogen levels.

ETIOLOGY Hyperbilirubinemia occurs as a result of (1) overproduction, (2) decreased hepatic uptake, (3) decreased hepatic conjugation (required for excretion), or (4) decreased biliary excretion (see Table 18-2). Disorders of liver transport mechanisms are often associated with pruritus, probably from decreased biliary excretion and increased skin deposition of bile salts; these include all causes of *conjugated* hyperbilirubinemia except Dubin-Johnson and Rotor syndromes and benign familial cholestasis (in which bilirubin excretion is disrupted exclusively).

HEPATOMEGALY

Definition Generally a span of greater than 12 cm in the right midclavicular line or a palpable left lobe in the epigastrium. It is important to exclude low-lying liver (e.g., with chronic obstructive pulmonary disease and lung hyperinflation) and other right upper quadrant masses. Independent assessment of size best obtained from ultrasound examination or radionuclide liver scan. Contour and texture are important: focal enlargement or rocklike consistency suggests tumor; tenderness suggests inflammation (e.g., hepatitis) or rapid enlargement (e.g., right-sided heart failure, Budd-Chiari syndrome, fatty infiltration). Cirrhotic livers are usually firm and nodular, often enlarged until late in course. Pulsations frequently connote tricuspid regurgitation. Arterial bruit or hepatic rub suggests tumor. Portal hypertension is occasionally associated with continuous venous hum (see Table 18-3).

TABLE 18-3   Important causes of hepatomegaly

Vascular congestion: Right-sided heart failure (including tricuspid valve disease), Budd-Chiari syndrome
Infiltrative disorders: Fatty liver (e.g., ethanol abuse, diabetes, parenteral hyperalimentation, pregnancy), lymphoma or leukemia, extramedullary hematopoiesis, amyloidosis, granulomatous hepatitis (e.g., TB, atypical mycobacterium, sarcoidosis, CMV), hemochromatosis, Gaucher's disease, glycogen storage diseases
Inflammatory disorders: Viral hepatitis, drug-induced hepatitis, cirrhosis
Tumors: Hepatocellular carcinoma, metastatic cancer, focal nodular hyperplasia, hepatic adenoma
Cysts (e.g., polycystic disease)

Modified from Isselbacher KJ, HPIM-12, p. 268.

For a more detailed discussion, see Isselbacher KJ: Jaundice and Hepatomegaly, Chap. 47, p. 264; Friedman LS, Needleman L: Hepatobiliary Imaging, Chap. 248, p. 1303; and Podolsky DK, Isselbacher KJ: Diagnostic Tests in Liver Disease, Chap. 249, p. 1308, in HPIM-12

19 ASCITES

DEFINITION

Accumulation of fluid within the peritoneal cavity. Small amounts may be asymptomatic; increasing amounts cause abdominal distention and discomfort, anorexia, nausea, early satiety, heartburn, frank pain, and respiratory distress.

DETECTION   Physical examination   (detects no less than several 100 mL): Bulging flanks, fluid wave, shifting dullness, "puddle sign" (dullness over dependent abdomen with patient on hands and knees). May be associated with penile or scrotal edema, umbilical or inguinal herniation, pleural effusion.

Ultrasonography/CT   Very sensitive; able to distinguish fluid from cystic masses.

EVALUATION   Diagnostic paracentesis (50–100 mL) essential; use 22-gauge needle in linea alba 2 cm below umbilicus or with "Z-track" insertion in LLQ or RLQ. Evaluation includes inspection, protein, cell count and differential, lactate dehydrogenase, amylase, pH, lipids, culture, cytology. Rarely, laparoscopy or even exploratory laparotomy may be required.

DIFFERENTIAL DIAGNOSIS   (More than 90% of cases due to cirrhosis, neoplasm, CHF, tuberculosis).

1. Diseases of peritoneum: Infections (bacterial, tuberculous, fungal, parasitic), neoplasms, vasculitis, miscellaneous (Whipple's disease, familial Mediterranean fever, endometriosis, starch peritonitis, etc.).

2. Diseases not involving peritoneum: Cirrhosis, CHF, Budd-Chiari syndrome, hypoalbuminemia (nephrotic syndrome, protein-losing enteropathy, malnutrition), miscellaneous (myxedema, ovarian diseases, pancreatic disease, chylous ascites).

Alternative classifications—serum-ascites albumin gradient   (difference in albumin concentrations between serum and ascites): *Exudative* (serum-ascites albumin gradient <1.1): 2° peritonitis, neoplasm, pancreatitis, vasculitis. *Transudative* (serum-ascites albumin gradient >1.1 suggesting increased hydrostatic pressure): cirrhosis, CHF, Budd-Chiari syndrome.

REPRESENTATIVE FLUID CHARACTERISTICS   (See Table 19-1.)

TABLE 19-1

Cause	Appearance	Protein, g/dL	Serum-ascites albumin gradient	Cell count, per mm³		Other
				RBC	WBC	
Cirrhosis	Straw-colored	<2.5	>1.1	Low	<250	—
Neoplasm	Straw-colored, hemorrhagic, mucinous, or chylous	>2.5	Variable	Often high	>1000 (>50% lymphs)	+ Cytology
2° bacterial peritonitis	Turbid or purulent	>2.5	<1.1	Low	>10,000	+ Gram's stain, culture (often multiple organisms)
Spontaneous bacterial peritonitis	Turbid or purulent	<2.5	>1.1	Low	>250 polys	+ Gram's stain, culture
Tuberculous peritonitis	Clear, hemorrhagic, or chylous	>2.5	<1.1	Occ. high	>1000 (>70% lymphs)	+ AFB stain, culture
CHF	Straw-colored	>2.5	>1.1	Low	<1000 (mesothelial)	—
Pancreatitis	Turbid, hemorrhagic, or chylous	>2.5	<1.1	Variable	Variable	Increased amylase

CIRRHOTIC ASCITES

PATHOGENESIS   Contributing factors: (1) portal hypertension, (2) hypoalbuminemia, (3) increased hepatic lymph formation, (4) renal sodium retention—secondary to hyperaldosteronism, increased sympathetic nervous activity (renin-angiotensin production); role of atrial natriuretic factor as yet unclear. Initiating event may be peripheral arterial vasodilation that leads to decreased "effective" plasma volume and activation of compensatory mechanisms to retain renal Na and preserve intravascular volume.

TREATMENT   Maximum mobilization $\simeq$ 700 mL/day (peripheral edema may be mobilized faster).

1. Initially bed rest, rigid salt restriction (400 mg Na/day).
2. Fluid restriction of 1–1.5 L only if hyponatremia.
3. Diuretics if no response after 1 week: spironolactone (mild, potassium-sparing, aldosterone-antagonist) 100 mg/day PO increased by 100 mg q 4–5 d to maximum of 600 mg/day; furosemide 40–80 mg/day PO or IV may be added if necessary (greater risk of hepatorenal syndrome, encephalopathy), can increase by 40 mg/d to maximum of 240 mg/d until effect achieved or complication occurs.
4. Monitor weight, urinary sodium and potassium, serum electrolytes and creatinine.
5. Repeated large-volume paracentesis (5 L) with IV infusions of albumin is an acceptable alternative to diuretic therapy for initial management of massive ascites and may be associated with fewer side effects.
6. In rare refractory cases, consider peritoneovenous (LeVeen, Denver) shunt (high complication rate—occlusion, infection, DIC) or side-to-side portacaval shunt (high mortality rate in end-stage cirrhotic patient).

COMPLICATIONS   Spontaneous bacterial peritonitis   Suspect in cirrhotic patient with ascites and fever, abdominal pain, worsening ascites, ileus, hypotension, worsening jaundice, or encephalopathy; suggested by ascitic fluid PMN cell count >250/mm³ or ascitic pH <blood pH; confirmed by positive culture (usually Enterobacteriaceae, group D streptococci, *Streptococcus pneumoniae, S. viridans*). Initial treatment: Cefotaxime 2 g IV q 6 h; efficacy demonstrated by marked decrease in ascitic PMN count after 48 h; treat 10–14 days.

Hepatorenal syndrome   Progressive renal failure characterized by azotemia, oliguria with urinary sodium concentration <10 mmol/L, hypotension, and lack of response to volume challenge. May be spontaneous or precipitated by bleeding, excessive diuresis, paracentesis, or drugs (aminoglycosides, NSAIDs). Thought to result from altered renal hemodynamics and decreased urinary prostaglandin levels. Prognosis poor. Treatment: Trial of plasma expansion; liver transplantation in selected cases.

For a more detailed discussion, see Glickman RM, Issel-bacher KJ: Abdominal Swelling and Ascites, Chap. 48, in HPIM-12, p. 269

---

20 ABNORMALITIES IN URINARY FUNCTION

AZOTEMIA Retention of nitrogenous waste normally cleared by the kidney, with marked (>50%) reduction in GFR; ↑ plasma creatinine (Cr) and urea (BUN).

OLIGURIA/ANURIA Oliguria results with urine output less than the minimal amount necessary to remove waste products. When maximally concentrated, 400–500 mL urine/d must be formed to excrete the daily osmolar load. Smaller volumes result in azotemia. Anuria occurs with less than 100 mL urine daily. Bilateral urinary obstruction and renal arterial occlusion are treatable causes. May also be due to cortical necrosis, crescentic glomerulonephritis, and severe acute tubular necrosis.

The approach to the patient with oliguria/anuria is given in Table 20-1. Consider *prerenal* azotemia, due to hypovolemia or CHF. Also consider *postrenal* failure due to lower urinary tract obstruction. Acute intrinsic renal failure (Chap. 93) is the cause in the remainder.

POLYURIA Urine volume >3 L/d; reflects renal water loss due either to an increase in obligatory excretion or a decrease in tubular reabsorption of water (Table 20-2).

Obligate water loss is due to increased intake in *primary polydipsia,* a psychogenic disorder commonly associated with other mental illness and occurring most often in middle-aged women. Diuretic or cathartic abuse is frequently present. Obligate water loss also may be due to *solute diuresis* after infusion of glucose, saline, or mannitol; glucosuria in the poorly controlled diabetic; and urea from high-protein feedings. Polyuria also occurs in the recovery phase of acute tubular necrosis, after renal transplantation, in salt-wasting conditions, after relief of urinary obstruction, and in diuretic abuse.

Decreased tubular reabsorption of water is due to *diabetes insipidus* (DI). Causes are inadequate secretion of vasopressin (central DI) or renal tubular unresponsiveness to the hormone (nephrogenic DI) (see Chap. 97). Nephrogenic DI may be congenital but is usually acquired, due to tubulointerstitial diseases (obstructive uropathy, hypercalcemia, hypokalemia, analgesic abuse, pyelonephritis) or to drugs (lithium, ethanol, propoxyphene, phenytoin, methoxyflurane).

Polydipsia and DI are best evaluated by water deprivation test and administration of exogenous vasopressin. During water deprivation polydipsic patients will concentrate urine

TABLE 20-1   Approach to the oliguric patient

1. Obtain Hx for volume depletion, i.e., prerenal oliguria (diarrhea, diuresis, poor intake) or postrenal factors (bladder, prostate, anticholinergic or opioid drugs, recent catheter).
2. Evaluate physical exam for prerenal (low BP, tachycardia, flat neck veins, poor skin turgor) or postrenal (large bladder, CVA tenderness, pelvic mass) factors.
3. Search for potential causes of ARF (hypotension, nephrotoxins, sepsis, systemic disease).
4. Obtain urine tests:

	Prerenal	ARF	Postrenal*
U_{Na} (mmol/L)	<20	>40	Variable
U_{osmol} (mosmol/kg)	>500	<350	Variable
FENA†	<1	>1	Variable
Urinalysis	Normal	Muddy brown casts	Crystals, WBCs, RBCs, bacteria
U/P Cr	>40	>20	Variable

5. Echo to rule out obstruction.
6. Fluid challenge if prerenal cause is suspected

---

* In acute obstruction values resemble prerenal.

† $FENA = \dfrac{U_{Na} (mmol/L)}{S_{Na} (mmol/L)} \times \dfrac{S_{Cr} (\mu mol/L)}{U_{Cr} (\mu mol/L)} \times 100$

where FENA = fraction of filtered Na which is excreted; U = urine; S = serum.

to 600–800 mosmol/kg, not lose weight, and exhibit little further response to vasopressin. Patients with complete central DI will lose weight and continue to form a dilute urine, which improves with vasopressin. Patients with nephrogenic DI will lose weight and elaborate a dilute urine during water deprivation and improve very little after vasopressin. Responses may overlap among milder cases of these disorders.

PROTEINURIA   An important indicator of renal parenchymal disease. Normal urine contains <150 mg protein/d. Concentrated urine may contain trace to 1 + proteinuria by dipstick. Alkaline urine may cause false-positive dipstick for protein. Dipstick will not detect light-chain proteinuria or small proteins from damaged renal tubules.

Conditions causing mild proteinuria (<1 g/d) include CHF, hypertensive nephrosclerosis, and polycystic kidney disease; also, orthostatic proteinuria, vigorous exercise, and fever. Interstitial nephritis, analgesic abuse, sickle cell anemia, and some glomerulonephritides are typically associated with moderate (1–3.5 g/d) proteinuria. Massive proteinuria (>3.5 g/d)

TABLE 20-2 Major causes of polyuria

Obligate water excretion	Decreased water reabsorption
Psychogenic polydipsia	**Central DI:**
	Idiopathic
Solute diuresis:	Hypophysectomy
Glucose	Head trauma
Saline	Tumors
Diabetes mellitus	Sarcoidosis
Protein feeding	Infection
Contrast agents	
Recovery ATN	**Nephrogenic DI:**
Renal transplant	Hypokalemia
Salt-wasting nephropathy	Hypercalcemia
Postobstruction	Obstructive uropathy
Diuretics	Analgesic abuse
	Pyelonephritis
	Drugs

with hypoalbuminemia, edema, and hyperlipidemia is characteristic of the nephrotic syndrome (Chap. 96).

Evaluation Given a reliable dipstick indicating proteinuria ≥1 +, a 24-h urine collection is done to quantify urine protein. If ≥150 mg of protein is present, electrophoresis should be done. Proteinuria due to activity or upright posture can be excluded by analyzing a first morning urine collection. Renal biopsy is often necessary in moderate to severe cases.

HEMATURIA Definition The presence of gross blood or RBCs (>1–2 per hpf) in the spun urine sediment. The dipstick does *not* distinguish among intact RBCs, Hb, and myoglobin. *Hemoglobinuria* may be due to lysis of urine red cells in hypotonic urine or to filtered plasma Hb. *Myoglobinuria* originates from circulating myoglobin due to injured muscle. Both hemoglobinuria and myoglobinuria cause + dipstick even in presence of a negative sediment.

Hematuria may originate at any site from glomerulus to urethra. Concomitant proteinuria and impaired renal function suggest a renal parenchymal source. RBC casts support a diagnosis of glomerulonephritis.

Isolated hematuria (without RBC casts or proteinuria) suggests bleeding from a site between renal pelvis and urethra, such as neoplasm of urinary tract, tuberculosis, renal calculi, trauma, papillary necrosis, analgesic nephropathy, hemoglobinopathies, IgA nephropathy, prostatitis, and acute cystitis. Menstrual contamination may be mistaken for hematuria in the female.

Hematuria is common with infection of the upper and lower urinary tracts. Hematuria associated with casts containing red blood cells or hemoglobin pigment connotes significant renal disease such as glomerulonephritis, tubulointerstitial injury, or vasculitis.

Diagnosis   Exclude coagulation disorders, UTI, tuberculosis, and sickle cell disease. The *pattern* of hematuria may suggest a specific source, e.g., bladder (hematuria throughout voiding), urethra (hematuria at start of voiding), or prostate (terminal hematuria). IVP, ultrasound, and cystoscopy are often useful.

If renal disease is evident, serologic tests (ANA, complement, hepatitis B, VDRL) should be performed. A renal biopsy may be required to make a specific diagnosis.

DYSURIA, FREQUENCY, AND URGENCY   Dysuria is a painful or burning sensation during urination. Frequency means voiding at abnormally brief intervals prompted by a sense of bladder fullness. Urgency is an exaggerated desire to urinate. Dysuria on urination may result from cystitis, prostatitis, radiation, chemicals, foreign bodies (catheters, stones), and bladder tumors.

Appropriate workup should include pelvic exam in women, rectal exam in both sexes, and if indicated prostatic massage for collection of prostatic fluid in men. Further evaluation may require urine or prostatic fluid cultures, radiographic studies, and cystoscopy.

INCONTINENCE   Incontinence is the inability to retain urine in the bladder. *Detrusor instability* is common in elderly pts with CNS disease. Other causes include bladder or pelvic infection or tumor, fecal impaction, uterine prolapse, and prostatic hyperplasia. The underlying cause must be treated. Imipramine, 25 mg qhs or calcium channel blockers may improve continence. *Stress incontinence*, the escape of small amounts of urine with increased intraabdominal pressure, is common in postmenopausal, parous women. Surgical elevation of the urethrovesical angle and/or estrogen replacement may be helpful. In men, causes include prostate surgery and prostate cancer. *Mechanical incontinence* from congenital abnormalities (exstrophy of the bladder, patent urachus, or ectopic uretral openings) may be surgically correctable. Alternatively, prostate or pelvic surgery or irradiation may be the cause. *Overflow incontinence* results from large residual volumes of urine secondary to bladder neck obstruction, urethral obstruction (stricture, BPH), or neurologic damage (spinal cord disease, peripheral neuropathy, collagen-vascular disease, toxic neuropathies).

Enuresis is the involuntary passage of urine at night or during sleep. Most bedwetting stops by the age of 3. Organic disease (UTI, obstructive lesions, neurovesical dysfunction, polyuric conditions) must be ruled out when enuresis persists beyond this age. Organic disease usually causes daytime incontinence as well. Imipramine (75 mg qhs) may be useful.

For a more detailed discussion, see Coe FL: Alterations in Urinary Function, Chap. 49, in HPIM-12, p. 271

Detrusor instability - 60-70%

AKA - unstable, uninhibited, spastic

Sx - frequency, urgency, day + night, volume moderate
Sns - residual <100ml
    - normal neuro

Tx - 1) treat cause
     2) toilet training, pads
     3) Rx - BEWARE - urine retention - hypotension, confusion

Overflow incontinence - 10%
  Sx - small volumes, day + night, hesitancy, etc.
  Sns - palpable bladder, residual >100 ml, +/- neuro signs
  Cause - outlet obstruction - prostate
        - detrusor inadequacy
  Tx - Obstruction - surgery, drugs (α-blocker), intermittent catheter,
              sepsis prophylaxis
       Detrusor inadeq. - decompress bladder, augment voiding,
              bethanecol

Sphincter insufficiency (Stress incontinence)
  Sx - stress, dry at night, low volume, normal residuals
  Sn - pelvic, neurological, NB - COPD

21 ELECTROLYTES/ACID-BASE BALANCE

SODIUM

HYPONATREMIA (Serum Na <135 mmol/L)   Due to excess body H_2O relative to Na and occurs in conditions in which total extracellular fluid Na may be normal, ↑, or ↓. Hypoosmolality is present unless non-Na solutes are ↑↑, as in diabetes mellitus, severe hyperlipidemia, or severe hyperproteinemic states, such as multiple myeloma. For interpretation of these disorders, assessment of volume status is essential (Fig. 21-1).

Hypovolemic hyponatremia   Results when Na losses, usually from GI tract, exceed losses of H_2O, often associated with partial volume replacement with H_2O and/or impaired H_2O diuresis. Clinical features reflect volume depletion; urinary Na <10 mmol/L, except when vomiting produces metabolic alkalosis and obligates renal $NaHCO_3$ losses. Hypovolemic hyponatremia may also result from renal losses (diuretics, Addison's disease, or osmotic diuresis); urinary Na >20 mmol/L.

Hypervolemic hyponatremia   Occurs when increase in total body H_2O exceeds increase of Na; may occur in severe CHF, cirrhosis, and nephrotic syndrome. Urinary Na <10 mmol/L except in renal failure.

Euvolemic hyponatremia   Occurs in syndrome of inappropriate vasopressin (AVP) secretion (also termed syndrome of inappropriate antidiuretic hormone, SIADH) in which excessive AVP-mediated H_2O reabsorption causes dilutional hyponatremia, urine is relatively hypertonic to plasma, and urinary Na is lost despite normal renal and adrenal function. Common causes are ectopic production of AVP by tumors (e.g., oat cell cancer of lung), endogenous overproduction due to pulmonary diseases (pneumonia, abscess, tuberculosis, positive end-expiratory pressure), CNS disorders (tumors, meningitis, encephalitis, trauma, subarachnoid hemorrhage, stroke), and stressful conditions. Drugs may impair water excretion by releasing AVP (e.g., morphine, tricyclics, cyclophosphamide, nicotine), enhancing its action (NSAIDs), or both (sulfonylureas). Hypothyroidism and cortisol deficiency may also cause euvolemic hyponatremia.

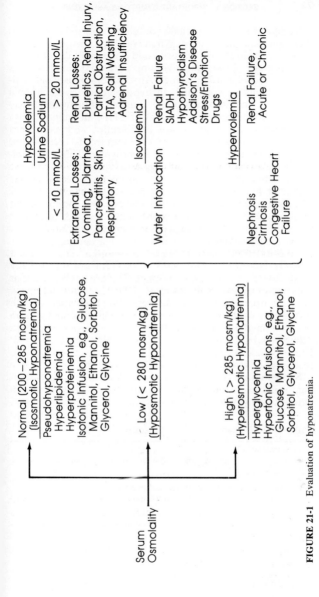

FIGURE 21-1 Evaluation of hyponatremia.

Serum Osmolality

Normal (200–285 mosm/kg)
(Isosmotic Hyponatremia)
Pseudohyponatremia
Hyperlipidemia
Hyperproteinemia
Isotonic Infusion, eg, Glucose,
Mannitol, Ethanol, Sorbitol,
Glycerol, Glycine

Low (< 280 mosm/kg)
(Hyposmotic Hyponatremia)

High (> 285 mosm/kg)
(Hyperosmotic Hyponatremia)
Hyperglycemia
Hypertonic Infusions, e.g.,
Glucose, Mannitol, Ethanol,
Sorbitol, Glycerol, Glycine

Hypovolemia
Urine Sodium

< 10 mmol/L

> 20 mmol/L

Extrarenal Losses:
Vomiting, Diarrhea,
Pancreatitis, Skin,
Respiratory

Renal Losses:
Diuretics, Renal Injury,
Partial Obstruction,
RTA, Salt Wasting,
Adrenal Insufficiency

Isovolemia

Water Intoxication

Renal Failure
SIADH
Hypothyroidism
Addison's Disease
Stress/Emotion
Drugs

Hypervolemia

Nephrosis
Cirrhosis
Congestive Heart
Failure

Renal Failure,
Acute or Chronic

Symptoms These include confusion, anorexia, lethargy, disorientation, and cramps. When Na drops abruptly to <120 mmol/L, seizures, hemiparesis, and coma may develop.

Treatment First, assess volume status. Hypovolemic pts should receive normal saline. Any mineralocorticoid deficiency should be corrected. In hypervolemic hyponatremia H_2O intake should be restricted. Further improvement may occur with appropriate treatment of CHF, albumin infusion in nephrosis, or cautious use of diuretics and sometimes albumin in cirrhosis. Pts with SIADH require H_2O restriction; demeclocycline, which induces nephrogenic diabetes insipidus (DI), may be helpful for long-term therapy. Hypertonic saline infusion is reserved for situations where there is profound hyponatremia (serum Na <120 mmol/L) and/or when neurologic status is compromised. The sodium deficit must be calculated, and half of the deficit required to correct Na to 120 mmol/L is replaced over 24 h (Table 21-1). Hypertonic solutions are always given via central veins.

HYPERNATREMIA (Serum Na >150 mmol/L) Due to deficit of H_2O relative to Na. May result from: (1) loss of H_2O, usually insensible losses (from skin or lungs) that are not replaced; or *renal* losses from diabetes insipidus (DI) caused by head injury, or neurosurgery; (2) H_2O losses exceeding Na losses: (a) with fever, burns, or exposure to high temperature; or (b) from renal losses during osmotic diuresis, as in severe hyperglycemia, in which urine is hypo- or isotonic with Na >20 mmol/L; (3) Na excess may occur in pts who ingest NaCl or are resuscitated with hypertonic $NaHCO_3$ (see Fig. 21-2).

Symptoms These include altered mental status, twitching, seizures, coma. Acute severe hypernatremia (>160 mmol/L) dehydrates cerebral cells and may rupture cerebral

TABLE 21-1　Guides for design of therapy

Hyponatremia:
　Calculated Na deficit (mmol) = 0.6 × wt (kg) × (140-Na) + 140 × volume deficit (L)

Corrections for serum triglycerides and protein:
　% serum water = 99 − 1.03 × lipids (g/L) − 0.073 × protein (g/L)
　Corrected Na = measured Na × $\dfrac{0.93}{\%\ \text{serum water}}$

Corrections for serum glucose:
　Corrected Na = glucose (mmol/L) + serum Na (mmol/L)

Hypernatremia:
　Calculated water deficit = 0.6 × wt (kg) × $\dfrac{(Na - 1)}{140}$

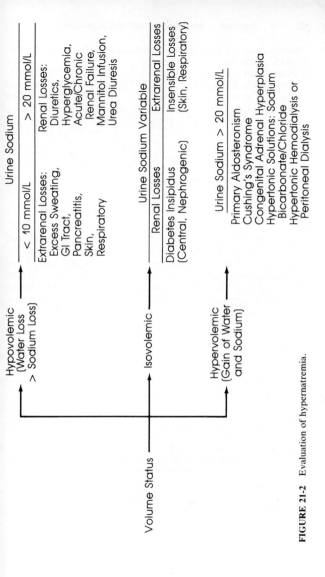

FIGURE 21-2 Evaluation of hypernatremia.

75

vessels, causing irreversible neurologic sequelae and substantial mortality.

Treatment   Correct osmolality by replacing H_2O slowly. Hypovolemic hypernatremia is initially treated with isotonic saline until volume is repleted, then with 0.45% saline. When manifestations of hypertonicity predominate, hypotonic saline may be initial therapy. Hypervolemic hypernatremia is best treated with hypotonic fluids and loop diuretics or, when indicated, dialysis. Pts with central DI should receive aqueous vasopressin or the intranasal analogue, desmopressin. In pts with partial central DI, chlorpropamide may suffice. Nephrogenic DI frequently responds to thiazides and Na restriction.

POTASSIUM

EXTERNAL K BALANCE   This is determined by oral intake and renal excretion. 90% of K intake is excreted by the kidney, most secreted by the distal nephron, a process augmented by aldosterone, high cell K content, and alkalosis. Factors that modulate *internal K balance* include insulin, beta$_2$-adrenergic agonists, and alkalosis, which promote K uptake by cells. Acidosis shifts K out of cells.

TABLE 21-2 **Causes of potassium depletion and hypokalemia**

 I. Gastrointestinal
   A. Deficient dietary intake
   B. Gastrointestinal disorders (vomiting, diarrhea, villous adenoma, fistulas, ureterosigmoidostomy)
 II. Renal
   A. Metabolic alkalosis
   B. Diuretics, osmotic diuresis
   C. Excessive mineralocorticoid effects
     1. Primary aldosteronism
     2. Secondary aldosteronism (including malignant hypertension, Bartter's syndrome, juxtaglomerular cell tumor)
     3. Licorice ingestion
     4. Glucocorticoid excess (Cushing's syndrome, exogenous steroids, ectopic ACTH production)
   D. Renal tubular diseases
     1. Renal tubular acidosis
     2. Leukemia
     3. Liddle's syndrome
     4. Antibiotics
   E. Magnesium depletion
 III. Hypokalemia due to shift into cells (no depletion)
   A. Hypokalemic periodic paralysis
   B. Insulin effect
   C. Alkalosis

HYPOKALEMIA (K <3.5 mmol/L) (Table 21-2) May result from: (1) inadequate intake and/or (2) excessive losses: (a) GI (vomiting, nasogastric suction, diarrhea, villous adenoma, and laxative abuse) and associated alkalosis, secondary hyperaldosteronism, and bicarbonaturia; (b) renal losses of K may result from alkalosis of any cause, from diuretics (except K-sparing agents), osmotic diuresis, as in hyperglycemia, primary and secondary hyperaldosteronism, renal tubular disorders, drugs (amphotericin, gentamicin, and carbenicillin), and Mg depletion; (3) hypokalemia due to *internal* imbalance occurs when cellular uptake of K from extracellular fluid is increased, as in alkalosis, after insulin therapy, or in periodic paralysis.

Clinical features Muscle weakness, ileus, polyuria, and ECG changes (U-waves, ↑ Q-T interval, and flat T-waves). Severe hypokalemia causes flaccid paralysis and cardiac arrest.

The cause of hypokalemia is usually evident on presentation (see Table 21-2). Inadequate intake or diarrhea is suggested when urinary K excretion <25 mmol/d. Greater urinary K losses suggest vomiting, current diuretic use, or renal tubular losses. Acidosis suggests diarrhea, renal tubular acidosis, or diabetic ketoacidosis. Mineralocorticoid excess is suggested by increased renal K losses and hypertension.

Treatment Dietary supplements, using KCl, suffices in mild cases. In edematous pts on diuretics, dietary supplementation and addition of K-sparing agents (e.g., aldactone) are useful. GI losses should be replaced with IV KCl (≤20 mmol/h). Severe symptomatic hypokalemia requires larger doses (20–40 mmol/h), with cardiac monitoring and frequent plasma K levels. Hypokalemia with digitalis toxicity also requires urgent correction.

HYPERKALEMIA (Serum K >5.5 mmol/L) (Table 21-3) May be due to *impaired K excretion,* as in oliguric acute renal failure, in chronic renal failure when GFR <10 mL/min, when dietary K is excessive, and/or with administration of K-sparing diuretics.

Hyporeninemic hypoaldosteronism Occurs in diabetes mellitus and the elderly. Acidosis and mild renal failure are frequent concomitants. Hypoaldosteronism also causes hyperkalemia in Addison's disease, in pts treated with NSAIDs, angiotensin converting enzyme inhibitors, heparin, and cyclosporine. Renal K retention is also provoked by spironolactone, triamterene, and amiloride.

Hyperkalemia due to *internal K imbalance* (release of K from cells) occurs in acidosis and in diabetics with deficient insulin-mediated K uptake. Cellular necrosis may release

TABLE 21-3   Causes of hyperkalemia

I. Inadequate excretion
  A. Renal failure
    1. Acute renal failure
    2. Severe chronic renal failure (GFR <10 mL/min)
    3. Tubular disorders
  B. Adrenal insufficiency
    1. Hypoaldosteronism
    2. Addison's disease
  C. Diuretics which inhibit potassium secretion (spironolactone, triam-terene, amiloride)
II. Shift of potassium from tissues
  A. Tissue damage (muscle crush, hemolysis, internal bleeding)
  B. Drugs: succinylcholine, arginine, digitalis poisoning, beta-adrenergic antagonists
  C. Acidosis
  D. Hyperosmolality
  E. Hyperkalemic periodic paralysis
III. Excessive intake
IV. Pseudohyperkalemia
  A. Thrombocytosis
  B. Leukocytosis
  C. Poor venipuncture technique
  D. In vitro hemolysis

---

excess K into the circulation, from muscle (e.g., rhabdomyolysis), tumor cells (tumor lysis syndrome), and RBCs (hemolytic states). Arginine HCl, used to correct metabolic acidosis, may elevate serum K in pts with renal and/or liver failure.

The most important *clinical effects* of hyperkalemia are cardiac conduction changes (Fig. 21-3) and arrhythmias, which are exaggerated by ↓ Na, ↓ Ca, acidosis, and ↑ Mg. Hyperkalemia may also cause an ascending muscle weakness.

Treatment   This is summarized in Table 21-4.

ACID-BASE DISORDERS   (Figure 21-4)

Regulation of normal pH (7.35–7.45) depends on lungs and kidneys. By the Henderson-Hasselbalch equation, pH is a function of the ratio of HCO_3 (regulated by the kidney) to P_{CO_2} (regulated by the lungs). The HCO_3/P_{CO_2} relationship is useful in classifying disorders of acid-base balance. *Acidosis* is due to gain of acid or loss of alkali; causes may be metabolic (fall in serum HCO_3) or respiratory (rise in P_{CO_2}). *Alkalosis* is due to loss of acid or addition of base, and is either metabolic (↑ serum HCO_3) or respiratory (↓ P_{CO_2}).

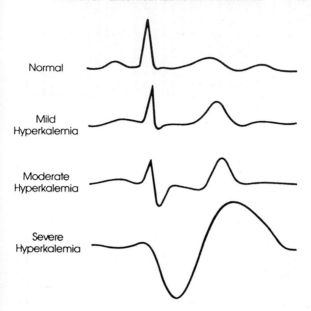

FIGURE 21-3   Diagrammatic ECGs at normal and high serum K. Peaked T waves (precordial leads) are followed by diminished R wave, wide QRS, prolonged P-R, loss of P wave, and ultimately a sine wave.

To limit the change in pH, metabolic disorders evoke an immediate compensatory response in ventilation; compensation to respiratory disorders by the kidneys takes days. *Simple* acid-base disorders consist of one primary disturbance and its compensatory response. In *mixed* disorders, a combination of primary disturbances is present.

METABOLIC ACIDOSIS   The low HCO_3 results from the addition of acids (organic or inorganic) or loss of HCO_3. The *causes* of metabolic acidosis are categorized by the anion gap, which equals $Na - (Cl + HCO_3)$ (Table 21-5). *Increased* anion gap acidosis (>12 mmol/L) is due to addition of acid (other than HCl) and unmeasured anions to the body. Causes include ketoacidosis (diabetes mellitus, starvation, alcohol), lactic acidosis, poisoning (salicylates, ethylene glycol, and ethanol) and renal failure. Diagnosis may be made by measuring BUN, creatinine, glucose, lactate, serum ketones, serum osmolality and obtaining a toxic screen.

Normal anion gap acidoses result from HCO_3 loss from the GI tract or from the kidney, e.g., renal tubular acidosis, urinary

TABLE 21-4 Management of hyperkalemia

Treatment	Indication	Dose	Onset	Duration	Mechanism	Note
Calcium gluconate*	K >6.5 mmol/L with advanced ECG changes	10 mL of 10% solution IV over 2–3 min	1–5 min	30 min	Lowers threshold potential. Antagonizes cardiac and neuromuscular toxicity of hyperkalemia.	Fastest action. Monitor ECG. Repeat in 5 min if abnormal ECG persists. Hazardous in presence of digitalis. Correct hyponatremia if present. Follow with other treatment for K.
Insulin + Glucose	Moderate hyperkalemia, peaked T waves only	10 U reg, IV + 50 mL, 50% IV	15–45 min	4–6 h	Moves K into cells.	Glucose unnecessary if blood sugar elevated. Repeat insulin q 15 min with glucose infusion if needed.
NaHCO$_3$	Moderate hyperkalemia	90 mmol (2 ampules, IV push over 5 min)	Immediate	Short	Moves K into cells.	Most effective when acidosis is present. Of more risk in CHF or hypernatremia. Beware of hypocalcemic tetany.
Kayexalate + Sorbitol	Moderate hyperkalemia	Oral: 30 g, with 50 mL 20% sorbitol; Rectal: 50 g in 200 mL 20% sorbitol enema, retain 45 min	1 h	4–6 h	Removes K.	Each gram Kayexalate removes about 1 mmol K orally or about 0.5 mmol K rectally. Repeat every 4 h. Use with caution in CHF.
Furosemide	Moderate hyperkalemia, serum creatinine <265 nmol/L (<3 mg%)	20–40 mg IV push	15 min	4 h	Kaliuresis.	Most useful if inadequate K excretion contributes to hyperkalemia.
Dialysis	Hyperkalemia with renal failure		Immediate after start-up	Variable	Removes K.	Hemodialysis most effective. Also improves acidosis.

* Calcium chloride may be preferable in presence of circulatory instability or liver impairment.

80

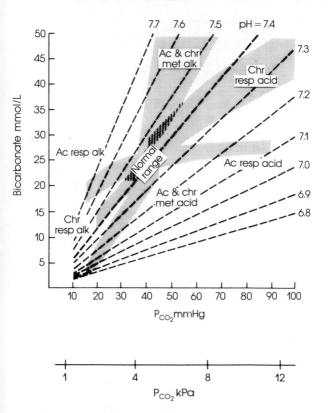

FIGURE 21-4 Nomogram, showing bands for uncomplicated respiratory or metabolic acid-base disturbances in intact subjects. Each "confidence" band represents the mean ±2 SD for the compensatory response of normal subjects or patients to a given primary disorder. Ac = acute; chr = chronic, resp = respiratory; met = metabolic; acid = acidosis; alk = alkalosis. *(From Levinsky NG: HPIM-12, p. 290; modified from Arbus GS: Can Med Assoc J 109:291, 1973.)*

obstruction, rapid volume expansion, and administration of NH_4Cl, lysine HCl, or arginine HCl. Calculation of urinary anion gap may be helpful in evaluation of hyperchloremic metabolic acidosis. A negative anion gap suggests GI losses; a positive anion gap suggests altered urinary acidification.

TABLE 21-5 Metabolic acidosis

Non-anion gap acidosis		Anion gap acidosis	
Cause	Clue	Cause	Clue
Diarrhea	Hx; ↓ K	DKA	Hypergly-cemia, ketones
Enterostomy	Drainage		
RTA		RF	Uremia, ↑ BUN, ↑ CR
Proximal	↓ K		
Distal	↓ K; UpH > 5.5	Lactic acidosis	Clinical setting + ↑ serum lactate
Dilutional	Volume expansion	Alcoholic ke-toacidosis	Hx; weak + ketones; + osm gap
Ureterosig-moidostomy	Obstructed ileal loop	Starvation	Hx; mild acidosis; + ketones
Hyperalimenta-tion	Amino acid infusion	Salicylates	Hx; tinnitus; high serum level; + ketones
Acetazola-mide, NH_4Cl, lysine HCl, arginine HCl	Hx of administration of these agents	Methanol	Large AG; retinitis; + toxic screen; + osm gap
		Ethylene glycol	RF, CNS; + toxic screen; crystalluria; + osm gap

RTA = renal tubular acidosis; UpH = urinary pH; DKA = diabetic ketoacidosis; RF = renal failure; AG = anion gap; osm gap = osmolar gap

Clinical features Include hyperventilation, cardiovascular collapse, and nonspecific symptoms ranging from anorexia to coma.

Treatment Depends on cause and severity. Always correct the underlying disturbance. Administration of alkali is controversial. It may be reasonable to treat lactic acidosis with intravenous HCO_3 at a rate sufficient to maintain a plasma HCO_3 of 8 to 10 mmol/L and a pH >7.10.

Chronic acidosis is treated when HCO_3 <15 mmol/L or symptoms of anorexia or fatigue are present. Na citrate may be more palatable than oral $NaHCO_3$. Oral therapy with $NaHCO_3$ usually begins with 1 g tid and is titrated *upward* to maintain desired serum HCO_3.

METABOLIC ALKALOSIS A primary increase in serum HCO_3. Most cases originate with volume concentration and loss of acid from the stomach or kidney. Less commonly, HCO_3 administered or derived from endogenous lactate is the cause and is perpetuated when renal HCO_3 reabsorption continues. In vomiting, Cl loss reduces its availability for renal reabsorption with Na. Enhanced Na avidity due to volume depletion then accelerates HCO_3 reabsorption and sustains the alkalosis. Urine Cl is typically low (<10 mmol/L) (Table 21-6). Alkalosis may also be maintained by hyperaldosteronism, due to enhancement of H secretion and HCO_3 reabsorption. Severe K depletion also causes metabolic alkalosis by increasing HCO_3 reabsorption; urine Cl >20 mmol/L.

Vomiting and nasogastric drainage cause HCl and volume loss, kaliuresis, and alkalosis. Diuretics are a common cause of alkalosis due to volume contraction, Cl depletion, and hypokalemia. Pts with chronic pulmonary disease, high P_{CO_2} and serum HCO_3 levels, whose ventilation is acutely improved, may develop alkalosis.

Excessive mineralocorticoid activity due to Cushing's syndrome (worse in ectopic ACTH or primary hyperaldosteronism) causes metabolic alkalosis not associated with volume or Cl depletion and not responsive to NaCl.

Severe K depletion also causes metabolic alkalosis.

Diagnosis The Cl on a random urine is useful (Table 21-6) unless diuretics have been administered.

Therapy Correct the underlying cause. In cases of Cl depletion, administer NaCl; and in hypokalemia, add KCl. Pts with adrenal hyperfunction require treatment of the underlying disorder.

Severe alkalosis may require, in addition, treatment with acidifying agents such as NH_4Cl, HCl, or acetazolamide. The initial amount of H needed (in mmol) should be calculated from $0.5 \times$ (body wt in kg) $\times$ (serum $HCO_3 - 24$).

RESPIRATORY ACIDOSIS Characterized by CO_2 retention due to ventilatory failure. Causes include sedatives, stroke,

TABLE 21-6 Metabolic alkalosis

NaCl responsive (low U_{Cl})	NaCl resistant (high U_{Cl})
Gastrointestinal causes:	Adrenal disorders:
Vomiting	Hyperaldosteronism
Nasogastric suction	Cushing's syndrome (1°, 2°, ectopic)
Chloride-wasting diarrhea	
Villous adenoma of colon	Exogenous steroids:
Diuretic therapy	Gluco- or mineralocorticoid
Posthypercapnia	Licorice ingestion
Carbenicillin or penicillin	Carbenoxolone
	Bartter's syndrome
	Refeeding alkalosis
	Alkali ingestion

chronic pulmonary disease, airway obstruction, severe pulmonary edema, neuromuscular disorders, and cardiopulmonary arrest.

Symptoms   These include confusion, asterixis, and obtundation.

Therapy   The goal is to improve ventilation through pulmonary toilet and reversal of bronchospasm. Intubation may be required in severe acute cases. Acidosis due to hypercapnia is usually mild.

RESPIRATORY ALKALOSIS   Excessive ventilation causes a primary reduction in CO_2 and $\uparrow$ pH in pneumonia, pulmonary edema, interstitial lung disease, asthma. Pain and psychogenic causes are common; other etiologies include fever, hypoxemia, sepsis, delirium tremens, salicylates, hepatic failure, mechanical overventilation, and CNS lesions. Severe respiratory alkalosis may cause seizures, tetany, cardiac arrhythmias, or loss of consciousness.

Therapy   Should be directed at the underlying disorders. In psychogenic cases, sedation or a rebreathing bag may be required.

"MIXED" DISORDERS   In many circumstances, more than a single acid-base disturbance exists. Examples include combined metabolic and respiratory acidosis with cardiogenic shock; metabolic alkalosis and acidosis in pts with vomiting and diabetic ketoacidosis; metabolic acidosis with respiratory alkalosis in pts with sepsis. The diagnosis may be clinically evident or suggested by relationships between the P_{CO_2} and HCO_3 that are markedly different from those found in simple disorders.

In simple anion-gap acidosis, anion gap increases in proportion to fall in HCO_3. When increase in anion gap occurs despite a normal HCO_3, simultaneous anion-gap acidosis and metabolic alkalosis are suggested. When fall in HCO_3 due to metabolic acidosis is proportionately larger than increase in anion gap, mixed anion gap and non-anion gap metabolic acidosis is suggested.

For a more detailed discussion, see Levinsky NG: Fluids and Electrolytes, Chap. 50, p. 278; and Levinsky NG: Acidosis and Alkalosis, Chap. 51, p. 289, in HPIM-12

22 LYMPHADENOPATHY AND SPLENOMEGALY

LYMPH NODE STRUCTURE AND FUNCTION

Lymph nodes are peripheral lymphoid organs populated by many cell types and connected to the circulation by afferent and efferent lymphatic vessels and postcapillary venules. Fibroblasts and fibroblast-derived reticular cells are supporting cells. Tissue macrophages, dendritic cells, and Langerhans cells are important antigen-presenting cells. Lymphoid follicles consist chiefly of B lymphocytes. Primary lymphoid follicles are aggregates of IgM- and IgD-bearing B cells as well as CD4$^+$ helper (inducer) T lymphocytes and arise prior to antigenic stimulation. Secondary lymphoid follicles result from antigenic stimulation and contain an inner zone (germinal center) of activated B cells, macrophages, reticular cells, and CD4$^+$ helper T cells. Interfollicular zones and paracortical areas are populated largely by T lymphocytes.

Juxtaposition of large numbers of macrophages, dendritic cells, Langerhans cells, and lymphocytes allows the lymph node to serve its major function as specialized structure for interaction of these cell types in efficient generation of cellular and humoral immune responses.

Lymph node enlargement can be due to (1) an increase in number of benign lymphocytes and macrophages during response to antigens, (2) infiltration of inflammatory cells during infections involving the node (lymphadenitis), (3) malignant proliferation of lymphocytes or macrophages arising in the node, (4) infiltration by metastatic malignant cells, or (5) infiltration by metabolite-laden macrophages in various storage diseases.

DISEASES ASSOCIATED WITH LYMPHADENOPATHY

For a complete list, see HPIM-12, Table 63-1, p. 355.
Infectious diseases

- Viral infections: Infectious hepatitis, mononucleosis syndromes, AIDS and AIDS-related complex, rubella, varicella zoster virus

- Bacterial infections: Streptococci, staphylococci, *Salmonella, Brucella, Francisella tularensis, Listeria monocytogenes, Pasteurella pestis, Haemophilus ducreyi,* cat-scratch disease
- Fungal infections
- Chlamydial infections
- Mycobacterial infections: Tuberculosis, leprosy
- Parasitic infections
- Spirochetal diseases

Immunologic diseases

- Rheumatoid arthritis, SLE, dermatomyositis
- Serum sickness
- Drug reactions: Diphenylhydantoin, hydralazine, allopurinol
- Angioimmunoblastic lymphadenopathy

Malignant diseases

- Hematologic: Hodgkin's disease, non-Hodgkin's lymphomas, acute and chronic leukemias
- Metastatic tumors to lymph nodes

Endocrine diseases   Hyperthyroidism.

Lipid storage diseases   Gaucher's and Niemann-Pick diseases.

Miscellaneous diseases   Giant follicular lymph node hyperplasia, sinus histiocytosis, dermatopathic lymphadenitis, sarcoidosis, amyloidosis, mucocutaneous lymph node syndrome (Kawasaki's disease), multifocal Langerhans cell (eosinophilic) granulomatosis.

SPLEEN STRUCTURE AND FUNCTION

The spleen is a lymphoreticular organ that serves at least four important functions: (1) major organ of immune system, involved in generation of cell-mediated and humoral responses to antigens, and major site of removal of microorganisms and particulate antigens from blood; (2) instrumental in sequestration and removal of normal and abnormal blood cells; (3) helps regulate portal blood flow; and (4) may be major site of extramedullary hematopoiesis in states of marrow stress or replacement.

DISEASES ASSOCIATED WITH SPLENIC ENLARGEMENT

For complete list, see HPIM-12, Table 63-2, p. 357.

Infections   Mononucleosis, septicemia, endocarditis, tuberculosis, parasites, AIDS, viral hepatitis, splenic abscess, histoplasmosis.

Disordered immunoregulation   Rheumatoid arthritis, SLE, immune hemolytic anemias, immune thrombocytopenias and neutropenias.

Disordered splenic blood flow   Portal or splenic venous hypertension with resultant splenic congestion.

Abnormal erythrocytes   Spherocytosis, sickle cell disease (before autosplenectomy occurs), ovalocytosis, thalassemia.

Infiltrative diseases   Benign and malignant.

Miscellaneous   Idiopathic splenomegaly, thyrotoxicosis, iron-deficiency anemia, sarcoidosis, berylliosis.

EVALUATION OF THE PATIENT WITH LYMPHADENOPATHY AND/OR SPLENOMEGALY

In normal adults, inguinal lymph nodes may be easily palpable, ranging from 0.5–2 cm in size. Smaller nodes may be palpable elsewhere due to past infections. Enlargement of lymph nodes requires investigation when there are one or more new nodes present ≥1 cm in diameter and not known to arise from a previously recognized cause. Important factors to consider: (1) pt's age, (2) physical characteristics of the node, (3) node locations, and (4) the clinical setting associated with the lymphadenopathy.

Normal sized spleen is about 12 cm in length and 7 cm in width; located along tenth left rib in mid-axillary line; inaccessible to palpation when normal in size and shape. Dullness can be percussed between ninth and eleventh ribs with pt lying on right side. Palpation best performed with lying to the right and inspiring deeply.

CLINICAL APPROACH TO THE PATIENT WITH LYMPHADENOPATHY AND/OR SPLENOMEGALY

1. Complete history and physical exam, with special attention to defining the presence and extent of adenopathy and presence of any systemic or localizing symptoms/signs, characterizing the illness as acute or chronic, eliciting any history of risk factors for HIV infection, and defining the size of the spleen.

2. If adenopathy is regional, search for infection or malignancy.

3. Laboratory studies should include (when appropriate): CBC, cultures of blood and other sites, CXR, PPD and

control skin testing, serologies (fungal, viral, HIV, parasitic, VDRL), mononucleosis screen (heterophile antibody and EBV titers), blood smear for cellular morphology and parasites, bone marrow aspiration and biopsy.

4. When necessary or appropriate, imaging techniques may prove useful: ^{99m}Tc-colloid liver/spleen scan, CT, abdominal ultrasound.

5. If adenopathy persists and remains unexplained, lymph node biopsy should be performed. Tissue should be processed for histologic exam, cultured for appropriate organisms, and frozen for lymphocyte studies and staining for other cell types.

6. Occasionally, laparotomy and splenectomy may be necessary for the diagnosis of persistent unexplained splenomegaly.

For a more detailed discussion, see Haynes BF: Enlargement of Lymph Nodes and Spleen, Chap. 63, in HPIM-12, p. 353

SECTION 2 MEDICAL EMERGENCIES

23 CARDIOVASCULAR COLLAPSE AND SUDDEN DEATH

Unexpected cardiovascular collapse and death most often results from ventricular fibrillation in pts with underlying coronary artery disease, with or without acute MI. Other common causes are listed in Table 23-1. The arrhythmic causes may be provoked by electrolyte disorders (primarily hypokalemia), hypoxemia, acidosis, or massive sympathetic discharge, as may occur in CNS injury. Immediate institution of cardiopulmonary resuscitation ˙(CPR) followed by advanced life support measures (see below) are mandatory. Ventricular fibrillation, or asystole, without institution of CPR within 4–6 min usually brings about death.

MANAGEMENT OF CARDIAC ARREST

Basic life support (BLS) commences immediately (Fig. 23-1):

TABLE 23-1 Differential diagnosis of cardiovascular collapse and sudden death

1. Ventricular fibrillation due to:
   Myocardial ischemia (severe coronary artery disease, acute MI)
   Congestive heart failure
   Dilated or hypertrophic cardiomyopathy
   Myocarditis
   Valvular disease [aortic stenosis, mitral valve prolapse (rare)]
   Preexcitation syndromes (Wolff-Parkinson-White)
   Prolonged QT syndromes (congenital, drug-induced)
2. Asystole or severe bradycardia
3. Sudden marked decrease in LV stroke volume from:
   Massive pulmonary embolism
   Cardiac tamponade
   Severe aortic stenosis
4. Sudden marked decrease in intravascular volume, e.g.:
   Ruptured aortic aneurysm
   Aortic dissection

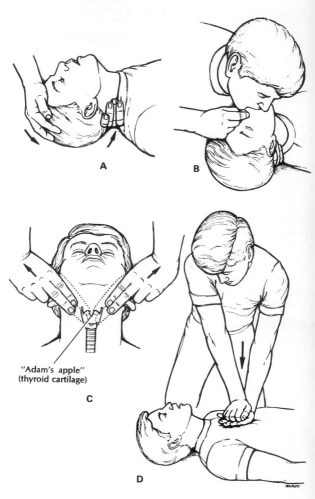

"Adam's apple"
(thyroid cartilage)

FIGURE 23-1 Major steps in cardiopulmonary resuscitation. *A*. Make certain the victim has an open airway. *B*. Start respiratory resuscitation immediately. *C*. Feel for the carotid pulse in the groove alongside the "Adam's apple" or thyroid cartilage. *D*. If pulse is absent, begin cardiac massage. Use 60 compressions/min with one lung inflation after each group of 5 chest compressions. (*From J Henderson, Emergency Medical Guide, 4th ed, New York, McGraw-Hill, 1978.*)

1. Open mouth of pt and remove visible debris or dentures. If there is respiratory stridor, consider possible aspiration of a foreign body and perform Heimlich maneuver.

2. Tilt head backward, lift chin, and begin mouth-to-mouth respiration if rescue equipment is not available (pocket mask is preferable to prevent transmission of infection). The lungs should be inflated once every 5 s when two persons are performing resuscitation, or twice in rapid succession every 15 s when one person performs both ventilation and chest compression.

3. If carotid pulse absent, perform chest compressions (depressing sternum 3–5 cm) at rate of 80–100 per min. For one rescuer, 15 compressions are performed before returning to ventilating twice.

As soon as resuscitation equipment is available, begin advanced life support (Fig. 23-2) with continued chest compressions and ventilation. Although performed as simultaneously as possible, defibrillation takes highest priority, followed by placement of intravenous access and intubation. 100% O_2 should be administered by endotracheal tube or, if rapid intubation cannot be accomplished, by bag-valve-mask device; respirations should not be interrupted for more than 30 s while attempting to intubate. Initial intravenous access should be through the antecubital vein, but if drug administration is ineffective, a central line (internal jugular or subclavian) should be placed. Intravenous $NaHCO_3$ should be administered only if there is persistent severe acidosis (pH <7.15) despite adequate ventilation. Calcium is *not* routinely administered but should be given to pts with known hypocalcemia, those who have received toxic doses of calcium channel antagonists, or if acute hyperkalemia is thought to be the triggering event for resistant ventricular fibrillation.

FOLLOW-UP

If cardiac arrest was due to ventricular fibrillation in initial hours of an AMI, follow-up is standard post-MI care (Chap. 74). For other survivors of a ventricular fibrillation arrest, extensive evaluation, including evaluation of coronary anatomy, left ventricular function, and invasive electrophysiologic testing, is recommended. Long-term antiarrhythmic drug therapy, implantation of an automatic defibrillator, and/or cardiac surgery (CABG, aneurysmectomy, or resection/ablation of arrhythmic foci) may be necessary.

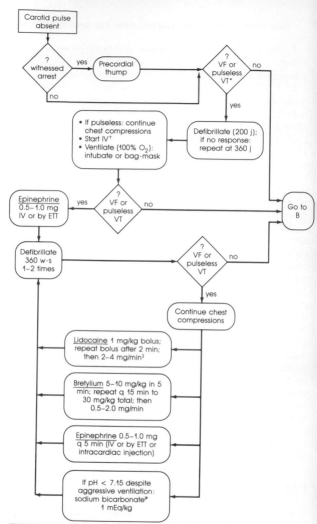

FIGURE 23-2 Advanced life support algorithm.

* Rhythm observed by "quick-look" defibrillator paddles; if monitored paddles are not available and patient is pulseless, do blind defibrillation.

\+ Antecubital route preferred; if infusions are not effective, place central (internal jugular, subclavian) line.

‡ Procainamide may be added if lidocaine is ineffective but loading is prolonged: 500–800 mg, no faster than 20 mg/min, followed by continuous infusion (2–5 mg/min).

¶ Do not infuse sodium bicarbonate in same IV line as calcium, epinephrine, or dopamine.

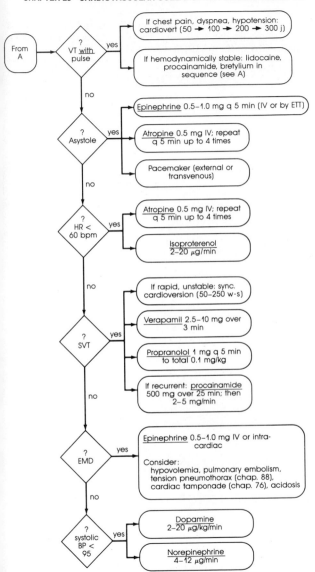

ETT = endotracheal tube. VT = ventricular tachycardia. HR = heart rate. SVT = supraventricular tachyarrhythmias. EMD = electromechanical dissociation.

For a more detailed discussion, see Myerburg RJ, Castellanos A: Cardiovascular Collapse, Cardiac Arrest, and Sudden Death, Chap. 40, in HPIM-12, p. 237

24 SHOCK

DEFINITION Condition of severe impairment of tissue perfusion. Rapid recognition and treatment are essential to prevent irreversible organ damage. Common etiologies are listed in Table 24-1.

CLINICAL MANIFESTATIONS Hypotension (systolic BP <90), tachycardia, tachypnea, pallor, restlessness, and altered sensorium; signs of intense peripheral vasoconstriction; weak pulses; cold clammy extremities (*note:* in septic shock, vasodilatation predominates and extremities are warm). Oliguria (<20 mL/h) and metabolic acidosis common.

APPROACH TO PATIENT Tissue perfusion must be restored immediately (see below); also obtain history for underlying cause, including

- Known cardiac disease (coronary disease, CHF, pericarditis)

TABLE 24-1 Common forms of shock

CARDIOGENIC SHOCK

Myopathic (acute MI, dilated cardiomyopathy)
Mechanical (acute mitral regurgitation, ventricular septal defect, severe aortic stenosis, idiopathic subaortic stenosis)
Arrhythmic

EXTRACARDIAC OBSTRUCTIVE SHOCK

Pericardial tamponade
Massive pulmonary embolism
Tension pneumothorax

OLIGEMIC SHOCK

Hemorrhage
Volume depletion (e.g., vomiting, diarrhea, diuretic overusage, ketoacidosis)
Internal sequestration (ascites, pancreatitis, intestinal obstruction)

DISTRIBUTIVE SHOCK (PROFOUND DECREASE IN SYSTEMIC VASCULAR TONE)

Sepsis
Toxic overdoses
Anaphylaxis
Neurogenic (e.g., spinal cord injury)
Endocrinologic (Addison's disease, myxedema)

- Recent fever or infection (leading to sepsis)
- Drugs, i.e., excess diuretics or antihypertensives
- Predisposing conditions for pulmonary embolism (Chap. 85)
- Possible bleeding from any site, particularly GI tract.

PHYSICAL EXAMINATION

- Jugular veins are flat in oligemic or distributive shock; jugular venous distention (JVD) suggests cardiogenic shock; JVD in presence of paradoxical pulse may reflect cardiac tamponade (Chap. 76).
- Look for evidence of CHF (Chap. 68), murmurs of aortic stenosis, acute regurgitation (mitral or aortic), ventricular septal defect.
- Check for asymmetry of pulses (aortic dissection).
- Tenderness or rebound in abdomen may indicate peritonitis or pancreatitis; high-pitched bowel sounds suggest intestinal obstruction. Perform stool guaiac to rule out GI bleeding.
- Fever and chills usually accompany septic shock.

LABORATORY   Obtain hematocrit, WBC, electrolytes. If actively bleeding, check platelet count, PT, PTT, DIC screen. Arterial blood gas usually shows metabolic acidosis (in septic shock, respiratory alkalosis precedes metabolic acidosis). If sepsis suspected, draw blood cultures, perform urinalysis, and obtain Gram stain and cultures of sputum, urine, and other suspected sites.

Obtain ECG (myocardial ischemia or acute arrhythmia), chest x-ray (CHF, tension pneumothorax, aortic dissection, pneumonia). Echocardiogram may be helpful (cardiac tamponade, CHF). Central venous pressure or pulmonary capillary wedge (PCW) pressure measurements may be necessary

TABLE 24-2   Vasopressors used in shock states*

Drug	Dose	Notes
Dopamine	1–5 µg/kg/min	Facilitates diuresis
	5–10 µg/kg/min	Positive inotropic effect
	10–20 µg/kg/min	Generalized vasoconstriction (decreases renal perfusion)
Norepinephrine	2–8 µg/kg/min	Potent vasoconstrictor; moderate inotropic effect; may result in myocardial ischemia/arrhythmias
Dobutamine	1–10 µg/kg/min	Primarily for cardiogenic shock (Chap. 74): positive inotrope; lacks vasoconstrictor activity

* Isoproterenol not recommended in shock states because of potential hypotension and arrhythmogenic effects.

to distinguish between the different categories of shock: mean PCW <6 mmHg suggests oligemic or distributive shock; PCW >20 mmHg suggests left ventricular failure. Cardiac output is decreased in patients with cardiogenic and oligemic shock, and usually increased initially in septic shock.

TREATMENT   Aimed at rapid improvement of tissue hypoperfusion and respiratory impairment:

1. Serial measurements of BP (intraarterial line preferred), heart rate, continuous ECG monitor, urine output, blood studies: HCT, electrolytes, creatinine, BUN, ABGs, urine Na concentration (<20 mmol/L suggests volume depletion). Continuous monitoring of CVP and/or pulmonary artery pressure, with serial PCW pressures.

2. Augment systolic BP to >100 mmHg: (a) place in reverse Trendelenburg position; (b) IV volume infusion (500 mL bolus), unless PCW >20 mmHg (begin with normal saline, then whole blood, dextran, or packed RBCs, if anemic); (c) vasoactive drugs are added after intravascular volume is optimized; administer vasopressors (Table 24-2) if systemic vascular resistance is decreased; vasodilators (Table 68-1) if systemic vascular resistance is elevated, as long as systolic BP >90 mmHg; (d) If CHF present, add inotropic agents (Chap. 68).

3. Administer 100% O_2; intubate with mechanical ventilation if P_{O_2} <70 mmHg.

4. If severe metabolic acidosis present (pH <7.15), administer $NaHCO_3$ (44.6–89.2 mmol).

5. Identify and treat underlying cause of shock. Cardiogenic shock in acute MI is discussed in Chap. 74.

In septic shock, antibiotic therapy is begun immediately after blood and potential sites of infection are cultured, and may be guided by Gram stain of infected site/fluid. If etiology unknown, therapy must cover enteric gram-negative bacilli and gram-positive cocci and should include an aminoglycoside (gentamicin or tobramycin) and a cephalosporin or semisynthetic penicillin (Chaps. 38 and 49). Septic foci (abscess, necrotic bowel, infected gallbladder) require surgical excision.

For a more detailed discussion, see Perillo JE: Shock, Chap. 39, in HPIM-12, p. 232

---

25 ACUTE PULMONARY EDEMA

Life-threatening, acute development of alveolar lung edema due to: (1) elevation of hydrostatic pressure in the pulmonary capillaries (left heart failure, mitral stenosis) or (2) increased permeability of the pulmonary alveolar-capillary membrane. Specific precipitants (Table 25-1) result in cardiogenic pulmonary edema in pts with previously compensated CHF or without previous cardiac history.

PHYSICAL FINDINGS Patient appears severely ill, sitting bolt upright, tachypneic, dyspneic, with marked perspiration; cyanosis may be present. Bilateral pulmonary rales; third heart sound may be present. The sputum is frothy and blood-tinged.

LABORATORY DATA In early stages, arterial blood gas measurements demonstrate reductions of both Pa_{O_2} and Pa_{CO_2}; later, with progressive respiratory failure, hypercapnia develops with progressive acidemia. CXR shows pulmonary vascular redistribution, diffuse haziness in the lung fields with perihilar "butterfly" appearance.

TREATMENT OF CARDIOGENIC PULMONARY EDEMA Immediate, aggressive therapy is mandatory for survival. The following measures should be instituted nearly simultaneously:

1. Sit patient upright to reduce venous return.
2. Administer 100% O_2 by mask to achieve Pa_{O_2} >60 mmHg.
3. Intravenous loop diuretic (furosemide 40–100 mg or bumetanide 1 mg); use lower dose if patient does not take diuretics chronically.
4. Morphine 2–5 mg IV (repetitively); assess frequently for hypotension or respiratory depression; naloxone should be available to reverse effects of morphine, if necessary.

TABLE 25-1 Precipitants of acute pulmonary edema

Acute tachy- or bradyarrhythmia
Infection, fever
Acute MI
Severe hypertension
Acute mitral or aortic regurgitation
Increased circulating volume (Na ingestion, blood transfusion, pregnancy)
Increased metabolic demands (exercise, hyperthyroidism)
Pulmonary embolism
Noncompliance (sudden discontinuation) of chronic CHF medications

5. Afterload reduction [IV sodium nitroprusside (20–300 μg/min) if systolic BP >100 mmHg]; arterial line should be placed for continuous BP monitoring.

Additional therapy may be required if rapid improvement does not ensue:

1. If patient does not take digitalis chronically, 75% of a full loading dose is administered intravenously (Chap. 68).
2. Aminophylline (6 mg/kg IV over 20 min, then 0.2–0.5 mg/kg/h) reduces bronchospasm and augments myocardial contractility and diuresis; can be used as initial therapy, in place of morphine, if not clear whether dyspnea is due to pulmonary edema or severe obstructive lung disease, before CXR is obtained.
3. If rapid diuresis does not follow diuretic administration, intravascular volume can be reduced by phlebotomy (removal of ~250 mL through antecubital vein) or by placement of rotating tourniquets on the extremities.
4. For persistent hypoxemia or hypercapnia, intubation may be required.

The precipitating cause of pulmonary edema (Table 25-1) should be sought and treated, particularly acute arrhythmias or infection.

Several noncardiogenic conditions may result in pulmonary edema (Table 25-2) in the absence of left heart dysfunction; therapy is directed toward the primary condition.

TABLE 25-2 Non-cardiogenic pulmonary edema

1. Excessive capillary permeability
   Diffuse pulmonary infection
   Gram-negative sepsis
   Aspiration pneumonia
   Thermal lung injury
   Toxic exposures (SO_2, N_2O, NH_3)
   Following cardiopulmonary bypass
   Hemorrhagic pancreatitis
2. Unknown mechanism
   Narcotic overdose
   High-altitude exposure
   Acute CNS disorders

For a more detailed discussion, see Ingram RH Jr., Braunwald E: Dyspnea and Pulmonary Edema, Chap. 36, in HPIM-12, p. 220

26 INCREASED INTRACRANIAL PRESSURE AND HEAD TRAUMA

INCREASED INTRACRANIAL PRESSURE

A limited volume of extra tissue, blood, CSF, or edema fluid can be added to the intracranial contents without raising the intracranial pressure (ICP). Pts will deteriorate and may die when ICP reaches levels that compromise cerebral perfusion or causes a shift in intracranial contents that distorts vital brainstem centers.

CLINICAL MANIFESTATIONS Symptoms that occur in pts with high ICP include headache (especially a constant ache that is worse upon awakening), nausea, emesis, drowsiness, diplopia, and blurred vision. Papilledema and sixth nerve palsies are common. If not controlled, then pupillary dilatation, coma, decerebrate posturing, abnormal respirations, systemic hypertension, and bradycardia may result.

A posterior fossa mass, which may initially cause ataxia, stiff neck, and nausea, is especially dangerous because it can compress vital brainstem structures and cause obstructive hydrocephalus. Masses that cause raised ICP also displace brain tissue against fixed intracranial structures and into spaces not normally occupied. These herniation syndromes include (1) medial cortex displaced under the midline falx → anterior or posterior cerebral artery occlusion and stroke; (2) uncus displaced through the tentorium, compressing the third cranial nerve and pushing the cerebral peduncle against the tentorium, → ipsilateral pupillary dilatation and contralateral hemiparesis; (3) cerebellar tonsils displaced into the foramen magnum, causing medullary compression, → cardio-respiratory collapse; and (4) downward displacement of the diencephalon through the tentorium, causing miotic pupils and drowsiness.

MANAGEMENT Cerebral perfusion pressure (CPP) = BP − ICP. Global cerebral ischemia occurs when CPP <45 mmHg. Hypertension should be treated carefully, if at all. Careful intubation (without causing gagging or coughing) allows controlled hyperventilation to lower ICP quickly. The arterial P_{CO_2} should be maintained around 30 mmHg. Mannitol (1 g/kg) lowers ICP by decreasing interstitial brain fluid. Lasix is somewhat less effective. Free H_2O should be restricted. Pt's head should be elevated to 45 degrees. Treat fever aggressively.

EVALUATION OF PATIENT After stabilization and initiation of the above therapies, a CT scan (or MRI, if feasible) is performed to delineate the cause of the elevated ICP. Emergency surgical intervention is sometimes necessary to decompress the intracranial contents. Hydrocephalus, cerebellar stroke with edema, surgically accessible cerebral hemorrhage or tumor, and subdural or epidural hemorrhage often require lifesaving neurosurgery. ICP monitoring can guide medical and surgical decisions in pts with cerebral edema due to stroke, head trauma, Reye's syndrome, and intracerebral hemorrhage. High doses of barbiturates may decrease ICP in otherwise refractory pts, and in these pts ICP monitoring is obligatory.

TRAUMA TO THE CENTRAL NERVOUS SYSTEM

Head trauma can cause immediate loss of consciousness. If transient and unaccompanied by other serious brain pathology, it is called *concussion*. Prolonged alterations in consciousness may be due to parenchymal, subdural, or epidural hematoma or to diffuse shearing of axons in the white matter. Skull fracture should be suspected in pts with CSF rhinorrhea, hemotympanum, and periorbital or mastoid ecchymoses. Spinal cord trauma can cause transient loss of function or a permanent myelopathy with loss of motor, sensory, and autonomic function below the damaged spinal level. (See also Chap. 4.)

MANAGEMENT The neck should be immobilized and spine kept straight; vital functions should be stabilized. An initial neurologic exam should determine the level of consciousness, visual acuity, cranial nerve palsies, gross motor and sensory deficits, presence of blood in the middle ear, visible evidence of head trauma, and presence of pain over spine. Cervical spine films should be evaluated before neck is freed. Dysfunction below a spinal level suggests cord injury; lesions at the C5 level or above can threaten respiratory function. If x-rays show aberration of vertebral alignment, then reduction should be quickly undertaken. Spinal CT scan, MRI, or myelography may show evidence of reversible cord compression.

The pt with minor head injury who is alert and attentive after short period of unconsciousness (<1 min) sometimes has headache with a single episode of emesis or mild vertigo. Head injury of intermediate severity causes more prolonged loss of consciousness followed by persistent emesis and change in mental state. CT scan or MRI is required to exclude

subdural or epidural hematoma and to define extent of
contusions and posttraumatic edema. CT scan may be normal
in comatose pts with axonal shearing lesions in cerebral
white matter. Pts with intermediate head injury require
medical observation to detect increasing drowsiness, respiratory dysfunction, and pupillary enlargement, as well as to
ensure fluid restriction. Management of pts with raised ICP
due to head injury is outlined above.

For a more detailed discussion, see Ropper AH: Trauma of
the Head and Spinal Cord, Chap. 352, in HPIM-12, p. 2002

---

27 STATUS EPILEPTICUS

DEFINITION Prolonged or repetitive seizures without a period of recovery between individual seizures. Condition may occur with all kinds of seizures: grand mal (clonic-tonic) status, petit mal status, and temporal lobe (complex partial) status. The condition is life-threatening when clonic-tonic seizures result in hyperpyrexia and acidosis (from prolonged muscle activity) or less commonly cause hypoxia and cerebral injury due to respiratory or cardiovascular compromise. Absence and temporal lobe status may continue for hours undetected (pts present with confusion, inattentiveness, or depressed level of consciousness—rarely, with coma but without convulsive movements). Focal status epilepticus (usually focal motor, rarely focal sensory) is called *epilepsia partialis continua*.

TREATMENT Generalized tonic-clonic status epilepticus is a medical emergency. Pts must be evaluated promptly and appropriate therapy instituted expeditiously. However, care must also be taken to avoid overmedication of pts with status where seizures are not life-threatening.

1. Assess pt carefully for evidence of respiratory or cardiovascular insufficiency. Protect the airway (intubation may be difficult before seizures are at least partially controlled), protect the tongue (with a large, soft object that cannot be swallowed), establish IV and administer 50 mL 50% dextrose in water, 100 mg thiamine, and 0.4 mg naloxone (Narcan).

2. Administer diazepam 10 mg IV over 2 min (see Table 27-1).

3. Administer 1000–1500 mg phenytoin (18–20 mg/kg) IV slowly over 30 min. Monitor BP, ECG, and, if possible, EEG during infusion. Phenytoin does not cause respiratory arrest but if given too quickly, can cause precipitous fall in BP.

TABLE 27-1 Treatment of status epilepticus

Drug	Initial dose	Administration rate	Maximum per 24 h
Diazepam, IV adults	5–10 mg	1–2 mg/min	100 mg
Phenytoin, IV adults	18–20 mg/kg	30–50 mg/min	1.5 g
Phenobarbital, IV adults	300–800 mg	25–50 mg/min	1–2 g

(Do not administer with 5% dextrose in water—phenytoin precipitates in this low pH solution.)

4. If seizures continue and are life-threatening, repeat diazepam 10 mg IV slowly. Diazepam may depress respiratory function.

5. If seizures persist consider administering phenobarbital 300 mg IV over 30 min and repeat two or three times with careful attention to respiratory and cardiac function.

6. If seizures remain refractory after 60 min, consider placing pt in pentobarbital coma or under general anesthetic. Consultation with an anesthesiologist is advised when this treatment is considered.

After the seizures have stopped, it is imperative to determine their cause in order to prevent recurrence. In most adults the cause is tumor, vascular disease, infection (meningitis, encephalitis, or cerebral venous thrombosis), or precipitous withdrawal from alcohol, drugs, or antiepileptic medication. In children the cause is idiopathic (unknown) in about 50% of pts with status.

PROGNOSIS The mortality rate is 10% in severe tonic-clonic status, and the incidence of permanent neurologic sequelae is another 10–30%.

For a more detailed discussion, see Dichter M: The Epilepsies and Convulsive Disorders, Chap. 350, HPIM-12, p. 1968

28 POISONING AND ITS MANAGEMENT

In the U.S. poison exposures result in an estimated 5 million requests for medical advice or treatment annually. Suicide attempts account for most serious or fatal poisonings. About 5% of ICU admissions and up to 30% of psychiatric admissions are poison victims. The diagnosis must be considered in any pt who presents with coma, seizure, or acute renal, hepatic, or bone marrow failure.

DIAGNOSIS

The correct diagnosis can usually be reached by history, physical exam, and laboratory evaluation (Table 28-1). Vital signs, cardiopulmonary and neurologic assessment are the initial focus of the exam to determine the need for immediate supportive treatment. Use all available sources to determine the exact nature of the ingestion or exposure. The Physicians

TABLE 28-1 Initial assessment of suspected poisoning

Class of poison	Pupils	Skin	Other signs and symptoms
Stimulants: Amphetamines, phencyclidine, cocaine	Dilated	Warm, sweaty	Agitation, headache, psychosis, seizures, hypertension, tachyarrhythmias
Anticholinergics: Antihistamines; tricyclic antidepressants; various plants	Dilated	Dry, hyperthermic	Hallucinations, delirium, coma, tachycardia, hypertension, decreased bowel sounds, urinary retention
Cholinergic drugs: Organophosphate insecticides	Small	Excessive sweating	Anxiety, agitation, seizures, coma, paralysis, bradycardia (muscarinics), tachycardia (nicotinics), excessive salivation, hyperactive bowel sounds, weakness, fasciculations
Narcotics	Small	Cold, clammy	Respiratory depression, somnolence, stupor, coma, flaccid muscles, bradycardia, hypotension

Desk Reference, a regional poison control center, or a local/ hospital pharmacy may be used to identify ingredients and potential effects of toxins.

TREATMENT

Goals of therapy include support of vital signs, prevention of further absorption, enhancement of elimination, administration of specific antidotes, and prevention of reexposure. Fundamentals of poisoning management are listed in Table 28-2. Treatment will likely be initiated before routine and toxicologic data are known. All symptomatic pts need large-bore IV access, supplemental O_2, cardiac monitoring, and continuous observation. All pts with altered mental status should receive 100 mg thiamine (IM or IV), 1 ampule of 50% dextrose in water, and 4 mg of naloxone along with specific antidotes as indicated. Intubate any pt who is unconscious or has questionable airway integrity. Activated charcoal may be given PO or via a large-bore orogastric or nasogastric tube. Gastric lavage must be performed with an orogastric tube. Disposition from the emergency department depends upon severity of poisoning. Suicidal pts require constant observation by qualified personnel.

SUPPORTIVE CARE   *Airway protection* is mandatory. Gag reflex alone is not a reliable indicator of the need for intubation. Need for O_2 supplementation and ventilatory support can be assessed by ABGs. Drug-induced pulmonary edema is usually secondary to hypoxia, but myocardial depression may contribute. Measurement of pulmonary artery pressure may be necessary to establish etiology.

Electrolyte imbalances should be corrected as soon as possible.

Supreventricular tachycardia (SVT) with hypertension and CNS excitation is almost always due to sympathetic, anticholinergic, or hallucinogenic stimulation or to drug withdrawal. Treatment is indicated if associated with hemodynamic instability, chest pain, or ischemia or ECG. Treatment with combined alpha and beta blocker or combination of beta blocker and vasodilator is indicated in severe sympathetic hyperactivity. For those with anticholinergic hyperactivity, physostigmine is the choice. SVT without hypertension usually responds to IV fluid administration.

Ventricular tachycardia (VT) can be caused by sympathetic stimulation, myocardial membrane destabilization, or metabolic derangements. Lidocaine and phenytoin are generally safe. *Do not* use any drug that prolongs the QT interval (quinidine, procainamide) in cases of *tricyclic antidepressant* overdose; sodium bicarbonate loading may be effective. In

TABLE 28-2   **Fundamentals of poisoning management**

I. Supportive care
    A. Airway protection
    B. Oxygenation/ventilation
    C. Treatment of arrhythmias
    D. Hemodynamic support
    E. Treatment of seizures
    F. Correction of temperature abnormalities
    G. Correction of metabolic derangements
    H. Prevention of secondary complications
II. Prevention of further poison absorption
    A. Gastrointestinal decontamination
        1. Syrup of ipecac–induced emesis
        2. Gastric lavage
        3. Activated charcoal
        4. Whole bowel irrigation
        5. Catharsis
        6. Dilution
        7. Endoscopic/surgical removal
    B. Decontamination of other sites
        1. Eye decontamination
        2. Skin decontamination
        3. Body cavity evacuation
III. Enhancement of poison elimination
    A. Multiple-dose activated charcoal
    B. Forced diuresis
    C. Alteration of urinary pH
    D. Chelation (see Table 28-3)
    E. Extracorporal removal
        1. Peritoneal dialysis
        2. Hemodialysis
        3. Hemoperfusion
        4. Hemofiltration
        5. Plasmapheresis
        6. Exchange transfusion
    F. Hyperbaric oxgenation
IV. Administration of antidotes
    A. Neutralization by antibodies
    B. Neutralization by chemical binding
    C. Metabolic antagonism
    D. Physiologic antagonism
V. Prevention of reexposure
    A. Adult education
    B. Child-proofing
    C. Notification of regulatory agencies
    D. Psychiatric referral

Modified from Lovejoy FH, Linden CH: HPIM-12, p. 2165.

pts with torsade de pointes, isoproterenol and magnesium sulfate should be given, or a temporary pacemaker should be inserted for overdrive pacing of the heart. Arrhythmias may be resistant to therapy until underlying acid-base, electrolyte derangements, hypoxia, and hypothermia are corrected. If pt is hemodynamically stable it is acceptable to observe without pharmacologic intervention.

Seizures are best treated with γ-aminobutyric acid agonists such as benzodiazepines or barbiturates. Do not administer barbiturates until pt is intubated. Seizures caused by isoniazid overdose may respond only to large doses of pyridoxine IV. Seizures from beta blockers or tricyclic antidepressants may require phenytoin and benzodiazepines.

PREVENTION OF ABSORPTION *Syrup of ipecac* is administered orally in doses of 30 mL for adults, 15 mL for children, and 10 mL for infants. Vomiting should occur within 20 min. Ipecac is contraindicated in pts with recent GI surgery, CNS depression, seizures, corrosive ingestion (lye), petroleum hydrocarbon ingestion, and rapidly acting CNS poisons (camphor, cyanide, tricyclic antidepressants, propoxyphene, strychnine).

Gastric lavage is performed using a 28F orogastric tube in children, and a 40F orogastric tube in adults. Saline or tap water may be used in adults or children (use saline in infants). Place pt in Trendelenburg and left lateral decubitus position to minimize aspiration (occurs in 10% of pts). Lavage is contraindicated with corrosives and petroleum distillate hydrocarbons because of risk of aspiration-induced hydrocarbon pneumonia and gastroesophageal perforation.

Activated charcoal is given orally or by nasogastric or orogastric tube in doses of 1–2 g/kg body weight, using 8 mL of diluent per gram of charcoal. Premixed formulations are usually available in emergency rooms. It may be given with a cathartic (sorbitol) to speed elimination. In pts treated within 1 h, lavage followed by charcoal is more effective than charcoal alone. Charcoal may inhibit absorption of other orally administered agents and is contraindicated in pts with corrosive ingestion.

Whole-bowel irrigation may be useful in cases of foreign-body, drug packet, and slow-release medication ingestions. Golytely is given orally or by gastric tube up to a rate of 0.5 L/h. Cathartic salts (magnesium citrate) and saccharides (sorbitol, mannitol) promote rectal evacuation. *Dilution* of corrosive acids and alkali is accomplished by having pt drink water, 5 mL/kg. *Endoscopy or surgical intervention* may be required in large foreign-body ingestion, heavy metal ingestion, and in cases where ingested drug packets leak or rupture.

Decontamination of skin or eyes is done by washing with copious amounts of water or saline.

ENHANCEMENT OF ELIMINATION   *Activated charcoal in repeated doses* of 1 g/kg q 2–4 h is useful for ingestions of carbamazepine, dapsone, diazepam, digoxin, glutethimide, meprobamate, methotrexate, phenobarbital, phenytoin, salicylate, theophylline, and valproic acid.

Forced alkaline diuresis enhances the elimination of chlorphenoxyacetic acid herbicides, chlorpropamide, phenobarbital, and salicylates. Sodium bicarbonate, 1–2 ampules per liter of 0.45% NaCl, is given at a rate sufficient to maintain urine pH ≥7.5 and urine output at 3–6 (mL/kg)/h. Acid diuresis is no longer recommended. *Saline diuresis* may enhance elimination of bromide, lithium, and isoniazid. Contraindications include CHF, renal failure, and cerebral edema.

Dialysis should be considered in severe poisoning due to bromide, chloral hydrate, ethanol, ethylene glycol, isopropyl alcohol, lithium, heavy metals, methanol, and salicylate. *Hemoperfusion* may be indicated for chloramphenicol, disopyramide, and hypnotic sedative overdose.

SPECIFIC POISONS

ACETAMINOPHEN   A dose of ≥140 mg/kg saturates the sulfate and glucuronide pathways, resulting in increased fraction of acetaminophen metabolized to mercapturic acid. Early manifestations are nonspecific (and not predictive of hepatic toxicity) and include nausea, vomiting, diaphoresis, and pallor 2–4 h after ingestion. Laboratory evidence of hepatotoxicity includes elevation of AST, ALT, and, in severe cases, PT and bilirubin, with ultimate hyperammonemia. A serum acetaminophen level drawn 4–24 h after ingestion is compared to the Rumack-Matthew nomogram (Fig. 28-1). Initial therapy consists of lavage and activated charcoal, then *N*-acetylcysteine therapy, which is indicated up to 24 h after ingestion. Loading dose is 140 mg/kg PO, followed by 70 mg/kg PO q 4 h for 17 doses. Start therapy immediately; it may be discontinued if serum level is below toxic range.

ACIDS AND ALKALI   Common acids include toilet bowl cleaners, soldering fluxes, antirust compounds, and automobile battery fluid. Common alkalis include bleach, drain cleaners, and surface cleaners. Clinical signs include burns, pain, drooling, vomiting of blood or mucus, and ulceration. Lack of oral manifestation does not rule out esophageal involvement. Perforation of esophagus or stomach can occur, and aspiration may cause fulminant trachitis.

Endoscopy is safe within 48 h to document site and severity of injury. Treatment consists of immediate dilution with

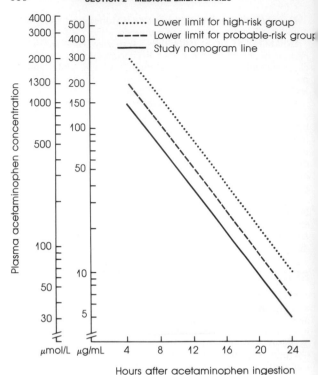

Hours after acetaminophen ingestion

FIGURE 28-1 Nomogram to define risk according to initial plasma acetaminophen concentration. (*After Rumack BH, Matthew H: Pediatrics 55:871, 1975.*)

water or saline. Glucocorticoids should be given within 48 h to pts with alkali (not acid) burns of the esophagus and continued for 3 weeks. Antacids may be used for stomach burns.

ANTIARRYTHMIC DRUGS　Acute ingestion of >2 × usual daily dose is potentially toxic, with onset of symptoms within 1 h. Manifestations include nausea, vomiting, diarrhea, lethargy, confusion, ataxia, bradycardia, hypotension, and cardiovascular collapse. Anticholinergic effects are seen with disopyramide ingestion. Quinidine and class IB agents can cause agitation, dysphoria, and seizures. VT, ventricular fibrillation (including torsade de pointes), and QT prolongation are characteristic of Class IA and IC poisonings. Myocardial depression may precipitate pulmonary edema. Treatment consists of GI decontamination and supportive therapy. Arrhythmias are treated with lidocaine, phenytoin, and bretylium. Sodium bicarbonate or lactate may be useful in class IA or IC overdoses. Torsade de pointes is treated with magnesium sulfate (4 g or 40 mL of 10% solution IV over 10–20 min) or overdrive pacing (with isoproterenol or pacemaker).

ARSENIC (See Table 28-3)

BARBITURATES Overdose may result in confusion, lethargy, coma, hypotension, pulmonary edema, and death. Treatment consists of GI decontamination and repetitive charcoal administration for long-acting barbiturates. Hemoperfusion and hemodialysis can be used in severe poisoning with short-acting or long-acting barbiturates.

BENZODIAZEPINES The major effects include weakness, ataxia, drowsiness, coma, and respiratory depression. Pupils are constricted and do not respond to naloxone. Treatment includes GI decontamination and support of vital signs.

BETA-ADRENERGIC BLOCKING AGENTS Toxicity is usually manifest 30 min after ingestion. Symptoms include nausea, vomiting, diarrhea, bradycardia, hypotension, and CNS depression. Agents with intrinsic sympathomimetic activity can cause hypertension and tachycardia. Bronchospasm and pulmonary edema may occur. Hyperkalemia, hypoglycemia, metabolic acidosis, all degrees of AV block, bundle branch block, QRS prolongation, VT, ventricular fibrillation, torsade de pointes, and asystole may occur. Treatment includes GI decontamination, supportive measures, and administration of calcium (10% chloride or gluconate salt solution, IV 0.2 mL/kg, up to 10 mL) and glucagon (5–10 mg IV, then infusion of 1–5 mg/L). Cardiac pacing or an intraaortic balloon pump may be required. Bronchospasm is treated with inhaled beta agonists.

CADMIUM (See Table 28-3)

CALCIUM CHANNEL BLOCKERS Toxicity usually develops within 30–60 min following ingestion of 5–10 × usual dose. Manifestations include confusion, drowsiness, coma, seizure, hypotension, bradycardia, cyanosis, and pulmonary edema. ECG findings include all degrees of AV block, prolonged QRS and QT intervals, ischemia, infarction or asystole. Metabolic acidosis and hyperglycemia may result. Treatment consists of GI decontamination, supportive care, calcium and glucagon (as above). Intraaortic balloon pump may be required.

CARBON MONOXIDE (CO) CO binds to hemoglobin (forming carboxyhemoglobin) with an affinity 210 times that of O_2 and

TABLE 28-3 Heavy metal poisons

Sources	Clinical toxicity	Laboratory	Treatment
ARSENIC			
Insecticides, rodenticides, fungicides, wood preservatives, smelting (arsine gas), galvanizing	*Arsine gas:* Severe hemolysis, jaundice, hemoglobinuria, renal failure, nausea, vomiting, diarrhea *Arsenic:* Lethal dose 130–300 mg; burning in throat, dysphagia, nausea, vomiting, diarrhea, garlic breath, cyanosis, dyspnea, hypotension, delirium, coma, seizures, hemolysis, ATN *Chronic exposure:* Erythroderma, hyperkeratosis, Aldrich-Mees lines on fingernails, laryngitis,	Radiopaque on x-ray, abnormal LFTs, anemia, leukocytosis, leukopenia, hemoglobinemia, proteinuria, hematuria, hemoglobinuria, cellular urinary casts tracheitis, bronchitis, polyneuritis, Bowen's disease of skin, lung cancer, basal cell carcinoma	*Acute:* If pt alert, ipecac; if obtunded, gastric lavage; no charcoal or cathartic; dimercaprol 2–3 mg/kg IM q 6 h × 24 h then q 12 h × 10 d until urine level <67 nmol/d (<5 µg/d); dimercaprol 3–5 mg/kg for more severe toxicity; also penicillamine (100 mg/kg) 1 g/d in 4 divided doses × 5 d may be used. If renal failure, hemodialysis. Exchange transfusions and hemodialysis for arsine gas poisoning
CADMIUM			
Occupational exposure (smelting, mining, battery manufacturing, ceramics industry)	*Ingestion:* Vomiting, abdominal pain, diarrhea, shock *Inhalation:* Dyspnea, weakness, chest pain, shortness of breath, cough, pulmonary edema (noncardiogenic), respiratory failure *Chronic exposure:* Emphysema, renal tubular damage with	Serum levels not useful; urinary excretion of >0.1 µmol (>10 µg)/L is associated with renal disease proteinuria; itai-itai (ouch-ouch) disease, renal tubular acidosis, and osteomalacia	*Acute exposure:* Edetate 1 g/m² surface area q several days; DMSA (succimer) *Inhalation:* Glucocorticoids and diuretics *Chronic exposure:* Large doses of vitamin D

112

LEAD			
Pica (paint, soil), household dust, drinking water, industry	**Childhood:** *Acute:* Abdominal pain, irritability, lethargy, anorexia, pallor (anemia), ataxia, slurred speech, seizure, coma, death (associated with pica, malnutrition) *Subclinical:* Mental retardation, language and cognitive deficits, behavior abnormalities **Adult:** Abdominal pain, anemia, renal disease, headache, peripheral neuropathy, ataxia, memory loss, encephalopathy, wrist drop, foot drop	Serum level >1.2 µmol/L; free erythrocyte protoporphyrin (FEP) >0.6 µmol/L, hemolysis (acute), microcytic anemia (chronic), azotemia, Fanconi syndrome, pyuria, lead lines on x-ray in children *Lead mobilization test:* Edetate is given; positive if 5 nmol lead found in urine per mg chelating agent	Edetate, dimercaprol, penicillamine. For acute encephalopathy use dimercaprol and edetate until blood levels <2 µmol/L. Fluids must be given to cause diuresis even in presence of cerebral edema; edetate 0.5–1 g/m²/d up to 1.5 g/m²; dimercaprol 12–24 mg/kg/d × 5 d. Wait 48–72 h between courses of therapy. Penicillamine: 20–40 mg/kg/d up to 1 g/d for 3–6 mos.
MERCURY			
Inorganic (elemental and mercuric) and organic	*Acute vapor poisoning:* Inflammation of large and small airways, pneumonitis *Chronic vapor poisoning:* Affects CNS: lassitude, anorexia, weight loss, intention tremor, mercurial erethism (timidity, memory loss, insomnia, excitability, delirium) *Chronic inorganic poisoning:* Same as above plus excessive salivation, loose teeth, gingivitis, stomatitis, dermatitis, nephrotic syndrome *Pink's disease* (acrodynia): Generalized rash, irritability, photophobia, hypertrichosis, profuse perspiration, swelling and desquamation of feet and hands *Acute inorganic:* Nausea, vomiting, abdominal pain, tenesmus, bloody diarrhea, shock, death, ATN	*Asymptomatic:* blood level >180 nmol/L (>3.5 µg/dL); urine level >0.7 µmol/L (>150 µg/L). Symptoms seen with blood levels >1 µmol/L and urinary levels >3 µmol/L	Polythiol resins bind mercury in the GI tract. Chelation therapy is indicated if blood or urine levels elevated *Acute inorganic:* Dimercaprol, up to 24 mg/kg/24 h IM in divided doses for up to 5 d; penicillamine can also be used 30 mg/kg/d in 2–3 divided doses; peritoneal dialysis in presence of renal failure; chronic inorganic poisoning: use penicillamine only

TABLE 28-3 Heavy metal poisons (Continued)

Sources	Clinical toxicity	Laboratory	Treatment
THALLIUM			
Insecticide, rodenticide, manufacturing of fireworks and jewelry, cardiac imaging	Severe poisoning with single-dose >1 g or 8 mg/kg; death at 15 mg/kg has occurred. *At 3-4 h:* Nausea, vomiting, abdominal pain, diarrhea, hematochezia *Within 1 week:* Confusion, psychosis, choreoathetosis, organic brain syndrome, seizure, coma, motor and sensory neuropathy, neuritis, ophthalmoplegia ptosis, strabismus, cranial nerve palsies	Radiopaque; serum levels 1.5–10 μmol/L (30–200 μg/dL) with severe ingestion; urine levels 0.5–1 μmol/L (10–20 μg/dL) *Late (2–4 weeks):* Diffuse hair loss with sparing of pubic and body hair and lateral one-third of eyebrows *Long-term:* Memory loss, tremor, foot drop, ataxia	GI decontamination—gastric lavage or ipecac within 4–6 h of ingestion; Prussian blue 250 mg/kg administered PO once. Activated charcoal also effective. Use cathartics; forced diuresis with furosemide; peritoneal dialysis; charcoal hemoperfusion. Ditiocarb contraindicated

hence causes cellular anoxia. Once exposure is discontinued, CO is excreted via the lungs with a half-life of 4–6 h. The half-life decreases to 40–80 min with 100% O_2 therapy and to 15–30 min with hyperbaric O_2. Manifestations include shortness of breath, dyspnea, tachypnea, headache, nausea, vomiting, emotional lability, confusion, impaired judgment, and clumsiness. Pulmonary edema, aspiration pneumonia, arrhythmias, and hypotension may occur. The "cherry red" color of skin and mucous membranes is rare; cyanosis is usual. 100% O_2 is administered by tightly fitting mask until CO levels are less than 10% and all symptoms have resolved. Hyperbaric O_2 is recommended for comatose pts with CO levels ≥40%, for pts with CO levels ≥25% who also have seizures or intractible arrhythmias, and for pts with delayed onset of sequelae.

CYANIDE   Cyanide blocks electron transport, resulting in decreased oxidative metabolism and oxidative utilization, decreased ATP production, and lactic acidosis. Lethal dose is 200–300 mg of sodium cyanide and 500 mg of hydrocyanic acid. Early effects include headache, vertigo, excitement, anxiety, burning of mouth and throat, dyspnea, tachycardia, hypertension, nausea, vomiting, and diaphoresis. Breath may have a bitter almond odor. Later effects include coma, seizures, opisthotonus, trismus, paralysis, respiratory depression, arrhythmias, hypotension, and death. Treatment is based upon history and begins immediately. General supportive measures, 100% O_2, and GI decontamination are provided concurrently with specific therapy. Amyl nitrite is inhaled for 30 s each min, with a new ampule broken q 3 min. (Nitrite produces methemoglobinemia, which has a higher affinity for cyanide, thus promoting release from peripheral sites.) Sodium nitrite is then given as a 3% solution IV at a rate of 2.5–5.0 mL/min up to a total dose of 10–15 mL. Finally, sodium thiosulfate is given to remove and bind circulating cyanide from its methemoglobin sites, producing sodium thiocyanate that is excreted in urine; 50 mL of a 25% solution is given over 1–2 min. (Children should be given 0.33 mL/kg sodium nitrite and 1.65 mL/kg sodium thiosulfate.) If symptoms persist, repeat half the dose of sodium nitrite and sodium thiosulfate.

DIGOXIN   Manifestations include vomiting, confusion, delirium, hallucinations, blurred vision, disturbed color perception (yellow vision), photophobia, all types of arrhythmias, and all degrees of AV block. The combination of SVT and AV block is highly suggestive of digitalis toxicity. Hypokalemia is common with chronic intoxication, while hyperkalemia is seen with acute overdosage. GI decontamination is done carefully to avoid vagal stimulation, repeated doses of activated charcoal are given, and hyperkalemia is treated with Kayexalate, insulin, and glucose. Atropine and electrical pacing may be required. Cardiac glycoside antibodies are available for treatment of severe poisoning. Dosage (in 40-mg vials) is calculated by dividing ingested dose of digoxin (mg) by 0.6 mg/vial. If dose and serum levels are unknown give 5–10 vials to an adult.

ETHYLENE GLYCOL Antifreeze contains 95% ethylene glycol. As little as 120 mg or 0.1 mL/kg can be hazardous. Manifestations include nausea, vomiting, slurred speech, ataxia, nystagmus, lethargy, sweet breath odor, coma, seizures, cardiovascular collapse, and death. Hypocalcemia occurs in half of pts. Anion gap metabolic acidosis, elevated serum osmolality, and oxalate crystalluria suggest the diagnosis. Renal failure may result from glycolic acid production. GI lavage, followed by activated charcoal, and supportive measures including airway protection are initiated immediately. Correct hypocalcemia with IV calcium salts at a dose of 7–14 mL (10% solution diluted 10:1 with IV fluids and given at rate of 1 mL/min). Correct metabolic acidosis with sodium bicarbonate. Treat seizures with phenytoin and benzodiazepines. Indications for ethanol treatment include ethylene glycol level >3 mmol/L (>20 mg/dL) and acidosis regardless of the level. A serum ethanol level of ≥20 mmol/L (≥100 mg/dL) is required to inhibit alcohol dehydrogenase. Ethanol therapy is as follows: Loading dose is 10 mL/kg of 10% ethanol IV or 1 mL/kg of 95% ethanol PO; maintenance dose is 1.5 (mL/kg)/h of 10% ethanol IV and 3 (mL/kg)/h of 10% ethanol during dialysis. Hemodialysis is indicated in cases not responding to above therapy, when serum levels are ≥8 mmol/L (≥50 mg/dL), and for renal failure. Give thiamine and pyridoxine supplements.

HALLUCINOGENS Mescaline, LSD, psilocybin cause disorders of mood, thought, and perception lasting 4–6 h. Psilocybin may cause fever, hypotension, and seizures. Symptoms include mydriasis, conjunctival injection, piloerection, hypertension, tachycardia, tachypnea, anorexia, tremors, and hyperreflexia. Treatment is limited: a calm environment, benzodiazepines for acute panic reactions, and haloperidol for psychotic reactions.

HYDROCARBONS All are CNS depressants. Other manifestations include nausea, vomiting, diarrhea, abdominal pain, renal tubular acidosis, bone marrow suppression, respiratory distress, rhabdomyolysis, psychosis and cerebral atrophy, and mucosal burns. Prompt gastric lavage is required for *aromatic* hydrocarbons (xylene, toluene). Gastric lavage, ipecac, and activated charcoal are *contraindicated* for petroleum distillate hydrocarbon ingestion. Mainstay of therapy is supportive care.

HYDROGEN SULFIDE A "rotten eggs" odor characterizes this chemical. It is irritative, producing rhinitis, conjunctivitis, and pharyngitis. Headache, vertigo, nausea, confusion, seizures, and coma may result. Respiratory depression causes hypoxia, cyanosis, and metabolic acidosis. Treatment includes maintenance of airway, 100% O_2, nitrite therapy (as for cyanide), and hyperbaric O_2 in refractory cases.

IRON Free iron injures mitochondria, causes lipid peroxidation, and results in renal, tubular, and hepatic necrosis and occasionally in myocardial and pulmonary injury. Manifestations include vomiting, diarrhea (often blood), fever, hyperglycemia, leukocytosis, lethargy, hypotension, metabolic acidosis, seizures, coma, vascular collapse, jaundice, elevated liver enzymes, prolongation of PT, and hyperammonemia. X-ray may identify iron tablets in stomach. Serum iron greater than binding capacity indicates serious toxicity. A positive urine deferoxamine provocative test (50 mg/kg IV or IM up to 1 g) is a vin rosé color that indicates presence of ferrioxamine. Ipecac or lavage is administered, followed by x-ray to check adequacy of decontamination. Charcoal is ineffective. Continuous deferoxamine infusion at 10–15 (mg/kg)/h (up to 1–2 grains) is given if iron exceeds binding capacity. If iron level >180 μmol/L (>1000 μg/dL), larger doses of deferoxamine can be given, then exchange transfusion or plasmapheresis to remove iron-desferal complex.

ISONIAZID Acute overdose decreases synthesis of γ-aminobutyric acid, resulting in CNS stimulation. Symptoms include nausea, vomiting, dizziness, slurred speech, coma, seizures, and metabolic acidosis. Prompt GI decontamination is followed by activated charcoal. Pyridoxine (vitamin B_6) should be given slowly IV in weight equivalency to ingested dose of isoniazid. If dose is not known, give 5 g pyridoxine IV over 30 min as a 5–10% solution.

ISOPROPYL ALCOHOL Manifestations include vomiting, abdominal pain, hematemesis, myopathy, headache, dizziness, confusion, coma, respiratory depression, hypothermia, and hypotension. Hypoglycemia, anion gap (small) metabolic acidosis, and elevated serum osmolality are found, as well as falsely elevated serum creatinine and hemolytic anemia. Treatment consists of GI decontamination, and supportive measures. Activated charcoal is not effective. Dialysis may be used in severe cases.

LEAD (See Table 28-3)

LITHIUM Manifestations include nausea, vomiting, diarrhea, weakness, fasciculations, twitching, ataxia, tremor, myoclonus, choreoathetosis, seizures, confusion, coma, and cardiovascular collapse. Laboratory abnormalities include leukocytosis, hyperglycemia, albuminuria, glycosuria, nephrogenic diabetes insipidus, ECG changes (AV block, prolonged QT), and ventricular arrhythmias. If seen within 2–4 h following ingestion, GI decontamination is indicated. Charcoal is not effective. Serial serum lithium levels should be measured until trend is downward. Supportive care includes alkaline diuresis for levels >2–3 mmol/L. Hemodialysis is treatment of choice for acute or chronic intoxication with symptoms and/or a serum level >4 mmol/L.

MONOAMINE OXIDASE (MAO) INHIBITORS Manifestations include CNS stimulation, fever, tachycardia, tachypnea, hypertension, nausea, vomiting, dilated pupils with nystagmus, and papilledema. GI decontamination should be followed by activated charcoal and cathartics. Dantrolene (2.5 mg/kg PO or IV q 6 h) may be effective for hyperthermia. Control of hypertension may require nitroprusside, and tachycardia may require propranolol. Hypotension should be treated with fluids and cautious use of pressors. Seizures are treated with benzodiazepines and phenytoin.

MERCURY (See Table 28-3)

METHANOL Metabolism to formic acid results in metabolic acidosis. Early manifestations include nausea, vomiting, abdominal pain, headache, vertigo, confusion, obtundation, coma, seizures, and death. A serum HCO_3 >12 mmol/L is associated with a large anion gap. Ophthalmic manifestations 15–19 h after ingestion include clouding, diminished acuity, dancing and flashing spots, dilated or fixed pupils, hyperemia of the disc, retinal edema, and blindness. GI decontamination is indicated. Activated charcoal is not effective. Systemic acidosis is corrected with sodium bicarbonate. Seizures respond to diazepam and phenytoin. Ethanol therapy (as described for ethylene glycol) is indicated in pts with visual symptoms or a methanol level >6 mmol/L (>20 mg/dL). Therapy with ethanol is continued until level falls below 6 mmol/L. Hemodialysis is indicated when visual signs are present or when metabolic acidosis is unresponsive to sodium bicarbonate.

METHEMOGLOBINEMIA This results from chemical exposure that oxidizes ferric hemoglobin (Fe^{2+}) to its ferric (Fe^{3+}) state. Oxidizing agents include nitrites, nitroglycerin, nitrates, aniline, paints, varnishes, inks, phenacetin, sulfonamides, pyridium, dapsone, primaquine, lidocaine, benzocaine, nitrophenol, toluidine, nitrobenzene, and isobutyl nitrate. Cyanosis occurs with methemoglobin levels >15%. Pts are asymptomatic until levels exceed 30%, at which point they develop fatigue, headache, dizziness, tachycardia, and weakness. At levels >55%, dyspnea, bradycardia, hypoxia, acidosis, seizures, coma, and arrhythmias occur. Death usually occurs with levels >70%. Hemolytic anemia may lead to hyperkalemia and renal failure 1–3 d after exposure. Cyanosis in conjunction with a normal Pa_{O_2} and decreased O_2 saturation (measured by oximeter) and with "chocolate brown" blood suggest the diagnosis. The chocolate color does not redden with exposure to O_2 but does fade when exposed to 10% potassium cyanide. Ingested toxins should be removed by lavage, then charcoal and cathartics. Methylene blue is indicated for methemoglobin level >30 g/L or methemoglobinemia with hypoxia. Dosage is 1–2 mg/kg as a 1% solution over 5 min. Additional doses may be needed. Methylene blue is contraindicated in glucose-6-phosphate dehydrogenase deficiency. Packed red blood cell transfusion to a hemoglobin of 150 g/L can enhance O_2 carrying capacity of the blood, along with 100% O_2 administration. Exchange transfusions may be indicated in G6PD-deficient pts.

MUSCLE RELAXANTS Manifestations of poisoning by carisoprodol, chlorphenesin, chlorzoxazone, and methocarbamol are nausea, vomiting, dizziness, headache, nystagmus, hypotonia, and CNS depression. Excess cyclobenzaprine produces anticholinergic effects coupled with agitation, hallucinations, seizures, stupor, coma, and hypotension. Baclofen causes CNS depression, hypothermia, excitability, delirium, myoclonus, seizures, conduction abnormalities, arrhythmias, and hypotension. Orphenadrine causes anticholinergic effects, tachycardia, arrhythmias, agitation, and depression. Manage with prompt GI decontamination and single-dose activated charcoal (repeated for baclofen overdose). Cathartics are indicated. Physostigmine is useful for anticholinergic effects.

NSAIDs All NSAIDs may cause gastroenteritis. Ibuprofen toxicity is mild, including nausea, vomiting, abdominal pain, drowsiness, nystagmus, and obtundation. Diflunisal produces, in addition, hyperventilation, tachycardia, and diaphoresis; fenoprofen is nephrotoxic. The enolic acid group (e.g., phenylbutazone and piroxicam) produces coma, metabolic acidosis, seizures, and renal failure. Hepatic injury has been reported. Manage with gastric lavage, activated charcoal, and cathartics. Repeated doses of charcoal are beneficial with indomethacin, phenylbutazone, and piroxicam ingestions.

ORGANOPHOSPHATE AND CARBAMATE INSECTICIDES Organophosphates (malathion, parathion, dichlorvos, diazinon, chlorothion) irreversibly inhibit acetylcholinesterase, resulting in accumulation of acetylcholine at muscarinic and nicotinic synapses. Carbamates (carbaryl, aldicarb, propoxur) reversibly inhibit acetylcholinesterase. Both types produce nausea, vomiting, abdominal cramps, urinary and fecal incontinence, increased bronchial secretions, coughing, sweating, salivation, lacrimation, and miosis, but carbamates are shorter acting. Bradycardia, conduction blocks, hypotension, twitching, fasciculations, weakness, respiratory depression, seizures, confusion, and coma may result. A reduction of cholinesterase activity by 50% in plasma or red cells is diagnostic. Management includes washing exposed surfaces with soap and water and GI decontamination in cases of ingestion, then activated charcoal. Atropine 0.5–2 mg is given IV q 15 min until complete atropinization is achieved (dry mouth). Pralidoxime (2-PAM), 1–2 g IV over several minutes, can be repeated q 8 h until nicotinic symptoms resolve. Use of 2-PAM in carbamate poisoning is controversial.

PHENOTHIAZINES   These CNS depressants cause lethargy, obtundation, respiratory depression, and coma. Pupils are often constricted. Hypothermia, hypotension, SVT, AV block, arrhythmias (including torsade de pointes), prolongation of PR, QRS, and QT intervals, and T-wave abnormalities are seen. Malignant neuroleptic syndrome may occur rarely. Acute dystonic reactions are common with symptoms of rigidity, opisthotonos, stiff neck, hyperreflexia, irritability, dystonia, fixed speech, torticollis, tremors, trismus, and oculogyric crisis. Management of overdose includes GI decontamination, then a single dose of activated charcoal. Seizures should be treated with phenytoin; hypotension with volume expansion and alpha agonists. Sodium bicarbonate is given for metabolic acidosis. Avoid the use of procainamide, quinidine, or any agent that prolongs cardiac repolarization. Neuroleptic malignant syndrome is treated with dantrolene and bromocriptine. Extrapyramidal signs respond well to IV diphenhydramine (1–2 mg/kg).

SALICYLATES   Clinical manifestations of poisoning include vomiting, tachycardia, hyperpnea, fever, tinnitus, lethargy, and confusion. More severe poisoning can result in seizures, coma, respiratory and cardiovascular failure, cerebral edema, and renal failure. Respiratory alkalosis is commonly coupled with metabolic acidosis (40–50%), but respiratory alkalosis (20%), metabolic acidosis (20%), and mixed respiratory and metabolic acidosis (5–10%) occur. Lactic and other organic acids are responsible for the increased anion gap. PT may be prolonged. Salicylates can be detected by ferric chloride test on either blood or urine. Management includes GI decontamination, then repeated administration of activated charcoal. Forced alkaline diuresis (urine pH >8.0) increases excretion and decreases serum half-life. Seizures can be controlled with diazepam or phenobarbital. Hemodialysis should be considered in pts who fail conventional therapy or have cerebral edema or hepatic or renal failure.

STIMULANTS   Amphetamines, phenylpropanolamines, and cocaine are the most commonly used agents. Manifestations include nausea, vomiting, diarrhea, abdominal cramps, irritability, confusion, delirium, euphoria, auditory and visual hallucinations, tremors, hyperreflexia, seizures, palpitations, tachycardia, hypertension, and arrhythmias. Cardiovascular collapse can occur. Sympathomimetic symptoms include dilated pupils, dry mouth, pallor, flushing of skin, and tachypnea. Gastric lavage should be followed by activated charcoal and a cathartic. Supportive care includes treatment of seizures with benzodiazepines; hypertension with nitroprusside; fever with salicylates; and agitation with sedatives. Rhabdomyolysis may occur, as can intracranial hemorrhage.

THALLIUM (See Table 28-3)

THEOPHYLLINE   Vomiting, restlessness, irritability, agitation, tachypnea, tachycardia, and tremors are common. Coma and respiratory depression are rare. Generalized tonic-clonic seizures and partial seizures occur in severe poisoning and may be difficult to treat. Atrial arrhythmias, ventricular arrhythmias and fibrillation can occur. Rhabdomyolysis with acute renal failure develops occasionally. Laboratory abnormalities include ketosis, metabolic acidosis, elevated amylase, hyperglycemia, and decreased potassium, calcium, and phosphorus. Prompt GI decontamination is followed by repeated activated charcoal administration every 2–4 h for 12–24 h after ingestion. Metoclopramide is useful to control vomiting. Tachycardia is treated with propranolol or esmolol; hypotension with volume expansion. Seizures are treated with benzodiazepines and barbiturates; phenytoin is ineffective. Indications for hemodialysis and hemoperfusion with acute ingestion include a serum level >500 μmol/L (>100 mg/L) and with chronic ingestion a serum level >200–300 μmol/L (>40–60 mg/L). Dialysis is also indicated in pts with lower serum levels who have refractory seizures or arrhythmias.

TRICYLIC ANTIDEPRESSANTS   These agents block reuptake of synaptic transmitters (norepinephrine, dopamine) and have central and peripheral anticholinergic activity. Manifestations include anticholinergic symptoms (fever, mydriasis, flushing of skin, urinary retention, decreased bowel motility). CNS manifestations include excitation, restlessness, myoclonus, hyperreflexia, disorientation, confusion, hallucinations, coma, and seizures. Cardiac effects include prolongation of the QRS complex, other AV blocks and arrhythmias. QRS duration ≥ 0.10 ms is correlated with seizures and life-threatening cardiac arrhythmias. Serum levels >3300 nmol/

L (>1000 ng/mL) indicate serious poisoning. Ipecac is contraindicated. Gastric lavage is followed by activated charcoal every 2–4 h (with cathartics). Metabolic acidosis should be corrected with sodium bicarbonate. Hypotension should be treated with volume expansion, norepinephrine, or high-dose dopamine. Seizures are treated with phenytoin or diazepam. Treatment of arrhythmias may involve sodium bicarbonate (0.5–1 mmol/kg), lidocaine, and phenytoin. Physostigmine reverses anticholinergic signs but is of unproven efficacy in the presence of coma, seizures, or ventricular arrhythmias. Hemodialysis or hemoperfusion has no benefit because of the large volume of distribution.

For a more detailed discussion, see Lovejoy FH, Linden CH: Acute Poison and Drug Overdosage, Chap. 374, p. 2163; and Graef JW, Lovejoy FH: Heavy Metal Poisoning, Chap. 375, p. 2182, in HPIM-12

29 DRUG OVERDOSE AND DRUG ABUSE

Drug abuse is defined as use of a chemical substance for more than a month resulting in impairment of social or occupational functioning or both. Overdose of drugs is a common medical emergency. Diagnosis and treatment depend on recognizing the symptoms and signs of specific drug effects.

SPECIFIC DRUGS

OPIATES   Opioid drugs (see Chap. 1) include morphine, heroin, hydromorphone, methadone, and meperidine.

Signs of intoxication   Hypotension, bradycardia, miosis, slurred speech, respiratory depression (shallow: 2–4 per min), hypothermia, stupor, and coma. Seizures may occur with meperidine. Pulmonary edema can occur with any opiate. An "allergic-type" response to adulterants can occur, with decreased alertness, pulmonary edema, and elevated eosinophil count.

Treatment   Naloxone 0.4 mg every 3–10 min until evidence of a clinical response. Duration of action is prolonged by SC or IM administration. With methadone overdose, the effects of naloxone wear off long before the effects of methadone; may require many repeated doses of naloxone over 6–8 h. Withdrawal symptoms develop in addicted individuals approximately 2–4 h after meperidine, 4–8 h after heroin, and 12–48 h after the last dose of methadone. Symptoms of drug withdrawal include anxiety, drug craving, irritability, insomnia, diaphoresis, lacrimation, abdominal cramping, diarrhea, fever, hypertension, and tachycardia. These symptoms may be attenuated by methadone 10–20 mg followed by 5–10 mg qid. Clonidine (0.1–0.2 mg bid) is also used for acute withdrawal symptoms.

SEDATIVES AND HYPNOTICS   This group includes the barbiturates, non-barbiturate sedatives, and the benzodiazepines.

Signs of intoxication   Drowsiness, nystagmus, ataxia, dysarthria, hyporeflexia, respiratory depression, confusion, stupor, and coma. Profound hypothermia (with an isoelectric EEG) is a common manifestation of severe overdose with barbiturates. Seizures and coma may occur with glutethimide (now rarely encountered) and methaqualone (non-barbiturate hypnotics). Dilated pupils occur with glutethimide; psychosis, myoclonus, and cardiovascular collapse occur with methaqualone.

Treatment   Respiratory and cardiovascular support are critical. Emesis should be induced only if pt is awake. Gastric lavage and administration of a cathartic and of activated charcoal should be considered. Hemoperfusion and hemodialysis are effective for short-acting barbiturates, but their use is advised only for severely intoxicated pts. Renal elimination of phenobarbital is enhanced by alkalinization of the urine with sodium bicarbonate administration.

STIMULANTS   This group includes amphetamine (Benzedrine), dextroamphetamine (Dexedrine), methamphetamine, phenmetrazine (Preludin), and cocaine and its alkaloid derivative "crack." The amphetamines, but not cocaine, are effective when taken orally and all produce a rapid effect, "a rush," when taken intravenously. Cocaine is usually taken intranasally, or intravenously, or smoked ("free-based"). Crack, when smoked, has a profound rapid surge of stimulation that is brief in duration. Combinations of crack and heroin are often taken to even out the stimulant effect and to prolong the period of euphoria. The rapid descent from euphoria ("crash") often results in intense craving leading to a high addiction rate among users.

Symptoms and signs of overdose.   Elation, hyperactivity, excess talking, and hypomania are characteristic of amphetamine overdose. Tachycardia, mydriasis, insomnia, anorexia, and hypertension are often present. Severe overdose accentuates these signs with psychosis, paranoia, hyperthermia, fever, extreme agitation, seizures, hallucinations, coma, and death. Cocaine can cause cardiac arrythmias with sudden death and tonic-clonic seizures.

Treatment   Benzodiazepines, haloperidol, and other antipsychotics are the drugs of choice. Parenteral administration together with general life support measures are required in severe cases. Hyperthermia and status epilepticus require aggressive treatment. Death from combinations of drug effects are becoming more common.

ANTIDEPRESSANTS   Included in this group of drugs are the tricyclic antidepressants and the monoamine oxidase (MAO) inhibitors (see also Chap. 178).

Symptoms and signs of overdose   The tricyclics cause symptoms 1–2 h after ingestion; anticholinergic effects predominate. In low doses agitation and hypertension are common. In high overdose myocardial function is depressed and cardiac arrhythmias (ventricular tachyarrhythmias, atrial fibrillation, or conduction blocks) occur. Fever, tachycardia, flushing of the skin, urinary retention, and decreased bowel function are prominent. CNS manifestations include restlessness, excitation, hyperreflexia, mydriasis, myoclonus, confusion, and hallucinations. Seizures and coma occur with the largest doses. MAO inhibitor overdose causes symptoms 6–12 h after ingestion and the peak effects may not occur for 24 h. CNS manifestations are hyperpyrexia, mydriasis, agitation, hyperactivity with confusion, twitching, tremor, and rigidity.

Treatment Ipecac-induced emesis is contraindicated. Gastric lavage is indicated for recent ingestion, and activated charcoal and cathartics for removal. Hyperthermia may require aggressive treatment. No specific antidote exists for either form of antidepressants.

HALLUCINOGENS This group of drugs includes lysergic acid diethylamide (LSD), 2,5-dimethoxy-4-methylamphetamine (STP), trimethoxytryptamine (TMA), mescaline, phencyclidine ("angel dust," PCP), psilocybin, thiocyclodine (TCP), delta-9-tetrahydrocannabinol (THC), and marijuana (cannibis). Many of these agents cause an altered perceptual state (hallucinations, euphoria, illusions).

Clinical manifestations of overdose Symptoms and signs include tachycardia, hypertension, dilated pupils, tremor, hyperreflexia, ataxia, and incoordination. PCP can cause a "dissociative reaction" with sensation of depersonalization. Higher doses can cause rigidity, paranoia, catatonic states, seizures, coma, and death. Toxicity to PCP includes hepatic necrosis, muscle necrosis with myoglobinuria, and severe hypertension. THC causes conjunctival injection, dry mouth, tachycardia, anxiety, and psychosis.

Therapy All drugs in this class can cause fatal reactions; the drugs most useful in counteracting their effects are the benzodiazepines and butyrophenones (haloperidol).

CLINICAL APPROACH TO A PATIENT WITH SUSPECTED OVERDOSE

Confirm that the problem is metabolic, consider the differential diagnosis, and initiate treatment. Drug intoxications are metabolic encephalopathies, and therefore pts have a symmetrical neurologic exam and reactive pupils. If these criteria are not met (unilateral weakness, hyperreflexia, asymmetric pupils), then the possibility of a mass lesion or stroke must be ruled out.

An acute overdose of a stimulant or hallucinogen presents clinically as an agitated confusional state and therefore requires differentiation from delirium tremens (sedative or alcohol withdrawal), acute disturbance of language function (fluent aphasias from dominant hemisphere stroke), acute amnestic states (posttraumatic transient global amnesia), or acute psychosis.

The sedatives and hypnotics present as an intoxication that may rapidly progress to obtundation and coma. In alert pts the sedative drugs produce nystagmus on lateral gaze; with stupor or coma the characteristic sign of these exogenous depressants is paralysis of inducible eye movements on passive head rotation (absent oculocephalic—doll's eyes—reflex). The differential diagnosis is that of endogenous metabolic disorders such as meningitis (the most critical consideration), uremia, osmolar disturbances, hyponatremia, or hypercalcemia. These endogenous disorders preserve reflex eye movements until deep coma supervenes.

For a more detailed discussion, see Schuckit MA: Opioid Drug Use, p. 2151; and Mendelson JH, Mello NK: Commonly Abused Drugs, p. 2155, in HPIM-12

30 DROWNING

EPIDEMIOLOGY 5400 fatalities per year; second most common cause of accidental death between 5 and 44 years of age.

PATHOPHYSIOLOGY 10–20% of deaths due to asphyxia. Most important is anoxia or hypoxia, also bronchospasm, laryngospasm, aspiration of particulate matter. Aspiration of salt H_2O → pulmonary edema → intrapulmonary right-to-left shunt. Aspiration of fresh H_2O → alveolar collapse → altered ventilation-perfusion ratio → hypoxia. Hemolysis is rarely important.

CLINICAL MANIFESTATIONS Cough, tachypnea, pulmonary edema, ARDS, CNS—organic brain syndromes; fever <24 h following aspiration; later, complicating infections.

LABORATORY FINDINGS ABGs show ↓ P_{O_2}, acidosis; CXR: 25% normal; perihilar infiltrates → pulmonary edema; increased WBC; decreased Hct; look for bleeding.

THERAPY

- On scene: mouth-to-mouth respiration; closed chest massage.
- Do not waste time draining H_2O from lungs.
- Establish airway, 100% O_2 stat and continuously.
- In hospital, ABGs, pH, hemogram, electrolytes, CXR.
- If alert, observe for several hours.
- Treat metabolic acidosis with $NaHCO_3$ and supplemental O_2.
- If pulmonary edema and no response to $F_{I_{O_2}}$ ≥40%, intubate and use positive end-expiratory pressure; continue PEEP until ABGs stable (48–72 h).
- Comatose pts often have ICP >15–20 mmHg; institute cerebral resuscitation (controlled hyperventilation, hypothermia, barbiturates, glucocorticoids, and osmotic and loop diuretics).
- Other measures: treat pulmonary infection; maintain fluid and electrolyte balance; plasma expanders (if ↓ BP); transfusion if blood volume ↓.

PROGNOSIS Depends on hypoxia, CNS status; good if CXR normal and pt alert.

For a more detailed discussion, see Wallace JF: Drowning and Near Drowning, Chap. 378, in HPIM-12, p. 2200

31 ANAPHYLAXIS AND TRANSFUSION REACTIONS

ANAPHYLAXIS

Definition A life-threatening systemic hypersensitivity reaction to contact with an allergen; may appear within minutes of exposure to offending substance. Manifestations include respiratory distress, pruritus, urticaria, mucous membrane swelling, GI disturbances (including nausea, vomiting, pain, and diarrhea), and vascular collapse. The more common inciting allergens are proteins such as antisera, hormones, pollen extracts, *Hymenoptera* venom, foods, drugs (especially antibiotics), and diagnostic agents.

Clinical manifestations Time to onset is variable, but symptoms may occur within seconds to minutes.

- *Respiratory:* Mucous membrane swelling, hoarseness, stridor, wheezing
- *Cardiovascular:* Tachycardia, hypotension
- *Cutaneous:* Pruritus, urticaria, angioedema

Diagnosis History of exposure to offending substance with subsequent development of characteristic complex of signs and symptoms.

Prevention and therapy • Epinephrine 0.2–0.5 mL of 1:1000 solution SC with repeat doses at 3-min intervals as necessary. • Epinephrine IV infusion of 1:50,000 solution to treat hypotension. • IV fluids and volume expanders. • Antihistamines such as diphenhydramine 50–80 mg IM or IV. • Aminophylline 0.25–0.5 g IV for bronchospasm. • Oxygen. • Glucocorticoids IV; not useful for acute manifestations but may help control persistent hypotension or bronchospasm. • *Prevention:* avoidance of offending antigen, where possible; skin testing and desensitization to materials such as penicillin and *Hymenoptera* venom, if necessary.

TRANSFUSION REACTIONS

Transfusion reactions may be classified as *immune* or *non-immune*.

IMMUNOLOGICALLY MEDIATED REACTIONS Reaction may be directed against red or white blood cells, platelets, or IgA;

proteins — allergic
wbc — febrile rxns

in addition, other, less well characterized reactions may occur.

Intravascular hemolysis: Usually due to ABO incompatibility; very rapid and massive hemolysis; symptoms and signs may include restlessness, anxiety, flushing, chest or back pain, tachypnea, tachycardia, nausea, shock, renal failure, coagulation disorders (including DIC).

Extravascular hemolysis: Usually due to antibodies of Rh system, but antibodies of Kell, Duffy, and Kidd systems may also be involved; clinical manifestations are less severe, often simply with malaise and fever; shock and renal failure are rare; initial red cell survival may be normal followed by delayed destruction in reticuloendothelial system.

Laboratory investigation of immune-mediated reactions

- Careful check on identity of donor and recipient; samples of recipient blood to blood bank for analysis and further crossmatching.
- Documentation of hemolysis—plasma and urine hemoglobin, haptoglobin, Hct, bilirubin.
- Check renal status—UA, BUN, creatinine.
- Check coagulation status—platelet count, PT, PTT.

Treatment

- Avoid further transfusion unless absolutely necessary.
- Management of shock and renal failure in intravascular hemolysis; osmotic diuresis and volume expansion may be indicated in certain cases; if renal failure ensues, adjust drug doses and closely monitor fluid/electrolyte status.
- Factor replacement if needed to control coagulation abnormalities; platelet infusion if thrombocytopenia severe.

NONIMMUNE REACTIONS

- *Circulatory overload*—especially in infants and pts with renal or cardiac insufficiency.
- *Effects of massive transfusion*—hyperkalemia, ammonia and citrate toxicity, dilutional coagulopathy, thrombocytopenia.
- *Infection*—hepatitis, syphilis, CMV, malaria, babesiosis, toxoplasmosis, brucellosis, AIDS can all be transmitted by transfused blood.
- *Iron overload*—with repeated transfusions; may require chelation therapy.

• *Complications related to intravenous access*—air embolism, thrombophlebitis.

For a more detailed discussion, see Austen KF: Diseases of Immediate Type Hypersensitivity, Chap. 267, p. 1422; and Giblett ER: Blood Groups and Blood Transfusion, Chap. 286, p. 1494, in HPIM-12

SNAKE BITE

EPIDEMIOLOGY AND ETIOLOGY

- In U.S., poisonous snakes are coral snake, rattlesnake, water moccasin, copperhead.
- 8000 snake bites/year; most in S.E. and Gulf States (esp. Texas); <20 fatal.
- Factors affecting severity of snake bite: age, size, health; location (trunk, face worse than extremities), size of snake, bacteria (*Clostridium*) in mouth of snake, exercise after bite (running promotes absorption of toxin).

SIGNS AND SYMPTOMS Burning at site, local swelling, gangrene of skin. Systemic—fever, nausea and vomiting, circulatory collapse, bleeding, muscle cramping, pupillary constriction, delirium, convulsions.

LABORATORY FINDINGS If severe, anemia, ↑ WBC, ↓ platelets, DIC.

THERAPY Verify fang marks, local edema.

First aid Rest, immobilize limb, tourniquet.

Hospital care Antivenin vital in severe bites. In treatment with polyvalent crotaline antivenin, reconstitute 1 vial with 10 mL H_2O; 5 vials usually sufficient; test for horse serum sensitivity.

No antivenin except above available in U.S., but antiserum against various types available at Oklahoma Zoo and Poison Info Center [(405) 271 5454].

Other Maintain respiration; provide tetanus toxoid or TIG, antibiotics for wound infection (gram-negative pathogens), debridement (fasciotomy), pain relief; combat shock and bleeding; glucocorticoids may or may not be useful.

PREVENTION Long pants, gloves. For first aid, carry sharp knife, constriction band, antiseptic, antivenin.

LIZARD BITE

EPIDEMIOLOGY AND ETIOLOGY Only poisonous lizards are Gila monster and Mexican beaded lizard.

SIGNS AND SYMPTOMS Tissue injury, pain, edema, erythema, nausea, vomiting, blurred vision, dyspnea, dysphonia, weakness.

THERAPY Constriction band, cooling of bitten area; prevent or treat infection; provide pain relief.

SPIDER BITES

WIDOW SPIDER   In U.S., black widow spider; bites between April and October; victims often males using privies; after bite, cramping pain from extremities → trunk (boardlike abdomen); pain is severe.

Treatment   Relieve pain, give hot tub bath, 10 mL of 10% calcium gluconate for cramps; if severe 1 vial (2.5 mL) *Latrodectus* antivenin in 50 mL saline over 15 min IV.

LOXOSCELES SPIDER   In the South and Southwest as well as California; bite—initially mild burning → severe pain → necrosis and bullae formation; some pts have systemic symptoms.

Treatment   If pain is not intense and there are no bullae, no treatment; if pain is severe, provide steroids, Dapsone (experimental), debridement.

OTHER ANIMALS

SCORPIONS   One dangerous species (*Centruroides*) in Arizona, New Mexico, southern California, Texas; most mild; rarely fatal: numbness → hyperexcitable state → coma and convulsions → death.

Treatment   Cold compresses and mild analgesics; severe: goat serum antivenin, diazepam; combat shock and dehydration.

BEE, WASP, HORNET, AND YELLOW JACKET STINGS

- Most severe and lethal reactions: allergic.
- Symptoms: sharp pain → wheal and erythema → itching.
- Danger if bee swallowed or inhaled → edema of glottis or larynx.
- In hypersensitive → acute anaphylaxis or serum sickness.
- Treatment: Remove stinger, apply tourniquet, icepacks.
- Anaphylaxis: Epinephrine 0.3–0.5 mL 1:1000 q 20–30 min, airway, vasopressors, O_2 as needed.

TICK BITE

- Vectors for Rocky Mountain spotted fever, Q fever, tularemia, borreliosis, babesiosis, Lyme disease.
- Local: papule, nodule.
- Remove tick intact.

Tick paralysis   Ascending, flaccid paralysis; victims mainly young girls with tick hidden in hair.

- Differential diagnosis: Poliomyelitis, diphtheria, Guillain-Barré, Eaton-Lambert, myasthenia gravis, botulism.
- Treatment: Remove tick.

MARINE ANIMALS

• Portuguese man-of-war and jellyfish: Local pain, swelling, erythema → muscle cramps, nausea and vomiting. *Treat* with saltwater bath, scrape off tentacles.
• Paralytic and neurotoxic shellfish: Coastal waters, "red tide"; humans infected by ingestion. *Treat* with purgation.

VENOMOUS FISH Dorsal fins of bullhead sharks, dogfish, ratfish, catfish. *Treat* by immersion in hot water. Most common in U.S. is tail of stringray resulting in local pain and occasional systemic absorption. *Treat* with constriction band, saltwater syringing of wound.

For a more detailed discussion, see Wallace JF: Disorders Caused by Venoms and Stings, Chap. 376, in HPIM-12, p. 2187

---

33 HYPER- AND HYPOTHERMIA

DISORDERS ASSOCIATED WITH HIGH TEMPERATURES

Heat cramps

- Body temp. usually normal; victim sweating.
- Painful spasms in voluntary muscles after strenuous exercise.
- Therapy: NaCl and H_2O.
- If abdominal muscles in spasm, do not operate!

Heat exhaustion

- Failure of cardiovascular responses to high external temperatures.
- Occurs in elderly receiving diuretics.
- Weakness, vertigo, anorexia, nausea; vomiting and faintness may precede collapse.
- Onset sudden; duration brief.
- Color gray; skin cold and clammy; BP low; body temp. normal or ↓.
- Therapy: Remove to cool place; recumbency.
- IV fluids rarely necessary.

Exertional heat injury

- Due to exertion at hot ambient temps. [≥27°C (≥80°F)] when relative humidity is high (≥60%).
- Common in runners who are insufficiently acclimatized, conditioned, and hydrated, or who are overweight.
- In contrast to heat stroke, these pts sweat freely and their temps. are lower [39–40°C (102–104°F)].
- Symptoms: headache, gooseflesh, chills, hyperventilation, nausea, vomiting, muscle cramps, ataxia, incoherent speech.
- Physical exam: Tachycardia, hypotension, sometimes loss of consciousness.
- Laboratory findings: ↑ Hct, ↑ Na^+, ↑ liver and muscle enzymes, ↓ Ca^{2+}, ↓ PO_4.
- Rarely, there are DIC, rhabdomyolysis, myoglobinemia.
- Therapy: Lower core temp. to 38–40°C (100–104°F) (wet sheets); massage extremities to improve blood flow; infuse hypotonic glucose/saline.
- Prevention for runner: Run races early in morning; enter race well-hydrated; place aid stations at intervals; do not increase pace at end; avoid alcohol before race.

Heat stroke

- Elderly, preexisting chronic disease; diuretics.
- Sometimes military recruits.
- Cardinal signs and symptoms: Hyperpyrexia [$\geq 41°C$ ($\geq 106°F$)] and prostration.
- Skin hot and dry; sweating ceases.
- Pulse rapid; respirations rapid and weak; BP low.
- Hemoconcentration; WBC $\uparrow$, BUN $\uparrow$; protein and casts in urine; respiratory alkalosis followed by metabolic acidosis.
- Lactic acidemia; $\downarrow Ca^{2+}$, $\downarrow PO_4$.
- ECG abnormal.
- Clotting abnormalities that may culminate in DIC.
- Early death or pt may die of acute complications such as renal failure.
- Therapy: *Emergency*—place pt in cool area; remove clothing; place in cool shower on a gurney; direct fan on pt; chill IV solutions; massage skin; phenothiazine to reduce shivering; Swan-Ganz catheter; ensure airway; avoid epinephrine and narcotics; hydrate but do not overhydrate.

Malignant hyperthermia

- Episodic rapid increase in temp. in response to inhalational anesthetic (halothane, methoxyflurane, or muscle relaxants such as succinyl choline).
- In autosomal dominant form, 50% have $\uparrow$ CK.
- In recessive form (King syndrome) in young boys there are a number of other congenital abnormalities.
- Symptoms: Decreased relaxation during induction of anesthesia; muscle fasciculations with succinyl choline, rapid rise in temp., muscle rigidity; hypotension and cyanosis.
- Laboratory findings: Respiratory and metabolic acidosis, $\uparrow K^+$, $\uparrow Mg$, $\uparrow$ blood lactate and pyruvate.
- Therapy: *Medical emergency*—stop surgery; cool with ice; 100% O_2; induce diuresis; give dantrolene sodium (1 mg/kg) rapidly IV until symptoms stop—up to maximum single dose of 10 mg/kg.
- Prevention: Family Hx; monitor temp. during anesthesia; prophylactic dantrolene 4–8 mg/kg PO beginning 1–2 d before surgery.

Neuroleptic malignant syndrome (NMS)

- Muscular rigidity, hyperthermia, altered consciousness; autonomic dysfunction.
- Leukocytosis (15,000–30,000); $\uparrow$ CK.
- Occurs after neuroleptics (haloperidol, thiothixene, or piperazine phenothiazine) in therapeutic doses.

- Primarily young adult males.
- Lasts 5–10 days after administration of neuroleptics is discontinued.
- Therapy: Bromocriptine 7.5–60 mg/d; or dantrolene as in malignant hyperthermia.

DISORDERS ASSOCIATED WITH LOW TEMPERATURES

Accidental hypothermia

- Winter months; after exposure; in alcoholics.
- Diagnosis often not made because thermometers do not register ≤35°C (≤95°F); use incubator thermometer or thermocouple.
- Associated with sepsis, myxedema, pituitary insufficiency, adrenal insufficiency, cerebrovascular disease, drug or alcohol ingestion.
- Pts appear cold, pale, stiff.
- If temp. <27°C (<80°F), pts are unconscious.
- Hemoconcentration, azotemia, metabolic acidosis (lactic acid).
- Therapy: *Medical emergency*—maintain airway; oxygenate well; monitor blood gases; expand blood volume; warm IV fluids; monitor K$^+$; watch for arrhythmias; give NaHCO$_3$ if pH ≤7.25; if severely hypothermic, rewarm in bath or Hubbard tank [40–42°C (104–108°F)].
- Watch for rewarming shock and treat with hemo- or peritoneal dialysis.
- Sepsis common; treat with broad-spectrum antibiotics unless specific organism and site identified.
- Do not cease resuscitation even in the face of asystole until pt has been rewarmed to 36°C (96.8°F) and remains unresponsive to CPR at that temperature.

Hypothermia of acute illness

- Differs from above in that it occurs at ambient temperatures.
- Degree of hypothermia modest [33–34°C (92–93°F)].
- Associated with CHF, uremia, diabetes mellitus, drug overdose, respiratory failure.
- Characterized by severe metabolic acidosis, cardiac arrhythmias, and loss of consciousness.
- Usually responds to rewarming with circulating blanket; otherwise, treat as above.

Immersion hypothermia

- Due to immersion in cold water for prolonged periods.

- Therapy: Rewarming in warm water.

Local cold injuries

- Frostnip (earlobes, nose, fingers, and toes).
- Immersion foot (feet wet but not freezing for prolonged periods; symptoms vary from ischemia to hyperemia); for ischemia, need to rewarm slowly (note: overheating of tissue may lead to gangrene); hyperemia requires careful cooling.
- Frostbite (differs from immersion foot because blood vessels are involved); rewarm frostbitten limb carefully in water at 10–15°C (50–59°F) and increase temperature every 5 min by 3°C (5°F) to maximum of 40°C (104°F); once rewarming has taken place, treatment is bed rest, elevation of injured part, tetanus toxoid, antibiotics, debridement of blebs and bullae, local antiseptic washes, early physiotherapy. Amputation usually not necessary; IV dextran of possible value; sympathectomy or intraarterial reserpine may decrease vasospasm.

For a more detailed discussion, see Petersdorf RG: Hypothermia and Hyperthermia, Chap. 377, in HPIM-12, p. 2194

DIABETIC KETOACIDOSIS (DKA)

DKA results from insulin deficiency with a relative or absolute increase in glucagon and may be caused by cessation of insulin therapy or by infection, surgery, or emotional stress. Anorexia, nausea and vomiting, and increased urine output herald the onset, and abdominal pain, altered consciousness, Kussmaul breathing, or frank coma may ensue. Volume depletion can lead to vascular collapse and renal shutdown. Leukocytosis is common. Body temperature is normal or $\downarrow$. Fever suggests infection, and a source must be actively sought.

Laboratory abnormalities include hyperglycemia and anion gap metabolic acidosis (with serum HCO_3 <10 mmol/L). The metabolic acidosis and anion gap are almost totally accounted for by the elevated level of acetoacetate and β-hydroxybutyrate. Despite a normal or elevated potassium level on initial assessment, there is actually a total body potassium deficit of several hundred mmol. Initial serum phosphorus may also be elevated despite depletion of body stores. Magnesium may be low. Serum sodium is decreased secondary to hyperglycemia. A very low serum sodium suggests an artifact due to hypertriglyceridemia.

Other forms of metabolic acidosis must be excluded: lactic acidosis, uremia, alcoholic ketoacidosis, and certain poisonings. If urine ketones are negative, another cause for acidosis is likely. If urine ketones are positive, plasma ketones should be measured; a strong test in undiluted plasma may be due to starvation whereas a strongly positive reaction beyond a 1:1 dulution is presumptive evidence for ketoacidosis.

Diabetic ketoacidosis cannot be reversed without insulin. Because pts with insulin resistance cannot be identified prospectively, it is preferable to administer 25–50 U/h of regular insulin IV until acidosis is reversed and lesser amounts for several hours thereafter (usually 0.1 U/kg/h). Therapy also requires IV fluids; the usual fluid deficit is 3–5 L. 1–2 L isotonic saline is given initially, and additional amounts are determined by clinical assessment. When plasma glucose falls to about 300 mg/dL, 5% glucose solutions should be started, both as source of free water and to prevent late cerebral edema and hypoglycemia. Potassium replacement is always necessary, but time of administration varies. Potassium replacement (as potassium phosphate) should be initiated early in therapy if initial levels are normal or low. If initial levels are elevated, potassium replacement should begin as soon as the measured level begins to fall with correction of acidosis and action of insulin shifting K^+ into intracellular water. Aggressive insulin and fluid therapy is not discontinued until the ketosis has cleared (correction of hyperglycemia is not an endpoint). Poor prognostic signs include hypotension, azotemia, deep coma, and associated illness. Bicarbonate should be given when acidosis is severe (pH ≤7.0), especially if hypotension is present. Most pts with diabetic ketoacidosis recover when properly treated. Causes of death include MI and infection, particularly pneumonia. See Table 34-1 for complications of DKA.

HYPEROSMOLAR NONKETOTIC COMA

Profound dehydration results from sustained osmotic diuresis when pt is unable to drink sufficient water to keep up with

TABLE 34-1 Complications of diabetic ketoacidosis

Complication	Clues
Acute gastric dilatation or erosive gastritis	Vomiting of blood or coffee-ground material
Cerebral edema	Obtundation or coma with or without neurologic signs, especially if occurring after initial improvement
Hyperkalemia	Cardiac arrest
Hypoglycemia	Adrenergic or neurologic signs; rebound ketosis
Hypokalemia	Cardiac arrhythmias
Infection	Fever
Insulin resistance	Unremitting acidosis after 4–6 h of adequate therapy
Myocardial infarction	Chest pain, appearance of heart failure; appearance of hypotension despite adequate fluids
Mucormycosis	Facial pain, bloody nasal discharge, blackened nasal turbinates, blurred vision, proptosis
Respiratory distress syndrome	Hypoxemia in the absence of pneumonia, chronic pulmonary disease, or heart failure
Vascular thrombosis	Strokelike picture or signs of ischemia in nonnervous tissue

Source: Adapted from DW Foster, in *Current Therapy in Endocrinology and Metabolism 1985–1986*, DT Krieger, CW Bardin (eds), Toronto/Philadelphia, Decker, 1985.

urinary fluid losses. Commonly, an elderly diabetic develops a stroke or infection, which worsens hyperglycemia and prevents adequate water intake so that volume depletion causes prerenal azotemia. Seizures may occur. Other causes include tube feedings of high-protein formulas, peritoneal dialysis, high carbohydrate intake, and osmotic agents such as mannitol or urea.

Plasma glucose is generally around 55 mmol/L (1000 mg/dL). Mild metabolic acidosis may be present. Serum bicarbonate <10 mmol/L and normal plasma ketones suggest lactic acidosis. The serum osmolality is high, but because of hyperglycemia, serum Na may be normal. Serum osmolality can be estimated:

Osmolality (mosm/kg) = 2([Na] + [K]) + glucose (mmol/L) + BUN (mmol/L)

The average fluid deficit is 10 L. Sufficient IV fluids must be given to support circulation and urine flow. While free water is ultimately needed, 2–3 L isotonic saline should be given over first 1–2 h. Subsequently, half-strength saline can be used. As plasma glucose approaches normal, 5% dextrose can be given as a vehicle for free water. Insulin should be given to control hyperglycemia. The mortality rate is >50%.

For a more detailed discussion, see Foster DW: Diabetes Mellitus, Chap. 319, in HPIM-12, p. 1739

SECTION 3 INFECTIOUS DISEASES

35 DIAGNOSTIC METHODS

MICROSCOPIC EXAMINATION

Direct examination Useful to diagnose *Borrelia* (relapsing fever) or *Plasmodium* (malaria) in blood smears.
Wet mounts
• Darkfield of genital lesions for syphilis.   • Superficial mycoses (tinea versicolor) from skin scrapings, hair, or nails in drop of 10% KOH.   • Diagnosis of systemic fungal infection (*Cryptococcus* in CSF, coccidioidomycosis spherules in sputum).   • Stool or duodenal drainage for protozoa (amebiasis, giardiasis, cryptosporidiosis).   • Stool for helminthic infections (ascariasis, trichuriasis, strongyloidiasis, hookworm).   • Blood smears for filariasis (microfilariae), sleeping sickness (trypanosomes).
Stains
• Gram's stain check for contaminating epithelial cells at low power under oil (blue: gram-positive; pink: gram-negative).   • Acid-fast (Ziehl-Neelsen, Kinyoun) to diagnose tuberculosis, *Cryptosporidium* in stool, *Nocardia* (mineral acid instead of acid-alcohol).   • Giemsa for *Chlamydia* from eye, urethra, cervix.   • Wright's or methenamine silver for *Pneumocystis carinii*   • Romanowsky for *Plasmodium, Leishmania*.   • Trichrome iron hematoxylin for intestinal protozoa.
Other stains
• Fluorescent antibody tests for herpes simplex or rabies on brain tissue.   • *Legionella* on lung tissue, pleural fluid, or sputum   • Influenza, parainfluenza, or respiratory syncytial virus (RSV) on nasal epithelial cells. Enzyme-linked chromogenic assays also useful (e.g., RSV).

OTHER DETECTION METHODS

Latex particle agglutination   Very sensitive test to detect pneumococcal, meningococcal, group B streptococcal, *H. influenzae*, or cryptococcal (CRAG) antigens in CSF.

In situ hybridization   Radiolabelled oligonucleotide probes hybridize to group- or species-specific sequences of several organisms, (e.g., CMV).

CULTURES

Collection
• Clean skin with 70% isopropyl alcohol and then iodophor; preferably transport to lab within 1 h.   • Aspirates in syringe with air expressed.   • Swabs in transport media except group A streptococci may be in dry sterile test tube.

Upper respiratory tract
• Cultures seldom useful except when looking for specific pathogen (*S. pyogenes, Bordetella pertussis, Corynebacterium diphtheriae*, meningococci, or gonococci).   • Single throat swab 90% positive for streptococcal pharyngitis.   • Throat cultures not indicated if no fever or cervical lymphadenopathy (<5%+).

Lower respiratory tract
• Should also culture blood.   • More likely to have lower tract flora if <10 epithelial cells and >25 leukocytes per low-power field.   • Bronchoscopy with brush biopsy or bronchoalveolar lavage (BAL) may be used for recovery of *Pneumocystis, M. tuberculosis*, CMV, and fungi.   • Percutaneous needle aspiration: high yield, 5% risk of pneumothorax.

Urine
• Periurethral cleaning important in females; first 25 mL discarded.   • Should refrigerate if not to lab within 1 h (can be held 4–6 h).   • Single specimen of >10^5 organisms/mL in male and 2 specimens in female suggest infection but ≥10^2 in symptomatic dysuric women and ≥10^3 in symptomatic men suggestive (may have lower counts if on antibiotics or specimens by catheterization or suprapubic aspiration).   • Even slight growth significant with suprapubic collection.   • With indwelling catheter, should disinfect catheter and collect directly with sterile needle and syringe.   • Gram's stain of unspun urine suggestive of infection if >1 bacterium per 20 oil fields.   • Never culture Foley drainage bag or tips.

Blood cultures
• Should culture all febrile patients with rigors, serious illness, possible endocarditis or vascular infection, or immunosuppression.   • Optimal: 2–3 blood cultures of 10–30

mL 1 h apart.   • With previous antibiotics, resin bottles may be useful and the number of cultures may need to be increased.   • Avoid collection from femoral vein, through indwelling intravascular cannula, or arterial blood cultures.

Cerebrospinal fluid

• Collect minimum of 2 mL for glucose (with simultaneous blood sugar), total protein, cell counts, cultures.   • With negative Gram's stain, consider latex particle agglutination.

Gastrointestinal tract

• Fecal cultures and/or toxin assays can detect diarrhea caused by *Salmonella, Shigella, Arizona, Vibrio parahemo-lyticus, Yersinia enterocolitica, Campylobacter jejuni, Clostridium difficile.*   • If not cultured in 1 h, preserve in phosphate-buffered glycerol.

Exudates and body fluids

• Optimal collection of pus by syringe and needle aspiration through disinfected skin.   • Sinus should be cultured through sterile plastic catheter but curettings or biopsy more definitive.

Skin, soft tissue

• Usually heavily contaminated with normal flora, so should aspirate with syringe or culture punch biopsy.   • Culture intravenous catheter tip (last 5 cm) after disinfecting skin to diagnose infected line.

Viral

• Throat swabs must be placed in buffered, high-protein transport medium.   • CSF cultures in pts with meningitis or encephalitis.   • Stool cultures for enteroviruses or adenoviruses.   • Urine cultures for rubella and CMV.   • Pericardial fluid to diagnose myocarditis or pericarditis.   • Buffy coat cultures for herpes and CMV infections.   • Brain biopsy culture best to diagnose herpes encephalitis.   • BAL or lung tissue cultures for CMV.   • Nasal wash for RSV antigen detection.

Serologic assays

• Measurement of IgM antibodies (e.g., hepatitis A, EBV, toxoplasma), other antibodies (e.g., HIV, hepatitis B and C), or antigens (e.g., HIV, hepatitis B, CRAG) useful to establish specific acute or chronic infections.   • Acute and convalescent (2- to 3-week) serum antibody response may establish diagnosis of brucellosis, Q-fever, other rickettsioses, or a variety of viral diseases.

For a more detailed discussion, see Plorde JJ: The Diagnosis of Infectious Diseases, Chap. 80, in HPIM-12, p. 454

36 INFECTIONS IN THE COMPROMISED HOST

A compromised host has a deficiency in one or more of the defenses against infection. These defenses include physical and chemical barriers, the inflammatory response, reticuloendothelial system, the complement system, and the specific immune response. Impairment in defenses may stem from congenital disorders, acquired diseases, or medications. Infections arise from either the endogenous or exogenous flora, which may be altered by antimicrobial therapy or other factors. In the compromised host, common pathogens may present atypically, and opportunistic organisms may be pathogenic. The nature of the infecting organism often provides insight into specific host defense defects. When possible, treatment or prevention of infection should include attempted correction of the abnormal host defense (e.g., immune serum globulin for hypogammaglobulinemic conditions).

Infections associated with common defects in inflammatory or immunologic response

Host defect	Examples of diseases or therapies associated with defects	Common etiologic agents of infections
INFLAMMATORY RESPONSE		
Neutropenia	Hematologic malignancies, cytotoxic chemotherapy, aplastic anemia	Gram-negative bacilli, *Staph. aureus, Candida* sp., *Aspergillus* sp.
Chemotaxis	Chédiak-Higashi syndrome	*Staph. aureus, Strep. pyogenes*
	Job's syndrome	*Staph. aureus, H. influenzae*
	Protein-calorie malnutrition	Gram-negative bacilli
Phagocytosis (cellular)	SLE, chronic myelogenous leukemia	*Strep. pneumoniae, H. influenzae*
Microbicidal defect	Chronic granulomatous disease	Catalase-positive bacteria and fungi: Staphylococci, *E. coli, Klebsiella* sp., *P. aeruginosa, Candida* sp., *Aspergillus* sp.

Host defect	Examples of diseases or therapies associated with defects	Common etiologic agents of infections
INFLAMMATORY RESPONSE (*continued*)		
	Chédiak-Higashi syndrome	*Staph. aureus, Strep. pyogenes*
COMPLEMENT SYSTEM		
C3	Congenital	*Staph. aureus*
	Liver disease	*Strep. pneumoniae*
	SLE	*Pseudomonas* sp., *Proteus* sp.
C5	Congenital	*Neisseria* sp., gram-negative rods
C6, C7, C8	Congenital	*N. meningitidis*
	SLE	*N. gonorrhoeae*
Alternate pathway	Sickle cell disease	*Strep. pneumoniae*
	Splenectomy	*Salmonella* sp.
IMMUNE RESPONSE		
T-cell deficiency or dysfunction	Thymic aplasia & hypoplasia, Hodgkin's disease, sarcoid, lepromatous leprosy	*L. monocytogenes, Mycobacterium* sp., *Candida* sp., *Aspergillus* sp., *Cryptococcus neoformans, H. simplex* & zoster
	AIDS	*P. carinii,* CMV, *H. simplex, M. avium intracellulare, C. neoformans, Candida* sp., *Salmonella, Shigella, Strep. pneumoniae, H. influenzae, Staph. aureus*
	Mucocutaneous candidiasis	*Candida* sp.
	Purine nucleoside phosphorylase deficiency	Fungi, viruses
B-cell deficiency or dysfunction	Bruton's X-linked agammaglobulinemia, common variable hypogammaglobulinemia, chronic lymphocytic leukemia, multiple myeloma, IgG subclass deficiency	*Strep. pneumoniae,* other streptococci, *H. influenzae, N. meningitidis, K. pneumoniae, E. coli, G. lamblia, P. carinii,* enteroviruses

Host defect	Examples of diseases or therapies associated with defects	Common etiologic agents of infections
IMMUNE RESPONSE (*continued*)		
	Selective IgA deficiency	*G. lamblia,* viral hepatitis, *Strep. pneumoniae, H. influenzae*
	Selective IgM deficiency	*Strep. pneumoniae, H. influenzae, E. coli*
Mixed T- and B-cell deficiency or dysfunction	Ataxia-telangiectasia	*Strep. pneumoniae, H. influenzae, Staph. aureus,* rubella, *G. lamblia*
	Severe combined immunodeficiency	*C. albicans, P. carinii,* varicella, rubella, CMV
	Wiskott-Aldrich	Infections seen in T- and B-cell abnormalities

From Masur H, Fauci AS: HPIM-12, p. 466.

For a more detailed discussion, see Masur H, Fauci AS: Infections in the Compromised Host, Chap. 82, HPIM-12, p. 464

37 HOSPITAL-ACQUIRED INFECTIONS

Important pathogens
• Gram-negative bacilli, especially in urinary tract; reservoirs in hospital environment; acquire and transfer antibiotic resistance by plasmids (R factors). • *Staphylococcus aureus:* Some strains in Europe and North America resistant to all β-lactam antibiotics. • Enterococcus: Nosocomial urinary tract infections; wound pathogen in pts who received broad-spectrum cephalosporins. • Opportunistic infections by low-virulence organisms: *S. epidermidis,* JK diphtheroid, fungi (*Aspergillus, Candida*).

Urinary tract infections
• Up to 40% of hospital-acquired infections, especially with indwelling catheters. • To prevent, should use indwelling catheters only for bladder obstruction or close monitoring of fluids; change after 5 to 7 days. Use intermittent catheterization when possible.

Wound infections
• Usually pt's flora introduced at the time of surgery. • Risk factors: Operations involving contaminated sites (bowel, vagina), lengthy surgery, foreign bodies, hematomas, advanced age, poor nutritional status, diabetes, renal failure, glucocorticoid therapy. • Early infections (24–48 h): Usually group A *Streptococcus* or *Clostridium* spp. • Staphylococcal infections: 4–6 d after surgery. • Gram-negative bacilli and anaerobic bacteria: At least 1 week. • Prophylactic antibiotics should be given immediately preoperatively and for only 24 to 48 h after surgery (especially colon surgery and vaginal hysterectomy).

Pneumonia
• Leading cause of mortality from hospital-acquired infections. • Especially gram-negative bacilli and *S. aureus* acquired by aspiration. • Risk factors: Obtundation with ineffective cough and gag reflex, underlying pulmonary disease or CHF with impaired pulmonary clearance mechanisms, respiratory tract instrumentation. • Prevention: Positioning obtunded pts in a swimmer's position, treatment of CHF.

Bacteremia
• Vascular cannulas infected by *S. epidermidis, S. aureus,* gram-negative bacilli, enterococci, *Candida* most important. • IV fluids (5% dextrose) may be contaminated by *Enterobacter, Klebsiella, Serratia, Pseudomonas cepacia, Citro-*

bacter freundii. • Prevention: Avoid use of legs; sterile insertion; change every 48 to 72 h.

Other

• Hepatitis B infection risk for hospital personnel who handle blood specimens and pts on dialysis or who receive blood products. Prevent with blood and needle precautions, labeling all blood and tissues from infected pts; hepatitis B immunization for hospital personnel at risk; prompt immunization with hepatitis B immune globulin after exposure. • AIDS: Universal blood and secretion precautions to protect other patients and hospital personnel; questionable role for AZT prophylaxis after needlestick or other blood exposure. • Legionnaires' disease: Can be prevented by hyperchlorination or superheating of hospital tap water. • *Clostridium difficile* colitis: Enteric precautions for infected pts.

For a more detailed discussion, see Gardner P, Klimek JJ: Hospital-Acquired Infections, Chap. 83, in HPIM-12, p. 468

---

38 ANTIMICROBIAL THERAPY

ANTIBACTERIAL THERAPY   See Table 38-1, p. 150.

ANTIVIRAL THERAPY   See Table 38-2, p. 157.

ANTIFUNGAL THERAPY   See Table 38-3, p. 159.

DRUGS FOR PARASITIC INFECTIONS   See Chap. 62.

TABLE 38-1 Antibacterial therapy

Drug	Organism/disease	Dosage	Comments
PENICILLINS			
Natural penicillins:			
Penicillin G	Pneumococcal pneumonia	600,000 U procaine IM bid	Dose adjustment needed for C_{cr} <30 mL/min
	Gonorrhea (β-lactamase negative)	2.4 million U procaine IM × 2 d + 1.0 g probenecid PO	3 million U → 115 µg/mL blood, 300 µg/mL urine, 6 µg/mL CSF
	Syphilis—primary, S. viridans endocarditis	2.4 million U benzathine IM	Other sensitive organisms: Erysipelothrix, Listeria monocytogenes, Pasteurella multocida, Streptobacillus, Spirillum, Fusospirochetes, Actinomyces israelii, Borrelia burgdorferi
	Pneumococcal and meningococcal meningitis	2 million U IV q 2 h*	
Penicillin VK	Streptococcal pharyngitis	250 mg PO qid × 10 d	60% absorbed; 0.25 g → 2 µg/mL blood, 300 µg/mL urine
Aminopenicillins:			
Ampicillin	Shigellosis	500 mg PO qid × 5 d*	0.25 g PO → 1.5 µg/mL blood, urine 50µg/mL
	Enterococcal endocarditis	2 g IV q 6 h + gentamicin 1 mg/kg IV q 8 h or streptomycin 1 g IM bid × 6 wks	90% rash with mono; 1 g IV → 35 µg/mL blood, 500 µg/mL urine, 10 µg/mL bile
Amoxicillin	UTI, bronchitis, otitis media with sensitive organisms	500 mg PO tid*	2 × oral absorption of ampicillin and should replace except for Shigella; 0.5 g → peak blood 10 µg/mL, urine 1000

Drug	Dose	Indications	Pharmacokinetics/Comments
Penicillinase-resistant penicillins:			
Nafcillin	4–9 g/d IV	Sensitive *S. aureus* and *S. epidermidis* infections: endocarditis, osteomyelitis, abscesses	1.0 g IV → 70 µg/mL blood, 2 µg/mL CSF
Dicloxacillin	0.25–0.5 g PO qid	Superficial *Staph.* infections	0.5 g → 15 µg/mL blood
Carboxy penicillins:			
Ticarcillin	200–300 mg/kg IV qd divided q 4–6 h*	Serious *Pseudomonas* infections	3.0 g IV → 190 µg/mL blood, >2000 µg/mL urine, 50 µg/mL bile; 4.7 mmol Na/g can precipitate CHF; high dose can precipitate hypokalemia, prolonged bleeding times
Indanyl carbenicillin	382 mg (1 tablet) PO qid × 7 d	*Pseudomonas* UTI or prostatitis only	1 g → 15 µg/mL blood, 600 µg/mL urine
Ureido penicillins:			
Azlocillin	3–4.5 g IV q 6 h†	*Pseudomonas* infections	3.0 g IV → 190 µg/mL blood; >2000 µg/mL urine, 50 µg/mL bile; less accumulation in renal failure than ticarcillin
Mezlocillin	3–4.5 g IV q 6 h†	*Pseudomonas* infections	Same levels as azlocillin, more active against streptococci
Piperacillin	3–4.5 g IV q 6 h†	*Pseudomonas* infections	Most active against *Pseudomonas*
PENICILLINS WITH β-LACTAMASE INHIBITORS			
Amoxicillin/clavulanate	250–500 mg PO tid	As amoxicillin; plus β-lactamase (+) *H. influenzae, E. coli, Branhamella, N. gonorrhoea, S. aureus, Klebsiella*	Each tablet contains amoxicillin & clavulanate in 2:1 ratio

TABLE 38-1 Antibacterial therapy (continued)

Drug	Organism/disease	Dosage	Comments
Ampicillin/sulbactam	As ampicillin; plus β-lactamase (+) H. influenzae, E. coli, S. aureus, Klebsiella, B. fragilis, Enterobacter, Acinetobacter	1.5–3 g IV/IM q 6 h	Each 1.5 g dose contains 1 g ampicillin and 0.5 g sulbactam
Ticarcillin/clavulanate	As ticarcillin; plus β-lactamase (+) Klebsiella, S. aureus, E. coli, H. influenzae, Enterobacter	3.1 IV/IM q 4–6 h; for UTI—3.2 g IV/IM q 8 h	Each dose contains 3 g ticarcillin and 0.1 or 0.2 g clavulanate
CEPHALOSPORINS			
1st generation:			
Cefazolin	Active against S. pneumoniae, S. aureus, S. epidermidis, ~80% of E. coli, P. mirabilis; prophylactic for surgery	0.5–1 g IV q 6–8 h†	1.0 g IV → 110 µg/mL blood, >1000 µg/mL urine, 50 µg/mL bile
Cephalexin/cephradine	Minor staphylococcal infections	0.25–0.5 g PO tid–qid†	0.25 g → 8 µg/mL blood, 500 µg/mL urine
Cefaclor	Respiratory infection	0.25–0.5 g PO q 8 h (adults)	—
2nd generation:			
Cefuroxime	H. influenzae, S. pneumoniae, N. meningitidis meningitis in children and young adults	750 mg q 8 h to 3 g q 8 h IV†	0.75 g IV → 40 µg/mL blood, >1000 µg/mL urine, 10–30 µg/mL bile, 1–20 µg/mL CSF
Cefoxitin, cefotetan	Mixed aerobic and anaerobic infections; prophylaxis for abdominal surgery	1–2 g IV q 6–8 h†	—
	Penicillinase-producing Neis-	2 g IM + probenecid 1 g PO	1.0 g IV → 70 µg/mL blood,

Drug	Spectrum / Uses	Dosage	Pharmacology / Comments
3rd generation:			
Cefotaxime	Meningitis due to group B Streptococcus, E. coli, H. influenzae, N. meningitidis, S. pneumoniae, infections with Enterobacteriaceae	1 g IV q 8 h to 2 g q 4 h†	1.0 g IV → 80 µg/mL blood, >1000 µg/mL urine, 15 µg/mL bile, 10 µg/mL CSF
Ceftizoxime	Gram-negative infections including meningitis	1 g IV q 8 h to 2 g q 4 h†	1.0 g IV → 80 µg/mL blood, >1000 µg/mL urine, 30 µg/mL bile, 1–10 µg/mL CSF
Ceftriaxone	Gram-negative meningitis; most gram-positive (except S. faecalis) and gram-negative infections (except Pseudomonas, anaerobes)	1 g IV or IM qd to 2 g bid†	1 g → 150 µg/mL blood, >1000 µg/mL urine, 200 µg/mL bile, 1–30 µg/mL CSF; may be given as once-daily IM injection
Cefoperazone	Active against most gram-positive, Enterobacteriaceae, and Pseudomonas infections	1–2 g IV q 12 h†	2.0 g IV → 250 µg/mL blood; disulfiram reactions
Ceftazidime	Very active against Pseudomonas and Enterobacteriaceae	1 g IV q 12 h to 2 g q 8 h	1 g IV → 80 µg/mL blood, >1000 µg/mL urine, 5–10 µg/mL bile
OTHER β-LACTAMS			
Imipenem	Active against aerobic gram-positive cocci and gram-negative bacilli, including S. faecalis; Pseudomonas; anaerobic species, B. fragilis	0.5 g IV q 8 h to 1 g q 6 h†	0.5 g IV → 30 µg/mL blood, 100 µg/mL urine, 10 µg/mL bile. Administered with dihydropeptidase inhibitor, cilastatin to prevent hydrolysis
Aztreonam	Active against aerobic gram-negative bacteria only	0.5 g IV q 12 h to 2 g q 6 h†	1 g IV → 160 µg/mL blood, >1000 µg/mL urine, 20 µg/mL bile

TABLE 38-1 Antibacterial therapy (continued)

Drug	Organism/disease	Dosage	Comments
AMINOGLYCOSIDES			
Streptomycin	*M. tuberculosis*, tularemia, plague, brucellosis	1 g IM twice weekly	—
	S. faecalis endocarditis	1 g IM qd	—
Gentamicin	Aerobic gram-negative infections	2 mg/kg loading; then 1.0–2 mg/kg q 8 h‡	1.5 g mg/kg → 6 μg/mL blood, 50 μg/mL urine, 2 μg/mL bile Desired serum levels: 5–10 μg/mL peak, 1–2 μg/mL trough All aminoglycosides may cause nephrotoxicity and ototoxicity
Tobramycin	More active against *Pseudomonas*	2 mg/kg loading; then 1.0–2 mg/kg q 8 h‡	Same levels as gentamicin
Amikacin	Aerobic gram-negative infections	8 mg/kg loading; then 5 mg/kg q 8 h‡	Less drug resistance but use should be restricted
TETRACYCLINES			
Tetracycline	*Rickettsia, Chlamydia, Mycoplasma, Brucella*, Lyme disease, gonorrhea	250–500 mg PO qid†	0.25 g PO → 2.2 μg/mL blood, 100 μg/mL urine, 15 μg/mL bile; absorption ↓ by milk, antacids
Doxycycline	*Rickettsia, Chlamydia, Mycoplasma, Brucella*, gonorrhea, traveler's diarrhea	100 mg PO bid	Avoid in pregnant women, children; 100 mg → 2.5 μg/mL blood, 100 μg/mL urine, 15 μg/mL bile

154

OTHER			
Vancomycin	Active against all gram-positives, including methicillin-resistant staphylococci	0.5–1.0 g IV q 8–12 h†	0.5 g IV → 30 μg/mL blood, 100 μg/mL urine, 3 μg/mL bile
	S. faecalis endocarditis in penicillin-allergic; infections in hemodialysis	0.5 g IV q 8 h + aminoglycoside	—
Chloramphenicol	Pseudomembranous colitis	125 mg PO qid × 10 d	1 g IV → 15 μg/mL blood, 100 μg/mL urine, 3 μg/mL bile, 10 μg/mL CSF; levels after oral dose equivalent to IV.; 1 in 25,000 develop aplastic anemia; ↑ half-life of tolbutamide, phenytoin, warfarin
	Anaerobic bacteria, Rocky mountain spotted fever, meningitis with H. influenzae, S. pneumoniae, N. meningitidis	12.5 mg/kg IV or PO q 6 h	0.25 g PO → 1.4 μg/mL blood
Erythromycin	Streptococcal infections in penicillin-allergic, Mycoplasma	250–500 mg PO qid	1 g IV → 10 μg/mL blood; ↑ blood levels of theophylline
	Legionella	500 mg–1 g IV q 6 h	Adjust dose for hepatic failure; 600 mg IV → 15 μg/mL blood
Clindamycin	Most Strep, Staph, and anaerobic infections	150–450 mg PO q 6 h; 300–900 mg IV q 6 h	8 mg/kg IV → 10 μg/mL blood, 50 μg/mL urine, 100 μg/mL bile, 0.5 μg/mL CSF; red discoloration of urine and tears; ↓ effect of steroids and birth control pills
Rifampin	Staphylococci with second drug	600 mg PO qid (10 mg/kg)	
	M. tuberculosis	600 mg PO qd (10 mg/kg)	
	Meningococcal prophylaxis	600 mg PO bid × 2 d	
	H. influenzae prophylaxis	600 mg PO qd × 4 d	
Metronidazole	Anaerobic infections	500 mg IV q 6–8 h	Disulfiram reaction with alcohol; potentiation of warfarin; should not be used in pregnancy
	Pseudomembranous colitis	250–500 mg PO qid × 10–14 d	
	T. vaginalis	2.0 gm PO	
	Amebic liver abscess, colitis	750 mg PO tid × 5–10 days	

155

TABLE 38-1 Antibacterial therapy (continued)

Drug	Organism/disease	Dosage	Comments
Sulfadiazine	Toxoplasmosis	75–100 mg/kg qd in 4 doses (combined with pyramethamine)	All sulfas can cause rash, fever, jaundice, hemolysis in G6PD-deficient, agranulocytosis, leukopenia
Trimethoprim-sulfamethoxazole	UTI, bronchitis, diarrhea *Pneumocystis carinii*	1 double-strength (DS) bid 20 mg trimethoprim + 100 mg sulfamethoxazole/kg/d (4 amps = 2 DS q 6 h)	Displaces warfarin, methotrexate, and chlorpropamide from albumin
QUINOLONES			
Ciprofloxacin	UTI, diarrhea, skin and bone infections. Most gram-positives and gram-negatives except enterococci, anaerobes; only fair against streptococci and pneumococcus	250–750 mg PO bid	Not to be used in pregnant women or children; cartilage lesions
Norfloxacin	UTI (including *Pseudomonas*)	400 mg PO bid × 7–10 d*	As for ciprofloxacin

* Minor adjustments necessary in renal failure.

† Major adjustments necessary in renal failure.

‡ Adjustment for creatinine clearance: $C_{cr} = \dfrac{(140 - \text{age}) \times \text{wt (kg)}}{\text{Cr (mg/dL)} \times 72}$. For $C_{cr} < 100$ mL/min, dose given q 8 h multiplied by $C_{cr} \times 0.01$.

TABLE 38-2 Antiviral therapy

Infection	Antiviral drug	Administration	Dosage	Comment
Influenza A (prophylaxis)	Amantadine	Oral	Adults: 200 mg/d for period at risk Children ≤9 y: 4.4-8.8 (mg/kg)/d not to exceed 150 mg/d	Needs to be administered for the duration of the outbreak. Dosage should be reduced in renal failure and in the elderly. Can be administered along with vaccine.
	or rimantadine	Oral	As above	Not yet licensed by FDA. May be better tolerated than amantadine.
Influenza A (therapy)	Amantadine	Oral	As above for 5–7 d	Both amantadine and rimantadine are effective in uncomplicated influenza. Neither drug has been demonstrated to be effective in complicated influenza (e.g., pneumonia).
	or rimantadine	Oral	As above for 5–7 d	Under study for treatment of complicated influenza in placebo-controlled trials.
Respiratory syncytial virus	Ribavirin	Aerosol	Administered continuously by small-particle aerosol from a reservoir containing 20 mg/mL for 3–6 d	Utilized for treatment of infants and young children hospitalized with RSV pneumonia and bronchiolitis.
Herpes simplex encephalitis	Acyclovir	IV	10 mg/kg q 8 h for 10 d	Acyclovir is the drug of choice for this infection on the basis of comparative trials vs. vidarabine. Optimal results are obtained when therapy is initiated early in illness.
	or			

TABLE 38-2 Antiviral therapy *(continued)*

Infection	Antiviral drug	Administration	Dosage	Comment
Neonatal herpes simplex	vidarabine	IV	15 (mg/kg)/d as a continuous infusion for 12 h for 10 d	Vidarabine reduces mortality, but severe morbidity is frequent. Therapeutically equivalent to acyclovir.
	Vidarabine or	IV	30 (mg/kg)/d given as a continuous infusion over 12 h/d for 10 d	
Genital herpes simplex: primary infection	acyclovir Acyclovir	IV IV	10 mg/kg q 8 h for 10 d 5 mg/kg q 8 h for 5–10 d	IV route is preferred if infection is of sufficient severity to warrant hospitalization, or if neurologic complications are present. Preferred route of administration for pts who do not warrant hospitalization. Adequate hydration should be maintained.
		Oral	200 mg 5 times/d for 10 d	Largely supplanted by oral therapy. May be of use in pregnant women in order to avoid systemic therapy. Systemic symptoms and untreated areas are not affected.
		Topical	5% ointment; 4–6 applications/d for 7–10 d	
Genital herpes simplex: recurrent infections (therapy)	Acyclovir	Oral	200 mg 5 times/d for 5 d	Clinical effect is modest and is enhanced if therapy is initiated early. No effect on subsequent recurrence rates.

Modified from Dolin R, IIPIM 12, p 404.

Agent	Organism/disease	Dosage	Comments
TOPICAL AGENTS			
Imidazoles and triazoles:			
Clotrimazole, econazole, miconazole, butoconazole, terconazole	Cutaneous/vaginal/oral candidiasis, tinea versicolor, dermatophytoses	Topically bid, 1 troche 5 times daily	Oral—dissolve troche in mouth slowly
Polyene macrolides:			
Nystatin	Cutaneous/vaginal/oral candidiasis	Topically bid; orally qid	Oral—swish then swallow
Amphotericin B cream	Cutaneous/vaginal/oral candidiasis	Topically bid	
SYSTEMIC AGENTS			
Griseofulvin	Dermatophytoses	500 mg PO qd	Photosensitive rash
Ketoconazole	Blastomycosis, histoplasmosis, paracoccidioidomycosis, candidiasis, some disseminated coccidioidomycosis, pseudallescheriasis	200–800 mg PO daily	Hepatotoxicity, decreased serum testosterone, adrenal glucocorticoids; requires gastric acid for absorption
Flucytosine (5-FC)	Cryptococcosis, candidiasis, chromomycosis	37.5 mg/kg PO qid	Monitor serum levels (50–100 µg/mL). Reduce dose in renal failure
Amphotericin B	Blastomycosis, histoplasmosis, paracoccidioidomycosis, mucormycosis, coccidioidomycosis, aspergillosis, sporotrichosis	0.3–0.6 (mg/kg)/d IV for 6–10 weeks	Begin with 1 mg test dose; may double dose and administer qod; follow electrolytes and creatinine.
Fluconazole	Candidiasis, cryptococcosis	100–400 mg/d PO or IV	Well-absorbed orally

159

For a more detailed discussion, see Neu HC: Therapy and Prophylaxis of Bacterial Infections, Chap. 85, p. 478; Dolin R: Antiviral Chemotherapy, Chap. 86, p. 493; Bennett JE: Antifungal Therapy, Chap. 87, p. 497; Plorde JJ: Therapy of Parasitic Infections, Chap. 88, p. 498, in HPIM-12

39 PREVENTION OF INFECTION BY IMMUNIZATION

PRINCIPLES OF IMMUNIZATION

- Inactivated vaccines can be given simultaneously at separate sites.
- Multiple doses of live vaccine should be separated by at least 1 month; live vaccine should be delayed 3 months after passive immunization.
- Live vaccines are contraindicated in immunosuppressed, febrile, or pregnant pts.

ACTIVE IMMUNIZATION   See Tables 39-1 and 39-2.
PASSIVE IMMUNIZATION   See Table 39-3.

For a more detailed discussion, see Finn A, Plotkin SA: Immunization, Chap. 84, in HPIM-12, p. 472

TABLE 39-1 Active immunization of normal adults

Vaccine and type	Administration and target group	Comments
Diphtheria and tetanus toxoids (Td)	IM at least q 10 years; also after tetanus-prone wounds if >5 years since last Td.	Reduced dose of diphtheria toxoid in Td compared to DTP for children. Give previously unimmunized adults passive immunization plus Td at time of injury.
Influenza, inactivated vaccine	IM or SC yearly in autumn. For all adults >65 years or with chronic disease (see Table 39-2).	Acute febrile illness is a contraindication. Most pts with egg allergy can be immunized with special precautions.
Pneumococcal 23-valent polysaccharide vaccine	SC once. For all adults >65 years or with increased risk of severe infection (see Table 39-2).	May be given simultaneously with influenza vaccine at separate sites.
Measles, live attenuated vaccine	SC once. For all adults born after 1956 without previous history of infection or immunization.	Serologic testing for immunity not necessary since previous infection or immunization not a contraindication to revaccination.
Mumps, live attenuated vaccine	SC once. For all adults, especially males, without history of prior infection or immunization.	To prevent orchitis in susceptible males. A combined measles-mumps vaccine is available.
Rubella, live attenuated vaccine	SC once. For all seronegative females, especially those of childbearing age.	Only to women who are antibody (HI) negative and if pregnancy can be prevented for 3 months.

Modified from Finn A, Plotkin SA: HPIM-12, p. 474.

TABLE 39-2 Active immunization of individuals at high risk of acquiring or developing severe infections

Vaccine and type	Administration and target group	Comments
Influenza, inactivated vaccine	IM or SC yearly. For pts with chronic cardiac, pulmonary, renal, metabolic (e.g., diabetes) diseases, severe anemia, immunosuppression (including AIDS); healthcare personnel caring for these pts; residents of institutions with these pts.	To reduce morbidity and mortality in these pts at risk for complications of influenza. Children should only be given "split" vaccine. (See also Table 39-1.)
Pneumococcal 23-valent polysaccharide vaccine	SC once. Same population as for influenza vaccine or pts with cirrhosis, alcoholism, functional/anatomic asplenia (e.g., sickle cell), myeloma, nephrotic syndrome, CSF leaks, immunosuppression (e.g., from HIV infection).	See also Table 39-1.
Hepatitis B, inactivated or recombinant subunit vaccine	3 doses IM in deltoid at 0, 1, and 6 months. For healthcare personnel exposed to blood products, household and sexual contacts of carriers, clients and staff of institutions for mentally handicapped, pts receiving hemodialysis or clotting factors, pts with multiple sexual partners, IV drug abusers, prisoners, groups with highly endemic infection, infants of HBsAg-positive mothers.	Pregnancy is not a contraindication for vaccination in women at high risk of acquiring hepatitis B virus infection.
Meningococcal 4-valent polysaccharide vaccine	SC once. For control of epidemics and adjunct to chemoprophylaxis of household contacts; pts with functional/anatomic asplenia (e.g., sickle cell), defects in terminal complement components.	Type B infection is most common; no vaccine against type B infection. Give rifampin to contacts also.
Haemophilus influenzae B polysaccharide vaccine	SC once. For all children 18–24 months and unimmunized young adults at high risk of infection.	

163

TABLE 39-2 Active immunization of individuals at high risk of acquiring or developing severe infections *(continued)*

Vaccine and type	Administration and target group	Comments
BCG, live attenuated vaccine (tuberculosis)	SC or intradermally once. For groups with high endemic infection; personnel caring for such pts.	Immunodeficiency (e.g., HIV infection) is a contraindication to BCG vaccination.
Adenovirus, bivalent live attenuated vaccine	PO once. For military recruits only.	
Rabies, human diploid cell vaccine (HDCV)	Preexposure prophylaxis: 3 IM doses at 0, 7, 28 days. Postexposure prophylaxis: 5 IM doses at 0, 3, 7, 14, 28 days with HRIG (see Table 39-3).	Preexposure prophylaxis for individuals with a high risk of exposure (veterinarians, laboratory workers).
Polio:		
Live attenuated vaccine (OPV)	4 oral doses at 0, 1–2, 3–4, and 9–16 months. For unimmunized adults at immediate risk of exposure.	Routine immunization against polio of adults in U.S. is not recommended.
Inactivated vaccine (IPV)	3 SC doses at 0, 1–2 months, 6–12 months. For unimmunized pts with immunosuppression and their household contacts, healthcare providers, and travelers exposed to wild-type virus.	Rapid protection: 2 doses 4 weeks apart. Immediate protection (including in pregnancy): administer oral polio vaccine (OPV).
Typhoid, killed bacilli vaccine	SC in two half doses 4 weeks apart.	Household contact of *S. typhi* carrier; traveler.
Yellow fever, live attenuated vaccine	SC once every 10 years. Administered at registered vaccination centers.	Contraindicated in immunosuppressed or pregnant pts, or infants <6 months.
Cholera, killed bacilli vaccine	SC every 6 months. Only if a requirement for entry into country of destination.	Infection is more effectively prevented by taking precautions in handling food and drink.
Japanese B encephalitis, inactivated virus vaccine	For travelers to rural areas of the Far East, including China and Korea.	Routinely given to children in endemic areas.

Modified from Finn A, Plotkin SA: HPIM-12, p. 475.

TABLE 39-3   Passive immunization

Disease	Preparation of choice	Target group and schedule	Comment
POSTEXPOSURE PROPHYLAXIS OF CONTACTS			
Hepatitis A	Immune globulin (human) (IG)	Contacts in day care centers, households, and custodial institutions. 0.02 mL/kg IM.	Up to 0.06 mL/kg IM for preexposure prophylaxis for foreign travel.
Hepatitis B	Hepatitis B immune globulin (HBIG)	1. Infants of HBsAg-positive mothers. 0.5 mL IM. 2. Possible percutaneous or sexual contact with hepatitis B. 0.06 mL/kg IM.	HBIG is usually given with appropriate doses of hepatitis B vaccine.
Varicella	Varicella-zoster immune globulin (VZIG)	1. Exposed infants and children at high risk of severe infection. 2. Exposed susceptible adults. 125 units (1 vial)/10 kg IM (minimum 125, maximum 625).	
Tetanus	Tetanus immune globulin (TIG)	Pts with wounds (other than clean minor wounds) without a clear history of full, up-to-date tetanus immunization 500–3000 units IM, part of dose infiltrated around wound.	Tetanus with diphtheria toxoids (Td) normally given as well.
Rabies	Human rabies immune globulin (HRIG)	Individuals thought to have had significant exposure to a rabid or potentially rabid animal. Pts known to be immune and/or fully immunized against rabies do not require HRIG but only 2 doses of rabies vaccine on days 0 and 3. 20 IU/kg, half infiltrated around wound, half IM.	Given early and follow with a 5-dose course of rabies vaccine on days 0, 3, 7, 14, and 28.
Measles	Immune globulin (human) (IG)	Susceptible household and close contacts, within 6 d of exposure, particularly immunosuppressed individuals (including those with HIV infection) and infants. 0.25 mL/kg IM.	Routine measles vaccination should be postponed until 3 months after IG administration.
Rubella	Immune globulin (human) (IG)	Pregnant women exposed in early pregnancy, where termination is not an option. 0.55 mL/kg IM.	Passive immunization does not ensure protection of the fetus.

165

TABLE 39-3 Passive immunization (continued)

Disease	Preparation of choice	Target group and schedule	Comment
TREATMENT OF ESTABLISHED DISEASE			
Botulism	Equine trivalent antitoxin*	Pts with food-borne or wound botulism.	Not used to treat infant botulism.
Diphtheria	Equine diphtheria antitoxin*	Pts with clinical diagnosis of diphtheria.	Probably of no value in cutaneous diphtheria.
Tetanus	Tetanus immune globulin (TIG)	Pts with clinical diagnosis of tetanus.	

* Tests for sensitivity and if necessary desensitization should be undertaken for these products.
Modified from Finn A, Plotkin SA: HPIM-12, p. 476.

40 SEXUALLY TRANSMITTED DISEASES

APPROACH

Male urethritis

- Diagnose by ≥5 WBC per oil field of discharge.
- PMNs with intracellular gram-negative diplococci → *N. gonorrhoeae* (confirm by culture); treat as for uncomplicated gonococcal infection (see below); always treat sexual partners.
- PMNs only—culture or antigen detection for *Chlamydia*; treat with tetracycline 0.5 g PO qid or doxycycline 100 mg bid × 7 d.

Epididymitis

- Rule out testicular torsion (Doppler exam or ^{99m}Tc scan), tumor, trauma.
- Pts up to 35 years of age—usually *C. trachomatis*; treat with doxycycline 100 mg bid × 10 d.
- *N. gonorrhoeae*; treat with ceftriaxone 250 mg IM then doxycycline 100 mg bid × 10 d.
- Older men or following urinary tract instrumentation—*E. coli* or *Pseudomonas*—mild: treat with trimethoprim/sulfamethoxazole (TMP/SMX) DS 1 bid; severe: tobramycin or gentamicin 1.5 mg/kg then 1.0 mg/kg q 8 h IV.

Lower GU tract infection in women

- Cystitis: ≥20 WBC/400× field spun midstream urine; ≥10^2 bacteria/mL on culture.
- Urethritis: pyuria and symptoms with negative urine cultures, probably chlamydial.
- Vaginitis: *T. vaginalis*—profuse, yellow, purulent discharge, motile trophozoites on wet mount; treat with a single dose of 2.0 g metronidazole PO; bacterial vaginosis—vaginal malodor with ↑ white or gray discharge, ''clue cells'' on wet-mount; treat with metronidazole 500 mg bid × 7 d; candidiasis—marked vulvar itching with thick white discharge, fungal elements on 10% KOH; treat with intravaginal miconazole or clotrimazole 100 mg qd × 7 d.

Mucopurulent cervicitis

- Yellowish discharge from cervical os with ≥10 PMN/oil field.
- ~50% chlamydial, but also treat for gonococcal cervicitis (GC) (see male urethritis); treat partners.

Ulcerative genital lesions

- Exclude syphilis by dark-field exam and VDRL.
- Painful vesicles or pustules: culture for herpes.
- Painful, nonvesicular ulcer: culture for herpes or chancroid, test for syphilis.
- Painless ulcerative lesions: test for syphilis.
- Treatment: If herpes and syphilis ruled out and lesions persist, consider ceftriaxone 250 mg IM or erythromycin 500 mg qid or TMP/SMX DS 1 bid × 7 d.

Proctitis, proctocolitis, enteritis

- Proctitis: tenesmus, constipation, anorectal pain, mucopurulent or bloody rectal discharge; herpes simplex virus and lymphogranuloma venereum (*C. trachomatis*); culture for *N. gonorrhoeae.*
- Proctocolitis and enterocolitis: in homosexual men, especially *Campylobacter* and *Shigella.*
- Enteritis: diarrhea, abdominal bloating, cramps without anorectal symptoms; in homosexuals, *Giardia lamblia, Campylobacter, Shigella, E. histolytica.*

Acute arthritis

- Gonococcal arthritis-dermatitis syndrome; most common infectious arthritis in sexually active; culture from synovial fluid, blood, skin lesions, or CSF; diagnosis: (1) culture + from mucosal site or from sex partner, (2) typical pustular or hemorrhagic skin lesions on extremities, and (3) prompt response to antibiotics; treat as for disseminated gonococcal infection (see below).
- Reiter's syndrome: 80% HLA-B27 + ; *C. trachomatis* most often associated with sporadic form; others: *Shigella, Campylobacter, Salmonella, Yersinia, N. gonorrhoeae*; diagnose by acute, noninfectious arthritis persisting at least 1 month; ↑ sacroiliitis; acute conjunctivitis or uveitis, painless ulcers of oral mucosa, circinate balanitis, keratoderma blenorrhagicum.

PELVIC INFLAMMATORY DISEASE

Clinical manifestations

- Tuberculous salpingitis: abnormal vaginal bleeding, pain, infertility; 50% postmenopausal; diagnose by endometrial biopsy → granulomas and/or positive culture.
- Nontuberculous salpingitis: evolves from cervicitis → endometritis → salpingitis (bilateral lower abdominal and pelvic pain); IUD-associated; cervical motion tenderness, uterine fundal and adnexal tenderness; gonococcal or chlamydial PID onset at time of menses in younger women with mucopurulent cervicitis.
- Perihepatitis and periappendicitis.

Diagnosis

- Associations: onset with menses, recent abnormal menstrual bleeding, IUD, previous salpingitis, exposure to male with urethritis.
- Laparoscopy most specific.
- Endometrial biopsy sensitive and specific for endometritis.
- Culture endocervical swabs, endocervical aspiration, culdocentesis, specimens at laparoscopy for *Chlamydia* and GC.

Treatment

- Exclude surgical emergencies (appendicitis, ectopic pregnancy); rule out pelvic abscess.
- Treatment regimens: doxycycline 100 mg q 12 h + cefoxitin 2 g q 6 h IV for 48 h after defervesence, then doxycycline 100 mg PO bid for 14 d total; clindamycin 600 mg q 6 h + gentamicin 2.0 mg/kg, then 1.5 mg/kg q 8 h for at least 4 d, then clindamycin 450 mg PO qid for 14 d total.
- Outpatients: ceftriaxone 250 mg single IM dose (or cefoxitin 2 g IM and probenicid 1 g PO single dose) + doxycycline 100 mg bid × 14 d with reevaluation in 48–72 h.
- Examine all sexual partners; remove IUD.

GONOCOCCAL INFECTIONS

Clinical manifestations

- Males: urethritis after incubation of 2 to 7 d; complications uncommon with therapy (epididymitis, inguinal lymphadenitis, fistulas); rectal GC in homosexuals with pain, pruritus, tenesmus, bloody, mucopurulent rectal discharge; pharyngeal infection frequently asymptomatic.
- Females: acute uncomplicated urethritis and endocervicitis → dysuria, frequency, increased vaginal discharge, infec-

tion extends from endocervix to fallopian tubes (PID) in 15%; acute inflammation of Bartholin's glands usually unilateral; asymptomatic infection of endocervix, urethra, rectum, or pharynx common.
- Children: during childbirth; conjunctiva, pharynx, respiratory tract, or anal canal may be infected; prophylaxis for ophthalmia—1% silver nitrate drops, erythromycin ophthalmic preparation (advantage: prophylaxis for *Chlamydia*, too).
- Disseminated gonococcal infection (DGI): two-thirds of women at time of menses; present with gonococcemia (fever, polyarthralgias, papular, petechial, or necrotic skin lesions usually on distal extremities, tenosynovitis of several asymmetrical joints) or septic arthritis (purulent arthritis in usually one joint).

Diagnosis Gram's stain of urethral or endocervical exudate diagnostic with gram-negative diplococci within PMNs, but need to confirm identity and determine susceptibility to penicillin with culture on Thayer-Martin medium with ↑ CO_2.

Treatment

- Should check VDRL and follow-up cultures for GC 3–7 d after therapy in all pts.
- Uncomplicated infection in nonpregnant adult: ceftriaxone 250 mg single IM dose + doxycycline 100 mg PO bid × 7 d; if pregnant, substitute erythromycin 500 mg PO qid for doxycycline.
- Treatment failures with the above regimen rare. Evaluate for reinfection, alternative diagnosis.
- Disseminated gonococcal infection: ceftriaxone 1 g IV or IM qd until 1–2 d after symptoms resolve then complete a total of 7–10 d of therapy with amoxicillin 500 mg PO tid (if organism is penicillin-sensitive); or cefuroxime axetil 500 mg PO bid, amoxicillin 500 mg with clavulanic acid 125 mg PO tid, or ciprofloxacin 500 mg PO bid (if pt not pregnant).

SYPHILIS

Clinical manifestations

- Primary syphilis: single painless papule → eroded and indurated; usually on penis, cervix, or labia, but rectum or mouth also; painless inguinal lymphadenopathy within 1 week; chancre heals in 4–6 weeks.
- Secondary: skin—pink, nonpruritic macules on trunk and extremities, may progress to papules ± superficial scaling

or necrotic lesions; intertriginous area—broad, moist, pink or gray lesions (condylomata lata, very infectious); mucous patches—painless silver-gray erosion with red periphery in mouth or on genitals; may have constitutional symptoms.
- Latent syphilis: positive VDRL, normal CSF and physical exam; early <1 year, late latent >1 year.
- Symptomatic neurosyphilis: meningovascular—stroke syndrome, may have prodrome of headache, vertigo, insomnia, psychological abnormalities; general paresis—20 years incubation, ↓ memory, ↑ reflexes, Argyll-Robertson pupils; tabes dorsalis (25–30 years)—demyelinization of posterior columns with ataxic wide-based gait, bladder disturbances, areflexia, trophic joint degeneration, optic atrophy.
- Cardiovascular syphilis (10–40 years): aortitis, aortic regurgitation, saccular aneurysm of ascending and transverse aortic arch.
- Gummas.
- Congenital syphilis.

Diagnosis

- Dark-field exam of all cutaneous lesions and saline aspirates of lymph nodes of secondary disease; repeat on three successive days before considering negative.
- Direct fluorescent antibody may be as sensitive and specific as dark-field microscopy.
- Nontreponemal serology: VDRL, RPR (rapid plasma reagin); used for initial screening and titers; fall in titer correlates with response to therapy; approximately one-third negative in primary or late (false positives in acute infections).
- Treponemal tests (FTA-ABS, MHA-TP) to confirm diagnosis of syphilis in pt with positive VDRL or RPR; remain positive.
- Asymptomatic neurosyphilis: CSF exam necessary in any seropositive pt with neurologic signs or untreated syphilis or >1 year's duration; CSF VDRL very specific but relatively insensitive.

Treatment

- Early syphilis: primary, secondary, or early latent—benzathine penicillin 1.2 million U IM in each buttock once (inadequate treatment for GC); tetracycline 500 mg PO qid × 14 d if allergic.
- Latent, late and unknown (late latent with normal CSF, cardiovascular, gummas)—benzathine penicillin 2.4 million U every week × 3; if allergic: tetracycline 2 g PO qd × 30.

Follow-up : RPR   3, 6 months
                      1, 3, 6, 9, 12 - in HIV⊕

↱ Follow-up CSF exam q6months until wbc ↓

- Neurosyphilis (asymptomatic or symptomatic): penicillin G 12–24 million U qd × 10–14 d or procaine penicillin 2.4 million U IM qd + probenecid 500 mg PO qid × 10 d, then benzathine penicillin 2.4 million U weekly × 3.
- Pregnant: treat with penicillin according to stage.
- Jarisch-Herxheimer reaction: fevers, chills, myalgias, headache, mild hypotension 2–8 h after treatment; treat with aspirin and bed rest.
- Follow-up: follow quantitative VDRL at 1, 3, 6, 12 months; should re-treat if does not ↓ 4-fold in 1 year. Pts with neurosyphilis: repeat LP q 3–6 mos. × 3 years.

CHLAMYDIAL INFECTIONS (See Chap. 61.)

Lymphogranuloma venereum (LGV)

- Clinical: primary lesion (painless vesicle or papule) → painful inguinal adenopathy and/or draining fistulas with fever, chills, meningismus; proctitis in homosexual men (mucopurulent rectal discharge with tenesmus).
- Diagnosis: culture from aspirated bubo, rectum, urethra, cervix; complement fixation (CF) titer ≥1:64 suggestive.
- Treatment: tetracycline 0.5 g qid × 3 weeks; aspirate fluctuant buboes to prevent rupture.

For a more detailed discussion, see Holmes KK, Handsfield HH: Sexually Transmitted Diseases, Chap. 93, p. 524; Holmes KK: Pelvic Inflammatory Disease, Chap. 94, p. 533; Holmes KK, Morse SA: Gonococcal Infections, Chap. 110, p. 593; Ronald AR, Plummer FA: Chancroid, Chap. 117, p. 623; Holmes KK: Donovanosis (Granuloma Inguinale), Chap. 118, p. 624; Lukehart SA, Holmes KK: Syphilis, Chap. 128, p. 651; and Stamm WE, Holmes KK: Chlamydial Infections, Chap. 155, p. 765, in HPIM-12

LP indications in late latent syphilis

① Neurologic Sx + Sn.
② Treatment failure
③ non-treponemal Ab titre (RPR) ≥ 1:32
④ other evidence of syphilis (aortic, gumma, iritis)
⑤ non-penicillin tx planned
⑥ HIV ⊕

_41_ INFECTIOUS DIARRHEAS

APPROACH TO THE PATIENT WITH DIARRHEA

- History: Inquire about fever, abdominal pain, nausea/vomiting, character of stools (water, bloody, volume), recent foods ingested (seafood, common source such as picnic), travel, sexual exposure, other diseases/medications (immunosuppressives, antibiotics).
- Complete physical exam.
- Examine stool specimen (gross and microscopic). Culture for _Salmonella, Shigella, Campylobacter_ if fecal leukocytes present.
- Other diagnostic tests (e.g., culture for _Yersinia_ or vibrios, examination for ova and parasites) if warranted.

NONINVASIVE BACTERIAL PATHOGENS

Enterotoxigenic _E. coli_

- Epidemiology: causes majority of traveler's diarrhea in S. America, Africa, and Asia.
- Clinical: 24–72 h incubation; mild, watery diarrhea to severe cholera-like; occasional low fever; vomiting in <50%.
- Treatment: fluid replacement; antibiotics may decrease duration of illness [tetracycline 7.5 mg/kg qid × 2 d, trimethoprim/sulfamethoxazole (TMP/SMX) 160/800 (DS) mg bid × 5 d]; symptomatic relief with bismuth subsalicylate 60 mL qh × 4; prophylaxis: doxycycline 100 mg qd or TMP/SMX 1 DS qd.

Clostridium perfringens
- Epidemiology: incubation 6–12 h after ingestion of contaminated meat, poultry, or legumes. • Clinical: diarrhea and crampy abdominal pain; rarely lasts >24 h. • Treatment: fluid replacement; no antibiotics.

Staphylococcus aureus
- Ingestion of preformed enterotoxin. • Epidemiology: institutional outbreaks; short incubation (2–6 h); short duration (<10 h); high attack rates (>75%). • Clinical: prominent vomiting. • Treatment: fluid replacement.

Bacillus cereus
• Two syndromes: one like *E. coli* enterotoxin, one like staphylococcal enterotoxin.   • Epidemiology: reheated boiled rice.   • Treatment: fluids.

INVASIVE PATHOGENS

Campylobacter jejuni
• Epidemiology: second to *Giardia* for waterborne outbreaks in U.S.; raw milk, contaminated water.   • Clinical: incubation 2–6 d with fever, cramping abdominal pain, diarrhea; lasts 2–5 d (up to 3–4 weeks); associated with acute reactive arthritis.   • Diagnosis: culture from stool at 42°C on special media.   • Treatment: erythromycin 30 mg/kg qd may shorten course.   • *C. fetus* especially associated with bacteremia in pts with chronic renal, hepatic, neoplastic, or alcoholic disease; requires 4 weeks of gentamicin because of infection of intravascular sites.

Vibrio parahemolyticus
• Epidemiology: present in coastal waters worldwide, but especially in Japan with ingestion of raw seafood.   • Clinical: incubation 6–48 h; moderately severe abdominal cramps; chills and fever in about half; lasts ~24 h.   • Diagnosis: stool with many PMNs; culture.   • Treatment: fluids.

Vibrio mimicus   Acute diarrheal illness, especially following raw oyster ingestion along Gulf Coast. Similar to *V. parahemolyticus*.

Invasive E. coli   Rare in U.S., E. Europe, S.E. Asia; symptoms similar to *Shigella* (see below) except less vomiting and shorter duration; treatment: symptomatic.

Enterohemorrhagic E. coli   Epidemiology: strain 0157:H7, undercooked meat, especially hamburger. Hemolytic-uremic syndrome may develop.

Salmonella typhi (typhoid fever)

• Epidemiology: ingestion of contaminated food, water, or milk; humans only reservoir; ↑ risk of infection with malnutrition, prior antibiotic therapy.
• Clinical: average incubation 10 d (3–60); insidious onset with headache, malaise, anorexia, fever for 2–3 weeks; rose spots (2–4 mm erythematous macules upper abdomen); ↑ liver and spleen by second week; fever abates after third week.
• Complications: intestinal hemorrhage or perforation, localized infection (meningitis, chondritis, periostitis, osteomyelitis, arthritis, pyelonephritis), relapse, chronic carriage.

- Diagnosis: leukopenia; 90% positive BC (first week); 75% positive stool culture (third week); 3% stools positive >1 year; serology less specific.
- Treatment: if sensitive, chloramphenicol 50 mg/kg qd orally (divided q 6–8 h) →30 mg/kg qd when afebrile for 2 weeks or ampicillin 1 g q 6 h IV or TMP/SMX 1 DS bid × 2 weeks; life-threatening toxemia—prednisone 60 mg or dexamethasone 3 mg/kg tapered over 24 to 48 h; chronic carriers: normal gallbladder—ampicillin 6 g PO qd + probenecid 1 g PO qd × 6 weeks; cholecystectomy if abnormal gallbladder plus ampicillin 2–3 weeks.

Other salmonella

- Epidemiology: acquired by ingestion of contaminated drink or food (especially egg or egg products); ↑ risk with antacids, antimotility drugs, antibiotics, immunosuppression, AIDS, sickle cell.
- Gastroenteritis: fever, crampy abdominal pain, diarrhea, fecal leukocytes.
- Enteric or paratyphoid fever: clinically indistinguishable from typhoid fever.
- Bacteremia: usually prolonged; BC intermittently +; 1/4 local infection; associated with *Schistosoma* infections
- Local pyogenic infections: with or without previous gastroenteritis or bacteremia; localization at site of preexisting disease—aneurysms, bone adjacent to aortic aneurysms, hematomas, tumors.
- Diagnosis: stool or BC.
- Treatment: antibiotics not indicated for gastroenteritis (may prolong excretion) unless documented bacteremia, prolonged fever, >50 years old with aneurysms or vascular prostheses; treat with chloramphenicol 3 g qd for at least 2 weeks; other: ampicillin (if sensitive), TMP/SMX, third generation cephalosporin.

Shigellosis

- Epidemiology: *S. sonnei* most common in U.S.; *S. flexneri* in developing countries; increased in children <10 years old, in day-care centers, in homosexuals.
- Clinical: symptoms 1–7 d after exposure; mild watery diarrhea to severe dysentery; severity increased in infants, elderly, *S. dysenteriae* type 1; without treatment, fever resolves in 3–4 d, diarrhea up to 1–2 weeks.
- Diagnosis: WBC normal to increased; stool cultures.
- Treatment: fluid replacement; antibiotics decrease fever, carriage; TMP/SMX 1 DS bid × 5–6 d; ampicillin 50 mg/kg qd if sensitive; antimotility drugs contraindicated.

Cholera

- Epidemiology: Ganges delta, S.E. Asia, coastal Texas and Louisiana; epidemics waterborne.
- Clinical: incubation 12–48 h, then abrupt onset of watery, painless diarrhea, severe vomiting → severe dehydration.
- Diagnosis: direct plating of stool on TCBS (thiosulfate-citrate-bile salt-sucrose) agar.
- Treatment: fluid replacement IV or oral (20 g glucose + 2.5 g $NaHCO_3$ + 3.5 g NaCl + 1.5 g KCl per liter H_2O); tetracycline 500 mg q 6 h × 2 d.

VIRAL GASTROENTERITIS

Rotavirus   Most important cause of severe dehydrating diarrhea in children under 3 years of age worldwide; vomiting (<24 h), diarrhea, and low-grade fever; replace fluids.

Norwalk and related viruses   Occurs year-round; a third of epidemics of nonbacterial diarrhea in developed countries; cause of food- and waterborne epidemics.

ACUTE PROTOZOAL DIARRHEAS

(See Chap. 62)

For a more detailed discussion, see Carpenter CCJ: Acute Infectious Diarrheal Diseases and Bacterial Food Poisoning, Chap. 92, p. 519; Keusch GT: Salmonellosis, Chap. 113, p. 609; Keusch GT: Shigellosis, Chap. 114, p. 613; Keusch GT: Cholera, Chap. 122, p. 632; and Greenberg HB: Viral Gastroenteritis, Chap. 145, p. 714, in HPIM-12

PNEUMOCOCCAL PNEUMONIA

Manifestations
• Distribution usually segmental or lobar in adults, but may be patchy bronchopneumonia. • Often preceded by coryza, followed by abrupt shaking chill, fever with subsequent severe pleuritic pain, and cough. • If untreated, high fever and cough continue for 7–10 d with defervescence; abdominal distention and herpes labialis frequent complications. • Physical exam: Tactile fremitus may be ↓ early but ↑ with consolidation, tubular breath sounds, fine crepitant rales. • Defervescence usually within 12–36 h of instituting therapy, but may take up to 4 d.

Complications
• Atelectasis can occur before or during treatment with sudden recurrence of pleuritic pain; usually clears with coughing and deep breathing, but bronchoscopy may be required. • Delayed resolution: physical exam usually normal within 2–4 weeks, with x-ray resolution as long as 8–18 weeks. • Lung abscess rare; may be associated with type 3. • Pleural effusion ~50%; usually sterile and absorbed spontaneously. • Empyema: <1% of treated cases; may have few cells early but progress to thick greenish pus; can cause extensive pleural scarring if not drained; may be complicated by brain abscess. • Pericarditis: Precordial pain and friction rub may be present, but consider in any seriously ill pt. • Arthritis, especially in children. • Paralytic ileus may occur in severely ill pts. • Impaired liver function: Abnormal LFTs and mild jaundice common.

Laboratory findings
• Gram's stain of sputum shows PMNs and lancet-shaped gram-positive organisms singly and in pairs. • Blood culture positive in 20–30%. • WBC usually 12,000–25,000 cells/μL; if normal or ↓, may have overwhelming infection with bacteremia. • Organisms may be seen in Wright's stained buffy coat; think of asplenia, multiple myeloma. • CXR: Usually homogeneous density, but may be >1 lobe or atypical with underlying pulmonary disease.

EXTRAPULMONARY PNEUMOCOCCAL INFECTION

Pneumococcal meningitis

• Second to meningococcus in adults and *Haemophilus influenzae* in children as cause of bacterial meningitis.   • May be only site of infection or associated with otitis, mastoiditis, sinusitis, skull fracture with CSF leak, multiple myeloma, sickle cell disease.   • CSF cloudy, ↑ protein, ↓ glucose, Gram's stain usually positive for bacteria.   • Latex agglutination positive in 80% of culture-positive pts.   • 70% recover.

Pneumococcal endocarditis

• Usually complication of pneumonia or meningitis.   • Clinical: High fever, splenomegaly, metastatic infections.   • Can infect normal valves, especially aortic with rapid development of valvular destruction, heart failure, loud murmurs.   • BC always positive without previous therapy.

Pneumococcal peritonitis

• Secondary to transient bacteremia; ↑ in young girls.
• Associated with nephrotic syndrome, cirrhosis, liver cancer.
• Ascitic fluid and BC positive.

TREATMENT

Pneumonia

• Sensitivity testing important only with new resistant strains.   • 600,000 U penicillin G IV q 12 h until afebrile for 48–72 h.   • Cephalosporins 1–2 g qd effective; use with caution if pt is allergic to penicillin.   • With sensitive strains and uncomplicated disease, erythromycin 2.0 g qd, clindamycin 1.2 g qd, trimethoprim/sulfamethoxazole 1 DS bid.

Peritonitis   Penicillin 2–4 million U qd.

Pneumococcal meningitis   Penicillin G 18–24 million U IV qd; vancomycin (2 g qd) for resistant strains. Chloramphenicol 50 (mg/kg)/d; cefotaxime or ceftriaxone if penicillin allergy.

Pneumococcal endocarditis   Penicillin G 8–12 million U IV qd; risk of valvular injury or myocardial abscesses that may require surgery.

Pneumococcal arthritis   Systemic antibiotics usually sufficient, but may require aspiration.

Empyema   All pleural effusions should be tapped diagnostically; chest tube is indicated if bacteria and/or frank pus are present.

Prevention   Vaccinate all pts over 55 and with heart disease; pulmonary, hepatic, or renal disease; diabetes;

malignancies; patients with sickle cell disease >2 years of age. Dose is 0.5 mL IM given once.

For a more detailed discussion, see Austrian R: Pneumococcal Infections, Chap. 99, in HPIM-12, p. 553

43 STAPHYLOCOCCAL INFECTIONS

SUPERFICIAL INFECTIONS

• Folliculitis. • Furuncles. • Hidradenitis suppurativa. • Carbuncles. • Impetigo, which cannot easily be distinguished from disease caused by group A streptococcus. • Treatment: usually local heat, germicidal soaps; but for severe recurrent disease: dicloxacillin or cloxacillin 500 mg qid for 7–10 d. Treatment with rifampin 600 mg qd for 5 d can eliminate carrier state and prevent recurrences.

TOXIC SHOCK SYNDROME

• Diagnostic criteria: high fever, diffuse "sunburn" rash that desquamates on palms and soles over 1–2 weeks, hypotension, involvement of three or more organ systems (GI, renal, hepatic, mucous membrane hyperemia, ↓ platelets, myalgia with ↑ CK, disorientation with normal CSF).
• Onset acute at start of menses.
• Non-menstrual-associated: cutaneous infections, focal tissue infections, postpartum and surgical wound infections (minimal signs of infection with onset typically on second day after surgery).
• Vaginal discharge: culture positive for *S. aureus* but blood cultures negative.
• Treatment: correct shock; treat renal failure, pulmonary insufficiency, DIC; drain focal collections; begin parenteral nafcillin, oxacillin, or cefazolin.
• Up to 30% of women may have recurrences with subsequent menses.

BACTEREMIA AND ENDOCARDITIS

• A third of pts with bacteremia do not have identifiable focus; others have local infection, extravascular (skin, burns, cellulitis, osteomyelitis, arthritis) or intravascular (IV catheters, dialysis access sites, IV drug abuse) focus. Metastatic infections and endocarditis are major complications of bacteremia.
• Second most common cause of endocarditis and first among drug addicts.
• Nonaddicts: 30–60% involve normal mitral or aortic valves, often older pts with underlying disease; acute course with

high fever, progressive anemia, frequent embolic and extracardiac complications.
- Addicts: tricuspid valve, septic pulmonary emboli most common.
- Diagnosis with up to three blood cultures; culture skin lesions, urine (positive in up to a third with bacteremia).
- Treatment: nafcillin 1.5 g q 4 h or oxacillin 2 g q 4 h; may add gentamicin (1.5 mg/kg then 1 mg/kg q 8 h) for 48–72 h; penicillin-sensitive strains: 4 million U q 4 h; penicillin-allergic or methicillin-resistant: vancomycin 0.5 g q 6 h.
- Duration of therapy: isolated bacteremia with normal heart valves and removable primary focus of infection—2 weeks; right-sided endocarditis in drug addicts—2 weeks of IV therapy with aminoglycoside; all others—4–6 weeks parenteral antibiotics; prosthetic valve endocarditis—penicillin or vancomycin + gentamicin and/or rifampin 600 mg qd × 6 weeks (surgery usually required).
- *S. epidermidis* common isolate in primary nosocomial bacteremias, especially with IV catheters and prosthetic valves (40%); usually multiply antibiotic-resistant; treatment: vancomycin 0.5 g q 6 h for 6 weeks (plus gentamicin and/or rifampin with prosthetic valves).

OSTEOMYELITIS AND SEPTIC ARTHRITIS

- May be hematogenous or from contiguous infection. Hematogenous especially in children younger than 12 years; spine in adults; 50% preceding superficial staphylococcal infection.
- Acute in children; vertebral in adult is of slower onset, especially lumbar spine; increased bony fusion.
- Diagnosis: radionuclide scans may be abnormal first week; x-ray, CT, or MRI scan (vertebrae); needle aspiration or bone biopsy before therapy; sinus tract cultures not reliable in chronic osteomyelitis.
- Treatment: parenteral nafcillin or oxacillin for 4–6 weeks as for endocarditis (or cephalosporins, clindamycin, vancomycin for penicillin-allergic); surgery to remove devitalized bone, drain abscesses, relieve cord compression. Closed or open (e.g., hip) drainage of infected joints essential as an adjunct to antibiotics.

PNEUMONIA

- 1% of community-acquired, especially during influenza outbreaks.
- Older children and adults: usually preceded by influenza-like respiratory infection.

- Bronchopneumonia in cystic fibrosis; nosocomial infection in intubated or debilitated pts; obstructive pneumonia with bronchogenic cancer. Necrosis with cavitation and/or empyema complications.
- Diagnosis: Gram's stain of sputum → many PMNs and gram-positive cocci; culture sputum and blood.
- Treatment: parenteral therapy as for endocarditis for 2 weeks unless complications.

URINARY TRACT INFECTION

- After *E. coli, S. saprophyticus* most common cause of nonobstructive UTI in sexually active women.
- Treatment: sensitive to ampicillin, trimethoprim, sulfonamides, nitrofurantoin; if relapse, look for renal calculi.

For a more detailed discussion, see Locksley RM: Staphylococcal Infections, Chap. 100, in HPIM-12, p. 557

44 STREPTOCOCCAL INFECTIONS

GROUP A STREPTOCOCCAL INFECTIONS

Streptococcal pharyngitis

- Highest age 5–15 years; normally group A, occasionally C or G.
- Spread person-to-person, mostly by acutely ill.
- Incubation 2–4 d; abrupt sore throat, headache, malaise, fever; nausea, vomiting, abdominal pain in children.
- Physical exam: Temperature ≥38°C (≥101°F); diffuse erythema, edema, and lymphoid hyperplasia; tonsils enlarged and covered by off-white exudate; enlarged cervical nodes; fever usually abates within 1 week.
- Scarlet fever follows pharyngitis with lysogenic phage producing erythrogenic toxin in host without neutralizing antibody; rash develops within 2 d of sore throat: first neck, upper chest, and back, then over remainder of body, sparing palms and soles; rash diffuse, blanching erythema with 1- to 2-mm punctate elevations ("sandpaper" texture), increased along skin folds (linear confluence of petechiae = Pastia's lines); erythema and petechiae of soft palate; lasts 4–6 d followed by desquamation.
- Complications: Acute otitis media and sinusitis, peritonsillar cellulitis, or abscess; pre-antibiotic-era meningitis, brain abscess, thrombosis of cerebral venous sinuses, bacteremia with metastatic infections; delayed nonsuppurative sequelae: acute rheumatic fever (ARF), acute glomerulonephritis (AGN).
- Diagnosis: Should culture or use direct antigen-detection kit; extremely rare in children 3 years old or less or in older adults; ASO (antistreptolysin O) titer confirms recent streptococcal infection in pts with ARF or AGN but not with acute streptococcal infection.
- Treatment: To prevent ARF (if given within 9 d of onset): benzathine penicillin G 1.2 million units IM [(600,000 U if <27 kg (<60 lb)] or penicillin VK 125–250 mg qid × 10 d; in the penicillin-allergic pt: erythromycin 250 mg qid × 10 d (resistance in Japan); higher doses of penicillin required if suppurative complications.

Streptococcal skin infections

- Erysipelas: Acute skin infection with marked involvement of cutaneous lymphatic vessels with group A streptococcus;

especially infants, young children, and elderly on face; abrupt onset with fever, chills, malaise, headache, vomiting, spreading erythema → vesicles and bullae → crusts; central clearing; butterfly distribution; may have high fever and bacteremia. Treat with penicillin as for pharyngitis.

- Pyoderma: Localized purulent streptococcal skin infections (impetigo); peak 2–6 years of age, especially lower legs; papules → vesicles with surrounding erythema → thick crusts over 4–6 d; diagnose by culture of base of lesion; treat with penicillin as for pharyngitis; does not cause ARF but most commonly precedes AGN.
- Cellulitis: Acute inflammation of skin and subcutaneous tissues with pain, erythema, fever, and/or regional lymphadenopathy; margins not elevated or demarcated like erysipelas. Treat with penicillin as for pharyngitis, elevate if possible; severe infections may be treated with IV penicillin (nafcillin or cefazolin if *S. aureus* involved).

Lymphangitis and puerperal sepsis

- Red linear streaks from local trauma to enlarged regional lymph nodes with chills, fever, malaise (possible bacteremia). Treat as for cellulitis.
- Puerperal sepsis follows abortion or childbirth with streptococcal invasion of endometrium and then lymphatics and bloodstream.

Pneumonia and empyema

- Uncommon; usually follows influenza, measles, pertussis, or varicella.
- May be epidemic, with abrupt fever, chills, myalgia, cough, hemoptysis, bronchopneumonia.
- Early and rapid accumulation of serosanguinous empyema fluid; 10–15% bacteremia.
- Treatment: 4–6 million units penicillin G IM or IV.

GROUP B STREPTOCOCCAL INFECTIONS

Perinatal infections

- Maternal chorioamnionitis, septic abortion, puerperal sepsis.
- One of two most frequent causes of neonatal sepsis and meningitis; early onset (within 10 d of birth) from maternal genital tract with lung involvement, 2 per 1000 live births, high mortality; late onset >10 d from nosocomial transmission, meningitis, and bacteremia, lower mortality. Treat with high-dose penicillin; addition of gentamicin may be synergistic.

Adult infections

- Urinary tract infections in women and elderly men with prostatism.
- Suppurative gangrenous lesions in pts with adult-onset insulin-dependent diabetes and peripheral vascular insufficiency.
- Other: Endocarditis, pyogenic arthritis, pneumonia, empyema, meningitis, peritonitis.

OTHER STREPTOCOCCAL INFECTIONS

Group C
- Can cause pharyngitis, cervical adenitis, disseminated deep tissue infections. • Especially *S. equisimilis;* outbreak of *S. zooepidemicus* in unpasteurized milk.

Group G
- Bacteremia from cellulitis or decubitus ulcers with chronic lymphatic obstruction and venous insufficiency. • Often underlying malignancy, alcoholism, drug abuse.

Group D
- Urinary tract infections with structural abnormalities.
- Infected decubitus ulcers, intraabdominal abscesses. • Enterococcal endocarditis: Must use high-dose penicillin or ampicillin plus aminoglycoside for synergism. • Nonenterococcal group D streptococcus (*S. bovis*) causes bacteremia or endocarditis, associated with colon cancer; penicillin-sensitive.

Viridans streptococci
- Most frequent cause of subacute bacterial endocarditis.
- *S. milleri* may cause liver and brain abscesses, peritonitis, and empyema.

Anaerobic streptococci
- Found in abscess cavities with other bacteria. • Streptococcal myositis: Edema, crepitant myositis, pain, chains of gram-positive cocci in foul-smelling, seropurulent exudate.
- Hemolytic streptococcal gangrene: Necrosis of subcutaneous and dermal tissues with spread along fascial planes following trauma or surgery. • Progressive synergistic gangrene: Ulcerated lesion about surgical incision surrounded by gangrenous skin. • Chronic burrowing ulcer: Deep soft-tissue infection that erodes through subcutaneous tissue to form ulcer. • Treatment: Drainage of abscesses, debridement of dead tissue, high-dose penicillin.

For a more detailed discussion, see Bisno A: Streptococcal Infections, Chap. 101, in HPIM-12, p. 563

45 ANAEROBIC INFECTIONS

TETANUS

Epidemiology and pathogenesis

- In U.S., in incompletely immunized pts; may follow surgery, skin testing, IM injections, burn wounds, chronic skin ulcers, otitis media, dental infections, abortion, pregnancy, or narcotic injection; 10–20% without history of injury or detectable lesion.
- Neonatal tetanus from infection of umbilical stump.

Clinical manifestations

- Incubation period 2–56 d (avg. 7 d); shorter with more severe disease.
- Initial symptoms: pain and stiffness in jaw, abdomen, or back; difficulty swallowing.
- 24–72 h later: rigidity, especially trismus, and reflex spasms; alert; low-grade fever; sweating; tachycardia.
- Physical exam: may precipitate spasms, hyperactive deep tendon reflexes; evaluate wounds, severity of trismus, potential respiratory compromise.
- Symptoms increase in severity 3–5 days; improvement by 10 d; complete recovery usually in 4 weeks.
- Complications: hypoxia; aspiration; venous thrombosis; vasomotor instability; hypertension; tachycardia, arrhythymias; pneumonia; vertebral fractures, acute peptic ulceration, paralytic ileus, constipation.

Diagnosis

- Clinical; *C. tetani* recovered from wound in only 30%; can be isolated from wounds without tetanus.

Treatment

- Drainage of infected wound.
- Quiet room; prevent aspiration, contractures.
- Antiserum as early as possible: human tetanus immune globulin 3000–6000 U IM; if only equine antiserum available, give 10,000 U after testing for hypersensitivity.
- Primary immunization.
- Muscle relaxation: diazepam 40–120 mg qd.
- Tracheostomy if laryngospasm; ventilation.
- Penicillin G if treatment of wound necessary.

Prevention

- Immunization: children—DPT at 2, 4, 6, 18 months; adults—three doses Td (4–8 weeks, then 6 months to 1 year apart); boosters every 10 years.
- Wound prophylaxis: toxoid and antitoxin given simultaneously in separate syringes at separate sites.

BOTULISM

Etiology and pathogenesis   Absorption of toxin produced by *Clostridium botulinum*. *Food-borne botulism* is due to ingestion of preformed toxin in food. *Infant botulism* results from ingestion of spores and production of toxin in the intestine of infants. *Wound botulism* is caused by contamination with soil containing toxin-producing *C. botulinum;* also associated with chronic IV or subcutaneous drug abuse.

Clinical manifestations

- Symptoms usually 12–36 h after ingestion (extremes of 3 h to 14 d).
- Symptoms: bulbar dysfunction, symmetric paralysis of extremities (ascending or descending); weakness of respiratory muscles, constipation; urinary retention; ↓ salivation and lacrimation.
- Physical exam: alert; afebrile; ptosis, ↓ extraocular motion, sluggish pupils; symmetric flaccid weakness of palate, tongue, larynx, respiratory muscles, and extremities; paralytic ileus and bladder distention.

Laboratory findings   Examine blood, feces, gastric contents, and suspected food for toxin.

Treatment

- Intubation or tracheostomy before respiratory failure.
- Cathartics and enemas to remove unabsorbed toxin.
- Trivalent ABE antitoxin (following sensitivity testing to horse serum) for food-borne botulism; not of proven benefit in infant or wound botulism.
- Debride wound; administer penicillin.

OTHER CLOSTRIDIAL INFECTIONS

FOOD POISONING

- *C. perfringens* second or third most common cause in U.S.
- Food sources: recooked meat, meat products, poultry.
- Symptoms develop 8–24 h after ingestion with epigastric pain, nausea, watery diarrhea.

ANTIBIOTIC-ASSOCIATED COLITIS   Due to toxin-producing strains of *C. difficile*. May occur during or up to 4 weeks after all antibiotics except streptomycin or vancomycin (especially clindamycin, ampicillin, cephalosporins, aminoglycosides).

Clinical manifestations   Usually watery diarrhea, abdominal cramps and tenderness, fever, leukocytosis.

Laboratory findings   WBC may be ↑ to 50,000/μL; stool exam → WBCs.

Diagnosis   >95% positive stool toxin assay; characteristic pathology on sigmoidoscopy.

Treatment   Mild—stop antibiotics; severe—vancomycin 125 mg PO qid or metronidazole 500 mg PO tid × 7–10 d.

SUPPURATIVE TISSUE INFECTION

- *Clostridium* isolated from two-thirds of pts with intestinal perforation (esp. *C. ramosum*, *C. perfringens*, *C. bifermentans*).
- *C. perfringens* frequent isolate from tuboovarian and pelvic abscesses (mild local disease); up to 20% of diseased gallbladders; up to 50% in emphysematous cholecystitis (gas in biliary radicles, esp. in diabetics); empyema.

Treatment   Usually requires broad-spectrum antibiotics for mixed infection.

LOCALIZED SKIN AND SOFT TISSUE INFECTION

- Localized, indolent infection without systemic toxicity.
- Associated with cellulitis, perirectal abscesses, and diabetic foot ulcers.
- Localized suppurative myositis in heroin addicts.

Treatment   Debridement; antibiotics only necessary with systemic sepsis.

SPREADING CELLULITIS

- Abrupt presentation with diffuse, spreading cellulitis and fasciitis but no myonecrosis or massive hemolysis.
- Physical exam: subcutaneous crepitance with little localized pain.
- Association with carcinoma of sigmoid or cecum.

Treatment   Incision of infected area and broad-spectrum antibiotics; almost uniformly fatal within 48 h.

CLOSTRIDIAL MYONECROSIS (GAS GANGRENE)   Originates in deep, necrotic surgical or traumatic wounds.

Clinical manifestations   Sudden pain in wound → local swelling and edema, thin hemorrhagic exudate → rapid toxemia, hypotension, renal failure, increased awareness of surroundings.

Diagnosis Wound smear showing positive rods; frozen section biopsy of muscle.

Treatment Extensive debridement; penicillin G 20 million U qd; penicillin-allergic: check sensitivities to chloramphenicol (4 g qd), cefoxitin, clindamycin, metronidazole; consider hyperbaric oxygen.

CLOSTRIDIAL SEPTICEMIA Differentiate from transient bacteremia when often with other bacteria; associated with GI, biliary, or uterine disease.

Etiology Primarily following infection of uterus (esp. septic abortion), colon, or biliary tract.

Clinical manifestations Sepsis; fever; chills 1–3 d after abortion with malaise, headache, severe myalgias, hemolysis, foul pelvic discharge; often no localizing signs; 50% hemolysis.

Treatment Penicillin G 20 million U qd; drainage of infected sites.

MIXED ANAEROBIC INFECTIONS

ANAEROBIC INFECTIONS OF HEAD AND NECK Gingivitis; pharyngeal infections; facial infections (arise from diseases of mucous membranes, dental manipulations); sinusitis and otitis.

Complications Contiguous spread → osteomyelitis of skull or mandible, brain abscesses, subdural empyema; caudad → mediastinitis; pleuropulmonary infections.

CENTRAL NERVOUS SYSTEM INFECTIONS

- Anaerobic bacteria in >85% of brain abscesses (peptostreptococci > fusobacteria > *Bacteroides*).
- Direct extension of infection from sinuses, mastoids, or middle ear; or hematogenous.

PLEUROPULMONARY INFECTIONS

- Anaerobic aspiration pneumonia: slow onset, low-grade fever, malaise, sputum; at risk—elderly, impaired consciousness; Gram stain of sputum → mixed bacterial flora; CXR—infiltrates in basilar segments of lower lobes.
- Necrotizing pneumonitis: numerous small abscesses involving several segments.
- Anaerobic lung abscesses: CXR—single or multiple cavities in dependent segments; oral anaerobes.
- Empyema: from long-standing anaerobic pulmonary infection.

INTRAABDOMINAL INFECTIONS Subphrenic abscess; liver abscess (50% have anaerobes).

PELVIC INFECTIONS   Tuboovarian abscess, septic abortion, pelvic abscess, endometritis, postoperative wound infection.

SKIN AND SOFT TISSUE

- Synergistic gangrene: postoperative wound painful, red, and swollen for several days → erythema with central necrosis.
- Necrotizing fasciitis: rapidly spreading fascial infection by group A streptococcus or *Peptostreptococcus* and *Bacteroides;* anaerobic cellulitis of scrotum, perineum, anterior abdominal wall—Fournier's gangrene.

BONE AND JOINT INFECTIONS   Soft tissue infection adjacent to bone (maxilla and mandible); septic arthritis.

BACTEREMIA   Transient bacteremia; may present like gram-negative sepsis.

Diagnosis   Consider with avascular sites, no culture isolates despite positive Gram stain, failure to respond to antibiotics.

TREATMENT

- Drainage of abscesses; resection of dead tissue.
- Infections above diaphragm (*B. fragilis* unusual): 6–12 million U penicillin G qd × 4 weeks for lung abscess; if penicillin-resistant, clindamycin, chloramphenicol, cefoxitin.
- Colonic source (*B. fragilis*): clindamycin 600 mg IV q 8 h or metronidazole 500 mg IV q 8 h plus aminoglycoside; cefoxitin and an aminoglycoside, imipenem, ampicillin-sulbactam, or ticarcillin–clavulanic acid are alternatives.
- CNS: penicillin G 20 million U qd and metronidazole 500 mg IV q 8 h.

For a more detailed discussion, see Abrutyn E: Tetanus, Chap. 105, p. 577; Abrutyn E: Botulism, Chap. 106, p. 579; Kasper DL: Gas Gangrene and Other Clostridial Infections, Chap. 107, p. 580; and Kasper DL: Infections due to Mixed Anaerobic Organisms, Chap. 108, p. 584, in HPIM-12

46 DISEASES CAUSED BY OTHER GRAM-POSITIVE ORGANISMS

DIPHTHERIA

Epidemiology   *Corynebacterium diphtheriae;* in U.S. increased in Native Americans and in Pacific Northwest in indigent adults with symptomatic skin lesions—usually spread by droplet.

Clinical manifestations
• Incubation 1–7 d; temperature usually <38°C (<101°F).
• Naso- or oropharyngeal: pain on swallowing, with thick, gray membrane over tonsils and pharynx; laryngeal: extension of membrane with airway occlusion.   • Cutaneous: invades wounds, burns, or abrasions.

Complications
• Extension of membrane: airway obstruction and increased toxin absorption.   • Toxic: myocarditis; peripheral neuritis.

Diagnosis
• Demonstration of organism (club-shaped gram-positive rod) by Gram stain or methylene blue; culture on Loeffler's medium.   • Fluorescein-labeled antitoxin.   • Toxin production.

Treatment
• Antitoxin after checking for hypersensitivity to horse serum; 20,000–40,000 U if pharynx or larynx and ≤48 h; 40,000–60,000 U for nasopharyngeal infections; 80,000–100,000 U for severe disease or ≥3 d.   • Acute and chronic carrier state: erythromycin 2 g qd × 7 d.   • Immunization (DPT): 2, 4, 6, 12–18 months, 5–6 years, and every 10 years with Td (tetanus toxoid and diphtheria).

LISTERIA MONOCYTOGENES

Epidemiology and pathogenesis
• Reservoir of most pts unclear, but there are food-borne outbreaks (coleslaw, milk, Mexican cheese).   • Increased in pts with lymphomas, diabetes mellitus, alcoholism, cardiovascular disease, or steroid or cytotoxic therapy.

Clinical manifestations   Sepsis in newborns; meningitis; bacteremia.

Diagnosis   Culture.

Treatment
• Severe disease: penicillin G 240,000–320,000 U/kg qd in 6 doses + tobramycin or gentamicin 5–6 mg/kg qd in 3 doses; for 2 weeks in newborns, pregnant patients; 4 weeks in primary listeremia; 4–6 weeks in endocarditis and immuno-suppressed pts.   • CNS infection: penicillin G 320,000–480,000 U/kg qd in 6 doses; *not* cephalosporins; in penicillin-allergic, trimethoprim/sulfamethoxazole 15 and 75 mg/kg qd in 3 doses for 14–21 d.

ANTHRAX

Epidemiology
• Outbreaks in Southern Europe, Middle East, Africa; in U.S. in workers who handle imported and unprocessed wool, hair, or hides.   • Infection from germination of spores acquired by contact, inhalation, ingestion of contaminated meat, flies.

Clinical manifestations
• Cutaneous: 95% of cases in U.S.   • Inhalation: "Wool-sorter's disease"—mediastinitis, hemoptysis, sudden dyspnea, cyanosis, stridor, shock; usually fatal within 24 h • Meningeal: fulminant with hemorrhagic and/or purulent CSF.   • Intestinal: bloody diarrhea.

Diagnosis
• Gram stain or direct fluorescent antibody stain of fluid usually positive unless previous antibiotics.   • Cultures usually positive in 24 h.

Treatment
• Cutaneous: procaine penicillin 2 million U q 6 h until edema subsides then PO × 7–10 d.   • Inhalation or meningeal: penicillin G 20 million U IV qd (+300–400 mg hydrocortisone qd in meningeal).   • Effective vaccine.

For a more detailed discussion, see Holmes RK: Diphtheria, Chap. 102, p. 569; Hoeprich PD: Infections Caused by *Listeria monocytogenes* and *Erysipelothrix rhusiopathiae,* Chap. 103, p. 573; and Holmes RK: Anthrax, Chap. 104, p. 575, in HPIM-12

---

47 MENINGOCOCCAL INFECTIONS

Epidemiology
• Person-to-person spread through nasopharyngeal secretions; attack rate highest ages 6 months to 1 year. • Disease caused by group B (50–55%) > C > W135 > Y > A (except in Alaska and Pacific Northwest). • Increased risks in household contacts, alcoholics, Alaskan natives, military recruits, pts with terminal complement component deficiencies.

Meningococcemia
• 30–50% have meningococcemia without meningitis. • Usually nonspecific prodrome of cough, headache, sore throat with sudden fever, chills, arthralgias, muscle pains; 75% have petechial rash on axillae, flanks, wrists, ankles. • Fulminant meningococcemia (Waterhouse-Friderichsen syndrome): 10–20% of pts with meningococcal infection, vasomotor collapse, large petechiae, and purpuric lesions: high fatality. • Chronic meningococcemia: Intermittent fever, arthralgia, rash (maculopapular).

Meningitis
• Children 6 months to 10 years; young adults. • Usual URI symptoms with progression to fever, vomiting, headache, confusion (25% have abrupt onset). • Presumptive diagnosis with meningitis and petechial rash.

Other manifestations
• Purulent conjunctivitis or sinusitis. • Primary pneumonia. • Genital infections identical to gonococcus.

Complications
• After meningitis: Seizures or deafness acutely in 10–20%, peripheral neuropathy, cranial nerve palsies usually clear within 2–4 months. • Arthritis: 2–10% with meningococcemia; often multiple joints involved while on therapy.

Diagnosis
• WBC usually 12,000–40,000, but may be normal to decreased. • Meningitis: CSF with glucose <35 mg/dL, 50% have + Gram's stain for bacteria, 100–40,000 PMNs. • Culture blood, spinal fluid, skin lesions. • Antigen in spinal fluid by latex agglutination (not group B).

Treatment
• Adults: penicillin G 12–24 million U/d; children: 16 million U/m^2 qd for 7 d or 4–5 d past when afebrile. • Meningococcemia alone: 5–10 million U qd. Penicillin-allergic pts: chloramphenicol 4–6 g qd or cefotaxime or ceftriaxone.

Prevention
• Vaccine for outbreaks of A, C, Y, W135.   • Prophylaxis of close contacts: rifampin 600 mg bid (5–10 mg/kg) × 2 d.

For a more detailed discussion, see Griffiss JM: Meningococcal Infections, Chap. 109, in HPIM-12, p. 590

48 *HAEMOPHILUS* AND *BORDETELLA* INFECTION

HAEMOPHILUS INFLUENZAE

Epidemiology
• Primarily affects children 6 to 48 months. • Increased risk: close contacts of primary cases, sickle cell disease, splenectomy, agammaglobulinemia, Hodgkin's, alcoholics. • 95% of systemic disease is type b.

Clinical manifestations
• Meningitis: most common bacterial cause at 9 months to 5 years. • Pneumonia: broncho- or lobar pneumonia (75% with empyema). • Bacteremia: especially 6–24 months; increased risk in sickle cell disease, splenectomy, Hodgkin's. • Cellulitis: cheek or periorbital area, rhinorrhea, fever, and/or ipsilateral otitis media; BC usually positive. • Epiglottitis: mean 4 years old; *H. influenzae* b leading cause; 90% positive BC. • Pyarthrosis: ≤2 years old; single, large weight-bearing joints. • Other: second leading cause of childhood otitis media, sinusitis, chronic bronchitis, endocarditis, brain abscess.

Diagnosis
• 70% culture and Gram stain positive. • Antigen detection in serum, CSF, urine. • BC positive in up to 80%.

Treatment
• Chloramphenicol 100 mg/kg (up to 4 g qd) divided q 6 h and/or ampicillin 200–400 mg/kg qd (up to 6 g) given q 4 h with change to ampicillin if sensitive.
• For multiply resistant: cefotaxime, ceftriaxone, ceftazidime, cefuroxime, ceftizoxime (see Chap. 38). Also preferred by many as primary therapy for serious disease.
• Outpatient: amoxicillin 50 (mg/kg)/d up to 2 g qd; if resistant, cefaclor, trimethoprim/sulfamethoxazole.

Prevention
• Prophylaxis: rifampin 20 mg/kg (up to 600 mg) qd × 4 d for household contacts if other children <4 years old. • Capsular polyribose ribitol phosphate–diphtheria toxoid vaccine for children at 18 months.

BORDETELLA PERTUSSIS

Clinical manifestations   >50% of cases occur in infants; incubation 5–21 d, with sneezing, fever, rhinorrhea, anorexia

for 1–2 weeks → paroxysms of cough. Prolonged bronchitis in adults.

Diagnosis   Suggested by contact, "whooping cough," peripheral lymphocytosis; culture; fluorescent antibody.

Treatment   Erythromycin 40–50 (mg/kg)/d (maximum 2 g/d) divided q 6 h for 14 d.

Prevention   DTP vaccine at 2, 4, 6, 18 months.

For a more detailed discussion, see Waagner DC, McCracken GH Jr.: *Haemophilus* Infections, Chap. 115, p. 616; Freij BJ, McCracken GH Jr.: Whooping Cough, Chap. 116, p. 620, in HPIM-12

---

49 DISEASES CAUSED BY GRAM-NEGATIVE ORGANISMS

ESCHERICHIA COLI

• UTI: causes >75%. • Peritoneal and biliary infections. • Bacteremia: most often from urinary tract, biliary, or intraperitoneal source. • Abscesses: especially at site of insulin administration in diabetics (with gas formation); in ischemic extremities, surgical wounds, perirectal phlegmons in leukemics.

Diagnosis Cannot be differentiated on Gram stain; readily grows in culture.

Treatment Uncomplicated infection (if sensitive)—ampicillin 2–4 g qd IV, IM, or PO; severe infections—ampicillin up to 12 g qd; cefazolin 1 g q 6–8 h, gentamicin or tobramycin 1.5 mg/kg then 1 mg/kg q 8 h; for meningitis, ceftriaxone 1–2 g q 12 h, cefotaxime 1–2 g q 4 h (adults).

KLEBSIELLA-ENTEROBACTER-SERRATIA

• *Klebsiella:* complicated and obstructive UTI, biliary tract, peritoneal cavity, middle ear, mastoids, paranasal sinuses, meningitis, pneumonia (especially in alcoholics, diabetics, chronic pulmonary disease). • *Serratia* and *Enterobacter:* pneumonia, UTI; bacteremia (especially nosocomial).

Diagnosis Gram's stain may be suggestive of *Klebsiella* with large capsule. Grows readily in culture.

Treatment *Klebsiella* usually susceptible to aminoglycosides and third generation cephalosporins; *Serratia* frequently multiply resistant, so sensitivity testing important; empiric therapy in ill patient—tobramycin or gentamicin [3–5 (mg/kg)/d or amikacin 15 (mg/kg)/d] plus cephalothin or cefazolin 4–12 g qd for 10–14 d.

PROTEUS, MORGANELLA, PROVIDENCIA

• Cutaneous infections. • Ears and mastoid sinuses: very destructive; may extend to cause sinus thrombosis, meningitis, brain abscess, bacteremia. • Ocular infections: corneal ulcers, especially after trauma. • Peritonitis: isolated after perforation. • UTI: chronic bacteriuria, obstructive uropathy, renal stones. • Bacteremia: 75% from urinary tract; indistinguishable from other gram-negatives.

Diagnosis   Culture.

Treatment   *P. mirabilis* usually sensitive to penicillins; bacteriuria—ampicillin 0.5 g q 4–6 h; severe infection—6–12 g ampicillin IV + tobramycin or gentamicin 3–5 (mg/kg)/d. Third generation cephalosporins usually active as monotherapy.

PSEUDOMONAS

• Infections associated with local tissue damage (burns, wounds) or ↓ host resistance (cystic fibrosis, prematurity, leukemia, neutropenia).   • Skin and subcutaneous tissues. • Osteomyelitis.   • Ears, mastoids, paranasal sinuses: malignant otitis in diabetics.   • Eye: corneal ulceration.   • Urinary tract: obstructive uropathy and manipulation.   • Respiratory tract: pneumonia infrequent.   • Meningitis: following LPs, spinal anesthesia, head trauma.   • Bacteremia: debilitated pts, premature infants, neutropenics; malignancies, after surgery of biliary or urinary tract.   • Endocarditis: following open-heart surgery; IV drug abuse.

Treatment   Ticarcillin or piperacillin 16–20 g IV qd + tobramycin 3–5 (mg/kg)/d; ceftazidime + tobramycin; imipenem and tobramycin or amikacin if resistant.

BRUCELLOSIS

Epidemiology

• Four species: *B. melitensis* (goats), *B. suis* (hogs), *B. abortus* (cattle), *B. canis* (dogs).
• Exposure through infected tissues (slaughterhouse workers, butchers), milk, or milk products.

Clinical manifestations

• Acute brucellosis: incubation 7–21 d; usually insidious onset with low-grade fever, malaise, fatigue, sweats; 10–20% ↑ spleen.
• Localized: osteomyelitis of lumbosacral vertebrae; arthritis of knee; splenic abscesses; epididymoorchitis; endocarditis.
• Chronic: ill health for >1 year following onset.

Diagnosis   Positive culture of blood, lymph node, bone marrow; serology: IgG correlates with active infection; titers ≥1:160 suggestive.

Treatment   Tetracycline 500 mg qid × 3–6 weeks + streptomycin 1 g q 12 h × 2 weeks or trimethoprim/sulfamethoxazole 480/2400 mg qd × 4 weeks.

TULAREMIA

Epidemiology *Francisella tularensis* transmitted by contact with skin of rabbits, squirrels, muskrats, beavers, deer, cattle, or by tick bite; in U.S. by rabbit skin, bite of tick, or deer fly.

Clinical manifestations
• Incubation 2–5 d, then fever, chills, headache, myalgias.
• Ulceroglandular: 75–85% from skin inoculation; papule → punched-out ulcer with necrotic base; large, tender regional adenopathy. • Oculoglandular: purulent conjunctivitis with regional adenopathy. • Pulmonary: nonproductive cough, bilateral patchy infiltrates, high mortality. • Typhoidal: fever without skin lesions or adenopathy.

Diagnosis
• Serology: 4-fold rise over 2–3 weeks in agglutination titer; single titer ≥1:160 suggestive. • Gram stain usually negative; culture (glucose-cysteine blood agar) requires special isolation.

Treatment Streptomycin 7.5–10 mg/kg q 12 h IM × 7–10 d; if severe, 15 mg/kg q 12 h × 48–72 h or gentamicin 1.7 mg/kg q 8 h; fever responds within 2 d.

PLAGUE

Epidemiology Humans infected with *Yersinia pestis* by bite of rodent flea; concentrated in southwestern U.S.

Clinical manifestations Bubonic—painful, enlarged lymph nodes, fever, headache, prostration 2–7 d after flea bite; may proceed to sepsis; pneumonia with multilobar involvement.

Diagnosis Laboratory: WBC ↑ 15,000–20,000 (up to 100,000); ↑ SGOT; DIC; smear of aspirate of bubo on Wayson's or Giemsa's stain → bipolar, "safety pin" forms; culture usually positive but may require 48–72 h.

Treatment Streptomycin 7.5–15 mg/kg IM q 12 h and/or tetracycline 5–10 mg/kg q 6 h IV for 3–4 d after afebrile; treat contacts with tetracycline 250 mg qid.

For a more detailed discussion, see Schaberg DR, Turck M: Diseases Caused by Gram-Negative Enteric Bacilli, Chap. 111, p. 600; Sanford JP: Melioidosis and Glanders, Chap. 112, p. 606; Kaye D: Brucellosis, Chap. 119, p. 625; Kaye D: Tularemia, Chap. 120, p. 627; Palmer DL: Plague and Other *Yersinia* Infections, Chap. 121, p. 629; Plorde JJ: Bartonellosis, Chap. 123, p. 633; and MacGregor RR: Infections Caused by Animal Bites and Scratches, Chap. 98, p. 550, in HPIM-12

TUBERCULOSIS

CLINICAL MANIFESTATIONS

- Primary tuberculosis (TBC): Usually asymptomatic; lower or midlung zone pneumonitis with enlarged hilar lymph nodes.
- Reactivation: Chronic wasting disease with weight loss and low-grade fever. Pulmonary involvement most common, but extrapulmonary including widely disseminated disease may occur.
- Pulmonary TBC: Apical posterior segments of upper lobes and superior segments of lower lobes typical for reactivation disease; usually insidious onset; chronic cough with scant, nonpurulent sputum; hemoptysis with cavitary disease.
- Pleurisy with effusion: Abrupt pleuritic pain following formation of effusion next to peripheral primary lesion; usually in young patients but in U.S. half >35 years old and a third have simultaneous pulmonary TBC; fluid; >30 g/L (>3.0 g/dL) protein, ↑ lymphocytes; a third are PPD-negative; good response to treatment; empyema requires surgical drainage.
- Pericarditis: Usually from drainage of infected lymph node or extension of pleurisy; may develop tamponade or late chronic constrictive pericarditis.
- Peritonitis: Hematogenous seeding, abdominal lymphatic or GU source; insidious onset; diagnose by culture of paracentesis fluid or biopsy.
- Laryngeal and endobronchial: Usually with advanced pulmonary disease; laryngitis → hoarseness, bronchitis → cough and minor hemoptysis; highly infectious; respond well to therapy.
- Adenitis: Scrofula: chronic cervical adenitis, just below mandible, rubbery, nontender; diagnose by surgical biopsy for culture and histology, with therapy at or immediately before surgery to prevent fistulas; in children <5 years old, usually *M. scrofulaceum* and *M. intracellulare*.
- Skeletal: Pott's disease: infection of midthoracic spine with anterior erosion of vertebral bodies; may be large ab-

scesses; responds to chemotherapy alone unless neurologic compromise.
- Genitourinary: Renal TBC usually as microscopic pyuria and hematuria with sterile urine cultures; may cause cavitation of renal parenchyma and ureteral stricture; females: salpingitis and sterility; males: prostate and seminal vesicles.
- Meningeal: Meningeal and cranial nerve signs; CSF: ↑ protein, ↓ glucose, lymphocytosis.
- Ocular: Chorioretinitis, uveitis; choroid tubercles in miliary TBC.
- Gastrointestinal: Ileitis occurs with extensive pulmonary cavitary disease and swallowed organisms; chronic diarrhea and fistulas.
- Adrenal: Cortical involvement may cause insufficiency.
- Cutaneous: Lupus vulgaris.
- Miliary: Fever, anemia, splenomegaly; 4–6 weeks into illness: fine nodules on CXR; transbronchial, liver, and bone marrow biopsy positive in two-thirds; more fulminant in previously diseased individual with diffuse pulmonary infiltrates and positive sputum; PPD often negative.

DIAGNOSIS

- Detect in sputum, body fluids, or tissues by acid-fast stain or fluorescence with auramine-rhodamine (not specific for *M. tuberculosis*).
- Primary isolation may take up to 4–8 weeks; radiometric techniques with liquid media can detect growth in 1 or 2 weeks.
- CXR: Healed primary lesion with calcified hilar node and peripheral lesion—Ghon complex; multinodular infiltrates and/or cavitation in apical posterior segments of upper lobes.
- Skin testing: Positive reaction >10 mm induration to PPD-S; half of pts with miliary TBC and a third with new pleurisy are PPD-negative.

TREATMENT (See Table 50–1)

- Symptomatic improvement in 2–3 weeks; sputum conversion usually within 2 months.
- Renal failure: isoniazid and ethambutol 2–3 times per week or after each dialysis; rifampin dose unchanged.
- Suspect drug resistance from Haiti, Southeast Asia, Latin America, and begin therapy with isoniazid, rifampin, and ethambutol, with or without pyrazinamide.
- Prophylaxis: 1 year of isoniazid 300 mg qd for all pts with +PPD <35 years old and with any +PPD in pts with

TABLE 50-1   Treatment of tuberculosis

Regimen (adult drug dose)	Comment
Isoniazid 300 mg and rifampin 600 mg qd for 9–12 months	The usual regimen for initial treatment of all pts; if drug resistance suspected, add ethambutol 15 mg/kg
Isoniazid 300 mg and ethambutol 15 mg/kg qd for 12–18 months	The least toxic effective regimen; suitable for pts with minimal disease; regimen of choice for pregnant women
✳ Isoniazid 300 mg, rifampin 600 mg, pyrazinamide 2 g, and streptomycin 1 g or ethambutol 15 mg/kg qd for 2 months followed by one of the following: *1.* Isoniazid 300 mg and rifampin 600 mg qd for 4 months *2.* Isoniazid 900 mg, rifampin 600 mg, and streptomycin 1 g twice weekly for 6 months	Initial intensive phase for short-course regimens; short-course regimens have only been demonstrated to be effective under conditions of close pt supervision.
Isoniazid 300 mg and rifampin 600 mg qd for 1 month followed by isoniazid 900 mg and rifampin 600 mg twice weekly for 8 months	Effectiveness demonstrated in ambulatory treatment program in Arkansas. Has not been compared with other regimens.

Modified from Daniel TM, Chap. 125 in HPIM-12, p. 643.

AIDS, Hodgkin's, chronic steroids, renal failure, and abnormal CXR in untreated older pt.

OTHER MYCOBACTERIAL INFECTIONS

M. ulcerans   Cause of Buruli ulcer, small painless nodule → extensive granulomatous ulceration on extremities; occurs in Australia and Africa.

M. marinum   Infection from exposure to freshwater or saltwater fish; nodule with lymphatic spread or ulcer; sensitive to rifampin, ethambutol, and/or tetracycline, trimethoprim-sulfamethoxazole; must be cultured at 30–32°C.

M. kansasii   Pigment with light exposure, grows at 37°C, can be identified on initial stains by prominent transverse banding; pulmonary disease similar to tuberculosis but milder symptoms; disseminated disease with pancytopenia, hairy-cell leukemia, malignancies, organ transplants, AIDS; treat with rifampin and ethambutol or isoniazid.

M. scrofulaceum   Lymphadenitis in children with few systemic symptoms; treat surgically.

M. avium-intracellulare   Pulmonary disease like TBC, risk factors are underlying pulmonary disease, age; lymphadenitis in children; disseminated disease with fever, anemia, leukocytosis, hepatosplenomegaly. Overwhelming infection with no cellular response in AIDS pts; may cause severe diarrhea; blood cultures positive. Treatment: Poor; 3–6 drugs depending on sensitivity testing (isoniazid, rifampin, ethambutol, ethionamide, pyrazinamide, cycloserine, amikacin, capreomycin, clofazamine, ansamycin).

M. fortuitum and M. chelonei   Grow within 1–5 weeks on most media. *M. fortuitum:* Posttraumatic and postoperative skin and soft-tissue infection. *M. chelonei:* Pulmonary infections and disseminated disease. Often resistant; sensitivity testing more reliable: amikacin, cefoxitin, doxycycline, gentamicin, erythromycin, sulfonamides.

For a more detailed discussion, see Daniel TM: Tuberculosis, Chap. 125, p. 637; and Freedman SD: Other Mycobacterial Infections, Chap. 127, p. 649, in HPIM-12

---

51 INFLUENZA AND OTHER VIRAL RESPIRATORY DISEASES

INFLUENZA

Epidemiology
• Major outbreaks from "antigenic shifts": reassortment of genomic segments with expression of new neuraminidase (N) or hemagglutinin (H) of influenza A. • Influenza B less variation, with outbreaks in schools and military camps.

Clinical manifestations
• Abrupt onset of headache, fevers, chills, cough, sore throat, myalgias. • Acute illness usually resolves over 2–5 d.

Complications
• Primary influenza pneumonia: Persistent fever, dyspnea, scanty sputum; CXR: diffuse interstitial infiltrates; ↑ with cardiac disease, especially mitral stenosis. • Secondary bacterial pneumonia: Improvement 2–3 days after acute influenza, then fever, productive cough; *Streptococcus pneumoniae, S. aureus, H. influenzae.* • Reye's syndrome: Onset of nausea and vomiting, CNS symptoms (lethargy, delirium, seizures); ↑ SGOT, SGPT, and ammonia, especially after influenza B; normal CSF; association with aspirin therapy. • Myositis, rhabdomyolysis: Marked muscle tenderness with ↑ CPK and aldolase.

Diagnosis
• Isolation of virus from throat swabs, nasopharyngeal washes, or sputum in tissue culture within 48–72 h. • Serology: Fourfold rise in hemagglutination inhibition, complement fixation titers over 10–14 d.

Treatment/prophylaxis
• Symptomatic therapy but no salicylates for pts younger than 16 years. • Amantadine for influenza A will decrease systemic symptoms if started within 48 h—200 mg qd for 3–5 d; rimantadine has fewer CNS side effects (jitteriness, anxiety, insomnia). • Inactivated influenza vaccine for A and B yearly, especially for pts with chronic cardiovascular or pulmonary disease, those older than 65 years, medical personnel; amantadine can be given simultaneously during outbreaks until vaccine is effective (2 weeks).

OTHER VIRAL RESPIRATORY INFECTIONS

RHINOVIRUS **Epidemiology** Major cause of common cold; seasonal peaks in fall and spring; spread by contact with infected secretions.

Clinical manifestations Incubation 1–2 d, then rhinorrhea, sneezing, nasal congestion, sore throat; systemic symptoms unusual; in children may cause bronchitis, bronchiolitis, bronchopneumonia; exacerbation of asthma and chronic obstructive pulmonary disease.

CORONAVIRUS **Epidemiology** 10–20% of colds, especially late fall, early winter, spring.

Clinical manifestations Incubation 3 d, duration 6–7 d. Similar to rhinovirus.

RESPIRATORY SYNCYTIAL VIRUS **Epidemiology** Major respiratory pathogen of young children, peak 2–3 months; lower respiratory disease in young infants (20–25% of hospital admissions for pneumonia); nosocomial pathogen in adults.

Clinical manifestations Infants: rhinorrhea, low-grade fever and cough → lower respiratory tract involvement in 25–40%, especially severe with congenital cardiac disease; adults: common cold with moderate systemic symptoms; occasionally severe lower respiratory involvement in immunocompromised pts.

Diagnosis Isolation from respiratory secretions; rapid diagnosis by immunofluorescence or ELISA of nasal washings; serology (CSF) useful if >4 months old.

Treatment Aerosolized ribavirin in hospitalized infants.

PARAINFLUENZA VIRUS **Epidemiology** Major cause of lower respiratory illness, especially croup, in children.

Clinical manifestations Children: acute fever, coryza, sore throat, cough; may progress to barking cough and frank stridor; older children and adults: common cold.

Diagnosis Viral cultures.

ADENOVIRUS **Epidemiology** Children, military recruits; spread through aerosols, inoculation of conjunctival sac, or fecal-oral.

Clinical manifestations Acute URI with rhinitis; pharyngoconjunctival fever: bilateral conjunctivitis, low-grade fever, rhinitis, sore throat, cervical adenopathy; acute respiratory disease (ARD) in military recruits with fever, cough, coryza; acute diarrheal illness in young children; hemorrhagic cystitis; epidemic keratoconjunctivitis.

Diagnosis Culture, serology.

Treatment Live attenuated vaccine against types 4 and 7; stimulates protective antibodies against subsequent ARD.

TREATMENT/PROPHYLAXIS

For antimicrobial therapy and prevention of infection by immunization, see Chaps. 38 and 39.

For a more detailed discussion, see Dolin R: Influenza, Chap. 139, p. 695, and Common Viral Respiratory Infections, Chap. 140, p. 700, in HPIM-12

MEASLES (RUBEOLA)

Epidemiology Transmitted by droplets of nasopharyngeal secretions; highly contagious; increased outbreaks in teenagers and young adults.

Manifestations Incubation approximately 10 d; then malaise, irritability, high fever, conjunctivitis, severe cough, coryza; 3–4 d after prodromal symptoms—Koplik's spots in mouth, then 1–2 d later, rash on forehead → face → trunk.

Complications Croup, bronchitis, bronchiolitis, interstitial giant cell pneumonia (immunocompromised children); conjunctivitis; myocarditis; hepatitis; acute glomerulonephritis; bacterial pneumonia; encephalomyelitis: 1 in 1000 pts, usually 4–7 d after rash (high fever, drowsiness, coma, fatal in 10%); late complication—subacute sclerosing panencephalitis.

Diagnosis Leukopenia during prodrome; <2000 lymphocytes/μL is poor prognostic sign; multinucleated giant cells in secretions; viral culture; immunofluorescent staining of respiratory or urinary epithelial cells; serology.

Prophylaxis Passive immunization with 0.25 mL/kg γ-globulin (to 15 mL) especially for children <3 years old, pregnant women, pts with tuberculosis; live attenuated vaccine at 15 months. Immunocompromised individuals should not be vaccinated; if exposed, administer 0.5 mL/kg γ-globulin.

RUBELLA (GERMAN MEASLES)

Clinical manifestations

- Incubation 14–21 d; prodrome of malaise, headache, fever, mild conjunctivitis.
- Maculopapular rash begins on forehead and face → trunk and extremities; enlarged lymph nodes, especially postauricular and suboccipital; arthralgias.
- Congenital rubella: patent ductus, interventricular septal defect, pulmonic stenosis, corneal clouding, cataracts, chorioretinitis; microcephaly, mental retardation, deafness; associated with maternal infection in first trimester.

Diagnosis Viral cultures; serology; hemagglutinating antibodies by second day of rash.

Prevention Live attenuated vaccine should not be given to a woman who may become pregnant within 3 months or to immunosuppressed pt.

VARICELLA-ZOSTER

CHICKENPOX

- Incubation 10–21 d; 90% attack rate among susceptibles.
- Prodrome of fever and lassitude → maculopapules, vesicles, and scabs in varying stages of evolution; first on trunk and face.

Complications Bacterial superinfection (skin); pneumonitis in up to 20% of adults; myocarditis; corneal lesions; arthritis; acute glomerulonephritis, hepatitis, acute cerebellar ataxia, meningitis, encephalitis, Reye's syndrome.

HERPES ZOSTER

- Reactivation of latent virus from dorsal root ganglia.
- Pain within dermatome for 48–72 h → erythematous rash → vesicular lesions.

Complications Meningoencephalitis; granulomatous angiitis with contralateral hemiplegia; 40% cutaneous dissemination with lymphoma.

Diagnosis Tzanck smear—multinucleated giant cells at base of lesions; specific immunofluorescence; viral culture; antigen detection; serology.

Prophylaxis Varicella-zoster immune globulin (VZIG) to immunodeficient patients <15 years old within 72–96 h of exposure and to newborn of infected mother with onset between 5 d before and 2 d after delivery.

Treatment Zoster ophthalmicus—analgesics, atropine, topical antivirals (IUDR, ara-A, acyclovir); chickenpox or zoster in immunocompromised pt—acyclovir 10 mg/kg IV q 8 h × 10 d.

POXVIRUSES

SMALLPOX (VARIOLA) Epidemiology Last natural case in 1977; spread through airborne transmission.

Clinical manifestations Incubation 14–17 d with prodrome of fever, headache, myalgia, transient erythematous eruption → painful ulcers on buccal mucosa and papules on extremities → hemorrhagic vesicles; infectious until scabs fall off (3 weeks).

Diagnosis   Electron microscopy of vesicle fluid for viral particles or agar precipitation of antigen from vesicles; cell culture.

VACCINIA   Virus used to induce immunity to smallpox; only indicated for laboratory workers involved with smallpox (*not* to treat HSV, warts).

Complications   Vaccinia gangrenosum (destruction of large areas of skin), eczema vaccinatum (widespread infection in pt with eczema), generalized vaccinia.

For a more detailed discussion, see Ray CG: Measles (Rubeola), Chap. 141, p. 705; Ray CG: Rubella ("German Measles") and Other Viral Exanthems, Chap. 142, p. 707; Friedman HM: Smallpox, Vaccinia, and Other Poxviruses, Chap. 143, p. 709; and Whitley RJ: Varicella-Zoster Virus Infections, Chap. 136, p. 686, in HPIM-12

---

53 MUMPS

Epidemiology

- Paramyxovirus; only reservoir is in humans.
- Transmitted by infected salivary secretions or urine for 6 days prior to parotitis to up to 2 weeks later.
- Incubation 12–25 d; peak ages 10–19 years.

Clinical manifestations

- Salivary adenitis: usually sudden parotitis with marked pain; skin over gland not warm or red (vs. bacterial parotitis); fever 38–39°C (100–103°F), malaise, headache, anorexia.
- Epididymoorchitis: 20–35% of postpubertal males; usually 7–10 d after parotitis with recrudescence of malaise, chills, fevers; half followed by testicular atrophy; sterility if bilateral atrophy.
- Pancreatitis: abdominal pain and tenderness rarely complicated by shock or pseudocyst; may see increased amylase with parotitis alone (but increased lipase only with pancreatitis).
- CNS: half of pts with mumps show increased cells in CSF, usually 3–10 d after onset of parotitis; rare—true encephalitis, paralytic polio-like syndrome, transverse myelitis, cerebellar ataxia.
- Other: subacute thyroiditis, dacryoadenitis, optic neuritis, iritis, conjunctivitis, myocarditis, hepatitis, thrombocytopenic purpura, interstitial pneumonia, migratory polyarthritis (esp. males ages 20–30).

Diagnosis

- Laboratory findings: relative lymphocytosis in uncomplicated parotitis; marked leukocytosis with orchitis; increased amylase; CSF: 1000–2000 WBCs with PMNs early (higher than aseptic meningitis with polio-, coxsackie-, and echoviruses).
- Culture from blood, throat swabs, CSF, urine; in tissue culture, immunofluorescence positive in 2–3 d.
- Serology: fourfold increases in titer by ELISA, CF (S antigen early, V later).

Treatment

- Prednisone 60 mg qd tapered over 7–10 d may give symptomatic relief in orchitis.

• Prevention: Live attenuated vaccine (0.5 mL IM) after 1 year of age; contraindicated if hypersensitivity reaction, febrile illness, malignancy, pregnancy.

For a more detailed discussion, see Ray CG: Mumps, Chap. 146, in HPIM-12, p. 717

54 ENTEROVIRUS AND REOVIRUS INFECTIONS

ENTEROVIRUS

Characteristics Picornavirus: small, single-stranded RNA; can survive in sewage and chlorinated water with organic debris. Asymptomatic infection common; epidemics in summer and fall. Fecal-oral transmission; incubation 2–10 d. Two-thirds of isolates from children <9 years old.

Diagnosis Virus isolation from throat, stool, body fluids; CSF positive 10–85% (except polio), but may shed in stool for 4 months.

POLIOVIRUS INFECTIONS

Clinical manifestations

- 90% subclinical or mild; abortive poliomyelitis—nonspecific febrile illness for 2–3 d.
- Aseptic meningitis: usually complete recovery.
- Paralytic poliomyelitis: fever recurs 5–10 d later with meningeal irritation, asymmetric flaccid paralysis, absent deep tendon reflexes, normal sensation; 6–25% bulbar; recovery continues for up to 6 months.

Prevention

- OPV (oral poliovaccine): live attenuated virus; 2, 4, 12 months of age; advantages—ease of administration, secondary immunization of nonimmune contacts; risk of paralytic polio (1 in 3.7 million doses).
- IPV: inactivated; 4 doses (3 doses 4–8 weeks apart, then 1 dose 6–12 months later).

COXSACKIE AND ECHOVIRUS INFECTIONS

Aseptic meningitis

- Symptoms: fever, headache, stiff neck, confusion.
- Laboratory findings: <500 WBC in CSF (may be ↑ PMNs early), protein slightly ↑, normal glucose.
- CSF usually culture-positive early.
- >90% recover completely.

Other diseases

- Generalized disease of the newborn: overwhelming enteroviral infection.
- Myocarditis and pericarditis: 50% coxsackievirus B.
- Exanthems: coxsackievirus A16 hand-foot-mouth disease.
- Herpangina: acute fever, sore throat, small vesicles posterior half of palate; coxsackievirus A.
- Epidemic myalgia: sudden fever, upper abdominal pain; coxsackievirus B.

REOVIRUS

Characteristics Double-stranded RNA; sporadic upper respiratory infections, exanthems, pneumonia, hepatitis, encephalitis.

For a more detailed discussion, see Ray CG: Enteroviruses and Reoviruses, Chap. 144, in HPIM-12, p. 712

55 HERPES SIMPLEX VIRUSES

CLINICAL DISEASE

ORAL-FACIAL INFECTIONS

- Primary infection: pharyngitis and gingivostomatitis with fever, malaise, myalgias lasting 3–14 d.
- Reactivation: intraoral, labial, or nasolabial facial lesions.
- Immunosuppressed pts (including AIDS pts) can develop severe mucositis; with atopic eczema, severe oral-facial infections (eczema herpeticum) with dissemination to visceral organs; associated with erythema multiforme.

GENITAL INFECTIONS

- Primary: fever, headache, malaise, myalgias with local pain, itching, dysuria, tender inguinal adenopathy; 80% of women: cervix and/or urethra involvement.
- Recurrences: 90% with HSV-2 infection will have recurrence within 1 year vs. 55% with HSV-1 infection.
- Rectal and perianal: especially homosexual men; anorectal pain, discharge, tenesmus, constipation; autonomic dysfunction with sacral paresthesias, impotence, urinary retention.

HERPETIC WHITLOW Infection of finger with abrupt edema, erythema, vesicular or pustular lesions; may be indistinguishable from pyogenic infections, but surgery may exacerbate.

EYE INFECTIONS

- Most frequent cause of corneal blindness in U.S.
- Keratitis: acute-onset pain, blurring of vision, chemosis, conjunctivitis, dendritic lesions of cornea.

ENCEPHALITIS

- Most common cause of acute, sporadic viral encephalitis in U.S.; >95% HSV-1.
- Symptoms: acute onset of fever and focal temporal lobe symptoms.
- Diagnosis: brain biopsy.

PERIPHERAL NERVOUS SYSTEM

- Autonomic nervous system dysfunction with numbness, tingling of buttock, urinary retention, constipation resolving over days to weeks.

- Transverse myelitis with symmetrical paralysis of lower extremities or Guillain-Barré syndrome.
- Bell's palsy following reactivation of HSV-1.

VISCERAL INFECTIONS

- Esophagitis: dysphagia, substernal pain, weight loss; especially distal esophagus; diagnose by culture and cytologic exam of secretions from endoscopy.
- HSV pneumonitis: in severely immunosuppressed pts; extension of herpetic tracheobronchitis → focal necrotizing pneumonitis; hematogenous dissemination → bilateral interstitial pneumonitis; mortality >80%.
- Hepatitis: immunosuppressed; fever; increased bilirubin, SGOT.

NEONATAL INFECTION

- Neonates (<6 weeks of age) have highest rate of visceral or CNS infection.
- 70% HSV-2 from infected genital secretions at delivery.

DIAGNOSIS

Rapid diagnosis Demonstration of giant cells or intranuclear inclusions on Wright, Giemsa (Tzanck prep), or Pap stain of scrapings of base of lesions; HSV differentiated from HZV by immunofluorescence. Culture usually positive in 48–96 h; serology useful only during primary infection.

THERAPY

I. Mucocutaneous HSV infections
  A. Immunosuppressed pts
   1. Acute symptomatic first or recurrent episodes: IV acyclovir (5 mg/kg q 8 h) or oral acyclovir (400 mg PO qid 7–10 d) relieves pain and speeds healing. With localized external lesions 5% topical acyclovir ointment applied 4–6 times daily may be beneficial. Suppression of reactivation disease: IV (5 mg/kg q 8 h) or oral acyclovir (400 mg PO 3–5 times per d) will when taken daily prevent recurrences during high-risk period, e.g., immediate posttransplantation period.
  B. Immunocompetent pts
   1. Genital herpes
    a. First episodes: oral acyclovir (200 mg PO 5 times per d for 10–14 d) is the treatment of choice. IV acyclovir (5 mg/kg q 8 h for 5 d) is given for severe disease or neurologic complications such as aseptic meningitis. Topical 5% ointment or cream applied 4–6 times daily for 7–10 days may be beneficial in pts without cervical, urethral, or pharyngeal involvement.

(continued)

THERAPY *(continued)*

      b. Symptomatic recurrent genital herpes: Oral acyclovir (200 mg PO 5 times per d for 5 d) has modest benefit in shortening lesions and viral excretion time. Routine use for all episodes not recommended. Suppression of recurrent genital herpes: Daily oral acyclovir 200-mg capsules, bid/tid or 400 mg PO bid will prevent reactivation of symptomatic recurrences; use at present limited to 6-month course in frequent recurrers.

  2. Oral-labial HSV

      a. First episode: Oral acyclovir 200 mg 4–5 times per d.

      b. Recurrent episodes: Topical acyclovir ointment is of no clinical benefit.

      c. Oral acyclovir is not routinely recommended.

  3. Herpetic whitlow: Oral acyclovir 200 mg 5 times daily for 7–10 d.

  4. HSV proctitis: Oral acyclovir (400 mg PO 5 times per d) is useful in shortening course of infection. In immunosuppressed pts or in severe infection, IV acyclovir 5 mg/kg q 8 h may be useful.

  5. Herpetic eye infections

      a. Acute keratitis: Topical trifluorothymidine, vidarabine, idoxuridine, acyclovir, and interferon are all beneficial. Debridement may be required; topical steroids may worsen disease.

II. CNS HSV infection

  A. HSV encephalitis: intravenous acyclovir 10 mg/kg q 8 h [30 (mg/kg)/d] for 10 d or vidarabine [15 (mg/kg)/d] decrease mortality; acyclovir is the preferred agent.

  B. HSV aseptic meningitis: No studies of systemic antiviral chemotherapy. If therapy is to be given IV, acyclovir at 15–30 (mg/kg)/d should be utilized.

  C. Autonomic radiculopathy: No studies are available.

III. Neonatal HSV infection: Intravenous vidarabine [30 (mg/kg)/d] or acyclovir [30 (mg/kg)/d]. Neonates appear to tolerate this high dose of vidarabine.

IV. Visceral HSV infections

  A. HSV esophagitis: Systemic acyclovir [15 (mg/kg)/d] or vidarabine [15 (mg/kg)/d] should be considered.

  B. HSV pneumonitis: No controlled studies: systemic acyclovir [15 (mg/kg)/d] or vidarabine [15 (mg/kg)/d] should be considered.

V. Disseminated HSV: No controlled studies, intravenous acyclovir or vidarabine should be attempted. No definite evidence that therapy will decrease mortality.

THERAPY *(continued)*

VI. Erythema multiforme associated with HSV: Anecdotal observations
suggest oral acyclovir capsules bid/tid will suppress EM.

Modified from Corey L: HPIM-12, p. 685.

For a more detailed discussion, see Corey L: Herpes Simplex
Viruses, Chap. 135, in HPIM-12, p. 681

56 CYTOMEGALOVIRUS AND EPSTEIN-BARR VIRUS INFECTIONS

CYTOMEGALOVIRUS (CMV) INFECTION

Epidemiology and pathogenesis
• 1% of newborns in U.S. infected. • Spread by repeated or prolonged intimate contact: day-care centers, venereal transmission; 0.14–10% transmission per unit of blood with viable WBCs transfused. • Clinical disease in fetus or newborn from primary maternal infection. • Virus persists indefinitely in tissues of host and may be reactivated during immunosuppression.

Clinical manifestations

- Congenital CMV infection: cytomegalic inclusion disease in ~5% infected fetuses of mothers with primary infections; petechiae, hepatosplenomegaly, jaundice; 30–50% have microcephaly and/or cerebral calcifications; 20–30% mortality with severe disease; most congenital infections clinically inapparent at birth.
- Perinatal: acquired at delivery from infected birth canal or contact with maternal milk; rare cause of protracted interstitial pneumonia in premature infants.
- CMV mononucleosis: incubation 20–60 d; lasts 2–6 weeks; prolonged high fevers, profound fatigue, malaise, myalgias, headache, splenomegaly (exudative pharyngitis and cervical adenopathy rare, unlike EBV); lymphocytosis with >10% atypicals; moderate ↑ SGOT, alkaline phosphatase.
- Immunocompromised host: maximum risk 1–4 months after organ transplant, causing fever, leukopenia, hepatitis, pneumonia, colitis, retinitis; pneumonia in 20% of bone marrow recipients; very frequent in pts with AIDS.

Diagnosis

- Culture: may be positive in days with high titer (congenital infection, AIDS, or immunosuppressive therapy) or several weeks (CMV mononucleosis); urine or saliva may be culture positive for months to years.
- Shell vial assay: detection of early antigen in tissue culture in 1 d.

- Serology: antibody rises may not be detectable for up to 4 weeks after primary infection.

Treatment and prevention

- Retinitis, colitis: ganciclovir (DHPG) 5 mg/kg IV bid for 14 d then 5 mg/kg qd 5–7 d/wk.
- CMV pneumonitis in bone marrow transplant recipients: ganciclovir plus CMV immune globulin.
- Prevent by using seronegative blood and organs for seronegative recipients; CMV immune globulin and acyclovir in transplant recipients.

EPSTEIN-BARR VIRUS INFECTIONS

Epidemiology and pathogenesis

- Transmitted by saliva (rarely by blood transfusions).
- Shed from oropharynx for up to 18 months after primary infection; can be isolated from 25–50% of oropharyngeal washings from renal transplant pts and virtually all pts with AIDS.
- Infected B lymphocytes polyclonally stimulated to produce immunoglobulin.

Clinical manifestations

- Symptoms: incubation 4–8 weeks; malaise, anorexia, chills, then pharyngitis, fever, and lymphadenopathy.
- Physical exam: >90% febrile; diffuse pharyngitis; cervical adenopathy; 50% splenomegaly. Older adults often lack pharyngitis.
- Clinical course: pharyngitis persists 7–10 d; fever 7–14 d: malaise may persist more than 3–4 weeks.
- Complications: hematologic—autoimmune hemolytic anemia, thrombocytopenia, granulocytopenia; splenic rupture during second or third week of illness; neurologic—cranial nerve palsies, encephalitis; hepatitis; cardiac—pericarditis, myocarditis rare; may have overwhelming infection with X-linked lymphoproliferative syndrome.

Diagnosis

- Heterophile antibodies: antibodies to sheep red blood cells removed by absorption with beef red blood cells; 10–15% may be negative in first week; may be positive up to 9 months after onset of illness.
- Atypical lymphocytosis: activated T lymphocytes.
- Specific antibodies: IgM to VCA (viral capsid antigen) diagnostic of primary infection; IgG-VCA positive for life.

Sero conversion to EBNA (nuclear antigen) diagnostic of primary infection.

Management   Supportive therapy; glucorticoids for airway obstruction or severe hemolytic anemia or thrombocytopenia.

EBV-associated malignancy

- Burkitt's lymphoma, anaplastic nasopharyngeal cancer.
- B-cell lymphomas, especially in immunosuppressed (organ transplant, ataxia telangiectasia, AIDS).

For a more detailed discussion, see Hirsch MS: Cytomegalovirus Infection, Chap. 138, p. 692; and Schooley RT: Epstein-Barr Virus Infections, Including Infectious Mononucleosis, Chap. 137, p. 689, in HPIM-12

---

57 VIRAL ENCEPHALITIS, DENGUE, AND RABIES

ENCEPHALITIS DUE TO "ARBOVIRUSES"

"Arbovirus" infections are transmitted by mosquitoes, so spread in late spring through early fall.

Clinical manifestations Differ by age and virus; <1 year old—sudden fever and convulsions, rigidity of extremities, abnormal reflexes; 5–14 years old—headache, fever, drowsiness, nausea, vomiting, photophobia, nuchal rigidity; adults—abrupt fever, nausea with vomiting, severe headache, confusion; may have tremors, cranial nerve abnormalities, abnormal reflexes (suck and snout). (See Table 57-1.)

Laboratory findings Slight to moderate ↑ WBC; CSF: 100–1000 WBC, ↑ PMNs early, slightly ↑ protein, glucose normal.

Treatment Supportive therapy—parenteral diazepam for seizures; discharge on phenobarbital × 6–12 months if severe disease.

DENGUE

Epidemiology

- Transmitted by *Aëdes* mosquitoes in S.E. Asia, the South Pacific, Africa, the Caribbean, and Central America.
- Dengue hemorrhagic fever (DHF) almost exclusively in previously immune.

Clinical manifestations

- Dengue: prodrome of fever, pharyngitis, severe headache, ocular pain and tenderness on pressure, vomiting, abdominal pain, high fevers, myalgias, and bone pain. Maculopapular rash (day 3–5), usually in children and nonindigenous adults.
- DHF: fever (acute onset, continuous for 2–7 days); hemorrhagic manifestations (petechiae, purpura, epistaxis); thrombocytopenia; hemoconcentration (20% have ↑ Hct).
- Dengue shock syndrome: hypotension, pulse pressure ≤20 mmHg.

Diagnosis Rise in specific CF or hemagglutination inhibition antibodies. IgM antibodies in primary infections; immune complexes in DHF.

TABLE 57-1 "Arbovirus" encephalitides common in the United States

Etiology	Geographic predominance in the U.S.	Urban/rural	Age, years	Sex	Unique clinical features	Mortality, %	Residua
California encephalitis	Midwest	Rural	5–10	M	Seizures	2	Seizures (one-fourth who had them in acute phase), behavioral problems (15%)
Eastern equine encephalitis	Eastern seaboard	Both	<5 >55	=	CSF may have >1000 WBC/μL	50	Children <10 years have emotional lability, retardation, convulsions
St. Louis encephalitis	Eastern and midwest	Both	>35	=	Dysuria	2–12	Ataxia, speech difficulties (5%)
Western equine encephalitis	Entire	Both	<1 >55	=	None	3	Children <3 months have behavioral problems, convulsions

From Sanford JP: HPIM-12, p. 731.

Treatment Fluid replacement; questionable role of heparin with DIC.

RABIES

Epidemiology

- In U.S. human cases from skunks, bats, raccoons, or domestic animal bites outside of country.
- Highest prevalence: S.E. Asia, Philippines, Africa, Indian subcontinent.
- Human-to-human transmission through corneal transplants.

Clinical manifestations

- Prodrome: 1–4 d of fever, headache, malaise, myalgias, anorexia, sore throat; 50–80% have paresthesias and/or fasciculations at site of inoculation.
- Encephalitis: excessive motor activity, excitation, agitation, hallucinations, muscle spasms, seizures, focal paralysis, hyperesthesia, fever, autonomic dysfunction (dilated, irregular pupils, ↑ lacrimation and salivation).
- Brainstem dysfunction: cranial nerve palsies, 50% hydrophobia (involuntary contraction of respiratory muscles with swallowing liquids); prominence of early brainstem dysfunction distinguishes from other encephalitides.
- Late complications: median survival 4 d; with respiratory support survival prolonged and pts may develop syndrome of inappropriate secretion of antidiuretic hormone, diabetes insipidus, cardiac arrhythmias; rare survivors have received pre- or postexposure prophylaxis.

Diagnosis

- Isolation of virus from saliva or brain by mouse inoculation.
- Serology: 4-fold rise in neutralizing antibody or CSF antibody titers >1:64 (if received rabies vaccine).
- Antigen detection: fluorescent antibody staining of corneal impression smears; skin or brain biopsies.

Prevention and treatment

- Indications for postexposure prophylaxis: physical contact with saliva, exposure to escaped wild animal at risk (bats, skunks, coyotes, foxes, raccoons), or positive fluorescent antibody test of brain of captured animal.
- Local wound therapy: vigorous cleansing with soap and water, tetanus toxoid, antibiotics.

- Postexposure passive immunization: human rabies immune globulin (RIG), 20 U/kg (half locally in wound, half IM) or equine globulin 40 U/kg.
- Postexposure active immunization: human diploid cell vaccine (HDCV) 1 mL IM on days 0, 3, 7, 14, 28.
- Preexposure prophylaxis: at risk—veterinarians, spelunkers, laboratory workers, animal handlers—HDCV 1 mL IM on days 0, 7, 21; check for neutralizing antibody titer ≥1:5; and/or booster every 2 years.

For a more detailed discussion, see Corey L: Rabies, Rhabdoviruses, and Marburg-like Agents, Chap. 147, p. 720; and Sanford JP: Arbovirus Infections, Chap. 148, p. 725, in HPIM-12

---

58 FUNGAL AND RELATED INFECTIONS

CRYPTOCOCCOSIS

Etiology/pathogenesis Infection by inhalation of *Cryptococcus neoformans;* 50% underlying lymphoma, sarcoid, steroid therapy, AIDS.

Clinical manifestations

- Meningoencephalitis: fever and nuchal rigidity often absent; altered mental status, papilledema, cranial nerve palsies common.
- Pulmonary: 40% with chest pain, 20% with cough, ≥1 well-circumscribed dense infiltrate.
- Disseminated: with papular or ulcerated skin lesions and multiple organ and CNS involvement. Rarely isolated prostatitis, osteomyelitis, endophthalmitis, hepatitis, pericarditis, endocarditis, or renal abscess.

Diagnosis

- CSF: 50% india ink +, glucose ↓, protein ↑; 20–600 WBC/μL; 90% CSF cryptococcal antigen +; in AIDS, 99% serum cryptococcal antigen +.
- Pulmonary: sputum culture + in 10%; serum antigens + in 33%; requires biopsy for Dx.
- Biopsy and culture skin lesions. May be mistaken for molluscum contagiosum in AIDS pts.

Treatment Amphotericin B 0.3 (mg/kg)/d + flucytosine 37.5 mg/kg q 6 h (maintain serum levels between 50–100 μL/mL) × 6 weeks; amphotericin B 0.5–0.6 (mg/kg)/d alone × 6 weeks; fluconazole 200–400 mg qd × 10–12 weeks after CSF culture negative. AIDS pts: lifelong maintenance therapy with amphotericin B 1 mg/kg weekly or fluconazole 200 mg PO qd.

BLASTOMYCOSIS

Etiology/pathogenesis Inhalation of *Blastomyces dermatitidis;* Southeastern, central, mid-Atlantic states.

Clinical manifestations

- Acute self-limited pneumonia.
- Chronic: progressive fever, cough, weight loss, skin lesions (pimple → verrucous, crusted, or ulcerated lesion); two-thirds have abnormal CXR; osteolytic lesions.

Diagnosis   Wet smear, culture, and/or histologic demonstration.

Treatment   Progressive disease or meningitis: amphotericin B 0.5–0.6 mg/kg qd to a total of 2.0–2.5 g; indolent disease: ketoconazole 400–800 mg qd × 6–12 months.

HISTOPLASMOSIS

Etiology/pathogenesis   Inhalation of *Histoplasma capsulatum;* in U.S., southeastern, mid-Atlantic, central states.
Clinical manifestations

- Acute pulmonary disease: most asymptomatic or mild; hilar adenopathy; erythema nodosum and erythema multiforme.
- Chronic pulmonary disease: weight loss; CXR—fibronodular apical infiltrates; 33% stabilize or improve spontaneously.
- Acute disseminated disease: fever, hepatosplenomegaly, lymphadenopathy, jaundice, anemia, leukopenia; 25% have indurated ulcers of mouth, nose, or larynx; 50% of CXRs show discrete nodules or miliary pattern.
- Ocular: uveitis with + skin test; none with active disease.

Diagnosis

- Serology: CF >1:32 suggestive but not diagnostic; may cross-react with blastomycosis. Skin testing of no value in diagnosis of acute disease and may cause seroconversion.
- Culture (+ in 2–6 weeks) or histology.

Treatment   Same as for blastomycosis in pts with normal immune systems. Treat AIDS pts with amphotericin B (not ketoconazole); may require indefinite 1 mg/kg IV weekly maintenance therapy.

COCCIDIOIDOMYCOSIS

Etiology/pathogenesis   Infection from inhalation of arthrospores of *Coccidioides immitis;* California, Arizona, W. Texas, New Mexico.

Clinical manifestations

- Symptomatic pulmonary infection: CXR—infiltrate, hilar adenopathy, or pleural effusion; may have mild eosinophilia.
- Chronic progressive pulmonary infection: cough, sputum, ± fever, weight loss.
- Dissemination: persistence of fever, malaise, hilar or paratracheal adenopathy; lesions in bone, skin, meninges, joints.

Diagnosis

- Wet smear and culture (biohazard) of sputum, urine, pus.
- Serology: seroconversion may not occur for up to 8 weeks following onset of primary pulmonary disease, + CF in CSF diagnostic of infection.
- Skin test: converts between third and twenty-first day, but often negative in pts with cavitary or disseminated disease.

Treatment

- Seriously ill—amphotericin B 0.5–0.7 mg/kg qd × 10–12 weeks; meningitis—long-term intrathecal amphotericin.
- Nonmeningeal disease—ketoconazole 200–400 mg qd × 1 year.
- Single thin-walled cavity—tends to resolve spontaneously; responds poorly to antifungals.
- Fluconazole and itraconazole are promising new therapeutic agents for chronic coccidioidomycosis.

CANDIDIASIS

Etiology/pathogenesis   Increased risk: skin maceration, pregnancy, diabetes, AIDS, hematologic malignancy, antibiotic or steroid therapy.

Clinical manifestations

- Oral thrush: painless white plaques in mouth and on tongue.
- Cutaneous candidiasis: red, macerated intertriginous areas.
- Chronic mucocutaneous candidiasis: circumscribed hyperkeratotic skin lesions, dystrophic nails, partial alopecia, oral and vaginal thrush; may have hypofunction of parathyroid, adrenal, or thyroid glands, T-cell function defects.
- Gastrointestinal: ulcerations of distal esophagus.
- Hematogenous: fever; retinal abscesses; pulmonary nodular infiltrate; endocarditis.

Diagnosis   Demonstration of pseudohyphae on wet smear; culture; histology.

Treatment

- Cutaneous: nystatin, ciclopirox, imidazole creams topically bid.
- Oral: clotrimazole 1 troche, dissolved in mouth 5 times qd, nystatin suspension swish and swallow 4–6 qd, fluconazole 100 mg PO qd × 7–14 d.
- Esophageal: ketoconazole 200–400 mg PO qd, fluconazole 100–200 mg PO or IV qd × 14–21 d; severe—amphotericin B 0.3 (mg/kg)/d × 5–10 d.
- Bladder: irrigation with amphotericin B 50 mg in 1 L × 5 d.
- Disseminated: amphotericin B 0.4–0.5 mg/kg IV qd ± flucytosine 37.5 mg/kg PO qid × several weeks; fluconazole 200 mg PO or IV qd × 4 weeks.

ASPERGILLOSIS

Etiology/pathogenesis Inhalation of spores in immunosuppressed patients: <500 PMNs, high-dose steroids, cytotoxic drugs.

Clinical manifestations

- Allergic bronchial aspergillosis: preexisting asthma, eosinophilia, IgE Ab to *Aspergillus,* fleeting pulmonary infiltrates. *diff. from asthma – skin test, IgE (fungus)*
- Endobronchial pulmonary aspergillosis: chronic productive cough, hemoptysis, preexisting chronic lung disease.
- Aspergilloma: ball of hyphae within lung cyst or cavity.
- Invasive: acute pneumonia in immunosuppressed; occasionally widely disseminated with endocardial and multiple organ involvement.
- Sinusitis: chronic in nonimmunosuppressed; may spread to orbit and brain.

Diagnosis
- Repeated isolation from sputum suggestive of colonization or infection. • Fungus ball on CXR. • Histopathology and cultures (BC rarely +).

Treatment Lobectomy for severe hemoptysis with fungus ball. Invasive: amphotericin B or itraconazole can arrest or cure.

MUCORMYCOSIS

Etiology/pathogenesis Infection by *Rhizopus* or *Mucor* in pts with poorly controlled diabetes mellitus (paranasal sinuses and nose); hematologic malignancy or organ transplantation (lung); uremia, severe malnutrition, diarrhea (gastrointestinal).

Diagnosis Biopsy and histology of nonseptate hyphae; culture difficult.

Treatment Regulation of diabetes; decrease immunosuppressive drugs; extensive debridement + maximum tolerated doses of amphotericin B for at least 10–12 weeks: cure in ~50%.

SPOROTRICHOSIS

Etiology/pathogenesis Inoculation of *Sporothrix schenckii* into subcutaneous tissue by minor trauma; increased risk: nursery workers, florists, gardeners.

Clinical manifestations Painless red papule at site of inoculation with proximal extension along lymphatic channels.

Diagnosis Culture of pus, joint fluid, sputum, or skin biopsy.

Treatment

- Cutaneous: saturated potassium iodide in increasing doses up to 4.5–9 mL/d for 1 month after complete resolution.
- Extracutaneous: amphotericin B; itraconazole promising.

ACTINOMYCOSIS

Etiology/pathogenesis Infection by break in mucosa or aspiration of *Actinomyces,* anaerobic higher gram-positive branching bacteria.

Clinical manifestations Cervicofacial; thoracic; abdominal; pelvic: increased with IUD.

Diagnosis Culture and histologic evidence of tissue invasion (not acid-fast).

Treatment

- Mild cervicofacial: penicillin V, oral tetracycline, or erythromycin 500 mg qid × 2–4 months.
- Thoracic and abdominal: penicillin G 2–6 million U IV qd × 6 weeks, then penicillin or tetracycline 500 mg PO qid for 6–12 months; drainage of necrotic tissue and abscesses.

NOCARDIOSIS

Etiology/pathogenesis Infection through inhalation or local trauma by *N. asteroides*; increased risk: steroids, cancer, pulmonary alveolar proteinosis, AIDS, chronic granulomatous disease.

Clinical manifestations

- Pneumonia: fever and productive cough; infiltrate → cavitation.
- CNS: multiple abscesses; if abscess ruptures into ventricle → purulent meningitis.

Diagnosis   Branching, weakly acid-fast organisms in histologic sections or smear of pus or sputum.

Treatment

- Surgical drainage of abscesses or empyemas.
- Sulfisoxazole 25 mg/kg PO or IV q 6 h then to peak blood concentration of 10–15 mg/dL or trimethoprim-sulfamethoxazole PO or IV as 50 (mg/kg)/d of sulfamethoxazole in 2 doses per day × 6–12 months.

For a more detailed discussion, see Bennett JE: Fungal Infections, Chap. 151, p. 743; and Bennett JE: Actinomycosis and Nocardiosis, Chap. 152, p. 752, in HPIM-12

ROCKY MOUNTAIN SPOTTED FEVER (RMSF)

Epidemiology   Transmission of *Rickettsia rickettsii* by bite of infected tick; >50% of cases from south Atlantic and south central states.

Clinical manifestations

- Incubation 3–12 d: abrupt onset of severe headache, rigors, prostration, generalized myalgia, fevers to 39–40°C (103–104°F); occasionally only low-grade fever, anorexia, lethargy.
- Rash: pink macular lesions on extremities, including palms and soles on fourth day of fever → maculopapular → petechial → ecchymoses; rash spreads centripetally and involves face.
- Severe infection: shock with gangrene of extremities, buttocks, earlobes, nose.
- Neurologic manifestations: severe headache, restlessness, stiff back, insomnia; CSF normal.
- Course: in mild cases, all symptoms may abate within 2 weeks without therapy; deaths usually in second week.

Diagnosis

- Serology: Weil-Felix OX-19 >1:40, OX-2 >1:20 by tenth day; 4-fold rise in CF antibodies.
- Immunofluorescence of skin lesions may be positive by fourth day.

Treatment   Chloramphenicol 50 mg/kg or tetracycline 25 mg/kg loading, then divided q 6 h until afebrile 24 h.

MURINE (ENDEMIC) TYPHUS FEVER

Epidemiology   Infection by bite of rat flea with *Rickettsia typhi;* predominantly urban, late summer; prevalent in southeastern and Gulf Coast states.

Clinical manifestations

- Incubation 8–16 d: headache, backache, arthralgia, nausea, shaking chills; severe frontal headache, fever, nonproductive cough; fever usually lasts 12 d.
- Rash: early lesions in axilla and inner aspect of arm → sudden generalized red, discrete macular rash of upper

abdomen, shoulders, chest, arms, thighs → maculopapular; little involvement of extremities, palms, soles, or face.
• Neurologic manifestations: severe frontal headache.
• Course: rapid recovery after defervesence; fatalities unusual.

Diagnosis   Fourfold rise in specific CF antibodies by third week; Weil-Felix OX-19 >160 by tenth day.

Treatment   As for RMSF, but parenteral antibiotics rarely necessary.

EPIDEMIC (LOUSE-BORNE) TYPHUS FEVER

Epidemiology   Infection by exposure to feces of body louse with *Rickettsia prowazekii;* new epidemics from pts with recrudescent typhus (Brill-Zinsser disease) or flying squirrels.

Clinical manifestations

• Incubation 7 d: abrupt headache, chills, fever, malaise; symptoms more severe than murine typhus.
• Rash: macular in axillary folds, trunk, and extremities.
• Neurologic: headache, general spasticity to extreme agitation, stupor, coma.
• Complications: azotemia, thrombosis, cutaneous gangrene.
• Brill-Zinsser disease: recrudescent episode years after initial attack with good recovery.

Diagnosis   Rise in specific CF serology, positive OX-19; in Brill-Zinsser, specific IgG rise as early as fourth day.

Treatment   As for RMSF, usually afebrile after second day.

Q FEVER

Epidemiology   Inhalation of dust or drinking milk contaminated with *Coxiella burnetti;* contact with infected sheep or cattle.

Clinical manifestations

• Incubation ~19 d: headache, chills, fever, malaise, myalgia, anorexia; dry cough and chest pain after 5 d; 20% have protracted disease with fever for longer than 4 weeks.
• Hepatitis: a third of pts with protracted disease; granulomas on biopsy.
• Endocarditis: subacute endocarditis with negative BC.

Diagnosis   High CF titer to phase I antigen.

Treatment Tetracycline or chloramphenicol for at least 2 weeks; endocarditis may require therapy for 2–5 years plus surgery.

For a more detailed discussion, see Woodward TE: Rickettsial Diseases, Chap. 153, in HPIM-12, p. 753

60 *MYCOPLASMA* INFECTIONS

MYCOPLASMA PNEUMONIAE

Epidemiology 50% of pneumonia in college students; antibody only protective several years.

Clinical manifestations

- Pharyngitis, tracheobronchitis, bullous myringitis, pneumonia.
- Almost all have cough; fever may persist 1–2 weeks if untreated, with prolonged malaise and weakness.
- Physical findings may be minimal despite extensive changes seen on CXR films.
- Rare complications: meningoencephalitis, polyneuritis, monarticular arthritis, Stevens-Johnson syndrome, pericarditis, myocarditis, hepatitis, DIC, hemolytic anemia.

Diagnosis

- Laboratory: 25% WBC 10,000–15,000; ESR >40 in two-thirds.
- Fourfold rise in CF antibodies.
- Cold agglutinins: development of IgM to I antigen on type O RBC; positive in half in first week of illness to 6 weeks.

Treatment Erythromycin 500 mg qid or tetracycline 250 mg qid × 10–14 d if mild, 21 d if severe.

For a more detailed discussion see Clyde WA, Jr.: Mycoplasma Infections, Chap. 154, in HPIM-12, p. 763

C. TRACHOMATIS GENITAL INFECTIONS

Epidemiology   Most common sexually transmitted disease in U.S.; caused by serovars D through K; peak incidence late teens, early twenties.

Clinical manifestations

- Nongonococcal (NGU) and postgonococcal urethritis (PGU); up to one-third of pts asymptomatic.
- Epididymitis: major cause in men under 35.
- Reiter's syndrome: up to 70% of men with untreated nondiarrheal Reiter's with urethritis positive for *Chlamydia*.
- Proctitis: symptoms—mild rectal pain, tenesmus, mucus discharge; lymphogranuloma venereum (LGV) more severe.
- Mucopurulent cervicitis: often asymptomatic, yellow discharge on speculum examination.
- Pelvic inflammatory disease (PID), perihepatitis, infertility.
- Urethral syndrome: most common isolate from young women with acute dysuria, frequency, and pyuria with urine cultures negative for bacteria.

Diagnosis

- Antigen detection: direct immunofluorescence of infected secretions, ELISA.
- Culture: difficult to grow in tissue culture except for LGV stains.
- Serology: fourfold increase in CF or microimmunofluorescence antibodies useful in LGV, infant pneumonia, or perihepatitis.

Treatment

- Urethritis: tetracycline 500 mg PO qid, doxycycline 100 mg PO bid, or erythromycin 500 mg PO qid × 7 d.
- Cervicitis: tetracycline 500 mg PO qid × 14 d; if pt pregnant, erythomycin 500 mg PO qid × 14 d.
- Should treat all pts with gonorrhea and sexual partners for *Chlamydia*.

LYMPHOGRANULOMA VENEREUM (LGV)

Epidemiology   Sexually transmitted disease by strains L_1, L_2, or L_3; occasional nonsexual transmission.

Clinical manifestations

- Primarily genital lesion: in heterosexuals 3 d to 3 weeks after exposure; small painless vesicle or nonindurated ulcer that is often unnoticed.
- Primary rectal infection: women and homosexual men; proctitis.
- Inguinal syndrome: painful inguinal lymphadenopathy 2–6 weeks after exposure; two-thirds unilateral; may progress to matted nodes and fistulas.
- Constitutional symptoms: fever, chills, headache, meningismus, anorexia, arthralgias, myalgias.
- Complications: perirectal abscess, fistulas, strictures.

Diagnosis

- Laboratory findings: elevated WBC, ESR; may have elevated LFTs.
- Culture of bubo aspirate and rectum.
- Serology: CF titer ≥1:64 suggestive.

Treatment Tetracycline 500 mg qid or sulfonamide 4 g qd × 3 weeks; aspirate all buboes.

TRACHOMA AND ADULT INCLUSION CONJUNCTIVITIS

Epidemiology

- Trachoma: serovars A, B, and C; eye-to-eye spread in endemic areas.
- Inclusion conjunctivitis: sexually transmitted through infected genital secretions.

Clinical manifestations

- Endemic trachoma: conjunctivitis with small lymphoid follicles in children usually <2 years old; cornea with leukocytic infiltration and superficial vascularization (pannus) → conjunctival scarring → inturned eyelashes → corneal ulceration → blindness.
- Genital strains: acute unilateral follicular conjunctivitis and periauricular lymphadenopathy in sexually active young adults.

Diagnosis

- Clinical diagnosis of classical trachoma if two of following present: (1) lymphoid follicles on upper tarsal conjunctiva, (2) conjunctival scarring, (3) vascular pannus, (4) limbal follicles.

- Giemsa- or immunofluorescent-stained smears of conjunctiva; culture; antibody not diagnostic.

Treatment Topical tetracycline or erythromycin for 21–60 d or oral erythromycin for 3 weeks; alternatively, nonpregnant adults may be treated with oral tetracycline for 3 weeks.

PSITTACOSIS

Epidemiology Respiratory transmission of *C. psittaci* from any avian species, especially psittacine (parrots, parakeets).

Clinical manifestations Incubation 7–14 d: fever, chills, headache, dry cough, myalgias; splenomegaly 10–70%.

Diagnosis

- Laboratory findings: usually patchy infiltrate on CXR; WBC normal or elevated; LFTs usually normal.
- Diagnose by culture or serology (but may cross-react with *C. trachomatis* or *C. pneumoniae*).

Treatment Tetracycline 500 mg qid for at least 7 days after defervescence.

C. PNEUMONIAE (formerly TWAR)

Epidemiology Newly recognized species, common infection in young adults (up to 40% seroprevalence.)

Clinical manifestations

- Acute pharyngitis, sinusitis, bronchitis.
- Pneumonia—mild illness resembling pneumonia from *Mycoplasma* primarily in young adults; can be severe in older adults.

Diagnosis

- Difficult to culture.
- Antigen detection not available.
- Serology—fourfold increase in CF antibodies; does not distinguish from *C. trachomatis* or *C. psittaci*.

Treatment Tetracycline 500 mg PO qid or erythromycin 500 mg PO qid × 10–14 d.

For a more detailed discussion, see Stamm WE, Holmes KK: Chlamydial Infections, Chap. 155, in HPIM-12, p. 765

AMEBIASIS

Epidemiology   Infection caused by ingestion of cyst of
E. histolytica; risk: poor hygiene (poverty, poor sanitation,
mental retardation), homosexuals.

Clinical manifestations

- Asymptomatic cyst passage: common.
- Intestinal: intermittent diarrhea with watery stools and/or
  mucus and blood; fulminant dysentery less common.
- Hepatic abscess: insidious or abrupt onset with fever,
  sweats, weight loss, RUQ pain, nausea, ↑ WBCs; ↑
  SGOT and bilirubin with more severe disease.
- Pleuropulmonary: direct extension into right pleural cavity
  and lung in 10–20% with liver abscess.
- Other extraintestinal: pericarditis, peritonitis, brain ab-
  scess.

Diagnosis

- Identification: cysts in formed stools; motile trophozoites
  in liquid stools.
- Serology: + in >90% of pts with hepatic abscess and most
  with amebic dysentery.
- Liver abscess: liver scan, ultrasound, or CT very sensitive
  (must differentiate from pyogenic abscess or hydatid cyst).

Treatment

- Asymptomatic carrier: iodoquinol 650 mg PO tid × 20 d
  or diloxanide furoate (from CDC) 500 mg PO tid × 10 d.
- Intestinal disease: mild to moderate—metronidazole 750
  mg tid × 5–10 d + luminal agent (iodoquinol or diloxanide
  furoate as above, or tetracycline 500 mg PO qid × 5 d);
  severe—metronidazole + either dehydroemetine 1.0–1.5
  mg/kg IM daily × 5 d or emetine 1 mg/kg IM qd × 5 d.
- Extraintestinal: metronidazole + luminal agent, or chloroquine phosphate 1 g qd × 2, then 500 mg qd × 4 weeks
  + dehydroemetine or emetine for 10 d; aspirate if imminent
  rupture, failure to respond to medical therapy in 72 h.

MALARIA

Epidemiology

- Four species: *Plasmodium vivax, P. ovale, P. malariae, P. falciparum;* transmitted by bite of female *Anopheles* mosquito.
- Infection starts with attachment to specific receptor on red blood cell surface; most W. Africans resistant to *P. vivax*.
- Drug-resistant *P. falciparum* in areas of S. Asia, W. Pacific, Central America, S. America, Africa, India.
- Parasitemia limited in sickle cell trait, thalassemia, G6PD deficiency.

Clinical manifestations

- *P. vivax* or *P. ovale:* incubation 10–14 d; prodrome of myalgia, headache, chills before paroxysm of rigor, sudden fever, then defervesence; occur every other day with synchronized infection.
- *P. malariae:* paroxysms every third day; mildest and most chronic; immune-complex nephropathy.
- *P. falciparum:* onset insidious with irregular fever; splenomegaly, headache, confusion, hypotension, edema; GI symptoms common; encephalopathy, abnormal renal function.
- Complications of *P. falciparum:* acute pulmonary insufficiency third or fourth day of therapy; blackwater fever— massive intravascular hemolysis → hemoglobinuria → acute renal failure; cerebral malaria; hypoglycemia; aspiration pneumonia.

Diagnosis   WBC normal or ↓, ↑ ESR. Thin and thick blood smears on Wright or Giemsa stain: *P. vivax*—immature (enlarged) RBCs, diffuse red dots (Schuffner's dots); *P. ovale*—RBC often oval; *P. malariae*—"band" forms; *P. falciparum*—small rings, often two chromatin dots, banana-shaped gametocyte.

Treatment

- See Table 62-1.
- Severe falciparum malaria: exchange transfusion if >10% parasitemia; dexamethasone, mannitol, and heparin should be avoided.
- Prophylaxis (see Table 62-2).

LEISHMANIASIS

Epidemiology   Infection with *Leishmania* species transmitted by sandflies; course determined by cellular immunity and species.

TABLE 62-1 Treatment of acute malaria

Infection	Regimen
Chloroquine-sensitive *P. falci-parum* and *P. malariae*	Chloroquine 10 mg base/kg (600 mg max) PO stat then 5 mg/kg (600 mg max) at 6, 24, 48 h or 10 mg/kg qd × 3 d.
For severe infection	Chloroquine 10 mg base/kg (600 mg max) IV infusion over 8 h then 15 mg base/kg (900 mg max) IV infused over 24 h.
P. vivax and *P. ovale*	Same as for *P. malariae* plus primaquine phosphate 26.3 mg (15 mg base) PO qd × 14 d (screen for G6PD deficiency).
Chloroquine-resistant *P. falci-parum*	Quinine 10 mg salt/kg (650 mg max) PO q 8 h × 5–7 d + either tetracycline (not if pt pregnant or < 8 years) 4 mg/kg (250 mg max) PO q 6 h × 7 d, or pyrimethamine 1 mg/kg and sulfadoxine 20 mg/kg (75/1500 mg max) stat; *or* mefloquine 1250 mg PO single dose with 8 ounces water.
For severe infection	Quinine 7 mg salt/kg (400 mg max) IV infusion over 30 min, followed immediately by 10 mg salt/kg (600 mg max) IV q 8 h (infused over 2–6) × 7 d. If quinine unavailable, may use quinidine gluconate 10 mg salt/kg IV infusion over 1 h (monitor ECG) then continuous infusion of 0.02 (mg/kg)/min × 3 d.

Modified from White NJ, Plorde JJ: HPIM-12, p. 786.

Clinical manifestations

- Visceral leishmaniasis (kala azar)—*L. donovani*; incubation 3 months, may have primary cutaneous lesion; fever, diarrhea, cough, splenomegaly, lymphadenopathy, cirrhosis in 10%, pancytopenia, hypoalbuminemia, increased immunoglobulins; amyloidosis and hyperpigmentation, superinfections, GI hemorrhage late.
- Old world cutaneous leishmaniasis—*L. tropica*, *L. major*, *L. aethiopica*; incubation 2–24 months; papule developing into necrotic sore then hypopigmented scar on face or legs.
- New world cutaneous and mucocutaneous leishmaniasis—*L. mexicana*, *L. braziliensis*; nodular or ulcerating lesions on hands, ears, face that usually heal; ulcerative lesions

TABLE 62-2 **Prophylaxis for malaria**

Purpose	Regimen
Suppression in areas without chloroquine resistance	Chloroquine 5 (mg base/kg)/week (300 mg max) *or* proguanil 3 (mg/kg)/d (200 mg max). Administer either regimen 1 week before entering region through 6 weeks after leaving region.
Prevent relapse of *P. vivax* and *P. ovale*	Primaquine phosphate 26.3 mg (15 mg base) PO qd × 14 d during last 2 weeks of suppressive therapy.
Suppression in areas with chloroquine resistance	No safe and reliable regiment for all areas. Strategies include:
	1. Chloroquine 10 (mg base/kg)/week (600 mg max).
	2. Mefloquine 250 mg weekly × 4 weeks (beginning 1 week before travel), then 250 mg every other week through 4 weeks after leaving area.
	3. Doxycyline 1.5 (mg/kg)/d (100 mg max).
	4. Presumptive treatment with three 25/500 mg tablets pyrimethamine-sulfadoxine.

Modified from White NJ, Plorde JJ: HPIM-12, p. 786.

on legs from *L. braziliensis s.s. braziliensis* may heal or lead to metastatic lesions in nasopharynx months to years later.
• Diffuse cutaneous leishmaniasis—massive cutaneous dissemination without visceral involvement.

Diagnosis   Biopsy or aspiration of skin lesions, bone marrow, lymph node; buffy coat stain; direct agglutination test; leishmanin skin test is nonstandardized and not widely available.

Treatment

• Visceral—sodium antimony gluconate 10 mg/kg (adults) or 20 mg/kg (children) IV or IM qd × 20–30 d; for relapses, 20 mg/kg qd × 40–60 d; resistant cases—amphotericin B 0.5–1 mg/kg qod or pentamidine 3–4 mg/kg qod × 5–25 weeks; investigational—interferon gamma.
• Cutaneous—short course of regimens above (10 d); intralesional injections, local heat may speed healing.
• Mucocutaneous and diffuse—sodium antimony gluconate 20 (mg/kg)/d × 30 d.

CHAGAS' DISEASE

Epidemiology   Infection with *Trypanosoma cruzi* is transmitted by reduviid bugs, most commonly among the poor in rural areas of Central and South America.

Clinical manifestations

- Acute infection—indurated chagoma, lymphadenopathy, Romaña's sign (unilateral painless periocular edema) → malaise, fever, anorexia, facial edema; rarely myocarditis with heart failure.
- Asymptomatic indeterminate phase of chronic infection; may progress to symptomatic infection.
- Symptomatic chronic infection: myocarditis with heart failure, rhythm and conduction disturbances (RBBB most common); megaesophagus with dysphagia, aspiration, chest pain; megacolon with abdominal pain, constipation, obstruction, perforation, septicemia, and death.

Diagnosis   Acute infection—examine buffy coat, thick, or thin smears of blood; culture on media or in mice; xenodiagnosis by allowing uninfected reduviid bugs to feed on pt's blood then examining intestinal contents 30 d later. Chronic infection (with or without symptoms)—serology, e.g., CF, immunofluorescence assay (IFA), ELISA; high rate of false-positives, confirm with two other serologic tests.

Treatment   Acute infection—nifurtimox 8–10 (mg/kg)/d for adults, 12.5–15 (mg/kg)/d for adolescents, 15–20 (mg/kg)/d for children 1–10 years divided in 4 doses each day for 90–120 d (available from CDC). Chronic infection—no satisfactory medical therapy.

TOXOPLASMOSIS

Clinical manifestations

- Lymphadenopathy: acute acquired infection in immunocompetent host; cervical and postauricular nodes most commonly involved; less than half pts also have confusion, malaise, stiff neck, sore throat, macular rash sparing palms and soles, hepatosplenomegaly, reactive lymphocytes.
- Ocular involvement: 35% of all chorioretinitis; usually reactivation of congenital disease; systemic symptoms rare.
- Immunocompromised: increased reactivation of latent infection with immunosuppression for lymphoproliferative disorders, hematologic malignancy, organ transplants; >50% CNS involvement, CSF—slight increase in mononuclear cells and protein, normal glucose.

• Intracerebral toxoplasmosis in pts with AIDS: headache, seizures, decreased mental status, neurologic findings, may have fever or chills; usually no increased antibody titers, CSF normal or ↑ WBCs and protein, ↓ glucose; CT—contrast-enhancing mass lesions <2 cm diameter particularly in basal ganglia, rarely encephalitis; MRI—more sensitive than CT.

Diagnosis
• Tissue culture; intraperitoneal in mice.   • Histology: demonstration of tachyzoites in tissue sections (e.g., brain biopsy).   • Serology: Sabin-Feldman dye test and IFA measure IgG, positive 1–2 weeks (peak 4–8 weeks) after infection; CF positive for IgG at 3–8 weeks (peak 3–8 months) ocular toxo usually with low positive titers; acute disease in pregnant women— ↑ IgM.

Therapy   Pyrimethamine—loading 100 mg PO qd × 1–2 d then 1 mg/kg up to 25 mg qd (50 mg in immunodeficient) + folinic acid 5–20 mg qd + sulfadiazine 75 mg/kg PO loading dose, then 75–100 mg/kg qd (max 8 g/d) in 4 divided doses for 4–6 weeks with active chorioretinitis or 4–6 weeks after resolution of active disease in pts with reversible immunosuppression (e.g., glucocorticoid therapy). Treat AIDS pts for life. If toxicity from sulfonamide, give pyrimethamine 50–75 mg PO qd + clindamycin 2.7 g/d IV or 1.2–1.8 g/d PO.

PNEUMOCYSTIS CARINII PNEUMONIA

Epidemiology/pathogenesis   Airborne transmission of protozoa; most pneumonia reactivation. Increased risk: premature, malnourished infants; children with primary immunodeficiency diseases; immunosuppressive therapy (especially glucocorticords) for cancer, organ transplantation; AIDS.

Clinical manifestations   Pneumonia—dyspnea, fever, dry cough; symptoms may be subtle in AIDS pts.

Diagnosis   Histopathologic staining by methenamine silver or Wright-Giemsa of induced sputum, bronchoalveolar lavage and/or transbronchial biopsy, open lung biopsy.

Treatment
• Trimethoprim/sulfamethoxazole (TMP/SMX) 20/100 (mg/kg)/d PO or IV in four doses × 14 d in non-AIDS pts and × 21 d in AIDS pts; 60–80% AIDS pts develop rash, fever, leukopenia.
• Pentamidine: 4 (mg/kg)/d IM or slow IV infusion × 14 d in AIDS pts; 50% develop hypoglycemia, hyperglycemia, hypocalcemia, azotemia, hepatic dysfunction.

- Dapsone 100 mg PO qd + trimethoprim 5 mg/kg PO q 6 h × 14–21 d for mild-moderate disease; check G6PD.

Prophylaxis   TMP-SMX 5/25 mg/kg PO gd for non-AIDS pts; aerosolized pentamidine for AIDS pts and HIV+ pts with CD4+ T cells <200/μL.   *or if previous pcp infection*

GIARDIASIS

Epidemiology/pathogenesis

- Ingestion of cysts of protozoa, *Giardia lamblia*.
- Most frequent cause of outbreaks of waterborne diarrhea in U.S.
- Increased risk: contaminated water supplies, male homosexuals, children in day-care centers; Ig deficiencies (particularly IgA), achlorhydria.

Clinical manifestations   Diarrhea 1–3 weeks.

Diagnosis   Identification of cyst in feces or trophozoite in diarrheal stool, duodenal secretions (Enterotest), or jejunal biopsies.

Treatment

- Quinacrine 100 mg PO tid × 5 d; 70–95% effective; may produce GI disturbances.
- Metronidazole 2 g PO qd × 3 d or 750 mg PO tid × 5 d; 95% effective; fewer side effects; should not be used in pregnancy.
- Examine household contacts and sexual partners of pts.

CRYPTOSPORIDIOSIS

Epidemiology   Fecal-oral transmission of oocysts; increased risk—homosexuals, day-care centers, immunosuppression, ↓ Ig, AIDS.

Clinical manifestations   Abdominal cramps, diarrhea.

Diagnosis   Demonstration of oocysts in stool.

Treatment   Self-limited in immunocompetent pts; no proven therapy for immunosuppressed pts.

ISOSPORIASIS

Epidemiology   Ingestion of cysts of *Isospora belli;* increased in children in tropical areas, male homosexuals, and AIDS pts.

Clinical manifestations   Abdominal cramps, diarrhea.

Diagnosis   50% with increased eosinophils; acid-fast oocysts in stool, duodenal aspirates, jejunal biopsies.

Treatment TMP/SMX 160/800 mg PO qid × 10 d, then tid × 3 weeks.

TRICHINOSIS

Epidemiology/pathogenesis Ingestion of meat containing encysted larvae of *Trichinella spiralis,* especially pork or walrus; prevalent in Europe, New England, Louisiana, Hawaii, Alaska.

Clinical manifestations

- Asymptomatic → severe disease.
- Intestinal phase (begins 1–2 d after ingestion): diarrhea, abdominal pain, nausea, fever.
- Muscular invasion (begins 7 d after ingestion): fever, periorbital edema, conjunctivitis, subconjunctival hemorrhages, muscle pain and tenderness, subungual hemorrhages, maculopapular rash.
- Lung: hemoptysis, consolidation on CXR.
- CNS: polyneuritis, meningitis, encephalitis, normal CSF.
- Cardiac: myocarditis with persistent tachycardia, CHF; 20% ST-T wave abnormalities.

Diagnosis Eosinophilia; serology; demonstration of larvae in muscle biopsy.

Treatment Thiabendazole 25 mg/kg bid (max 3 g/d) × 5–7 d or mebendazole 400 mg PO tid × 14 d; prednisone 20–60 mg qd if myocardial, CNS, or allergic manifestations.

SCHISTOSOMIASIS

Epidemiology/pathogenesis

- Infection after contact with water containing infective stage (cercariae) → migrate to lungs → portal veins where mature to adult schistosomes; pathology due to granulomatous reaction to eggs, dependent on duration and intensity of exposure.
- *S. mansoni:* S. America (Brazil, Venezuela, Suriname), Caribbean Islands, Africa, Middle East.
- *S. japonicum:* China, Philippines.
- *S. haematobium:* Africa, Middle East.

Clinical manifestations

- Acute schistosomiasis (Katayama fever): *S. mansoni* and *japonicum;* intense itching; 2–6 weeks later fever, chills, headache, angioedema, weakness, abdominal pain, diarrhea; may last 2–3 months.

- Liver fibrosis: *S. mansoni* and *S. japonicum*.
- Glomerulonephritis and pulmonary hypertension.
- Urinary tract: *S. haematobium;* dysuria and hematuria, anatomic obstruction, hydroureter, hydronephrosis, renal failure rare.

Diagnosis   Acute schistosomiasis: eosinophilia >50%, positive serology; identification of ova in stool (*S. mansoni, S. japonicum*) or urine (*S. haematobium*).

Treatment   Praziquantel 40 mg/kg PO single dose or 20 mg/kg × 24 h apart for *S. mansoni* or *S. haematobium*; 20 mg/kg q 4 h × 3 doses for *S. japonicum*.

INTESTINAL NEMATODES

ENTEROBIASIS (PIN WORM)   Epidemiology   Ingestion of eggs of *Enterobius vermicularis;* most common helminthic infection.

Clinical manifestations   Pruritus ani at night.

Diagnosis   Identification of ova in perianal area using cellophane tape over end of tongue blade.

Treatment   Mebendazole 100 mg PO single dose (not for infants or pregnant women); or pyrantel pamoate 11 mg/kg (max 1 g) PO single dose.

TRICHURIASIS (WHIPWORM)   Epidemiology   Ingestion of embryonated eggs of *Trichuris trichiuria;* especially in tropics and southeastern U.S.; most common helminthic infection in Americans returning from tropics.

Clinical manifestations   Symptoms only with heavy infection, especially in children—nausea, abdominal pain, diarrhea.

Diagnosis   Identification of eggs in feces.

Treatment   Mebendazole 100 mg PO bid × 3 d.

ASCARIASIS   Epidemiology   Ingestion of embryonated eggs of *Ascaris lumbricoides* from contaminated food or soil; larvae migrate through intestinal wall → lungs → swallowed → jejunum.

Clinical manifestations   Fever, cough, dyspnea, ↑ eosinophils, migratory pulmonary infiltrates, abdominal pain with heavy infection, malabsorption.

Diagnosis   Ova in feces; passage of adult worm.

Treatment   Mebendazole 100 mg PO bid × 3 d or pyrantel pamoate 11 mg/kg PO single dose.

HOOKWORM DISEASE   Epidemiology   Infection through skin penetration of filariform larvae of *Ancylostoma duodenale* or *Necator americanus;* migrate through lungs to intestine.

Clinical manifestations   If severe, iron-deficiency anemia and hypoalbuminemia.

Diagnosis Identification of ova in feces.
Treatment Mebendazole or pyrantel pamoate as for ascariasis.

STRONGYLOIDIASIS Epidemiology Infection by penetration of skin by larvae of *Strongyloides stercoralis;* after migration through lung, adults mature in small intestine; may develop autoinfection where larvae invade intestinal mucosa or perianal skin without going through soil phase.

Clinical manifestations Transitory skin eruptions with blotchy erythema, urticaria, cough, dyspnea, bronchospasm, epigastric pain, tenderness, nausea; debilitated and immunodepressed pts—widespread dissemination of larvae to extraintestinal organs.

Diagnosis Identification of larvae in fresh fecal specimens, duodenal aspirates, or jejunal biopsies; ↑ eosinophils except in very severe cases.

Treatment Thiabendazole 25 mg/kg PO bid × 2–3 d (≥7 d with disseminated infection).

TREMATODES OR FLUKES (see HPIM-12, Chap. 171)

CESTODE (TAPEWORM) INFECTIONS (see HPIM-12, Chap. 171)

For a more detailed discussion, see Plorde JJ: Therapy of Parasitic Infections, Chap. 88, p. 498; Plorde JJ: Amebiasis, Chap. 158, p. 778; Plorde JJ, White NJ: Malaria, Chap. 159, p. 782; Locksley RM: Leishmaniasis, Chap. 160, p. 789; Kirchoff LV: Trypanosomiasis, Chap. 161, p. 791; Murray HW: Toxoplasmosis, Chap. 162, p. 795; Walzer PD: *Pneumocystis carinii* Pneumonia, Chap. 163, p. 799; Plorde JJ: Babesiosis, Chap. 164, p. 801; Plorde JJ: Giardiasis, Chap. 165, p. 802; Plorde JJ: Cryptosporidiosis, Chap. 166, p. 803; Plorde JJ: Trichomoniasis and Other Protozoan Infections, Chap. 167, p. 805; Plorde JJ: Trichinosis, Chap. 168, p. 807; Greene BM: Filariasis, Chap. 169, p. 809; Nash TE: Schistosomiasis, Chap. 170, p. 813; Plorde JJ, Ramsey PG: Nematodes, Cestodes, and Hermaphroditic Trematodes, Chap. 171, p. 817, in HPIM-12

---

63 LYME BORRELIOSIS

Epidemiology Spirochete *Borrelia burgdorferi,* worldwide distribution, transmitted by ixodid ticks during summer.

Clinical manifestations Incubation period 3–32 d. Three characteristic stages; however, pts may lack rash or present with stage 2 or 3 findings. Many pts do not recall tick bite.

- Stage 1: Erythema migrans—red macule or papule → large annular lesion with red border and central clearing at site of tick bite; severe headache, mild neck stiffness, fever, chills, malaise, fatigue, arthralgias. Lasts several weeks.
- Stage 2: After weeks to months, ~15% pts have frank neurologic abnormalities—meningitis, mild encephalitis, cranial neuritis, radiculopathy, mononeuritis multiplex, chorea, myelitis. CSF: ~100 lymphs, high protein, normal or low glucose. 8% with cardiac disease—AV block, myocarditis. Lasts a few weeks.
- Stage 3: After weeks to 2 years, 80% untreated pts develop oligoarticular arthritis of large joints, particularly knees, lasting weeks to months with recurrences.

Diagnosis Serology: ↑ specific IgG antibodies after 2–3 weeks; may cross-react with *T. pallidum.* Culture may be positive early in disease from blood, skin, CSF but difficult to perform.

Treatment

- Early (stage 1): Tetracycline 250 mg PO qid, penicillin V 500 mg PO qid, or erythromycin 250 mg PO qid × 10–30 d.
- Meningitis, neuropathies, AV block (stage 2): Penicillin G 20 million U IV qd in divided doses or ceftriaxone 2 g IV or IM qd × 14 d.
- Arthritis (stage 3): Doxycycline 100 mg PO bid or amoxicillin 500 mg with probenecid 500 mg PO qid × 30 d.

For a more detailed discussion, see Steere AC: Lyme Borreliosis, Chap. 132, in HPIM-12, p. 667

64 OTHER INFECTIONS OF CLINICAL IMPORTANCE

LEGIONELLA INFECTIONS

Etiology/epidemiology

- Aerobic gram-negative rods with complex growth requirements; thrive in hot water distribution systems of buildings, causing common-source outbreaks.
- Infection by respiratory inhalation of environmental aerosols; incubation 2–10 d.
- Increased risk with smoking, chronic renal failure, malignancy, immunosuppression.

Clinical manifestations

• Pneumonia: malaise, headache, nonproductive cough → cough productive of mucoid sputum, pleuritic chest pain, myalgia; may have GI symptoms, altered sensorium. May require 4–5 d to show clinical response despite antibiotics. Complications: 10–15% respiratory failure; hypotension, shock; lung abscess, empyema; DIC; renal failure.
• Pontiac fever: acute, self-limited flu-like illness lasting 2–5 d.

Diagnosis

• Laboratory findings: normal to ↑ WBCs (20% >20,000), ↑ ESR, mild proteinuria.   • CXR: 65% unilateral pulmonary parenchymal infiltrates → bilateral; a third show pleural effusions.   • Culture requires selective media. Immunofluorescent staining of specimens: less sensitive than culture. Detection of antigen in urine sensitive and specific, but antigenemia may persist for months after past infection.
• Serology: fourfold rise in titer to ≥1:128 or single titer ≥1:256.

Treatment   Erythromycin 0.5–1 g q 6 h IV or PO × 21 d. Add rifampin 600 mg qd for severe disease or immunocompromised pt.

LEPROSY

Etiology/epidemiology   Chronic granulomatous infection with *Mycobacterium leprae*; human-to-human transmission, probably from nasal secretions of untreated lepromatous patients.

Clinical manifestations

- Early leprosy: one or more hypopigmented or hyperpigmented macules or plaques, often anesthetic.
- Tuberculoid: early—hypopigmented macule; nerve involvement early; ulnar, peroneal, and greater auricular nerves may be palpable → muscle atrophy; contractures; trauma; corneal ulcerations.
- Lepromatous: hypopigmented macules, nodules, plaques, papules, especially face, ears, wrists, buttocks, knees; loss of lateral eyebrows; early nasal symptoms → nasal obstruction, laryngitis, hoarseness.
- Borderline: borderline tuberculoid—increased skin lesions and involvement of multiple peripheral nerves; borderline lepromatous—heterogeneous and symmetric skin lesions.
- Reactional states: erythema nodosum leprosum (ENL) in lepromatous; reversal reaction.
- Complications: most frequent cause of crippling of hand in world; trauma and secondary chronic infections → loss of digits; blindness.

Diagnosis   Demonstration of acid-fast bacilli in skin smears, skin or nerve biopsies, but may be negative in tuberculoid; 10–20% of lepromatous false-positive VDRL, serology 95% sensitive in lepromatous and 30% in tuberculoid.

Treatment

- Tuberculoid, borderline tuberculoid: dapsone 50–100 mg qd + rifampin 600 mg qd × 6–12 months, then dapsone alone × 18 months.
- Borderline, borderline lepromatous: dapsone + rifampin for minimum of 2 years if dapsone-sensitive.
- Lepromatous: dapsone + rifampin + clofazamine 50–200 mg qd for a minimum of 2 years to indefinitely.

LEPTOSPIROSIS

Epidemiology   Infection by contact with urine or tissue of infected animal through abrasions or mucous membranes; two-thirds by incidental exposure to contaminated water.

Clinical manifestations

- Incubation average of 10 d; leptospiremic phase—abrupt headache, severe myalgias, chills, high fevers, conjunctival

suffusion, pharyngeal infection, cutaneous hemorrhages, maculopapular rashes on trunk; lasts 4–9 d.
- "Immune phase": appearance of IgM; fever and/or meningismus (50–90% pleocytosis in CSF).
- Weil's syndrome: severe leptospirosis with jaundice, azotemia.
- Aseptic meningitis.
- Myocarditis.

Diagnosis

- Laboratory findings: >70% PMN common in leptospiremic phase; may have >70,000 WBCs; platelets may be <30,000; half show increased CK in first phase; mild proteinuria.
- Cultured from blood or CSF during first phase or urine during second on semisolid medium (Fletcher's). Leptospiras may be excreted in urine for months after the illness.
- Serology: fourfold rise in agglutination; 6–12th day of illness.

Treatment Doxycycline 100 mg PO bid × 7 d useful within 4 d of onset; penicillin G 1.5 million U q 6 h × 7 d even after fifth day; Jarisch-Herxheimer reaction may occur.
Prevention Doxycycline 200 mg PO weekly.

For a more detailed discussion, see Bernstein MS, Locksley RM: *Legionella* Infections, Chap. 124, p. 634; Miller RA: Leprosy (Hansen's Disease), Chap. 126, p. 645; Sanford JP: Leptospirosis, Chap. 130, p. 663, in HPIM-12

---

65 LOCALIZED PYOGENIC INFECTIONS, INFECTIOUS ARTHRITIS, AND OSTEOMYELITIS

ABSCESSES OF THE SKIN AND SOFT TISSUES

- Impetigo: multiple pruritic erythematous lesions that develop into vesicles, pustules and then crusts; group A streptococci, less often *Staph. aureus*; complications—metastatic abscesses, acute glomerulonephritis; local care, dicloxacillin 250–500 mg PO qid if severe.
- Skin abscesses: 25% *Staph. aureus* alone, rest mixed infection or anaerobes; incise and drain, dicloxacillin 250–500 mg PO qid.
- Paronychia: periungual infection, acute—*Staph. aureus;* chronic—*Candida;* drain.
- Suppurative tendinitis: swelling, tenderness over sheath, flexion of fingers, pain on extension of finger; incise immediately, IV antibiotics.
- Human bites: cleanse thoroughly, usually do not suture; amoxicillin–clavulanic acid 250–500 mg PO tid.
- Chronic cutaneous ulcers: colonized with bacteria, no need for routine cultures or antibiotics unless cellulitis, osteomyelitis, fever, or abscess present.

ABSCESSES OF THE HEAD AND NECK

- Suppurative parotitis: elderly and chronically ill pts with dry mouth; *Staph. aureus;* unilateral pain and swelling, fever, chills, pus expressed from duct; treat with systemic antistaphylococcal antibiotics.
- Peritonsillar abscess (quinsy): group A streptococci and anaerobes; fever, sore throat, cervical lymphadenopathy, unilateral pain radiating to ear on swallowing, enlargement of tonsil and soft palate; IV penicillin and needle aspiration.
- Ludwig's angina: cellulitis of sublingual and submaxillary spaces; elevation of tongue, edema, induration, apical abscess of mandibular molars; IV penicillin or clindamycin ± gentamicin; ensure airway.

- Retropharyngeal abscess: dysphagia, stridor, pain, fever, mass; may extend to mediastinum; incise and drain immediately, IV penicillin or clindamycin ± gentamicin.
- Lateral pharyngeal space infections: fever, leukocytosis, trismus if anterior; may lead to suppurative jugular venous thrombophlebitis with bacteremia, septic pulmonary emboli, thrombosis of intracranial venous sinuses; drainage and IV penicillin or clindamycin ± gentamicin.

INTRAABDOMINAL ABSCESSES

INTRAPERITONEAL ABSCESSES

- From perforated viscera, trauma, or postoperative infections. Most require drainage and systemic antibiotics against aerobic gram-negative rods, anaerobes, and enterococci.
- Subphrenic abscess: supra- and subhepatic spaces, left subphrenic space, lesser sac; fever may be mild, may have referred pain to shoulder, hiccups; 90% are complications of surgery, symptoms 3–6 weeks after surgery.
- Midabdominal abscess: in lower quadrants and between loops of bowel; from appendicitis, Crohn's disease, diverticulitis, surgery; fever, pain, palpable mass, air-fluid levels on upright films; appendideal abscesses are usually treatable with antibiotics alone.
- Pelvic abscess: from appendicitis, diverticulitis, salpingitis; fever and lower abdominal discomfort, may have diarrhea or urinary frequency, may have palpable mass on rectal or vaginal exam; surgical drainage although if from salpingitis, may resolve with antibiotics alone. (See Chap. 40.)

RETROPERITONEAL ABSCESS

- Anterior retroperitoneal abscess: between the posterior peritoneum and anterior renal fascia; from pancreatitis or perforation of ascending or descending colon, or duodenum; fever, abdominal or flank pain, tenderness, palpable mass.
- Perinephric abscess: between anterior and posterior renal fascia (contains kidney, adrenal, ureter); usually from rupture of renal abscess from pyelonephritis; aerobic gram-negatives, staphylococci, mixed infection; fever, chills, unilateral flank pain, dysuria, may have palpable mass; leukocytosis, pyuria, positive urine culture in 60% and blood culture in 20–40%; pts fail to become afebrile >5 d after beginning antibiotics for UTI; CT more sensitive than ultrasound; systemic antibiotics, drainage of pus percutaneously or by surgery.

VISCERAL ABSCESS

- Hepatic abscess: amebic (see Chap. 62) or pyogenic (from portal vein or systemic bacteremia, ascending cholangitis, direct extension, trauma, cryptogenic; aerobic gram-negatives, streptococci, anaerobes, staphylococci); most abscesses single, with subacute onset over weeks, fever, chills, nausea, anorexia, weight loss, 50% of pts have RUQ pain and hepatomegaly; if multiple abscesses, usually microscopic with more acute onset (from bacteremia or complete biliary obstruction); anemia, leukocytosis, increased alkaline phosphatase; ultrasound or CT usually shows fluid-filled masses; blood cultures positive in 50% of pts. Treat with antibiotics against isolated organisms; if bacteriology unknown, clindamycin (or metronidazole) and aminoglycoside; ampicillin may be added. Most pts also require percutaneous drainage or surgery.
- Splenic abscess: Most asymptomatic, multiple, small lesions; if symptomatic, usually single abscess from bacteremia, infected splenic infarct, contiguous infection; staphylococci, streptococci, anaerobes, gram-negative rods, *Candida* (in neutropenics); subacute onset, fever, leukocytosis, pain and tenderness (may be referred to left shoulder), splenomegaly; ultrasound and CT diagnostic. Treat with systemic antibiotics (as for hepatic abscess) and drain percutaneously or by surgery.
- Pancreatic abscess: 10–21 d after acute pancreatitis; fever, abdominal pain and tenderness, nausea, vomiting, ileus, palpable mass; leukocytosis and increased serum amylase; ultrasound and CT showing pancreatic gas are diagnostic. Treat with systemic antibiotics (as for hepatic abscess) and drain percutaneously or by surgery.
- Renal abscess: cortex—*Staph. aureus* (hematogenous); medulla—gram-negative rods (pyelonephritis). Acute onset of fever, chills, costovertebral pain and tenderness; pyuria only if medullary; leukocytosis; ultrasound or CT will show fluid-filled defect; treat with systemic antibiotics, analgesics, fluids; surgical drainage usually not necessary, percutaneous drainage may help.

MISCELLANEOUS ABSCESSES

- Retrofascial abscess: between transversalis and psoas fascias (contains psoas and quadratus lumborum muscles); from vertebrae, ilium and sacroiliac joints, hematogenous; abdominal pain, hip pain especially on extension or internal rotation; x-rays—loss of psoas shadow, displacement of ureter, CT or MRI to detect; systemic antibiotics with drainage necessary.

- Prostatic abscess: middle-aged men; most afebrile with frequency, retention, dysuria; may have hematuria, perineal pain, urethral discharge; rectal exam—prostatic tenderness and enlargement common but may be normal; pyuria and bacteriuria; aerobic gram-negative rods and staphylococci; treat with antibiotics; drainage if necessary by transurethral or perineal incision.
- Rectal abscess: most superficial and perirectal, may have fistula; painful, palpable, often visible; incise and drain, even if no fluctuance or neutropenic pt; antibiotics if extensive cellulitis. Evaluate for ulcerative colitis or Crohn's disease if nonhealing or recurrent.

INFECTIOUS ARTHRITIS

NONGONOCOCCAL SEPTIC ARTHRITIS   Etiology   75% gram-positive cocci—particularly *Staph. aureus,* also pneumococci, streptococci (groups A, G, and viridans; group B in neonates), *Staph. epidermidis* in prosthetic joints; 20% gram-negative rods—*Pseudomonas* in drug abusers and neonates, *H. influenzae* in children <5 years; usually hematogenous seeding of synovium.

Clinical manifestations   Monarticular synovitis, most often in large weight-bearing joints (knees > hips > ankle, wrist, shoulder, elbow, sternoclavicular, sacroiliac; interphalangeal joints rarely involved). Gram-positives—acute onset of swelling, pain, warmth, restricted motion of joint (septic hip—effusion may be difficult to detect, pain may be minimal or referred to groin, buttock, lateral thigh, or anterior knee); blood cultures positive in 50%. Gram-negatives—may be indolent over 3 weeks, osteomyelitis more frequent. Prosthetic joints—mild symptoms over weeks to months, may have draining fistula; infection occurs in 1–4% of prostheses over 10 years, increased after revision; concomitant osteomyelitis common.

Diagnosis   Turbid synovial fluid with >100,000/μL WBC (90% neutrophils) in 33–50% pts, gram stain positive in 79–95% of gram-positive and 50% gram-negative infections; joint fluid cultures usually positive; prosthetic joints—implant loosening and osteomyelitis on x-rays; CT or MRI for deep joints (hip, shoulder); radionuclide scan nonspecific.

Treatment   Intravenous antibiotics, joint drainage, immobilize joint, remove infected prosthetic joint. Gram-positives—IV nafcillin (penicillin for streptococci), cefazolin, or vancomycin initially followed by oral antibiotic; gram-negatives—two drugs IV initially (e.g., ampicillin or ticarcillin and an aminoglycoside) followed by oral antibiotic (e.g., quinolone or cephalosporin). Duration—streptococcal 2 weeks, other organisms 3–6 weeks. Drain purulent joint fluid via needle aspiration (daily × first 5–7 d), arthroscopy, or surgery (consider if hip, shoulder, sternoclavicular joint; persistent positive culture, purulent effusion present >7 d, loculations).

GONOCOCCAL ARTHRITIS   (See Chap. 40)

OTHER CAUSES OF SELF-LIMITED, ACUTE INFECTIOUS ARTHRITIS
Rubella, hepatitis B, mumps, coxsackieviruses, adenoviruses, parvoviruses, some arboviruses.

CHRONIC MONARTICULAR ARTHRITIS   Slowly progressive—*M. tuberculosis, Coccidioides, Sporothrix, Histoplasma*, syphilitic, Lyme disease; may also be acute—*Candida, Blastomyces.*

OSTEOMYELITIS

Etiology   Hematogenous or contiguous infection (e.g., trauma, infected prosthetic joint, chronic cutaneous ulcer); metaphyses of long bones in children, vertebrae and metaphyses of long bones in adults; *Staph. aureus* and *Staph. epidermidis* most common, gram-negative rods, anaerobes, polymicrobial especially from diabetic foot ulcers.

Clinical manifestations   50% of pts have vague pain in limb or back for 1–3 months, little or no fever; children may have acute onset of fever, irritability, lethargy, local inflammation <3 weeks duration; point tenderness, muscle spasms, may have draining sinus especially if infected prosthetic joint.

Diagnosis   Culture of blood (often negative in chronic osteomyelitis) and bone (deep bone biopsy, not sinus tract cultures); x-ray abnormalities occur ≥2 weeks after infection; radionuclide scans may be positive as early as 2 d after infection but may be difficult to interpret if overlying inflammation; CT or MRI most definitive.

Treatment

- Acute hematogenous osteomyelitis—IV antibiotics directed at organisms identified (nafcillin or cefazolin for empiric therapy) for at least 2 weeks followed by PO antibiotics for total of 4–6 weeks; debridement if poor response in 48 h, soft tissue abscess, septic arthritis.
- Chronic osteomyelitis—drainage, debridement of sequestra (necrotic bone), removal of prosthetic joint, bone grafts, coverage with muscle and skin flaps, IV antibiotics × 4–6 weeks after last surgery.
- Chronic osteomyelitis associated with vascular insufficiency—assess vascular status and tissue oxygen tension;

debridement plus broad-spectrum IV antibiotics × 4–6 weeks, *or* long-term suppressive antibiotics, *or* ablative surgery.

For a more detail discussion, see Hirschmann JV: Localized Infections and Abscesses, Chap. 91, p. 513; Rotrosen D: Infectious Arthritis, Chap. 96, p. 544; Mader JT: Osteomyelitis, Chap. 97, p. 548, in HPIM-12

SECTION 4 CARDIOVASCULAR DISEASES

66 PHYSICAL EXAMINATION OF THE HEART

General examination of a patient with suspected heart disease should include vital signs (respiratory rate, pulse, blood pressure), skin color, clubbing, edema, evidence of decreased perfusion (cool and sweaty skin), and hypertensive changes in optic fundi. Important findings on cardiovascular examination include:

CAROTID ARTERY PULSE (Fig. 66-1)

1. *Pulsus parvus:* Weak upstroke due to decreased stroke volume (hypovolemia, LV failure, aortic or mitral stenosis).
2. *Pulsus tardus:* Delayed upstroke (aortic stenosis).
3. *Bounding pulse:* Hyperkinetic circulation, aortic regurgitation, patent ductus arteriosus, marked vasodilatation.
4. *Pulsus bisferiens:* Double systolic pulsation in aortic regurgitation, hypertrophic cardiomyopathy.

A. Hypokinetic Pulse

B. Parvus et Tardus Pulse

C. Hyperkinetic Pulse

D. Bisferiens Pulse

E. Dicrotic Pulse + Alternans

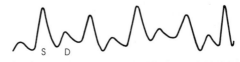

FIGURE 66-1

5. *Pulsus alternans:* Regular alteration in pulse pressure amplitude (severe LV dysfunction).
6. *Pulsus paradoxus:* Exaggerated inspiratory fall (>10 mmHg) in systolic BP (pericardial tamponade, obstructive lung disease).

JUGULAR VENOUS PULSATION (JVP) (Fig. 66-2) Jugular venous distention develops in right-sided heart failure, constrictive pericarditis, pericardial tamponade, obstruction of superior vena cava. JVP normally *falls* with inspiration, but may *rise* (Kussmaul's sign) in constrictive pericarditis. Abnormalities in examination include:

1. *Large "a" wave:* Tricuspid stenosis, pulmonic stenosis, AV dissociation (right atrium contracts against closed tricuspid valve).
2. *Large "v" wave:* Tricuspid regurgitation, atrial septal defect.
3. *Steep "y" descent:* Constrictive pericarditis.
4. *Slow "y" descent:* Tricuspid stenosis.

PRECORDIAL PALPATION Cardiac apical impulse is normally localized in the fifth intercostal space, midclavicular line. Abnormalities include:

1. *Forceful apical thrust:* Left ventricular hypertrophy.

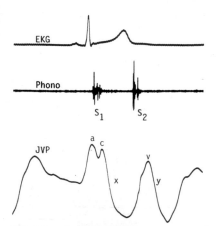

FIGURE 66-2. Normal jugular venous pressure recording.

2. *Lateral and downward displacement of apex impulse:* Left ventricular dilatation.
3. *Prominent presystolic impulse:* Hypertension, aortic stenosis, hypertrophic cardiomyopathy.
4. *Double systolic apical impulse:* Hypertrophic cardiomyopathy.
5. *Sustained "lift" at lower left sternal border:* Right ventricular hypertrophy.
6. *Dyskinetic (outward bulge) impulse:* Ventricular aneurysm, large dyskinetic area post MI, cardiomyopathy.

AUSCULTATION

HEART SOUNDS S_1 *Loud:* Mitral stenosis, short PR interval, hyperkinetic heart, thin chest wall. *Soft:* Long PR interval, heart failure, mitral regurgitation, thick chest wall, pulmonary emphysema.

S_2 Normally A_2 precedes P_2 and splitting increases with inspiration; abnormalities include:

- *Widened* splitting: Right bundle branch block, pulmonic stenosis, mitral regurgitation.
- *Fixed* splitting (no respiratory change in splitting): Atrial septal defect.
- *Narrow* splitting: Pulmonary hypertension.
- *Paradoxical* splitting (splitting *narrows* with inspiration): Aortic stenosis, left bundle branch block, CHF.
- *Loud* A_2: Systemic hypertension.
- *Soft* A_2: Aortic stenosis (AS).
- *Loud* P_2: Pulmonary arterial hypertension.
- *Soft* P_2: Pulmonic stenosis (PS).

S_3 Low-pitched, heard best with bell of stethoscope at apex, following S_2; normal in children; after age 30–35, indicates LV failure or volume overload.

S_4 Low-pitched, heard best with bell at apex, preceding S_1; reflects atrial contraction into a noncompliant ventricle; found in AS, hypertension, hypertrophic cardiomyopathy, and CAD.

Opening snap (OS) High-pitched; follows S_2 (by 0.06–0.12 s), heard at lower left sternal border and apex in mitral stenosis (MS); the more severe the MS, the shorter the OS–S_2 interval.

Ejection clicks High-pitched sounds following S_1; observed in dilatation of aortic root or pulmonary artery, congenital AS (loudest at apex) or PS (upper left sternal border); the latter *decreases* with inspiration.

Pericardial Knock - a loud diastolic sound in constrictive
pericarditis - related to the abrupt halt to diastolic filling which
occurs in this condition

Midsystolic clicks   At lower left sternal border and apex, often followed by late systolic murmur in mitral valve prolapse.

HEART MURMURS   Systolic murmurs   May be "crescendo-decrescendo" ejection type, pansystolic, or late systolic; right-sided murmurs (e.g., tricuspid regurgitation) typically increase with inspiration. A number of simple maneuvers produce characteristic changes depending on cause of murmur (Table 66-1).

Diastolic murmurs

1. Early diastolic murmurs: Begin immediately after S_2, are high-pitched, and usually are caused by aortic or pulmonary regurgitation.

2. Mid-to-late diastolic murmurs: Low-pitched, heard best with bell of stethoscope; observed in MS or TS; less commonly due to atrial myxoma.

3. Continuous murmurs: Present in systole and diastole (envelops S_2); found in patent ductus arteriosus and sometimes in coarctation of aorta; less common causes are systemic or coronary AV fistula, aortic septal defect, ruptured aneurysm of sinus of Valsalva.

TABLE 66-1

		Maneuver			
Lesion	Type of murmur	Valsalva	Hand grip	Squat	Stand
Aortic stenosis	Crescendo-decrescendo	↓	↓	↑	↓
Mitral regurgitation	Holosystolic	↓	↑	↑	↓
Ventricular septal defect	Holosystolic	↓	↑	↑	↓
Mitral valve prolapse	Late systolic (follows click)	↑	↓	↓	↑
Hypertrophic obstructive cardiomyopathy	Harsh, diamond-shaped at left sternal border; holosystolic at apex	↑	↓	↓	↑

For a more detailed discussion, see O'Rourke RA, Braunwald E: Physical Examination of the Cardiovascular System, Chap. 175, in HPIM-12, p. 843

↓ pressure of outflow --sitting, standing, amyl nitrate - less resistance more blood to leave

↑ pressure of outflow - handgrip, squatting, vasopressor - increased allows less blood to leave, and keeps wall apart

Valsalva - ↓ venous return

67 ELECTROCARDIOGRAPHY AND ECHOCARDIOGRAPHY

STANDARD APPROACH TO THE ECG

Normally, standardization is 1.0 mV per 10 mm, and paper speed is 25 mm/s (each horizontal small box = 0.04 s).

HEART RATE Beats/min = 300 divided by the number of *large* boxes (each 5 mm apart) between consecutive QRS complexes. For faster heart rates, divide 1500 by number of *small* boxes (1 mm apart) between each QRS.

RHYTHM *Sinus rhythm* is present if every P wave is followed by a QRS, PR interval ≥0.12 s, every QRS is preceded by a P wave, and the P wave is upright in leads I, II, and III. Arrhythmias are discussed in Chap. 70.

MEAN AXIS If QRS is primarily positive in limb leads I and II, then axis is *normal*. Otherwise, find limb lead in which QRS is most isoelectric (R = S). The mean axis is perpendicular to that lead (Fig. 67-1). If the QRS complex is *positive* in that perpendicular lead, then mean axis is in the direction of that lead; if *negative,* then mean axis points directly away from that lead.

Left-axis deviation (≤30°) occurs in diffuse left ventricular disease, inferior MI; also in left anterior hemiblock (small r, deep S in leads II, III, aVF).

Right-axis deviation (>90°) occurs in right ventricular hypertrophy (R > S in V_1) and left posterior hemiblock (small Q and tall R in leads II, III, and aVF). Mild right-axis deviation is seen in thin, healthy individuals (up to 110°).

INTERVALS (normal values in parentheses)

PR (0.12–0.20 s)

- *Short:* (1) preexcitation syndrome (look for slurred QRS upstroke due to "delta" wave), (2) nodal rhythm (inverted P in aVF).
- *Long:* first-degree AV block (Chap. 70).

QRS (0.06–0.10 s)

- *Widened:* (1) ventricular premature beats, (2) bundle branch blocks: *right* (RsR′ in V_1, deep S in V_6) and *left* (RR′ in V_6) (see Fig. 67-2), (3) toxic levels of certain drugs (e.g., quinidine), (4) severe hypokalemia.

QT (≤0.43 s; <50% of RR interval)

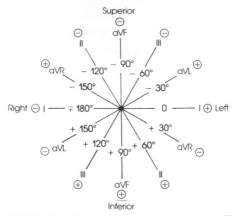

FIGURE 67-1 Electrocardiographic lead systems: The hexaxial frontal plane reference system to estimate electrical axis. Determine leads in which QRS deflections are maximum and minimum. For example, a maximum positive QRS in I which is isoelectric in aVF is oriented to 0°. Normal axis ranges from −30° to +90°. An axis >+90° is right axis deviation and <30° is left axis deviation. Normal ranges are described in the text, and applications are derived in Figs. 176-5 and 176-6 in HPIM-12. *(Reproduced from Myerburg RJ: HPIM-12.)*

- *Prolonged:* congenital, hypokalemia, hypocalcemia, drugs (quinidine, procainamide, tricyclics).

✳ HYPERTROPHY

- *Right atrium:* P wave ≥2.5 mm in lead II.
- *Left atrium:* P biphasic (positive, then negative) in V_1, with terminal negative force wider than 0.04 s.
- *Right ventricle:* R > S in V_1 and R in V_1 > 5 mm; deep S in V_6; right-axis deviation.
- *Left ventricle:* S in V_1 plus R in V_5 or V_6 ≥ 35 mm or R in aVL > 11 mm.

INFARCTION (Fig. 67-3 and 67-4) *Q-wave MI:* Pathologic Q waves (≥0.04 s and ≥25% of total QRS height) in leads shown in Table 67-1; acute *non-Q-wave MI* shows ST-T changes in these leads without Q wave development:
ST-T WAVES

- *ST elevation:* Acute MI, coronary spasm, pericarditis (concave upward), LV aneurysm.
- *ST depression:* Digitalis effect, strain (due to ventricular hypertrophy), ischemia, or nontransmural MI.

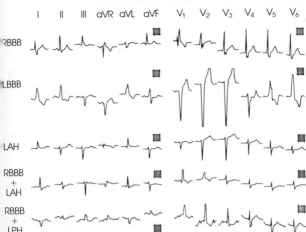

FIGURE 67-2 Intraventricular conduction abnormalities. Illustrated are right bundle branch block (RBBB); left bundle branch block (LBBB); left anterior hemiblock (LAH); right bundle branch block with left anterior hemiblock (RBBB + LAH); and right bundle branch block with left posterior hemiblock (RBBB + LPH). *(Reproduced from Myerburg RJ: HPIM-12.)*

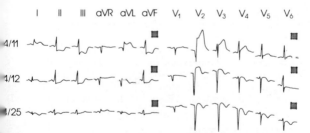

FIGURE 67-3 Acute anterior wall myocardial infarction. On 4/11, changes of a very early acute myocardial infarction in leads I, aVL, V_2, and V_3, with reciprocal changes in II, III, and aVF. On 4/12, ST segments remain elevated in the anterior leads, but T waves are inverted. On 4/25, a completed large anterior myocardial infarction is recorded—Q in I, aVL, V_1 to V_4. *(Reproduced from Myerburg RJ: HPIM-12.)*

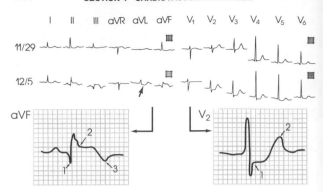

FIGURE 67-4   Acute inferior wall myocardial infarction. The ECG of 11/29 shows minor nonspecific ST-segment and T-wave changes. On 12/5 an acute myocardial infarction occurred. There are pathologic Q waves (1), ST-segment elevation (2), and terminal T-wave inversion (3) in leads II, III, and aVF indicating the location of the infarct on the inferior wall. Reciprocal changes in aVL (small arrow). Increasing R-wave voltage with ST depression and increased voltage of the T wave in V_2 is characteristic of true posterior wall extension of the inferior infarction. *(Reproduced from Myerburg RJ: HPIM-12.)*

TABLE 67-1

Leads with abnormal Q waves	Site of infarction
V_1–V_2	Anteroseptal
V_3–V_4	Apical
I, aVL, V_5–V_6	Anterolateral
II, III, aVF	Inferior
V_1–V_2 (tall R, *not* deep Q)	True posterior

- *Tall peaked T:* Hyperkalemia; acute MI ("hyperacute T").
- *Inverted T:* Non-Q-wave MI, ventricular "strain" pattern, drug effect (e.g., digitalis), hypokalemia, hypocalcemia, increased intracranial pressure (e.g., subarachnoid bleed).

INDICATIONS FOR ECHOCARDIOGRAPHY (Fig. 67-5)

VALVULAR STENOSIS   Both native and artificial valvular stenosis can be evaluated, and severity can be determined by Doppler [peak gradient = $4 \times$ (peak velocity)^2].

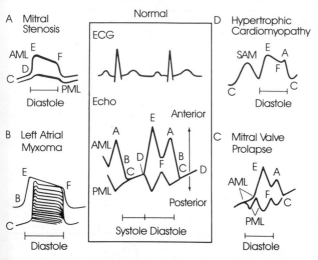

FIGURE 67-5 A schematic presentation of the normal M-mode echo-cardiographic (ECHO) recording of anterior (AML) and posterior mitral leaflet (PML) motion is shown in the center with the simultaneous ECG. Abnormal mitral echocardiograms which occur in (*A*) mitral stenosis, (*B*) left atrial myxoma, (*C*) mitral valve prolapse, and (*D*) obstructive hypertrophic cardiomyopathy are also depicted. In the ECHO, the A point represents the end of anterior movement resulting from left atrial contraction, the CD segment represents the closed position of both mitral leaflets during ventricular systole, and panel E ends the anterior movement as the leaflet opens. The slope EF results from posterior motion of the AML during rapid ventricular filling. In obstructive hypertrophic cardiomyopathy, SAM represents systolic anterior movement. (*Reproduced from Wynne J, O'Rourke RA, Braunwald E: HPIM-10, p. 1333.*)

VALVULAR REGURGITATION Structural lesions (e.g., flail leaflet, vegetation) resulting in regurgitation may be identified. Echo can demonstrate whether ventricular function is normal; Doppler (Fig. 67-6) can identify and estimate severity of regurgitation through each valve.

VENTRICULAR PERFORMANCE Global and regional wall-motion abnormalities of both ventricles can be assessed; ventricular hypertrophy/infiltration may be visualized; evidence of pulmonary hypertension may be obtained.

CARDIAC SOURCE OF EMBOLISM May visualize atrial or ventricular thrombus, intracardiac tumors, and valvular vegetations. Yield of identifying cardiac source of embolism is *low* in absence of cardiac history or physical findings.

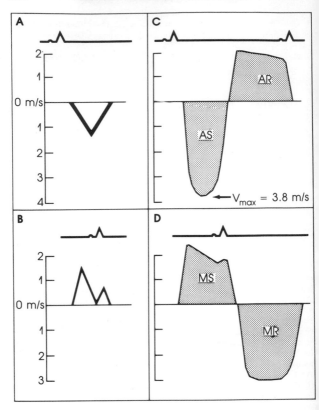

FIGURE 67-6 Schematic presentation of normal Doppler flow across the (*A*) aortic and (*B*) mitral valves. Abnormal continuous wave Doppler profiles are depicted in (*C*). Aortic stenosis (AS) [peak transaortic gradient $= 4 \times V_{max}^2 = 4 \times (3.8)^2 = 58$ mmHg] and regurgitation (AR); (*D*) Mitral stenosis (MS) and regurgitation (MR).

ENDOCARDITIS Vegetation visualized in more than half of pts, but management is generally based on clinical findings, not echo. Complications of endocarditis (e.g., valvular regurgitation) may be evaluated.

CONGENITAL HEART DISEASE Echo, Doppler, and contrast echo (rapid IV injection of saline) are noninvasive procedures of choice in identifying congenital lesions.

AORTIC ROOT Aneurysm and dissection of the aorta may be evaluated and complications (aortic regurgitation, tamponade) assessed (Chap. 78).

HYPERTROPHIC CARDIOMYOPATHY, MITRAL VALVE PROLAPSE, PERICARDIAC EFFUSION Echo is the diagnostic technique of choice for identifying these conditions.

For a more detailed discussion, see Myerburg RJ: Electro-cardiography, Chap. 176, in HPIM-12, p. 850, and Come PC, Wynne J, Braunwald E: Noninvasive Methods of Cardiac Examination, Chap. 177, in HPIM-12, p. 861

68 CONGESTIVE HEART FAILURE AND COR PULMONALE

HEART FAILURE

DEFINITION Heart is unable to pump the blood required by metabolizing tissues or can do so only from an abnormally elevated filling pressure. It is important to identify the *underlying* nature of the cardiac disease, and the factors which precipitate acute CHF.

UNDERLYING CARDIAC DISEASE Includes states that depress ventricular function (coronary artery disease, hypertension, dilated cardiomyopathy, valvular disease, congenital heart disease) and states that restrict ventricular filling (mitral stenosis, restrictive cardiomyopathy, pericardial disease).

ACUTE PRECIPITATING FACTORS Include (1) increased Na intake, (2) noncompliance with anti-CHF medications, (3) acute MI (may be silent), (4) exacerbation of hypertension, (5) acute arrhythmias, (6) infections and/or fever, (7) pulmonary embolism, (8) anemia, (9) thyrotoxicosis, (10) pregnancy, (11) acute myocarditis or infective endocarditis.

SYMPTOMS Due to inadequate perfusion of peripheral tissues (fatigue, dyspnea) and elevated intracardiac filling pressures (orthopnea, paroxysmal nocturnal dyspnea, peripheral edema).

PHYSICAL EXAM Jugular venous distention, S_3, pulmonary congestion (rales, dullness over pleural effusion, peripheral edema, hepatomegaly, and ascites).

LABORATORY CXR can reveal cardiomegaly, pulmonary vascular redistribution, Kerley B lines, pleural effusions. Left ventricular contraction can be assessed by *echocardiography* or *radionuclide ventriculography*. In addition, echo can identify underlying valvular, pericardial, or congenital heart disease, as well as regional wall-motion abnormalities typical of coronary artery disease.

CONDITIONS THAT MIMIC CHF   Pulmonary disease Chronic bronchitis, emphysema, and asthma (see Chaps. 81 and 83); look for sputum production and abnormalities on CXR and pulmonary function tests.

Other causes of peripheral edema Liver disease, varicose veins, and cyclic edema, none of which results in jugular venous distention. Edema due to renal dysfunction is often accompanied by elevated serum creatinine and abnormal urinalysis. (See Chap. 13.)

TREATMENT Aimed at symptomatic relief, removal of precipitating factors, and control of underlying cardiac disease:

1. Decrease cardiac workload: Reduce physical activity, including periods of bed rest for hospitalized pts (prevent deep venous thrombosis with heparin 5000 U SC bid).

2. Control excess fluid retention: (a) *Dietary sodium restriction* (eliminate salty foods, e.g., potato chips, canned soups, pork, salt added at table); more stringent requirements (<2 g NaCl/d) in advanced CHF. If dilutional hyponatremia present, restrict fluid intake (<1000 mL/d). (b) *Diuretics* (see Table 13-1): *Loop diuretics* (e.g., furosemide 20–120 mg/day PO or IV) are most potent and unlike thiazides remain effective when GFR <25 mL/min. Combine loop diuretic with thiazide or metolazone for augmented effect. Potassium-sparing diuretics are useful adjunct to reduce potassium loss. They should *not* be added in pts receiving ACE inhibitors, to avoid *hyper*kalemia.

During diuresis, obtain daily weights aiming for loss of 1–1.5 kg/d.

3. Vasodilators (Table 68-1): Recommended if symptoms persist despite diuretics. Venous dilators (e.g., nitrates) reduce pulmonary congestion; arterial dilators (e.g., hydralazine) augment forward stroke volume, particularly if systemic vascular resistance (SVR) is markedly elevated or mitral or aortic regurgitation is present. ACE inhibitors are mixed (arterial and venous) dilators and are particularly effective and well tolerated. They, and to a lesser extent the combination of hydralazine plus nitrates, have been shown to prolong life in pts with advanced CHF. Vasodilators may result in significant hypotension in pts who are volume depleted, so start at lowest dosage; pt should remain supine for 2–4 h after the initial doses.

In sicker, hospitalized pts, IV vasodilator therapy (Table 68-1) is monitored by placement of a pulmonary artery catheter and indwelling arterial line. Nitroprusside is a potent mixed vasodilator for pts with markedly elevated SVR. It is metabolized to thiocyanate, then excreted via the kidneys. To avoid thiocyanate toxicity (seizures, altered mental status, nausea), follow thiocyanate levels in pts with renal failure or if administered for more than 2 d.

4. Digoxin is useful in heart failure due to (a) marked systolic dysfunction (LV dilatation, low ejection fraction, S_3), and (b) heart failure associated with atrial fibrillation and rapid ventricular rate. Not indicated in CHF due to pericardial disease, restrictive cardiomyopathy, or mitral stenosis (unless atrial fibrillation is present). Digoxin is contraindicated in

TABLE 68-1 Vasodilators for treatment of congestive heart failure

Drug	Site of action (venous/arterial)	Usual dose	Comments and adverse effects
IV agents:			
Nitroprusside	V = A	0.5–5 µg/kg/min	Possible thiocyanate toxicity with prolonged use.
Nitroglycerin	V > A	10–200 µg/min	Hypotension if LV filling pressure is low.
Oral agents:			
Captopril	V = A	6.25–25 mg tid }	Angioedema, cough, rash, hyperkalemia. Monitor for proteinuria or leukopenia if creatinine >1.6.
Enalapril	V = A	2.5–10 mg bid }	
Hydralazine	A	50–200 mg tid	Precipitation of angina. Drug-induced lupus.
Nitrates (e.g., isosorbide dinitrate)	V		Tolerance may develop.
Prazosin	V = A	20–80 mg qid 1–5 mg qid	High rate of drug tolerance.

Note: Arteriolar dilator may be combined with venous dilator (e.g., hydralazine plus nitrate).

hypertrophic cardiomyopathy and in pts with AV conduction blocks.

Digoxin loading dose is administered over 24 h (0.5 mg PO/IV, followed by 0.25 mg q 6 h to achieve total of 1.0–1.5 mg). Subsequent dose (0.125–0.25 mg qd) depends on age, weight, and renal function and is guided by measurement of serum digoxin level. The addition of quinidine increases serum digoxin level; therefore, digoxin dosage should be halved. Verapamil, amiodarone, and spironolactone also increase serum digoxin level but to a lesser extent.

Digitalis toxicity may be precipitated by hypokalemia, hypoxemia, hypercalcemia, hypomagnesemia, hypothyroidism, or myocardial ischemia. Early signs of toxicity include anorexia, nausea, and lethargy. *Cardiac toxicity* includes ventricular extrasystoles, ventricular tachycardia, and fibrillation; atrial tachycardia with block; sinus arrest and sinoatrial block; all degrees of AV block. *Chronic* digitalis intoxication may cause cachexia, gynecomastia, "yellow" vision, or confusion. At first sign of digitalis toxicity, discontinue the drug; maintain serum K concentration between 4.0 and 5.0 mmol/L. Bradyarrhythmias and AV block may respond to atropine (0.6 mg IV); otherwise a temporary pacemaker may be required. Digitalis-induced ventricular arrhythmias are treated with lidocaine or phenytoin (Chap. 70). Antidigoxin antibodies are available for massive overdose.

5. *IV sympathomimetic amines* are administered to hospitalized patients for refractory symptoms or acute exacerbation of CHF. They are contraindicated in hypertrophic cardiomyopathy. *Dobutamine* (2.5–10 μg/kg/min), the preferred agent, augments cardiac output without significant peripheral vasoconstriction or tachycardia. *Dopamine* at low dosage (1–5 μg/kg/min) facilitates diuresis; at higher dosage (5–10 μg/kg/min) positive inotropic effects predominate; peripheral vasoconstriction is greatest at dosage greater than 10 μg/kg/min. *Amrinone* (5–10 μg/kg/min after a 0.75 mg/kg bolus) is a nonsympathetic positive inotrope and vasodilator. Vasodilators and inotropic agents may be used together for additive effect.

Patients with severe refractory CHF with less than 6 months expected survival, who meet stringent criteria, may be candidates for cardiac transplantation.

COR PULMONALE

Right ventricular enlargement resulting from *primary* lung disease; leads to RV hypertrophy and eventually to RV failure. Etiologies include the following:

Pulmonary parenchymal or airway disease   Chronic obstructive lung disease (COPD), interstitial lung diseases, bronchiectasis, cystic fibrosis (Chaps. 83 and 86).

Pulmonary vascular disease   Recurrent pulmonary emboli, primary pulmonary hypertension (PHT), vasculitis, sickle cell anemia.

Inadequate mechanical ventilation   Kyphoscoliosis, neuromuscular disorders, marked obesity, sleep apnea.

SYMPTOMS   Depend on underlying disorder, but include dyspnea, cough, fatigue, and sputum production (in parenchymal diseases).

PHYSICAL EXAM   Tachypnea, cyanosis, clubbing are common. RV impulse along left sternal border, loud P_2, right-sided S_4. If RV failure develops, elevated jugular venous pressure, hepatomegaly with ascites, pedal edema.

LABORATORY: ECG   RV hypertrophy and RA enlargement (Chap. 67); tachyarrhythmias are common.

CXR   RV and pulmonary artery enlargement; if PHT present, tapering of the pulmonary artery branches. Pulmonary function tests and arterial blood gases characterize intrinsic pulmonary disease.

Echocardiogram   RV hypertrophy; LV function typically normal. If pulmonary emboli suspected, obtain radionuclide lung scan.

TREATMENT   Aimed at underlying pulmonary disease and may include bronchodilators, antibiotics, and oxygen administration. If RV failure is present, treat as CHF, instituting low-sodium diet and diuretics; digoxin must be administered cautiously (toxicity increased due to hypoxemia, hypercapnia, acidosis). Supraventricular tachyarrhythmias are common and treated with digoxin, quinidine, or verapamil (*not* beta blockers). Chronic anticoagulation with warfarin is indicated when pulmonary hypertension is accompanied by RV failure.

For a more detailed discussion, see Braunwald E: Heart Failure, Chap. 182, in HPIM-12, p. 890, and Butler J: Cor Pulmonale, Chap. 191, in HPIM-12, p. 971

69 HYPERTENSION

DEFINITION Chronic elevation in BP >140/90; etiology unknown in 90–95% of patients ("essential hypertension"). Always consider a secondary correctable form of hypertension, especially in patients under age 30 or those who become hypertensive after 55. Isolated systolic hypertension (systolic >160, diastolic <90) most common in elderly pts, due to reduced vascular compliance.

SECONDARY HYPERTENSION

RENAL ARTERY STENOSIS Due either to atherosclerosis (older men) or fibromuscular dysplasia (young women). Presents with sudden onset of hypertension, refractory to usual antihypertensive therapy. Abdominal bruit often audible; mild hypokalemia due to activation of the renin-angiotensin-aldosterone system may be present.

RENAL PARENCHYMAL DISEASE Elevated serum creatinine and/or abnormal urinalysis, containing protein, cells, or casts.

COARCTATION OF AORTA Presents in children or young adults; constriction is usually present in aorta at origin of left subclavian artery. Exam shows diminished, delayed femoral pulsations; late systolic murmur loudest over the midback. CXR shows indentation of the aorta at the level of the coarctation and rib notching (due to development of collateral arterial flow).

PHEOCHROMOCYTOMA Catecholamine-secreting tumor, typically of the adrenal medulla, that presents as paroxysmal or sustained hypertension in young to middle-aged pts. Sudden episodes of headache, palpitations, and profuse diaphoresis are common. Associated findings include chronic weight loss, orthostatic *hypotension*, and impaired glucose tolerance. Pheochromocytomas may be localized to the bladder wall and may present with micturition-associated symptoms of cathecholamine excess. Diagnosis is suggested by elevated urinary catecholamine metabolites in a 24-h urine collection (see below); the tumor is then localized by CT scan or angiography.

HYPERALDOSTERONISM Due to aldosterone-secreting adenoma or bilateral adrenal hyperplasia. Should be suspected when hypokalemia is present in a hypertensive patient off diuretics (see Chap. 144).

OTHER CAUSES Oral contraceptive usage, Cushing's and adrenogenital syndromes (Chap. 144), thyroid disease (Chap.

143), hyperparathyroidism (Chap. 150), and acromegaly (Chap. 141).

APPROACH TO PATIENT

HISTORY   Most patients are asymptomatic. Severe hypertension may lead to headache, epistaxis, or blurred vision.
Clues to specific secondary forms of hypertension
Use of birth control pills or glucocorticoids; paroxysms of headache, sweating, or tachycardia (pheochromocytoma); history of renal disease or abdominal traumas (renal hypertension).
PHYSICAL EXAM   Measure BP with appropriately sized cuff (large cuff for large arm). Measure BP in both arms as well as a leg (to evaluate for coarctation). Signs of hypertension include retinal arteriolar changes (narrowing/nicking); left ventricular lift, loud A_2, S_4. Clues to secondary forms of hypertension include Cushinoid appearance, thyromegaly, abdominal bruit (renal artery stenosis), delayed femoral pulses (coarctation of aorta).
SCREENING TESTS FOR SECONDARY HYPERTENSION   Should be carried out on all patients with documented hypertension: (1) serum creatinine, BUN, and urinalysis (renal parenchymal disease); (2) serum K measured off diuretics (hypokalemia prompts workup for hyperaldosteronism or renal artery stenosis); (3) CXR (rib notching or indentation of distal aortic arch in coarctation of the aorta); (4) ECG (left ventricular hypertrophy suggests chronicity of hypertension), (5) other useful screening blood tests include CBC, glucose, cholesterol, triglycerides, calcium, uric acid.
FURTHER WORKUP   Indicated for specific diagnoses if screening tests are abnormal or BP is refractory to antihypertensive therapy: (1) renal artery stenosis: digital subtraction angiography, IVP, renal arteriography, and measurement of renal vein renin; (2) Cushing's syndrome: dexamethasone suppression test (Chap. 144); (3) pheochromocytoma: 24-h urine collection for catecholamines, metanephrines, and vanillylmandelic acid; (4) primary hyperaldosteronism: depressed plasma renin activity and hypersecretion of aldosterone, both of which fail to change with volume expansion; (5) renal parenchymal disease: see Section 6.

DRUG THERAPY OF ESSENTIAL HYPERTENSION

Goal is to control hypertension with minimal side effects using a single drug if possible. First-line agents include

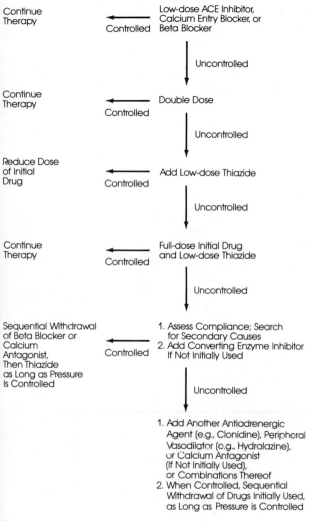

FIGURE 69-1 Schematic approach to the treatment of the patient with hypertension in whom a specific form of therapy is unavailable or unknown.

angiotensin converting enzyme inhibitors, calcium antagonists, beta blockers, or diuretics.

Beta blockers (Table 69-1): Particularly effective in young pts with "hyperkinetic" circulation. Begin with low dosage (e.g., atenolol 25 mg qd). Relative contraindications: bronchospasm, CHF, AV block, bradycardia, and "brittle" insulin-dependent diabetes.

ACE inhibitors (Table 69-2): Well tolerated with low frequency of side effects. May be used as monotherapy or in combination with beta blockers, calcium antagonists, or diuretics. Side effects are uncommon and include rash, angioedema, proteinuria, or leukopenia, particularly in pts with elevated serum creatinine. A nonproductive cough may develop in the course of therapy, requiring an alternative regimen. Note that renal function may deteriorate as a result of ACE inhibitors in pts with bilateral renal artery stenosis.

Potassium supplements and potassium-sparing diuretics should not be combined with ACE inhibitors, unless hypokalemia is documented. If pt is intravascularly volume depleted, hold diuretics for 2–3 d prior to initiation of ACE inhibitor, which should then be administered at very low dosage (e.g., captopril 6.25 mg bid).

Calcium antagonists (Table 69-3): Direct arteriolar vasodilators; all have negative inotropic effects (particularly verapamil) and should be used cautiously if LV dysfunction is present. Verapamil, and to a lesser extent diltiazem, can result in bradycardia and AV block so combination with beta blockers is generally avoided.

TABLE 69-1   Beta blockers*

Drug	Usual dosage (PO)	Features
Propranolol	10–120 mg q 6–12 h	
Metoprolol	25–150 mg q 12 h	Beta₁ selective
Nadolol	20–120 mg q 24 h	Once-a-day dosage
Atenolol	25–100 mg q 24 h	Beta₁ selective; once-a-day dosage
Timolol	10–30 mg q 12 h	
Pindolol	10–30 mg q 12 h	Partial beta-agonist activity
Labetolol	100–600 mg 12 h	Both alpha and beta blocker
Acebutolol	200–600 mg q 12 h	Once-a-day; partial beta-agonist

**Side effects:* Bradycardia (less common with pindolol and acebutolol), GI side effects, LV dysfunction, bronchospasm (less common with atenolol and metoprolol), exacerbation of diabetes or impaired response to insulin-induced hypoglycemia, impotence.

TABLE 69-2   **ACE inhibitors**

	Dose	Half-life
Captopril	PO: 12.5–75 mg bid	3 h
Enalapril	PO: 2.5–40 mg qd	11 h
Enalaprilat	IV: 0.625–1.25 mg q 6 h	
Lisinopril	PO: 5–40 mg qd	12 h

Diuretics (Table 13-1): Thiazides preferred over loop diuretics because of longer duration of action; however, the latter are more potent when GFR <25 mL/min. Major side effects include hypokalemia, hyperglycemia, and hyperuricemia, which can be minimized by using low dosage (e.g., hydrochlorothiazide 12.5–50 mg qd). Diuretics are particularly effective in elderly and black pts. Prevention of hypokalemia is especially important in pts on digitalis glycosides.

If BP proves refractory to drug therapy, workup for secondary forms of hypertension, especially renal artery stenosis and pheochromocytoma (see HPIM-12, p. 1010 for detailed list of antihypertensives).

SPECIAL CIRCUMSTANCES

PREGNANCY   Safest antihypertensives include methyldopa (250–1000 mg PO bid-tid), hydralazine (10–150 mg PO bid-tid), and a beta blocker (Table 69-1).

RENAL FAILURE   Standard thiazide diuretics may not be effective. Consider metolazone, furosemide, or bumetanide alone or in combination.

MALIGNANT HYPERTENSION   Diastolic BP >120 mmHg is a medical emergency. Immediate therapy is mandatory if there is evidence of cardiac decompensation (CHF, angina), encephalopathy (headache, seizures, visual disturbances), or deteriorating renal function. Drugs to treat hypertensive crisis are listed in Table 69-4. Replace with PO antihypertensive as patient becomes asymptomatic and diastolic BP improves.

TABLE 69-3   **Calcium channel antagonists**

	Dose	Adverse effects
Nifedipine	PO: 10–30 mg qid *or* Slow-release: 30–90 mg qd	Tachycardia, headache, flushing, edema, CHF
Diltiazem	PO: 30–120 mg qid *or* Slow release: 6–240 mg bid	Bradycardia, edema, CHF
Verapamil	PO: 40–120 mg tid *or* Slow release: 120–480 g qd	Bradycardia, AV block, CHF, constipation, increased digoxin level

TABLE 69-4 Treatment of malignant hypertension and hypertensive crisis

Drug	Dosage	Side effects
Diazoxide	IV: 150–300 mg	Na^+ retention,* hyperglycemia
Nitroprusside†	IV: 0.5–8.0 μg/kg/min	Hypotension; after 24 h watch for tinnitus, blurred vision, altered mental status
Trimethaphan†	IV: 1–10 μg/min	Urinary retention
Labetolol	IV: 20 mg bolus, then 1–2 mg/min	Hypotension, bradycardia, AV block, bronchospasm
Enalaprilat	IV: 1.25 mg q 6 h	Angioedema, hyperkalemia
Nifedipine	10–20 mg SL (pierce capsule)	Hypotension, flushing, headache

*Administer furosemide 20–80 mg IV to prevent Na^+ retention.
†Intraarterial BP monitoring is recommended to avoid rapid fluctuations in BP.

For a more detailed discussion, see Williams GH: Hypertension, Chap. 196, in HPIM-12, p. 1001

Arrhythmias may appear in the presence or absence of structural heart disease; they are more serious in the former. Conditions that provoke arrhythmias include (1) myocardial ischemia, (2) CHF, (3) hypoxemia, (4) hypercapnia, (5) hypotension, (6) electrolyte disturbances (especially involving K, Ca, and Mg), (7) drug toxicity (digoxin, antiarrhythmic agents that prolong QT interval), (8) caffeine, (9) ethanol.

DIAGNOSIS Examine ECG for evidence of ischemic changes (Chap. 67), prolonged QT interval, and characteristics of Wolff-Parkinson-White (WPW) syndrome (see below). See Fig. 70-1 for diagnosis of tachyarrhythmias; always identify atrial activity and relationship between P waves and QRS complexes. Aids in the diagnosis include the following:

- Obtain long rhythm strip of leads II, aVF, or V_1. Double the ECG voltage and increase paper speed to 50 mm/s to help identify P waves.
- Place accessory ECG leads (right-sided chest, esophageal, right-atrial) to help identify P waves. Record ECG during carotid sinus massage (Table 70-1) for 5 s. *Note:* Do not massage both carotids simultaneously.

Tachyarrhythmias with wide QRS complex beats may represent ventricular tachycardia or supraventricular tachycardia with aberrant conduction. Factors favoring *ventricular tachycardia* include (1) AV dissociation, (2) QRS >0.14 s, (3) LAD, (4) no response to carotid sinus massage, (5) morphology of QRS is similar to that of previous ventricular premature beats.

GUIDELINES FOR TREATMENT OF TACHYARRHYTHMIAS (Tables 70-1 and 70-2) Precipitating causes (listed above) should be corrected. If pt is hemodynamically compromised (angina, hypotension, CHF), proceed to immediate cardioversion. *Note:* Do not cardiovert sinus tachycardia; exercise caution if digitalis toxicity is suspected. Initiate drugs as indicated in the tables; follow drug levels and ECG intervals (especially QRS and QT). Reduce dosage for pts with hepatic or renal dysfunction as indicated in Table 70-2. Drug efficacy is confirmed by ECG monitoring (or Holter), stress testing, and in special circumstances, invasive electrophysiologic study.

Antiarrhythmic agents all have potential toxic side effects, including *provocation* of ventricular arrhythmias, especially in pts with LV dysfunction or history of sustained ventricular arrhythmias. Drug-induced QT prolongation and associated

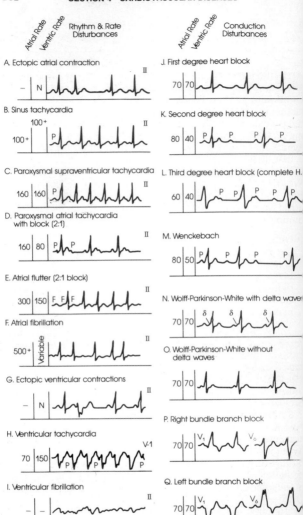

FIGURE 70-1. *(Reproduced from Sobel BE, Braunwald E: HPIM-9, p 1052.)*

torsade de pointes ventricular tachycardia (Table 70-1) is most common with group IA agents; the drug should be discontinued if the QTc interval (QT divided by square root of RR interval) increases by more than 25%. Flecainide and encainide should be avoided in pts with asymptomatic ventricular arrhythmias after MI, as mortality risk increases.

PREEXCITATION SYNDROME (WPW) Conduction occurs through an accessory pathway between atria and ventricles. Baseline ECG typically shows a short PR interval and slurred upstroke of the QRS ("delta" wave) (Fig. 70-1*N*). Associated tachyarrhythmias are of two types:

- *Narrow QRS complex tachycardia* (antegrade conduction through AV node): usually paroxysmal supraventricular tachycardia. Treat cautiously with IV verapamil, digoxin, or propranolol (Table 70-2).
- *Wide QRS complex tachycardia* (antegrade conduction through accessory pathway): often associated with AF with a very *rapid* (>250/min) ventricular rate (which may degenerate into VF). If hemodynamically compromised, immediate cardioversion is indicated; otherwise, treat with IV lidocaine or procainamide, *not* digoxin or verapamil.

AV BLOCK

FIRST DEGREE (Fig. 70-1*J*) Prolonged, constant PR interval (>0.20 s). May be normal or secondary to increased vagal tone or digitalis; no treatment required.

SECOND DEGREE Mobitz I (Wenkebach) (Fig. 70-1*M*) Narrow QRS, progressive increase in PR interval until a ventricular beat is dropped, then sequence is repeated. Seen with digitalis toxicity, increased vagal tone, inferior MI. Usually transient, no therapy required; if symptomatic, use atropine (0.6 mg IV, repeated × 3–4) or temporary pacemaker.

Mobitz II (Fig. 70-1*K*) Fixed PR interval with occasional dropped beats, in 2:1, 3:1, or 4:1 pattern; the QRS complex is usually wide. Seen with MI or degenerative conduction system disease; a dangerous rhythm—may progress suddenly to complete AV block; pacemaker is indicated.

Third degree (complete AV block) (Fig. 70-1*L*) Atrial activity is not transmitted to ventricles; atria and ventricles contract independently. Seen with MI, digitalis toxicity, or degenerative conduction system disease. Permanent pacemaker is indicated, except when associated transiently with inferior MI or in asymptomatic congenital heart block.

TABLE 70-1 Clinical and electrocardiographic features of common arrhythmias

Rhythm	Example (Fig. 70-1)	Atrial rate	Features	Carotid sinus massage	Precipitating conditions	Initial treatment
NARROW QRS COMPLEX						
Atrial premature beats	A	—	P wave abnormal; QRS width normal	—	Can be normal; or due to anxiety, CHF, hypoxia, caffeine, abnormal electrolytes (K^+, Ca^{2+}, Mg^{2+})	Remove precipitating cause; if symptomatic: beta blocker or group IA drug*
Sinus tachycardia	B	100–160	Normal P wave	Rate gradually slows	Fever, dehydration, pain, CHF, hyperthyroidism, COPD	Remove precipitating cause; if symptomatic: beta blocker
Paroxysmal SVT	C	140–250	P wave "peaked" or inverted in leads II, III, aVF	Abruptly converts to sinus rhythm (or no effect)	Healthy individuals; preexcitation syndromes (see text)	Vagal maneuvers; if unsuccessful: verapamil, beta blocker, group IA drug, cardioversion (150 J)
Paroxysmal atrial tachycardia with block	D	130–250	Upright "peaked" P; 2:1, 3:1, 4:1, block	No effect on atrial rate; block may ↑	Digitalis toxicity	Hold digoxin, correct [K^+]; phenytoin (250 mg IV over 5 min)

Arrhythmia		Rate	ECG findings	Response	Etiology	Treatment
Atrial flutter	L	250–350	"Sawtooth" flutter waves; 2:1, 4:1 block	↑ Block; ventricular rate ↓	Mitral valve disease, hypertension, pulmonary embolism, pericarditis, post-cardiac surgery, hyperthyroidism, obstructive lung disease, EtOH, idiopathic	1. Slow the ventricular rate: digoxin, beta blocker, or verapamil 2. Convert to NSR (after anticoagulation if chronic) with quinidine† or procainamide; may require electrical cardioversion (flutter: 50 J; fib: 100–200 J). Atrial flutter may respond to rapid atrial pacing
Atrial fibrillation	F	>350	No discrete P; irregularly spaced QRS	Ventricular rate ↓		
Multifocal atrial tachycardia		100–220	More than 3 different P wave shapes with varying P-P intervals	No effect	Severe respiratory insufficiency	Treat underlying lung disease; verapamil may be used to slow ventricular rate

285

TABLE 70-1 Clinical and electrocardiographic features of common arrhythmias *(Continued)*

Rhythm	Example (Fig. 70-1)	Atrial rate	Features	Carotid sinus massage	Precipitating conditions	Initial treatment
WIDE QRS COMPLEX						
Ventricular premature beats	G		Fully compensatory pause between normal beats	No effect	Coronary artery disease, myocardial infarction, CHF, hypoxia, hypokalemia, digitalis toxicity, prolonged QT interval (congenital or drugs: quinidine and other antiarrhythmics, tricyclics, phenothiazines)	May not require therapy;‡ use same drugs as ventricular tachycardia
Ventricular tachycardia	H		QRS rate 100–250; slightly irregular rate	No effect		If unstable: electrical conversion (100 J); otherwise: Acute (IV): lidocaine, procainamide, bretylium; chronic (PO) prevention: group IA, IB, IC, III drugs*

Arrhythmia	ECG features		Etiology	Treatment
Ventricular fibrillation	Erratic electrical activity only	No effect		Immediate defibrillation (200–400 J)
Torsade de pointes	Ventricular tachycardia with sinusoidal oscillations of QRS height	No effect	Prolonged QT interval (congenital or drugs: quinidine and other antiarrhythmics, tricyclics, phenothiazines)	Lidocaine; isoproterenol (unless CAD present); overdrive pacing; magnesium; bretylium. Drugs that prolong QT interval (e.g., quinidine) are contraindicated.
Supraventricular tachycardias with aberrant ventricular conduction	P wave typical of the supraventricular rhythm; wide QRS complex due to conduction through partially refractory pathways	No effect	Etiologies of the respective supraventricular rhythms listed above; atrial fibrillation with rapid, wide QRS may be due to preexcitation (WPW)	Same as treatment of respective supraventricular rhythm; if ventricular rate rapid (>200), treat as WPW (see text)

*Antiarrhythmic drug groups listed in Table 70-2.
†Decrease digoxin dose when starting quinidine.
‡Indications for treating VPCs listed in Chap. 74.
Note: J = joules.

TABLE 70-2 Antiarrhythmic drugs

Drug	Loading dose	Maintenance dose	Side effects	Excretion
Group IA:				
Quinidine sulfate	IV: 500–1,000 mg	PO: 200–400 mg q 6 h	Diarrhea, tinnitus, QT prolongation,	Hepatic
Quinidine gluconate	IV: 500–1000 mg	PO: 324–628 mg q 8 h	hypotension, anemia, thrombocytopenia	Hepatic
Procainamide		IV: 2–5 mg/min	Nausea, lupus-like syndrome,	Renal and hepatic
		PO: 500–1000 mg q 4 h	agranulocytosis, QT prolongation	
		PO: 500–1250 mg q 6 h		
Sustained-release:				
Disopyramide		PO: 100–300 mg q 6–8 h	Myocardial depression, AV block, QT prolongation, anticholinergic effects	Renal
Group IB:				
Lidocaine	IV: 20–50 mg/min to 1.4 mg/kg; repeat after 5 min	IV: 1–4 mg/min	Confusion, seizures, respiratory arrest	Hepatic
Tocainide		PO: 400–600 mg q 8 h	Nausea, confusion, tremors, lupus-like reaction	Hepatic and renal
Mexiletine		PO: 100–300 mg q 6–8 h	Nausea, tremor, gait disturbance	Hepatic
Group IC:				
Flecainide		PO: 50–200 mg q 12 h	Nausea, exacerbation of ventricular arrhythmia, prolongation of PR and QRS intervals	Hepatic and renal
Encainide		PO: 25–50 mg q 8 h		Hepatic and renal
Group II:				
Propranolol	IV: 0.5–1 mg/min to 0.15–0.2 mg/kg	PO: 10–200 mg q 6 h	CHF, bradycardia, AV block, bronchospasm	Hepatic

Group III:			
Amiodarone	PO: 800–1400 mg qd × 1–2 weeks PO: 200–600 mg qd	Thyroid abnormalities, pulmonary fibrosis, hepatitis, corneal microdeposits, bluish skin, QT prolongation	—
Bretylium	IV: 5–10 mg/kg	Hypertension, orthostatic hypotension, nausea, parotid pain	Renal
Group IV:			
Verapamil	IV: 2.5–10 mg PO: 80–120 mg tid-qid	AV block, CHF, hypotension, constipation	Hepatic
Other:			
Digoxin	IV, PO: 0.75–1.5 mg over 24 h IV, PO: 0.125–0.25 mg qd	Nausea, AV block, ventricular and supraventricular arrhythmias	Renal

For a more detailed discussion, see Josephson ME et al: The Bradyarrhythmias, Chap. 184, and The Tachyarrhythmias, Chap. 185, in HPIM-12, pp. 902 and 908

71 VALVULAR HEART DISEASE

MITRAL STENOSIS (MS)

ETIOLOGY Most commonly rheumatic, although history of acute rheumatic fever is now uncommon; congenital MS is an uncommon cause, observed primarily in infants.

HISTORY Symptoms most commonly begin in the fourth decade, but MS often causes severe disability by age 20 in economically deprived areas. Principal symptoms are dyspnea and pulmonary edema precipitated by exertion, excitement, fever, anemia, paroxysmal tachycardia, pregnancy, sexual intercourse, etc.

PHYSICAL EXAM Peripheral and facial cyanosis in severe MS. Right ventricular lift; palpable S_1; opening snap (OS) follows A_2 by 0.06 to 0.12 s; OS–A_2 interval inversely proportional to severity of obstruction. Diastolic rumbling murmur with presystolic accentuation in sinus rhythm. Duration of murmur correlates with severity of obstruction.

COMPLICATIONS Hemoptysis, pulmonary embolism, pulmonary infection, systemic embolization; endocarditis is *uncommon* in pure MS.

LABORATORY ECG Typically shows atrial fibrillation (AF) or left atrial (LA) enlargement when sinus rhythm is present. Right-axis deviation and RV hypertrophy in the presence of pulmonary hypertension.

CXR Shows LA and RV enlargement and Kerley B lines.

Echocardiogram Most useful noninvasive test; shows inadequate separation, calcification and thickening of valve leaflets, and LA enlargement. Doppler echocardiogram allows estimation of transvalvular gradient and mitral valve area (Chap. 67).

MANAGEMENT (Fig. 71-1) Pts should receive prophylaxis for rheumatic fever (penicillin) and infective endocarditis (Chap. 73). In the presence of dyspnea, medical therapy for heart failure: digitalis, verapamil, or beta blockers to slow ventricular rate in AF, diuretics, and sodium restriction. Anticoagulants for pts with AF and/or history of systemic and pulmonic emboli. Open mitral valvuloplasty in the presence of symptoms and mitral orifice ≤ approximately 1.2 cm². In selected pts, without mitral regurgitation, percutaneous balloon valvuloplasty is frequently a successful alternative to surgery.

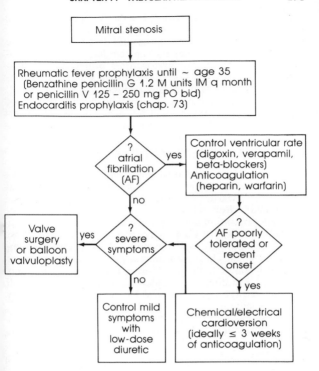

FIGURE 71-1 Management of mitral stenosis.

MITRAL REGURGITATION (MR)

ETIOLOGY Rheumatic heart disease in approximately 50%. Other causes: mitral valve prolapse, ischemic heart disease with papillary muscle dysfunction, LV dilatation of any cause, mitral annular calcification, hypertrophic cardiomyopathy, infective endocarditis, congenital.

CLINICAL MANIFESTATIONS Fatigue, weakness, and exertional dyspnea. Physical examination: sharp upstroke of arterial pulse, LV lift, S_1 diminished: wide splitting of S_2; S_3; loud holosystolic murmur and often a brief early–mid-diastolic murmur.

ECHOCARDIOGRAM Enlarged LA, hyperdynamic LV; Doppler echocardiogram helpful in diagnosing and assessing severity of MR.

MANAGEMENT   As for heart failure (see Chap. 68), including diuretics and digoxin. Afterload reduction (captopril, enalapril, hydralazine, or IV nitroprusside) decreases the degree of regurgitation, increases forward cardiac output, and improves symptomatology. Endocarditis prophylaxis is indicated, as is anticoagulation in the presence of atrial fibrillation. Surgical treatment, most commonly valve replacement, is indicated in the presence of symptoms and impairment of LV function. Operation should be carried out *before* development of severe chronic heart failure.

MITRAL VALVE PROLAPSE (MVP)

ETIOLOGY   Most commonly idiopathic; ?familial; may accompany rheumatic fever, ischemic heart disease, atrial septal defect, Marfan's syndrome.

PATHOLOGY   Redundant mitral valve tissue with myxedematous degeneration and elongated chordae tendineae.

CLINICAL MANIFESTATIONS   More common in females. Most pts are asymptomatic and remain so. Most common symptoms are atypical chest pain and a variety of supraventricular and ventricular arrhythmias. Most important complication is severe MR resulting in LV failure. Rarely, systemic emboli from platelet-fibrin deposits on valve. Sudden death is a *very rare* complication.

PHYSICAL EXAM   Mid or late systolic click(s) followed by late systolic murmur; exaggeration by Valsalva maneuver, reduced by squatting and isometric exercise (Chap. 66).

Echocardiogram   Shows posterior displacement of posterior (occasionally anterior) mitral leaflet late in systole.

MANAGEMENT   Asymptomatic pts should be reassured, but if systolic murmur is present, prophylaxis for infective endocarditis is indicated. Valve repair or replacement for pts with severe mitral regurgitation; anticoagulants for pts with history of embolization.

AORTIC STENOSIS (AS)

ETIOLOGY   Often congenital; rheumatic AS is usually associated with rheumatic mitral valve disease. Idiopathic, calcific AS is a degenerative disorder common in the elderly and usually mild.

SYMPTOMS   Dyspnea, angina, and syncope are cardinal symptoms; they occur late, after years of obstruction.

PHYSICAL EXAM   Weak and delayed arterial pulses with carotid thrill. Double apical impulse; A_2 soft or absent; S_4 common. Diamond-shaped systolic murmur $\geq$ grade 3/6, often with systolic thrill.

LABORATORY ECG and CXR   Often show LV hypertrophy, but not useful for predicting gradient.

Echocardiogram   Shows thickening of LV wall, calcification and thickening of aortic valve cusps. Dilatation and reduced shortening of LV indicate poor prognosis. Doppler useful for predicting gradient.

MANAGEMENT   Avoid strenuous activity in asymptomatic phase. Treat heart failure in standard fashion (see Chap. 68), but *avoid afterload reduction*. Valve replacement is indicated in adults with symptoms resulting from AS and hemodynamic evidence of severe obstruction. Operation should be carried out *before* frank failure has developed.

AORTIC REGURGITATION (AR)

ETIOLOGY   Rheumatic in 70%; may also be due to infective endocarditis, syphilis, aortic dissection, or aortic dilatation due to cystic medial necrosis; three-fourths of pts are males.

CLINICAL MANIFESTATIONS   Exertional dyspnea and awareness of heart beat, angina pectoris, and signs of LV failure. Wide pulse pressure, waterhammer pulse, capillary pulsations (Quincke's sign), A_2 soft or absent, S_3 common. Blowing, decrescendo diastolic murmur along left sternal border (along right sternal border with aortic dilatation). May be accompanied by systolic murmur of augmented blood flow.

LABORATORY ECG and CXR   LV enlargement.

Echocardiogram   Increased excursion of posterior LV wall, LA enlargement, LV enlargement, high-frequency fluttering of mitral valve. Doppler studies useful in detection and quantification of AR.

MANAGEMENT   Standard therapy for LV failure (see Chap. 68). Surgical valve replacement should be carried out in pts with severe AR soon after development of symptoms or in asymptomatic pts with LV dysfunction on radionuclide ventriculogram, angiogram, or echocardiogram.

TRICUSPID STENOSIS (TS)

ETIOLOGY   Usually rheumatic; most common in females; almost invariably associated with MS.

CLINICAL MANIFESTATIONS   Hepatomegaly, ascites, edema, jaundice, jugular venous distention with slow y descent (Chap. 66). Diastolic rumbling murmur along left sternal border increased by inspiration with loud presystolic component. Right atrial and superior vena caval enlargement on x-ray.

MANAGEMENT   In severe TS, surgical relief is indicated and usually requires valve replacement.

TRICUSPID REGURGITATION (TR)

ETIOLOGY   Usually functional and secondary to marked RV dilatation of any cause and often associated with pulmonary hypertension.

CLINICAL MANIFESTATIONS   Severe RV failure, with edema, hepatomegaly, and prominent *v* waves in jugular venous pulse with rapid *y* descent (Chap. 66). Systolic murmur along sternal edge is increased by inspiration.

pulsatile

MANAGEMENT   Intensive diuretic therapy. In severe cases (in absence of severe pulmonary hypertension), surgical treatment consists of tricuspid annuloplasty or valve replacement.

For a more detailed discussion, see Braunwald E: Valvular Heart Disease, Chap. 188, in HPIM-12, p. 938

ATRIAL SEPTAL DEFECT (ASD)

HISTORY Usually asymptomatic until third or fourth decades, when exertional dyspnea, fatigue, and palpitations may develop. Symptoms often associated with pulmonary hypertension (see below).

PHYSICAL EXAM Parasternal RV lift, wide fixed splitting of S_2, systolic flow murmur along sternal border, diastolic flow rumble across tricuspid valve, prominent jugular venous v wave.

ECG Incomplete RBBB. LAD common with ostium primum (lower septal) defect.

CXR Increased pulmonary vascular markings, prominence of RV and main pulmonary artery (LA enlargement *not* usually present).

ECHOCARDIOGRAM RA and RV enlargement; Doppler shows abnormal turbulent transatrial flow.

RADIONUCLIDE ANGIOGRAM Noninvasively estimates ratio of pulmonary flow to systemic flow (PF:SF).

MANAGEMENT Dyspnea and palpitations may respond to digitalis and mild diuretic (e.g., hydrochlorothiazide 50 mg/d). An ASD with PF:SF >1.5:1.0 should be surgically repaired. Surgery is contraindicated with significant pulmonary hypertension and PF:SF <1.2:1.0.

VENTRICULAR SEPTAL DEFECT (VSD)

Congenital VSDs may close spontaneously during childhood. Symptoms relate to size of the defect and pulmonary vascular resistance.

HISTORY CHF in infancy. Adults may be asymptomatic or develop fatigue and reduced exercise tolerance.

PHYSICAL EXAM Systolic thrill and holosystolic murmur at lower left sternal border, loud P_2, S_3; flow murmur across mitral valve.

ECG Normal with small defects. Large shunts result in LA and LV enlargement.

CXR Enlargement of main pulmonary artery, LA, and LV, with increased pulmonary vascular markings.

ECHOCARDIOGRAM   LA and LV enlargement; defect may be visualized; Doppler shows high-velocity flow in RV outflow tract, near the defect.

MANAGEMENT   Fatigue and mild dyspnea are treated with digitalis, mild diuretics, and afterload reduction (Chap. 68). Surgical closure is indicated if PF:SF>1.5:1. Antibiotic prophylaxis for endocarditis is important.

PATENT DUCTUS ARTERIOSUS (PDA)

Abnormal communication between the descending aorta and pulmonary artery; associated with birth at high altitudes and maternal rubella.

HISTORY   Asymptomatic or dyspnea on exertion and fatigue.

PHYSICAL EXAM   Hyperactive LV impulse; loud systolic-diastolic "machinery" murmur at upper left sternal border. If pulmonary hypertension develops, diastolic component of the murmur may disappear.

ECG   LV hypertrophy is common; RV hypertrophy with pulmonary hypertension.

CXR   Increased pulmonary vascular markings; enlarged main pulmonary artery, ascending aorta, LV; occasional calcification of ductus.

ECHOCARDIOGRAPHY   Hyperdynamic, enlarged LV; the PDA can often be visualized on 2-dimensional echo; Doppler demonstrates abnormal flow contained within it.

MANAGEMENT   In absence of pulmonary hypertension, PDA should be ligated to prevent infective endocarditis, LV dysfunction, and pulmonary hypertension.

PROGRESSION TO PULMONARY HYPERTENSION (PHT)

Patients with significant, uncorrected ASD, VSD, or PDA may develop progressive, irreversible PHT with shunting of desaturated blood into the arterial circulation (right-to-left shunting). Fatigue, light-headedness, and chest pain due to RV ischemia are common, accompanied by cyanosis, clubbing of digits, loud P$_2$, murmur of pulmonary valve regurgitation, and signs of RV failure. ECG and echocardiogram show RV hypertrophy. Surgical correction of congenital defects contraindicated with severe PHT and right-to-left shunting.

PULMONIC STENOSIS (PS)

A transpulmonary valve gradient <50 mmHg rarely causes symptoms, and progression tends not to occur. Higher gradients result in dyspnea, fatigue, light-headedness, chest pain (RV ischemia).

PHYSICAL EXAM Shows jugular venous distention with prominent *a* wave, RV parasternal impulse, wide splitting of S_2 with soft P_2, ejection click followed by "diamond-shaped" systolic murmur at upper left sternal border, S_4.

ECG RA and RV enlargement in advanced PS.

CXR Often shows poststenotic dilatation of the pulmonary artery and RV enlargement.

ECHOCARDIOGRAPHY RV hypertrophy and "doming" of the pulmonic valve. Doppler accurately measures transvalvular gradient.

TREATMENT Prophylaxis for infective endocarditis is mandatory. Moderate or severe stenosis (gradient >50 mmHg) requires surgical (or balloon) valvuloplasty.

COARCTATION OF THE AORTA

Aortic constriction just distal to the origin of the left subclavian artery is a surgically correctable form of hypertension (Chap. 69). Usually asymptomatic, but it may cause headache, fatigue, or claudication of lower extremities.

PHYSICAL EXAM Hypertension in upper extremities; delayed femoral pulses with decreased pressure in lower extremities. Pulsatile collateral arteries can be palpated in the intercostal spaces. Systolic (and sometimes diastolic) murmur is best heard over the mid-upper back.

ECG LV hypertrophy.

CXR Notching of the ribs due to collateral arteries; "figure 3" appearance of distal aortic arch.

TREATMENT Surgical correction, although hypertension may persist. Antibiotic prophylaxis against endocarditis is required even after correction.

For a more detailed discussion, see Friedman WF, Child JS: Congenital Heart Disease in the Adult, Chap. 186, HPIM-12, p. 923

73 INFECTIVE ENDOCARDITIS

EPIDEMIOLOGY

- Native valve endocarditis: most commonly in males >50 years; 60–80% pts with predisposing cardiac lesion—rheumatic heart disease in 30%, mitral valve > aortic; congenital heart disease in 10–20% pts (e.g., bicuspid aortic valve, pulmonary stenosis, ventricular septal defect, not atrial septal defect); mitral valve prolapse in 10–33% pts; calcific aortic stenosis; asymmetric septal hypertrophy; Marfan's syndrome.
- Endocarditis in IV abusers—tricuspid valve most commonly infected.
- Predisposing conditions may be associated with specific organisms (see Table 73-1).

MANIFESTATIONS

- *Native valve endocarditis:* symptoms—weakness, fatigue, fever, chills, night sweats, painful fingers, toes, or skin lesions; physical exam ± petechiae (mouth, conjunctiva), splinter hemorrhages under nails, erythematous or purple tender nodules on pads of toes or fingers (Osler nodes), retinal hemorrhages with pale centers (Roth spots), non-tender erythematous lesions on palms and soles (Janeway lesions); changes in cardiac murmur, splenomegaly, arthralgias, emboli (fungal emboli to large vessels); mycotic aneurysms in 10%, neurologic manifestations in 33%, heart failure, glomerulonephritis. *Subacute endocarditis*—insidious onset of symptoms, low-grade fever without chills, extracardiac manifestations common. *Acute endocarditis*—abrupt onset, high fever with chills, extracardiac manifestations may be absent (though Janeway lesions most common in acute endocarditis).
- *Right-sided endocarditis:* fever, pleuritic chest pain, dyspnea, malaise over several weeks; murmur may be absent or difficult to detect; pulmonary emboli; increased risk—IV drug addicts, infected venous catheters or pacing wires.
- *Prosthetic valve endocarditis:* symptoms indistinguishable from native valve endocarditis; increased risk of valve ring infection, myocardial abscess, conduction disturbances, valve stenosis secondary to vegetations or new regurgitant murmur from valve dehiscence.

TABLE 73-1

Predisposing condition	Organism	Comment
Dental manipulations	Viridans streptococci	
IV drug addicts	*S. aureus* Group A streptococcus Gram-negative rods *Candida* spp.	Septic phlebitis and septic pulmonary emboli common.
Prosthetic valve recipients:		
<2 months after surgery	*S. epidermidis* Diphtheroids Gram-negative rods *Candida* spp. Enterococcus *S. aureus*	Early-onset infections tend to be resistant to prophylactic antimicrobials administered at surgery.
>2 months after surgery	*Streptococcus* spp. *S. epidermidis* Diphtheroids Enterococcus *S. aureus*	Some low-virulence infections implanted at surgery are slow to develop.
Urinary tract instrumentation or disease	Enterococcus Gram-negative rods	Associated in older men with prostatism and in women with genitourinary tract infections.
Catheter-related phlebitis	*S. aureus* *S. epidermidis* *Candida* spp. Gram-negative rods	An increasingly common source of endocarditis in hospitalized patients.
Colonic lesions	*Streptococcus bovis*	Cancer, villous adenoma, or polyp in >33% of pts.

Modified from Pelletier LL Jr., Petersdorf RG: HPIM-11, p. 972.

LABORATORY FINDINGS

- ↑ WBC usually, normochromic normocytic anemia in subacute, ↑ ESR, proteinuria, microscopic hematuria, ↓ CH_{50} or C3, circulating immune complexes (positive rheumatoid factor).
- Echo: vegetation in up to 80% pts with native valve endocarditis but cannot differentiate active from healed lesions.
- Blood cultures: 3–5 sets of venous blood (arterial not necessary).

TABLE 73-2   Therapy of infective endocarditis caused by gram-positive cocci (regimens A to L)*

Streptococci† with MIC ≤0.1 mg/L (μg/mL) penicillin G

   A: Penicillin G, 10–20 million units/d IV in divided doses q 4 h × 4 weeks *or*

   B: Penicillin as in regimen A plus streptomycin, 7.5 mg/kg IM q 12 h or gentamicin, 1 mg/kg IV q 8 h, both × 2 weeks *or*

   C: Penicillin plus streptomycin or gentamicin × 2 weeks as in regimen B with penicillin continued 2 weeks longer *or*

   D: Cefazolin 1–2 g IV or IM q 6–8 h × 4 weeks *or*

   E: Vancomycin, 15 mg/kg IV q 12 h × 4 weeks

Enterococci, other streptococci with MIC >0.5 mg/L (μg/mL) penicillin G

   F: Penicillin G, 20–30 million units/d or ampicillin, 12 g/d IV in divided doses q 4 h plus gentamicin, 1 mg/kg IV q 8 h or streptomycin 7.5 mg/kg IM q 12 h, both × 4–6 weeks *or*

   G: Vancomycin, 15 mg/kg IV q 12 h plus gentamicin or streptomycin as in regimen F, both × 4–6 weeks

Streptococci other than enterococci with MIC >0.1 but <0.5 mg/L (μg/mL) penicillin G

   H: Use regimen C *or* regimen E if penicillin allergic

Methicillin-susceptible *S. aureus* or *S. epidermidis*

   I: Nafcillin, 2 g IV q 4 h × 4–6 weeks with or without gentamicin, 1 mg/kg IV q 8 h × the first 3–5 d *or*

   J: Cefazolin, 2 g IV q 6 h × 4–6 weeks with or without gentamicin as in regimen I *or*

   K: Vancomycin 15 mg/kg IV q 12 h × 4–6 weeks with or without gentamicin as in regimen I

Methicillin-resistant staphylococci or *Corynebacterium* sp.

   L: Vancomycin with or without gentamicin as in regimen K

Endocarditis on a prosthetic valve

   C but with 20 million units of penicillin qd and a longer duration of penicillin (a total of 6 weeks)

   D × 6 weeks with gentamicin or streptomycin × the first 2 weeks

   E × 6 weeks with gentamicin or streptomycin × the first 2 weeks

   F or G × 6 weeks

   H, but continue penicillin × 6 weeks

   I, J, or K × 6–8 weeks with gentamicin × the first 2 weeks

   L × 6–8 weeks with gentamicin × the first 2 weeks

   In the presence of *S. epidermidis* also add rifampin, 300 mg PO q 8 h × 6–8 weeks. The use of rifampin with *S. aureus* is controversial.

---

* Peak serum concentrations of gentamicin should be about 3 mg/L (μg/mL). Streptomycin peaks should be about 20 mg/L (μg/mL). The maximum dose of vancomycin is 1 g every 12 h.

† For Group A streptococci or *S. pneumoniae* use regimen A.

NOTE: MIC = minimal inhibitory concentration.

Modified from Kaye D: HPIM-12, p. 511.

TREATMENT

• Antibiotic therapy: see Table 73-2.
• Consider surgery in pts with fungal or prosthetic valve endocarditis, persistently positive blood cultures on therapy, recurrent emboli, valve ring or myocardial abscesses, heart failure, large vegetation.

PROPHYLAXIS

• At high risk: congenital (except uncomplicated atrial septal defect) or acquired valvular disease, prosthetic valves, ventriculoseptal patches, prior history of endocarditis; at lower risk—mitral valve prolapse with regurgitation, asymmetrical septal hypertrophy, tricuspid or pulmonary valve lesions. Not cost effective to give prophylaxis to all pts with mitral valve prolapse without systolic murmur for all procedures.
• Optimize oral hygiene in pts at risk, especially prior to implantation of prosthetic valves. For antibiotic regimens, see Table 73-3.

TABLE 73-3   Antimicrobial prophylaxis of endocarditis

Dental, oral, nasal, or other procedures involving or passing through the oropharynx

Low-risk pts:

Recommended:	Penicillin V 2 g PO 1 h before and 1 g PO 6 h after.
Alternative:	Amoxicillin 3 g PO 1 h before only.
Penicillin allergy:	Erythromycin 1 g PO 1 h before and 0.5 g 6 h after.

High-risk pts:

Recommended:	Ampicillin 2 g IV or IM and gentamicin 1.5 mg/kg IM or IV both 30 min before and penicillin V 1 g PO 6 h after.
Penicillin allergy:	Vancomycin 1 g IV over 1 h starting 1 h before.

Gastrointestinal or genitourinary procedures (in general, not for colonoscopy or barium enema)

Recommended:	Ampicillin 2 g IV or IM and gentamicin 1.5 mg/kg IM or IV both 30 min before and penicillin V 1 g PO 6 h after.
Penicillin allergy:	Vancomycin 1 g IV over 1 h starting 1 h before and gentamicin 1.5 mg/kg IV or IM 1 h after.

Low-risk pts with minor procedure:

Recommended:	Amoxicillin 3 g PO 1 h before and 1.5 g 6 h after.

TABLE 73-3   (Continued)

Cardiac surgery (not for coronary artery bypass grafts, transvenous pacemakers, cardiac catheterization)

Recommended:	Cefazolin 2 g IV and gentamicin 1.5 mg/kg IV starting immediately preoperatively; repeat doses q 8 h × 2.
Alternative:	Vancomycin 15 mg/kg IV over 1 h beginning 1 h before and gentamicin 1.5 mg/kg IV before then q 8 h × 2 followed by vancomycin 10 mg/kg at end of operation, then vancomycin 7.5 mg/kg q 6 h × 3 doses.

For a more detailed discussion, see Kaye D: Infective Endocarditis, Chap. 90, in HPIM-12, p. 508

74 ACUTE MYOCARDIAL INFARCTION

Early recognition and immediate treatment of acute MI are essential; diagnosis is based on characteristic history, ECG, and evolution of cardiac enzymes.

SYMPTOMS Chest pain similar to angina (Chap. 2), but more intense and persistent (>30 min); not fully relieved by rest or nitroglycerin, often accompanied by nausea, sweating, apprehension. However, 25% of MIs are clinically silent.

PHYSICAL EXAM Pallor, diaphoresis, tachycardia, S_4, dyskinetic cardiac impulse may be present. If CHF exists: rales, S_3. Jugular venous distention is common in right ventricular infarction.

ECG **Q-wave MI** ST elevation, followed by T-wave inversion, then Q-wave development (Chap. 67) over several hours.

Non-Q-wave MI ST depression followed by persistent ST-T wave changes *without* Q-wave development. Comparison with old ECG helpful.

CARDIAC ENZYMES Time course is important for diagnosis; creatine phosphokinase (CK) level should be checked every 8 h for first day: CK rises within 6–8 h, peaks at 24 h, returns to normal by 36–48 h. CK-MB isoenzyme is more specific for MI. Total CK (but not CK-MB) rises (two- to threefold) after IM injection, vigorous exercise, or other skeletal muscle trauma. CK-MB peaks earlier (about 8 h) following acute reperfusion therapy (see below). LDH peaks at day 3–4 and remains elevated as long as 14 days; LDH_1 isoenzyme is more specific for MI than total LDH.

NONINVASIVE IMAGING TECHNIQUES Useful when diagnosis of MI is not clear. *Thallium 201 scan* after MI shows "cold spot" within a few hours, but cannot distinguish from old infarction. *Echocardiogram* or *radionuclide ventriculogram* is used to characterize wall-motion abnormalities after acute MI. Echo is also useful in detecting RV infarction, LV aneurysm, LV dyskinesis, and LV thrombus.

INITIAL THERAPY

Goal is to relieve pain, minimize extent of infarcted tissue, and to prevent/treat arrhythmias and mechanical complications. Early thrombolytic therapy with streptokinase or tissue plasminogen activator (tPA) can reduce infarct size and mortality and limit left ventricular dysfunction. In appropriate

General selection criteria (with individual exceptions):

- Age < 75–80
- Chest pain < 6 h in duration
- ST elevation ($\geq$ 0.1 mV) in at least 2 leads in anterior, inferior, or lateral distribution

Check for contraindications:

- History of cerebrovascular accident
- Surgery or prolonged CPR within 2 weeks
- Severe hypertension (SBP > 180 or DBP > 100)
- Recent GI bleeding or active peptic ulcer

Thrombolytic drug	Dose
tPA	10 mg bolus, then 50 mg over 1st h, then 20 mg/h × 2 h
Streptokinase	1.5 mU over 1 h (premedication often used: hydrocortisone 100 mg IV plus diphenhydramine 25 mg IV)

Concurrent with thrombolytic therapy, administer:

- Aspirin 80–325 mg then qd
- Heparin 100 U/kg, then constant infusion (~ 1000 U/h) to maintain PTT = 2 × control for 2–5 days

Subsequent coronary arteriography reserved for:

- Spontaneous recurrent angina during hospitalization
- Positive exercise test prior to discharge

FIGURE 74-1 Approach to thrombolytic therapy of patients with acute MI.

candidates (Fig. 74-1) thrombolysis should be initiated as quickly as possible in the emergency room or coronary care unit (CCU); pts treated within 3 h of initial symptoms benefit the most. Complications include bleeding, reperfusion arrhythmias, and, in the case of streptokinase, allergic reactions. Anticoagulation (aspirin and heparin) is begun concurrently with the thrombolytic agent (Fig. 74-1). Subsequent coronary arteriography is reserved for pts with current angina or positive exercise test prior to discharge.

Additional standard treatment (whether or not thrombolytic therapy is administered):

1. Hospitalize in CCU with continuous ECG monitoring.

2. IV line for emergency arrhythmia treatment.

3. Pain control: (a) Morphine sulfate 2–4 mg IV q 5–10 min until pain is relieved or side effects develop [nausea, vomiting, respiratory depression (treat with naloxone 0.4–1.2 mg IV), hypotension (if bradycardic, treat with atropine 0.5 mg IV; otherwise use careful volume infusion)]; (b) nitroglycerin 0.3 mg SL if systolic BP >100 mmHg; for refractory pain: IV nitroglycerin (begin at 10 μg/min, titrate upward to maximum of 200 μg/min, monitoring BP closely); (c) beta-adrenergic antagonists (see below).

4. Oxygen 2–4 L/min by nasal cannula (maintain O_2 saturation >90%).

5. Mild *sedation* (e.g., diazepam 5 mg PO qid).

6. Soft diet and stool softeners (e.g., docusate sodium 100–200 mg/d).

7. Beta-adrenergic blockers (Chap. 69) reduce myocardial O_2 consumption, limit infarct size, and reduce mortality. Especially useful in pts with hypertension, tachycardia, or persistent ischemic pain; contraindications include CHF, systolic BP <95 mmHg, heart rate <50 beats/min, AV block, or history of bronchospasm. Administer IV (e.g., metoprolol 5 mg q 5–10 min to total dose of 15 mg), followed by PO regimen (e.g., metoprolol 25–100 mg bid).

8. Anticoagulation/antiplatelet agents: Pts who receive thrombolytic therapy are begun on heparin and aspirin. In absence of thrombolytic therapy, administer aspirin 80–325 mg qd and low-dose heparin (5000 U SC q 12 h). Full-dose IV heparin (PTT 2 × control) followed by oral anticoagulants is recommended for pts with severe CHF, presence of ventricular thrombus by echocardiogram, or large dyskinetic region in anterior MI. Oral anticoagulants are continued for 3 to 6 months.

COMPLICATIONS

VENTRICULAR ARRHYTHMIAS Isolated ventricular premature beats (VPBs) occur frequently. Precipitating factors should be corrected (hypoxemia, acidosis, hypokalemia, hypercalcemia, hypomagnesemia, CHF, arrhythmogenic drugs). For prophylaxis against serious ventricular arrhythmia, consider prophylactic IV lidocaine (Chap. 70); infusion rate should be lower (1 mg/min) in patients with CHF or liver disease, and in the elderly (>70 years).

More definitive indications for lidocaine: (1) more than 5 isolated VPBs per minute, (2) ventricular couplets or runs of ventricular tachycardia, (3) "R-on-T" VPBs. If lidocaine fails to suppress ventricular ectopy, add IV procainamide, a beta blocker, or bretylium (Chap. 70). Ventricular tachycardia with hemodynamic instability requires immediate cardioversion (Chap. 70).

VENTRICULAR FIBRILLATION VF requires immediate defibrillation (200–400 J). If unsuccessful, initiate CPR and standard resuscitative measures (Chap. 23). Ventricular arrhythmias which appear several days or weeks following MI often reflect pump failure and may warrant invasive electrophysiologic study.

ACCELERATED IDIOVENTRICULAR RHYTHM Wide QRS complex, regular rhythm, rate 60–100 beats/min is common and usually benign; if it causes hypotension, treat with atropine 0.6 mg IV.

Sinus tachycardia may result from CHF, hypoxemia, pain, fever, pericarditis, hypovolemia, administered drugs. If no cause identified, may treat with beta blocker (Table 69-1). For persistent sinus tachycardia (>120), use Swan-Ganz catheter to differentiate CHF from decreased intravascular volume. Other *supraventricular arrhythmias* (paroxysmal supraventricular tachycardia, atrial flutter, and fibrillation) are often secondary to CHF, in which digoxin (Chap. 68) is treatment of choice. In absence of CHF, may also use verapamil or propranolol (Chap. 70). If hemodynamically unstable, proceed with electrical cardioversion.

BRADYARRHYTHMIAS AND AV BLOCK (Chap. 70) In *inferior MI*, usually represent heightened vagal tone or discrete AV nodal ischemia. If hemodynamically compromised (CHF, hypotension, emergence of ventricular arrhythmias), treat with atropine 0.5 mg IV q 5 min (up to 2 mg). If no response, use temporary pacemaker. Isoproterenol should be avoided. In *anterior MI*, AV conduction defects usually reflect extensive tissue necrosis. Consider temporary pacemaker for (1) complete heart block, (2) Mobitz type II block (Chap. 70), (3) new bifascicular block (LBBB, RBBB + left anterior hemiblock, RBBB + left posterior hemiblock), (4) any bradyarrhythmia associated with hypotension or CHF. If a temporary pacemaker is not placed for these conditions, a reliable external temporary pacing device must be available.

CONGESTIVE HEART FAILURE   CHF may result from systolic "pump" dysfunction, increased left ventricular diastolic "stiffness," and/or acute mechanical complications.

Symptoms   Dyspnea, orthopnea, tachycardia.

Examination   Jugular venous distention, S_3 and S_4 gallop, pulmonary rales; systolic murmur if acute mitral regurgitation or ventricular septal defect (VSD) have developed.

Therapy   (Chaps. 25 and 68)   Initial therapy includes diuretics (begin with furosemide 10–20 mg IV), inhaled O_2, and vasodilators, particularly nitrates [PO, topical, or IV (Chap. 68) unless pt is hypotensive (systolic BP <100 mmHg)]; digitalis is usually of little benefit in acute MI unless supraventricular arrhythmias are present. Diuretic, vasodilator, and inotropic therapy best guided by invasive hemodynamic monitoring (Swan-Ganz pulmonary artery catheter, arterial line) particularly in patients with accompanying hypotension (see Table 74-1 and Fig. 74-2). In acute MI, optimal pulmonary capillary wedge pressure (PCW) is 15–20 mmHg; in the absence of hypotension, PCW >20 mmHg is treated with diuretic plus vasodilator therapy [IV nitroglycerin (begin at 10 μg/min) or nitroprusside (begin at 1–2 μg/kg/min)] and titrated to optimize BP, PCW, and systemic vascular resistance (SVR).

$$SVR = \frac{(\text{mean arterial pressure}) - (\text{mean RA pressure}) \times 80}{\text{cardiac output}}$$

Normal SVR = 900–1350 dyn · s/cm⁵. If PCW >20 mmHg and pt is hypotensive (Fig. 74-2), evaluate for VSD or acute mitral regurgitation, add dobutamine (begin at 1–2 μg/kg/min), titrate upward to maximum of 10 μg/kg/min; beware of drug-induced tachycardia or ventricular ectopy.

If CHF improves on parenteral vasodilator therapy, oral therapy follows with ACE inhibitor (captopril or enalapril—Chap. 69) or the combination of nitrates plus hydralazine (Chap. 68).

TABLE 74-1   Indications for Swan-Ganz catheter in acute myocardial infarction

1. Moderate to severe CHF
2. Hypotension not corrected by volume infusion
3. Unexplained sinus tachycardia or tachypnea
4. Suspected acute mitral regurgitation or ventricular septal rupture
5. To manage IV vasodilator therapy

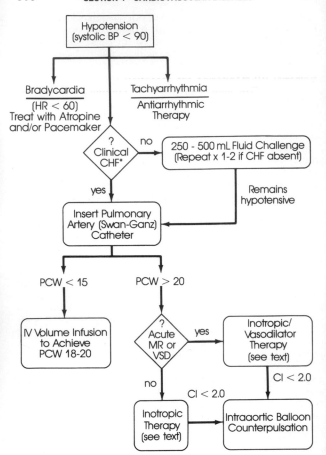

*CHF manifest by pulmonary rales, jugular venous distension

FIGURE 74-2 Approach to hypotension in patients with acute myocardial infarction.

CARDIOGENIC SHOCK Severe LV failure with hypotension (BP <80 mmHg) *and* elevated PCW (>20 mmHg), accompanied by oliguria (<20 mL/h), peripheral vasoconstriction, dulled sensorium, and metabolic acidosis.

Treatment (see Chap. 24) Swan-Ganz catheter and intraarterial BP monitoring are essential; aim for mean PCW of 18–20 mmHg with adjustment of volume (diuretics or infusion) as needed. Intraaortic balloon counterpulsation may be necessary to maintain BP and reduce PCW. Administer high concentration of O_2 by mask; if pulmonary edema coexists, intubation and mechanical ventilation should be considered. Acute mechanical complications (see below) should be sought and promptly treated.

If cardiogenic shock develops within 4 h of first MI symptoms, acute reperfusion [thrombolytic therapy and/or percutaneous coronary angioplasty (PTCA)] may markedly improve LV function.

Hypotension also may result from *RV MI,* which should be suspected in the setting of inferior or posterior MI, if jugular venous distention and elevation of right-heart pressures predominate (rales are typically absent and PCW may be normal); right-sided ECG leads typically show ST elevation, and echocardiography may confirm diagnosis. *Treatment* consists of volume infusion, gauged by PCW and arterial pressure. Noncardiac causes of hypotension should be considered (Fig. 74-2): hypovolemia, acute arrhythmia, or sepsis.

ACUTE MECHANICAL COMPLICATIONS Ventricular septal rupture and acute mitral regurgitation due to papillary muscle ischemia/infarct develop during the first week following MI and are characterized by sudden onset of CHF and new systolic murmur. PCW tracings may show large *v* waves in either condition, but an oxygen "step-up" as catheter is advanced from RA to RV suggests septal rupture. Acute medical therapy of these conditions includes vasodilator therapy (IV nitroprusside: begin at 10 μg/min and titrate to maintain systolic BP ≃ 100 mmHg); intraaortic balloon pump may be required to maintain cardiac output. Surgical correction is postponed for 4–6 weeks after acute MI if pt is stable; surgery should not be deferred if pt is unstable. Acute ventricular free-wall rupture presents with sudden loss of BP, pulse, and consciousness, while ECG shows an intact rhythm; emergent surgical repair is crucial, and mortality is high.

PERICARDITIS Characterized by *pleuritic, positional* pain and pericardial rub (Chap. 76); atrial arrhythmias are common; must be distinguished from recurrent angina. Often responds to aspirin 650 mg PO qid. Anticoagulants should be withheld when pericarditis is suspected.

VENTRICULAR ANEURYSM Localized "bulge" of LV chamber due to infarcted myocardium. *True aneurysms* consist of scar tissue and do not rupture. However, complications include CHF, ventricular arrhythmias, and thrombus formation. Typically, <u>ECG shows persistent ST segment elevation, longer than 2 weeks after initial infarct</u>; aneurysm is confirmed by echocardiography and by left ventriculography. The presence of thrombus within the aneurysm, or a large aneurysmal segment due to anterior MI, warrants oral anticoagulation for 3–6 months.

In contrast, *pseudoaneurysm* is a form of cardiac rupture contained by a local area of pericardium and organized thrombus; direct communication with the left ventricular cavity is present; surgical repair usually necessary to prevent rupture.

RECURRENT ANGINA Usually associated with transient ST-T wave changes; signals high incidence of reinfarction; when it occurs in early post-MI period (2 weeks), proceed directly to coronary arteriography in most pts, to identify those who would benefit from PTCA or coronary artery bypass surgery.

DRESSLER'S SYNDROME Syndrome of fever, pleuritic chest pain, pericardial effusion which may develop 2–6 weeks following acute MI; pain and ECG characteristic of pericarditis (Chap. 76); usually responds to aspirin or NSAIDs. Reserve glucocorticoid therapy (prednisone 1 mg/kg PO qd) for those with severe, refractory pain.

SECONDARY PREVENTION

Submaximal exercise testing should be performed prior to, or soon after discharge. A positive test (Chap. 75) suggests need for cardiac catheterization to evaluate myocardium at risk of recurrent infarction. *Beta blockers* (e.g., timolol 10 mg bid, metoprolol 25–100 mg bid) should be prescribed routinely commencing 7–14 days following acute MI (Table 69-1), unless contraindication present (asthma, CHF, bradycardia, "brittle" diabetes). Diltiazem (Chap. 69) may reduce infarct extension following non-Q-wave MI if LV function is not impaired. Aspirin (80–325 mg/d) is administered to reduce incidence of subsequent infarction, unless contraindicated (e.g., active peptic ulcer, allergy).

Modification of cardiac risk factors must be encouraged: discontinue smoking; control hypertension, diabetes, and serum lipids (Chap. 152); and pursue graduated exercise.

For a more detailed discussion, see Pasternak RC, Braunwald E: Acute Myocardial Infarction, Chap. 189, in HPIM-12, p. 953

75 CHRONIC CORONARY ARTERY DISEASE

Angina pectoris, the most common clinical manifestation of CAD, results from an imbalance between myocardial O_2 supply and demand, most commonly resulting from atherosclerotic coronary artery obstruction. Other major conditions that upset this balance and result in angina include aortic valve disease (Chap. 71), hypertrophic cardiomyopathy (Chap. 77), and coronary artery spasm (see below).

SYMPTOMS Angina is typically associated with exertion or emotional upset; relieved quickly by rest or nitroglycerin (TNG) (see Chap. 2). Major risk factors are cigarette smoking, hypertension, hypercholesterolemia (↑ LDL fraction; ↓ HDL), diabetes, and family history of CAD below age 55.

PHYSICAL EXAM Often normal; arterial bruits or retinal vascular abnormalities suggest generalized atherosclerosis; S_4 is common. During acute anginal episode other signs may appear: loud S_3 or S_4, diaphoresis, rales, and a transient murmur of mitral regurgitation due to papillary muscle ischemia.

ECG May be normal between anginal episodes or show old infarction (Chap. 67). During angina, ST- and T-wave abnormalities typically appear (ST-segment depression reflects subendocardial ischemia; ST-segment elevation may reflect acute infarction or transient coronary artery spasm). Ventricular arrhythmias frequently accompany acute ischemia.

STRESS TESTING Enhances diagnosis of CAD. Exercise is performed on treadmill or bicycle until target heart rate is achieved or pt becomes symptomatic (chest pain, lightheadedness, hypotension, marked dyspnea, ventricular tachycardia) or develops diagnostic ST-segment changes. Useful information includes duration of exercise achieved; peak heart rate and BP; depth, morphology, and persistence of ST-segment depression; and whether and at which level of exercise pain, hypotension, or ventricular arrhythmias develop. *Thallium 201* imaging increases sensitivity and specificity and is particularly useful if baseline ECG abnormalities prevent interpretation of test (e.g., LBBB). *Note:* Exercise testing should not be performed in pts with acute MI, unstable angina, or severe aortic stenosis.

Some pts do not experience chest pain during ischemic episodes with exertion ("silent ischemia"), but are identified by transient ST-T wave abnormalities during stress testing or Holter monitoring (see below).

CORONARY ARTERIOGRAPHY The definitive test for assessing severity of CAD; major indications are (1) angina refractory to medical therapy; (2) markedly positive exercise test ($\geq$2-mm ST-segment depression, or hypotension with exercise) suggestive of left main or three-vessel disease; (3) recurrent angina or positive exercise test after MI; (4) to assess for coronary artery spasm; (5) to evaluate pts with perplexing chest pain in whom noninvasive tests are not diagnostic.

MANAGEMENT

GENERAL

- Identify and treat risk factors: mandatory cessation of smoking, treatment of diabetes, hypertension, and lipid disorders (Chap. 152).
- Correct exacerbating factors contributing to angina: marked obesity, CHF, anemia, hyperthyroidism.
- Reassurance and pt education.

DRUG THERAPY Sublingual nitroglycerin (TNG 0.3–0.6 mg); may be repeated at 5-min intervals; warn pts of possible headache or light-headedness; teach prophylactic use of TNG prior to activity that regularly evokes angina. If chest pain persists for more than 10 min despite 2–3 TNG, pt should report promptly to nearest medical facility for evaluation of possible unstable angina or acute MI.

LONG-TERM ANGINA SUPPRESSION Three classes of drugs are used, frequently in combination:

Long-acting nitrates May be administered by many routes (Table 75-1); start at the lowest dose to limit tolerance and side effects of headache, light-headedness, tachycardia.

Beta blockers (Table 69-1) All have antianginal properties; β_1-selective agents are less likely to exacerbate airway or peripheral vascular disease. Dosage should be titrated to resting heart rate of 50–60 beats/min. *Contraindications* to

TABLE 75-1 **Examples of long-acting nitrate preparations**

Drug	Dosage
Isosorbide dinitrate	
Oral	10–60 mg tid-qid
Sublingual	5–20 mg q 3 h
Long-acting oral tembid	40–80 mg PO bid-qid
Nitroglycerin skin ointment	0.5–2.0 in qid
Transdermal nitroglycerin patch*	5–25 mg per day

* Removal at bedtime may prevent nitrate tolerance.

beta blockers include CHF, AV block, bronchospasm, "brittle" diabetes. Side effects include fatigue, bronchospasm, depressed LV function, impotence, depression, and masking of hypoglycemia in diabetics.

Calcium antagonists (Table 69-3)   Useful for stable and unstable angina, as well as coronary vasospasm. Combination with other antianginal agents is beneficial, but verapamil should be administered very cautiously or not at all to pts on beta blockers or disopyramide (additive effects on LV dysfunction).

Aspirin   80–325 mg/d may reduce the incidence of MI and is recommended in pts with CAD in absence of contraindications.

MECHANICAL REVASCULARIZATION   Percutaneous coronary angioplasty (PTCA)   Performed on anatomically suitable stenoses of native vessels and bypass grafts; pts should generally be sufficiently symptomatic to warrant consideration of bypass surgery. Initial relief of angina occurs in 85–90% of pts; however, stenosis recurs in 25–40% within 6 months (more commonly in pt with initial unstable angina or incomplete dilation). If restenosis occurs, PTCA can be repeated with similar success and risks as original procedure. Potential complications include dissection or thrombosis of the vessel and uncontrolled ischemia or CHF. Complications are most likely to occur in pts with CHF, long eccentric stenoses, calcified plaque, female gender, and dilation of an artery that perfuses a large segment of myocardium with inadquate collaterals. PTCA has also been successful in some pts with recent *total* coronary occlusion (<3 months).

Coronary artery bypass surgery (CABG)   For angina refractory to medical therapy or when the latter is not tolerated (and when lesions are not amenable to PTCA) or if severe CAD is present (left main, three-vessel disease with impaired LV function).

UNSTABLE AGINA

Includes (1) new onset (<2 months) of severe angina, (2) angina at rest or with minimal activity, (3) recent increases in frequency and intensity of chronic angina, (4) recurrent angina within several days of acute MI without reelevation of cardiac enzymes.

MANAGEMENT

- Admit to continuous ECG-monitored floor.   *S-T elev*
- Identify and treat exacerbating factors (hypertension, arrhythmias, CHF, acute infection).
- Rule out MI by ECG and cardiac enzymes.

stable - angina — ST depression

- Maximize therapy with oral nitrates, beta blockers, calcium antagonists.
- For refractory pain: IV TNG (begin at 5 μg/min); titrate dosage to maintain systolic BP ≥100 mmHg.
- Anticoagulation: IV heparin (aim for PTT 2× control) × 3–5 d; then aspirin 325 mg/d.
- Refractory unstable angina warrants coronary arteriography and possible PTCA or CABG. If symptoms are controlled on medical therapy, a predischarge exercise test should be performed to assess need for coronary arteriography.

CORONARY VASOSPASM

Caused by intermittent focal spasm of a coronary artery; often associated with atherosclerotic lesion near site of spasm. Chest discomfort is similar to angina but more severe and occurs typically at rest, with transient ST-segment elevation. Acute infarction or malignant arrhythmias may develop during spasm-induced ischemia. Evaluation includes observation of ECG (or ambulatory Holter monitor) for transient ST elevation; diagnosis confirmed at coronary angiography using provocative IV ergonovine testing. *Treatment* consists of long-acting nitrates and calcium antagonists. Prognosis is better in pts with anatomically normal coronary arteries compared to those with fixed coronary stenoses.

SILENT ISCHEMIA

Myocardial ischemia that develops without anginal symptoms; detected by Holter monitoring or exercise electrocardiography; occurs mainly in pts who also have *symptomatic* ischemia, but is sometimes demonstrated in totally asymptomatic individuals. *Management* is guided by exercise electrocardiography, often with thallium 201, to assess severity of myocardial ischemia. Pts with evidence of severe silent ischemia are candidates for coronary arteriography. It has *not* been demonstrated that pts with silent ischemia without marked abnormalities on exercise testing require chronic antiischemic therapy.

For a more detailed discussion, see Selwyn AP, Braunwald E: Ischemic Heart Disease, Chap. 190, in HPIM-12, p. 964

ACUTE PERICARDITIS (Table 76-1)

HISTORY   Chest pain, which may be intense, mimicking acute MI, but characteristically sharp, pleuritic, and positional (relieved by leaning forward); fever and palpitations are common.

PHYSICAL EXAM   Rapid or irregular pulse, coarse pericardial friction rub, which may vary in intensity and is loudest with pt sitting forward.

ECG (Table 76-2)   Diffuse ST elevation (concave upwards) usually present in all leads except aVR and V_1; PR-segment depression may be present; *days* later (unlike acute MI) ST returns to baseline and T-wave inversion develops. Atrial premature beats and atrial fibrillation may appear.

CXR   Increased size of cardiac silhouette if large (>250 mL) pericardial effusion present, with "water bottle" configuration.

ECHOCARDIOGRAM   Most sensitive test for detection of pericardial effusion, which commonly accompanies acute pericarditis.

TREATMENT   Aspirin 650–975 mg qid or NSAIDs; for *severe, refractory* pain, prednisone 40–60 mg/d is used and tapered over several weeks or months. Intractable, prolonged pain or frequently recurrent episodes may require pericardiectomy. Anticoagulants are relatively contraindicated in acute pericarditis because of risk of pericardial hemorrhage.

CARDIAC TAMPONADE

Life-threatening emergency resulting from accumulation of pericardial fluid under pressure; impaired filling of cardiac chambers and decreased cardiac output.

TABLE 76-1   Most common causes of pericarditis

Idiopathic
Infections (particularly viral)
Acute myocardial infarction
Metastatic neoplasm
Radiation therapy for tumor (up to 20 years earlier)
Chronic renal failure
Connective-tissue disease (rheumatoid arthritis, SLE)
Drug reaction (e.g., procainamide, hydralazine)
"Autoimmune" following heart surgery or myocardial infarction (several weeks/months later) *Dressler's syndrome*

TABLE 76-2   ECG in acute pericarditis vs. acute (Q-wave) MI

ST segment elevation	ECG lead involvement	Evolution of ST and T waves	PR segment depression
PERICARDITIS			
Concave upward	All leads involved except aVR and V_1	ST remains elevated for several days; after ST returns to baseline, T waves invert	Yes, in majority
ACUTE MI			
Convex upward	ST elevation over infarcted region only; reciprocal ST depression in opposite leads	T waves invert within hours, while ST still elevated; followed by Q wave development	No

ETIOLOGY   Previous pericarditis (most commonly metastatic tumor, uremia, acute MI, viral or idiopathic pericarditis), cardiac trauma, or myocardial perforation during catheter or pacemaker placement.

HISTORY   Hypotension may develop suddenly; subacute symptoms include dyspnea, weakness, confusion.

PHYSICAL EXAM   Tachycardia, hypotension, pulsus paradoxus (inspiratory fall in systolic blood pressure >10 mmHg), jugular venous distention with preserved x descent, but loss of y descent; heart sounds distant. If tamponade develops subacutely, peripheral edema, hepatomegaly, and ascites are frequently present.

ECG   Low limb lead voltage; large effusions may cause electrical alternans (alternating size of QRS complex due to swinging of heart).

CXR   Enlarged cardiac silhouette if large effusion present.

ECHOCARDIOGRAM   Swinging motion of heart within large effusion; prominent respiratory alteration of RV dimension with RA and RV collapse during diastole.

CARDIAC CATHETERIZATION   Confirms diagnosis; shows equalization of diastolic pressures in all four chambers; pericardial = RA pressure.

TREATMENT   Immediate pericardiocentesis and IV volume expansion.

CONSTRICTIVE PERICARDITIS

Rigid pericardium leads to impaired cardiac filling, elevation of systemic and pulmonary venous pressures, and decreased cardiac output. Results from healing and scar formation in some pts with previous pericarditis. Viral, tuberculosis, previous cardiac surgery, uremia, neoplastic pericarditis are most common etiologies.

HISTORY   Gradual onset of dyspnea, fatigue, pedal edema, abdominal swelling; symptoms of LV failure uncommon.

PHYSICAL EXAM   Tachycardia, jugular venous distention (prominent y descent) which increases further in inspiration (Kussmaul's sign); hepatomegaly, ascites, peripheral edema are common; sharp diastolic sound, "pericardial knock," following S_2 sometimes present.

ECG   Low limb lead voltage; atrial arrhythmias are common.

CXR   Rim of pericardial calcification in 50% of pts.

ECHOCARDIOGRAM   Thickened pericardium, normal ventricular contraction.

CT or MRI   More precise than echocardiogram in demonstrating thickened pericardium.

CARDIAC CATHETERIZATION   Equalization of diastolic pressures in all chambers; ventricular pressure tracings show "dip and plateau" appearance (to distinguish from restrictive cardiomyopathy; see Table 77-1). Patients with constrictive pericarditis should be investigated for tuberculosis.

TREATMENT   Surgical stripping of the pericardium. Progressive improvement ensues over several months.

APPROACH TO PATIENT WITH ASYMPTOMATIC PERICARDIAL EFFUSION OF UNKNOWN CAUSE

If careful history and physical exam do not suggest etiology, the following may lead to diagnosis:

- Skin test and cultures for tuberculosis (Chap. 50)
- Serum albumin and urine protein measurement (nephrotic syndrome)
- Serum creatinine and BUN (renal failure)
- Thyroid function tests (myxedema)
- ANA (SLE and other collagen-vascular disease)
- Search for a primary tumor (especially lung and breast)

For a more detailed discussion, see Braunwald E: Pericardial Disease, Chap. 193, in HPIM-12, p. 980

77 CARDIOMYOPATHIES AND MYOCARDITIS

DILATED CARDIOMYOPATHY (CMP)

Symmetrically dilated left ventricle (LV), with poor systolic contractile function; right ventricle (RV) commonly involved.

ETIOLOGY Previous myocarditis or "idiopathic" most common; also toxins (ethanol, doxorubicin), connective tissue disorders, muscular dystrophies,"peripartum." Severe coronary disease/infarctions or chronic aortic/mitral regurgitation may behave similarly.

SYMPTOMS Congestive heart failure (Chap. 68); advanced arrhythmias and peripheral emboli from left ventricular mural thrombus occur.

PHYSICAL EXAM Jugular venous distention (JVD), rales, diffuse and dyskinetic LV apex, S_3, hepatomegaly, peripheral edema; murmurs of mitral and tricuspid regurgitation are common.

LABORATORY ECG Left bundle-branch block and ST-T-wave abnormalities common.

CXR Cardiomegaly, pulmonary vascular redistribution, pulmonary effusions common.

Echocardiogram LV and RV enlargement with globally impaired contraction. *Regional* wall motion abnormalities suggest coronary artery disease rather than primary cardiomyopathy.

TREATMENT Standard therapy of CHF (Chap. 68); vasodilator therapy with ACE inhibitor or hydralazine-nitrate combination shown to improve longevity; chronic anticoagulation with warfarin, if no contraindications; antiarrhythmic drugs (Chap. 70) for symptomatic or sustained arrhythmias (guided by invasive electrophysiologic study). Possible trial of immunosuppressive drugs, if active myocarditis present on RV biopsy (controversial). In select patients, consider cardiac transplantation.

RESTRICTIVE CARDIOMYOPATHY

Increased myocardial "stiffness" impairs ventricular relaxation; diastolic ventricular pressures are elevated. Etiologies include infiltrative disease (amyloid, sarcoid, hemochromatosis, eosinophilic disorders), myocardial fibrosis, and fibroelastosis.

SYMPTOMS   Are of CHF, although right-sided heart failure often predominates with peripheral edema and ascites.

PHYSICAL EXAM   Signs of right-sided heart failure: JVD, hepatomegaly, peripheral edema, murmur of tricuspid regurgitation. Left-sided signs also may be present.

LABORATORY   ECG   Low limb lead voltage, sinus tachycardia, ST-T-wave abnormalities.

CXR   Mild LV enlargement.

Echocardiogram   Bilateral atrial enlargement; increased ventricular thickness ("speckled pattern") in infiltrative disease, especially amyloidosis. Systolic function is usually normal, but may be mildly reduced.

Cardiac catheterization   Increased LV and RV diastolic pressures with "dip and plateau" pattern; RV biopsy useful in detecting infiltrative disease (rectal biopsy useful in diagnosis of amyloidosis).

Note: Must distinguish restrictive cardiomyopathy from constrictive pericarditis, which is surgically correctable (see Table 77-1).

TREATMENT

- Salt restriction and diuretics for pulmonary and systemic congestion; digitalis is not indicated unless systolic function impaired or atrial arrhythmias present. *Note:* Increased sensitivity to digitalis in amyloidosis.
- Anticoagulation, particularly in patients with eosinophilic endomyocarditis.
- For specific therapy of hemochromatosis see HPIM-12, Chap. 327, and sarcoidosis see HPIM-12, Chap. 277.

TABLE 77-1   Restrictive cardiomyopathy vs. constrictive pericarditis

	Constrictive pericarditis	Restrictive cardiomyopathy
Prominent palpable cardiac apex	No	Often present
Cardiac size	Normal	May be enlarged
S_3, S_4	Absent (pericardial knock possible)	Often present
Calcification of pericardium on x-ray	Frequent	Absent
Systolic function	Normal	May be depressed
"Dip and plateau"	Yes	Yes
LV vs. RV diastolic pressure	Equal	LV usually higher
RV biopsy	Normal	Abnormal: may show infiltrative disease

HYPERTROPHIC OBSTRUCTIVE CARDIOMYOPATHY (HOCM)

Marked LV hypertrophy; often asymmetric, without underlying cause. Systolic function is normal; increased LV stiffness results in elevated diastolic filling pressures.

SYMPTOMS   Secondary to elevated diastolic pressure, dynamic LV outflow obstruction, and arrhythmias; dyspnea on exertion, angina, and presyncope; sudden death may occur.

PHYSICAL EXAM   Brisk carotid upstroke with pulsus bisferiens; S_4, harsh systolic murmur along left sternal border, blowing murmur of mitral regurgitation at apex; murmur changes with Valsalva and other maneuvers (see Chap. 66).

LABORATORY   ECG   LV hypertrophy with prominent "septal" Q waves in leads I, aVL, V_{5-6}. Periods of atrial fibrillation or ventricular tachycardia are often detected by Holter monitor.

Echocardiogram   LV hypertrophy, asymmetrical septal hypertrophy (ASH) and $\geq 1.3 \times$ thickness of LV posterior wall; LV contractile function excellent with small end-systolic volume. If LV outflow tract obstruction is present, systolic anterior motion (SAM) of mitral valve and midsystolic partial closure of aortic valve are present. Doppler shows early systolic accelerated blood flow through LV outflow tract. Carotid pulse tracing shows "spike and dome" configuration.

TREATMENT   Strenuous exercise should be avoided. Beta blockers, verapamil, or disopyramide used individually to reduce symptoms. Digoxin, other inotropes, diuretics, and vasodilators are *contraindicated*. Endocarditis antibiotic prophylaxis (Chap. 73) is necessary when outflow obstruction or mitral regurgitation is present. Antiarrhythmic agents, especially amiodarone, may suppress atrial and ventricular arrhythmias. Surgical myectomy in patients refractory to medical therapy.

Table 77-2 summarizes distinguishing features of the cardiomyopathies.

MYOCARDITIS

Inflammation of the myocardium most commonly due to acute viral infection; may progress to chronic dilated cardiomyopathy.

HISTORY   Fever, fatigue, palpitations; if LV dysfunction is present, then symptoms of CHF are present. Viral myocarditis may be preceded by URI.

PHYSICAL EXAM   Fever, tachycardia, soft S_1; S_3 common.

LABORATORY   CK-MB isoenzyme may be elevated in absence of MI. Convalescent antiviral antibody titers may rise.

ABLE 77-2 Characteristics of the cardiomyopathies

Dilated	Restrictive	Hypertrophic
ENTRICULAR CHARACTERISTICS		
V (and usually RV) chamber dilatation	Impaired relaxation (reduced compliance); often due to ventricular infiltration	Marked hypertrophy, often asymmetric with septal thickness > LV free wall
PHYSICAL EXAM		
Dyskinetic LV apex with biventricular CHF: rales, S_3, JVD, peripheral edema; may have murmurs of mitral and tricuspid regurgitation	Predominant right-sided CHF: JVD, hepatomegaly, peripheral edema	Brisk carotid upstroke; prominent S_4, harsh systolic murmur at left sternal border plus apical murmur of mitral regurgitation
CHEST X-RAY		
4-chamber cardiac enlargement; pulmonary vascular redistribution	Mild cardiac enlargement	Mild cardiac enlargement
ECHOCARDIOGRAM		
Ventricular dilatation and global contractile impairment	Systolic function usually normal or mildly decreased; increased ventricular wall thickness in infiltrative disease; marked biatrial enlargement typical	Left ventricular hypertrophy, often asymmetric (septal thickness ≥1.3 × LV free wall); systolic anterior motion of mitral valve; mitral regurgitation and outflow gradient by Doppler

ECG Transient ST-T-wave abnormalities.

CXR Cardiomegaly.

Echocardiogram Depressed LV function; pericardial effusion present if accompanying pericarditis present.

TREATMENT Rest; treat as CHF (Chap. 68); immunosuppressive therapy (steroids and azathioprine) may be considered if RV biopsy shows active inflammation. This treatment is experimental, and should not be given early in the course.

For a more detailed discussion, see Wynne J, Braunwald E: The Cardiomyopathies and Myocarditides, Chap. 192, in HPIM-12, p. 975

78 DISEASES OF THE AORTA

AORTIC ANEURYSM

Abnormal widening of the abdominal or thoracic aorta; in ascending aorta most commonly secondary to cystic medial necrosis or atherosclerosis; aneurysms of descending thoracic and abdominal aorta are primarily atherosclerotic.

HISTORY May be clinically silent, but thoracic aortic aneurysms often result in deep, diffuse chest pain, dysphagia, hoarseness, hemoptysis, dry cough; abdominal aneurysms result in abdominal pain or thromboemboli to the lower extremities.

PHYSICAL EXAM Abdominal aneurysms are often palpable, most commonly in periumbilical area. Patients with ascending thoracic aneurysms may show features of Marfan's syndrome (see HPIM-12, Chap. 333).

LABORATORY CXR Enlarged aortic silhouette (thoracic aneurysm); confirm abdominal aneurysm by *abdominal plain film* (rim of calcification), *ultrasound, CT scan,* or *MRI.* Contrast aortography is performed preoperatively. If clinically suspected, obtain serologic test for syphilis, especially if ascending thoracic aneurysm shows thin shell of calcification.

TREATMENT Control of hypertension (Chap. 69) is essential. Surgical resection of aortic aneurysms >6 cm in diameter, for persistent pain despite BP control, or for evidence of rapid expansion.

AORTIC DISSECTION (Fig. 78-1)

Potentially life-threatening condition in which disruption of aortic intima allows dissection of blood into vessel wall; may involve ascending aorta (type II), descending aorta (type III) or both (type I). Alternative classification: Type A—dissection involves ascending aorta; type B—limited to descending aorta. Involvement of the ascending aorta is most lethal form.

ETIOLOGY Ascending aortic dissection associated with hypertension, cystic medial necrosis, Marfan's syndrome (see HPIM-12, Chap. 333); descending dissections commonly associated with atherosclerosis or hypertension. Incidence is increased in pts with coarctation of aorta, bicuspid aortic valve, and rarely in third trimester of pregnancy in otherwise normal women.

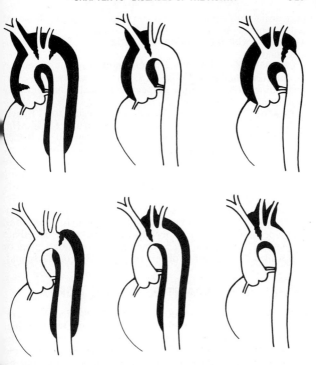

FIGURE 78-1   Classification of aortic dissections. Stanford classification: Top panels illustrate type A dissections that involve the ascending aorta independent of site of tear and distal extension; type B dissections (bottom panels) involve transverse and/or descending aorta without involvement of the ascending aorta. DeBakey classification: Type I dissection involves ascending to descending aorta (top left); type II dissection is limited to ascending or transverse aorta, without descending aorta (top center + top right); type III dissection involves descending aorta only (bottom left). *(From DC Miller, in RM Doroghazi, EE Slater (eds). Aortic Dissection. New York, McGraw-Hill, 1983, with permission.)*

SYMPTOMS   Sudden onset of severe anterior or posterior chest pain, with "ripping" quality; maximal pain may travel if dissection propagates. Additional symptoms relate to obstruction of aortic branches (stroke, MI), dyspnea (acute aortic regurgitation), or symptoms of low cardiac output due to cardiac tamponade (dissection into pericardial sac).

PHYSICAL EXAM   Sinus tachycardia common; if cardiac tamponade develops, hypotension, pulsus paradoxus, and pericardial rub appear. Asymmetry of carotid or brachial pulses, aortic regurgitation, and neurologic abnormalities associated with interruption of carotid artery flow are common findings.

LABORATORY   CXR   Widening of mediastinum; dissection can be confirmed by *CT scan, MRI,* or *ultrasound.* However, once dissection is strongly suspected clinically, aortography is indicated.

TREATMENT   Reduce cardiac contractility and treat hypertension to maintain systolic BP between 100 and 120 mmHg, using IV agents (Table 78-1), e.g., sodium nitroprusside accompanied by a beta blocker (or reserpine), followed by oral therapy. Direct vasodilators (hydralazine, diazoxide) are contraindicated as they may increase shear stress. Ascending aortic dissection (type A) requires surgical repair emergently or, if pt can be stabilized with medications, semielectively. Descending aortic dissections are stabilized medically (maintain systolic BP between 110 and 120 mmHg) with oral antihypertensive agents (especially beta blockers); immediate surgical repair is not necessary unless continued pain or extension of dissection is observed (serial MRI or CT scans).

OTHER ABNORMALITIES OF THE AORTA

ATHEROSCLEROSIS OF ABDOMINAL AORTA   Particularly common in presence of diabetes mellitus or cigarette smoking. Symptoms include intermittent claudication of the buttocks and thighs and impotence (Leriche syndrome); femoral and other distal pulses are absent. Diagnosis is established by

TABLE 78-1   Treatment of aortic dissection

Drug	Dose
PREFERRED REGIMEN	
Sodium nitroprusside *plus*	20–400 μg/min IV
A beta blocker:	
Propranolol *or*	0.5 mg IV; then 1 mg q 5 min, to total of 0.15 mg/kg
Esmolol	500 μg/kg IV over 1 min; then 50–200 μg/kg/min
Or (if beta blocker contraindicated):	
Reserpine	1–2 mg IM q 4–6 h
ALTERNATE REGIMENS	
Trimethaphan camsylate *or*	2 mg/min IV; then titrate to BP
Labetolol	1–2 mg/min IV

noninvasive leg pressure measurements and Doppler velocity analysis, and confirmed by aortography. Aortic-femoral bypass surgery is required for symptomatic treatment.

TAKAYASU'S ("PULSELESS") DISEASE   Arteritis of aorta and major branches in young women. Anorexia, weight loss, fever, and night sweats occur. Localized symptoms relate to occlusion of aortic branches (cerebral ischemia, claudication, and loss of pulses in arms). ESR is increased; diagnosis confirmed by aortography. Glucocorticoid and immunosuppressive therapy may be beneficial, but mortality is high.

For a more detailed discussion, see Dzau VJ, Creager MA: Diseases of the Aorta, Chap. 197, in HPIM-12, p. 1015

---

79 PERIPHERAL VASCULAR DISEASE

Occlusive or inflammatory disease that develops within the peripheral arteries, veins, or lymphatics.

ARTERIOSCLEROSIS OF PERIPHERAL ARTERIES

HISTORY *Intermittent claudication* is muscular cramping with exercise; quickly relieved by rest. Pain in buttocks and thighs suggests aortoiliac disease; calf muscle pain implies femoral or popliteal artery disease. More advanced arteriosclerotic obstruction results in pain at rest; painful ulcers of the feet (painless in diabetics) may result.

PHYSICAL EXAM Decreased peripheral pulses, blanching of affected limb with elevation, dependent rubor (redness). Ischemic ulcers or gangrene of toes may be present.

LABORATORY Doppler ultrasound of peripheral pulses before and during exercise localizes stenoses; contrast arteriography performed only if reconstructive surgery is planned.

TREATMENT Most pts can be managed medically with daily exercise program, careful foot care (especially in diabetics), low-cholesterol/low-saturated-fat diet, and local debridement of ulcerations. Abstinence from cigarettes is mandatory. Patients with severe claudication, rest pain, or gangrene are candidates for arterial reconstructive surgery; percutaneous transluminal angioplasty can be performed in selected pts.

Other conditions that impair peripheral arterial flow:

1. Arterial embolism: Due to thrombus or vegetation within the heart or aorta or paradoxically from a venous thrombus through a right-to-left intracardiac shunt. *History:* sudden pain or numbness in an extremity in absence of previous history of claudication. *Physical exam:* absent pulse, pallor and decreased temperature of limb distal to the occlusion. Lesion is identified by angiography and requires immediate anticoagulation and surgical embolectomy.

2. Vasospastic disorders: Manifest by Raynaud's phenomenon in which cold exposure results in triphasic color response: blanching of the fingers, followed by cyanosis, then redness. Usually a benign disorder. However, suspect an underlying disease (e.g., scleroderma) if tissue necrosis occurs, if disease is unilateral, or if it develops after age 50. *Treatment:* keep extremities warm; calcium channel blockers (nifedipine 10–40 mg PO tid-qid) may be effective.

3. *Thromboangiitis obliterans (Buerger's disease):* Occurs in young men who are heavy smokers and involves both upper and lower extremities; nonatheromatous inflammatory reaction develops in veins and small arteries leading to superficial thrombophlebitis and arterial obstruction with ulceration or gangrene of digits. Abstinence from tobacco is essential.

VENOUS OCCLUSION

SUPERFICIAL THROMBOPHLEBITIS Benign disorder characterized by erythema, tenderness, and edema along involved vein. Conservative therapy includes local heat, elevation, and antiinflammatory drugs such as aspirin. More serious conditions such as cellulitis or lymphangitis may mimic this, but these are associated with fever, chills, lymphadenopathy, and red superficial streaks along inflamed lymphatic channels.

DEEP VENOUS THROMBOSIS (DVT) More serious condition that may lead to pulmonary embolism (Chap. 85). Particularly common in pts on prolonged bed rest, those with chronic debilitating disease, and those with malignancies (Table 79-1).

History Pain or tenderness in calf or thigh, usually unilateral; may be asymptomatic, with pulmonary embolism as primary presentation.

Physical exam Often normal; local swelling or tenderness to deep palpation may be present over affected vein.

TABLE 79-1 Conditions associated with an increased risk for development of venous thrombosis

Surgery
  Orthopedic, thoracic, abdominal, and genitourinary procedures
Neoplasms
  Pancreas, lung, ovary, testes, urinary tract, breast, stomach
Trauma
  Fractures of spine, pelvis, femur, tibia
Immobilization
  Acute myocardial infarction, congestive heart failure, stroke, postoperative convalescence
Pregnancy
Estrogen use (for replacement or contraception)
Hypercoagulable states
  Deficiencies of antithrombin III, protein C, or protein S; circulating lupus anticoagulant; myeloproliferative disease; dysfibrinogenemia; disseminated intravascular coagulation
Venulitis
  Thromboangiitis obliterans, Behçet's disease, homocysteinuria
Previous deep vein thrombosis

Laboratory Noninvasive impedance plethysmography, ultrasound, and Doppler are useful in detecting DVT; definitive diagnosis is made by peripheral venography.

Treatment Systemic anticoagulation with heparin (5000 to 10,000 U bolus, followed by continuous IV infusion to maintain PTT at 2 × normal) for 7–10 days, followed by warfarin PO (for at least 3 months if proximal deep veins involved).

DVT can be prevented by early ambulation following surgery or with low-dose heparin during prolonged bed rest (5000 U SC bid-tid), supplemented by pneumatic compression boots. Following knee or hip surgery, warfarin (PTT to 1.5 × control) is most effective regimen.

LYMPHEDEMA

Chronic, painless edema, usually of the lower extremities; may be primary (inherited) or secondary to lymphatic damage or obstruction (e.g., recurrent lymphangitis, tumor, filariasis).

PHYSICAL EXAM Marked pitting edema in early stages; limb becomes indurated with *non*pitting edema chronically. Differentiate from chronic *venous* insufficiency, which displays hyperpigmentation, stasis dermatitis, and superficial venous varicosities.

LABORATORY Abdominal and pelvic ultrasound or CT to identify obstructing lesions. Lymphangiography or lymphoscintigraphy (rarely done) to confirm diagnosis. If *unilateral* edema, differentiate from DVT by noninvasive venous studies (above).

TREATMENT (1) Meticulous foot hygiene to prevent infection; (2) leg elevation; (3) compression stockings and/or pneumatic compression boots. Diuretics should be *avoided* to prevent intravascular volume depletion.

For a more detailed discussion, see Dzau VJ, Craeger MA: Vascular Diseases of the Extremities, Chap. 198, in HPIM-12, p. 1018

SECTION 5 RESPIRATORY DISEASES

80 RESPIRATORY FUNCTION AND DIAGNOSIS

DISTURBANCES OF RESPIRATORY FUNCTION

The respiratory system includes not only the lungs but also the central nervous system, chest wall (diaphragm, abdomen, intercostal muscles), and pulmonary circulation. Prime function of the system is to exchange gas between inspired air and venous blood.

DISTURBANCES IN VENTILATORY FUNCTION (Fig. 80-1) Ventilation is the process whereby lungs deliver fresh air to alveoli. Measurements of ventilatory function consist of quantification of air in the lungs [total lung capacity (TLC), residual volume (RV)] and the rate at which air can be expelled from the lungs [forced vital capacity (FVC), forced expiratory volume in 1 s (FEV_1)] during a forced exhalation from TLC. Expiratory flow rates may be plotted against lung volumes yielding a flow-volume curve (see HPIM-12, Fig. 201-4, p. 1035).

Two major patterns of abnormal ventilatory function are restrictive and obstructive patterns. In <u>obstructive</u> pattern:

- Hallmark is decrease in expiratory flow rate, i.e. FEV_1.
- Ratio FEV_1/FVC is reduced.
- TLC is normal or increased.
- RV is elevated due to trapping of air during expiration.

In <u>restrictive</u> disease:

- Hallmark is decrease in TLC.
- May be caused by pulmonary parenchymal disease or extraparenchymal (neuromuscular such as myasthenia gravis or chest wall such as kyphoscoliosis).
- Pulmonary parenchymal disease usually occurs with a reduced RV but extraparenchymal disease (with expiratory dysfunction) occurs with an increased RV.

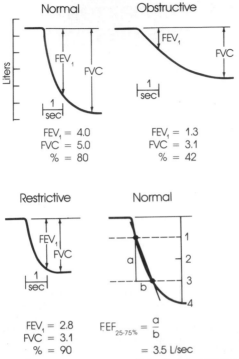

FIGURE 80-1 Measurement of the forced expiratory volume, FEV_1; forced vital capacity, FVC; and maximum midexpiratory flow, $FEF_{25-75\%}$. The patient makes a full inspiration and then exhales as hard and as fast as possible. As the patient exhales the pen moves down. The FEV_1 is the volume exhaled in 1 s; the FVC is the total volume exhaled. $FEF_{25-75\%}$ is the mean flow rate measured over the middle half of the FVC. Note the differences between the normal, obstructive, and restrictive patterns. *(Reproduced from West JB: HPIM-11, p. 1055.)*

DISTURBANCES IN PULMONARY CIRCULATION   Pulmonary vasculature handles the cardiac output, approximately 5 L/min. Low-pressure system with thin-walled vessels. Perfusion of lung greatest in dependent portion. Assessment requires measuring pulmonary vascular pressures and cardiac output to derive pulmonary vascular resistance. Pulmonary vascular resistance rises with hypoxia, intraluminal thrombi, scarring, or loss of alveolar beds.

All diseases of the respiratory system causing hypoxia are capable of causing pulmonary hypertension.

DISTURBANCES IN GAS EXCHANGE Primary functions of the respiratory system are to remove CO_2 and provide O_2. Normal tidal volume is about 500 mL and normal frequency is 15 breaths/min for a total ventilation of 7.5 L/min. Because of dead space, alveolar ventilation is 5 L/min.

Partial pressure of CO_2 in arterial blood (Pa_{CO_2}) is directly proportional to amount of CO_2 produced each minute ($\dot{V}_{CO_2}$) and inversely proportional to alveolar ventilation ($\dot{V}A$).

$$Pa_{CO_2} = 0.863 \times \dot{V}_{CO_2}/\dot{V}A$$

Gas exchange is critically dependent upon proper matching of ventilation and perfusion.

Assessment of gas exchange requires measurement of arterial blood gases. The actual content of O_2 in blood is determined by both P_{O_2} and hemoglobin.

Arterial P_{O_2} can be used to measure alveolar-arterial O_2 difference (A-a gradient). Increased A-a gradient (normal <15 mmHg rising by 3 mmHg each decade after age 30) indicates impaired gas exchange.

In order to calculate A-a gradient, the alveolar P_{O_2} (PA_{O_2}) must be calculated:

A-a =
$$PA_{O_2} = FI_{O_2} \times (PB - P_{H_2O}) - Pa_{CO_2}/R$$

where FI_{O_2} = fractional concentration of inspired O_2 (0.21 breathing room air); PB = barometric pressure (760 mmHg at sea level); P_{H_2O} = water vapor pressure (47 mmHg when air is saturated at 37°C); and R = respiratory quotient (the ratio of CO_2 production to O_2 consumption, usually assumed to be 0.8).

Adequacy of CO_2 removal is measured by the partial pressure of CO_2 in arterial blood.

Ability of gas to diffuse across the aolveolar-capillary membrane is assessed by the diffusing capacity of the lung (DL_{CO}). Carried out with low concentration of carbon monoxide during a single 10-s breath-holding period or during 1 min of steady breathing. Value depends on alveolar-capillary surface area, pulmonary capillary blood volume, degree of $\dot{V}/\dot{Q}$ mismatching, and thickness of alveolar-capillary membrane.

MECHANISMS OF ABNORMAL FUNCTION Four basic mechanisms of hypoxemia are: (1) ↓ inspired P_{O_2}; (2) hypoventilation; (3) shunt; (4) $\dot{V}/\dot{Q}$ mismatch. Diffusion block contributes to hypoxemia only under selected circumstances. Approach to the hypoxemic pt is shown in Fig. 80-2.

The essential mechanism underlying all cases of hypercapnia is inadequate alveolar ventilation. Potential contributing factors include: (1) increased CO_2 production; (2) decreased

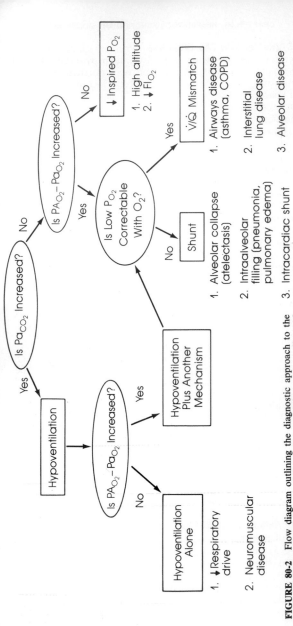

FIGURE 80-2 Flow diagram outlining the diagnostic approach to the patient with hypoxemia (Pa_{O_2} <80 mmHg). PA_{O_2}–Pa_{O_2} is usually <15 mmHg for subjects ≦30 years old, and increases ~3 mmHg per decade after that.[20]

ventilatory drive; (3) malfunction of the respiratory pump or increased airways resistance; and (4) inefficiency of gas exchange (increased dead space or $\dot{V}/\dot{Q}$ mismatch) necessitating a compensatory increase in overall minute ventilation.

DIAGNOSTIC PROCEDURES

NONINVASIVE PROCEDURES Radiography No CXR pattern is sufficiently specific to *establish* a diagnosis; instead, the CXR serves to *detect* disease, assess magnitude, and guide further diagnostic investigation. Fluoroscopy provides a dynamic image of the chest and is particularly helpful in localizing lesions poorly visible on the CXR. Both fluoroscopy and standard tomography have largely been supplanted by thoracic CT, which is now routine in evaluation of patients with pulmonary nodules and masses. CT is especially helpful in the assessment of pleural lesions. Contrast enhancement also makes thoracic CT useful in differentiating tissue masses from vascular structures. MRI has potential applications in evaluation of pulmonary diseases.

Skin tests Specific skin test antigens are available for tuberculosis, histoplasmosis, coccidioidomycosis, blastomycosis, trichinosis, toxoplasmosis, and aspergillosis. A positive delayed reaction (type IV) to a tuberculin test indicates only prior infection, not active disease. Immediate (type I) and late (type III) dermal hypersensitivity to *Aspergillus* antigen supports diagnosis of allergic bronchopulmonary aspergillosis in pts with a compatible clinical illness.

Sputum exam Sputum is distinguished from saliva by presence of bronchial epithelial cells and alveolar macrophages. Sputum exam should include gross inspection for blood, color, and odor, as well as microscopic inspection of carefully stained smears. Culture of expectorated sputum may be misleading owing to contamination with oropharyngeal flora. Sputum samples induced by inhalation of nebulized, warm, hypertonic saline can be stained for the presence of *Pneumocystis carinii*.

Pulmonary function tests May indicate abnormalities of airway function, alterations of lung volume, and disturbances of gas exchange. Specific patterns of pulmonary function may assist in differential diagnosis. PFTs also may provide objective measures of therapeutic response, e.g., to bronchodilators.

Pulmonary scintigraphy Scans of pulmonary ventilation and perfusion aid in the diagnosis of pulmonary embolism. Quantitative ventilation-perfusion scans also are used to assess surgical resectability of lung cancer in pts with diminished respiratory function. *Gallium scanning* may be used to identify inflammatory disease of the lungs or mediastinal lymph nodes. Inflammatory activity of the lungs detected with gallium may be associated with diffuse interstitial infections. Gallium uptake by the lungs also may occur in *P. carinii* pneumonia (PCP).

INVASIVE PROCEDURES Bronchoscopy Permits visualization of airways, identification of endobronchial abnormalities, and collection of diagnostic specimens by lavage, brushing, or biopsy. The fiberoptic bronchoscope permits exam of smaller, more peripheral airways than the rigid bronchoscope, but the latter permits greater control of the airways and provides more effective suctioning. These features make rigid bronchoscopy particularly useful in pts with central obstructing tumors, foreign bodies, or massive hemoptysis. The fiberoptic bronchoscope increases the diagnostic potential of bronchoscopy, permitting biopsy of peripheral nodules and diffuse infiltrative diseases as well as aspiration and lavage of airways and airspaces.

Bronchography Performed to outline congenital malformations or acquired forms of tracheobronchial distortion and to delineate bronchiectatic airways; now largely replaced by chest CT.

Transtracheal, catheter-brush, and percutaneous needle aspiration of the lung These procedures provide microbiologic specimens from lung while avoiding contamination with oropharyngeal flora. These procedures all involve risks and should be performed only by experienced individuals.

Bronchoalveolar lavage (BAL) An adjunct to fiberoptic bronchoscopy permitting collection of cells and liquid from distal air spaces. Useful in diagnosis of PCP, other infections, and some interstitial diseases.

Thoracentesis and pleural biopsy Thoracentesis should be performed as an early step in the evaluation of any pleural effusion of uncertain etiology. Analysis of pleural fluid helps differentiate transudate from exudate (Chap. 88). (Exudate: pleural fluid LDH >200 IU, pleural fluid/serum protein >0.5, pleural fluid/serum LDH >0.6.) Pleural fluid pH <7.2 suggests that an exudate associated with an infection is an empyema and will almost certainly require drainage. WBC count and differential; glucose, P_{CO_2}, amylase, Gram stain, culture, and cytologic exam should be performed on all specimens. Rheumatoid factor and complement may also be useful. Closed pleural biopsy also can be done when a pleural effusion is present; particularly useful when tuberculosis is suspected.

Pulmonary angiography The definitive test for pulmonary embolism; also may reveal AV malformations.

Bronchial arteriography Performed to identify and possibly embolize arterial sites in pts with massive hemoptysis.

Mediastinoscopy Diagnostic procedure of choice in pts with disease involving mediastinal lymph nodes. However, lymph nodes in left superior mediastinum must be approached via *mediastinotomy*.

Lung biopsy Closed biopsies are performed percutaneously with a cutting needle, aspiration needle, or with a fiberoptic bronchoscope; open biopsies require thoracotomy. The needle biopsies are favored over the bronchoscope for small peripheral lesions, whereas transbronchial biopsy is preferred for diffuse disease. Aspiration biopsies yield cytologic, but not histologic specimens. Open biopsy is favored when histologic diagnosis is difficult and when an accurate tissue diagnosis must be made rapidly.

For a more detailed discussion, see Weinberger S, Drazen G: Disturbances of Respiratory Function, Chap. 201, p. 1033; Moser KM: Diagnostic Procedures in Respiratory Diseases, Chap. 203, p. 1044, and Friedman PJ: Imaging in Pulmonary Disease, Chap. 202 p. 1040, in HPIM-12

ASTHMA

DEFINITION Disease characterized by increased responsiveness of lower airways to multiple stimuli; episodic, and with reversible obstruction; may range in severity from mild without limitation of pt's activity to severe and life-threatening. Obstruction persisting for days or weeks is known as *status asthmaticus.*

EPIDEMIOLOGY AND ETIOLOGY Five percent of adults and up to 10% of children are estimated to experience episodes of asthma. Basic abnormality is airway hyperresponsiveness to both specific and nonspecific stimuli. All pts demonstrate enhanced bronchoconstriction in response to inhalation of methacholine or histamine (nonspecific bronchoconstrictor agents). Some pts may be classified as having *allergic asthma;* these experience worsening of symptoms on exposure to pollens or other allergens. They characteristically give personal and/or family history of other allergic diseases, such as rhinitis, urticaria, and eczema. Skin tests to allergens are positive; serum IgE may be ↑. Bronchoprovocation studies may demonstrate positive responses to inhalation of specific allergens.

A significant number of asthmatic pts have negative allergic histories and do not react to skin or bronchoprovocation testing with specific allergens. Many of these develop bronchospasm after an upper respiratory infection. These pts are said to have *idiosyncratic* or *intrinsic asthma.*

Some pts experience worsening of symptoms on *exercise* or exposure to *cold air* or *occupational* stimuli. Many note increased wheezing following *viral URI* or in response to *emotional stress.*

PATHOGENESIS Common denominator underlying the asthmatic diathesis is nonspecific hyperirritability of the tracheobronchial tree. Airway reactivity may fluctuate, and fluctuations correlate with clinical symptoms. Airway reactivity may be increased by a number of factors: allergenic, pharmacologic, environmental, occupational, infectious, exercise-related, and emotional. Among the more common are airborne allergens, aspirin, beta-adrenergic blocking agents (e.g., propranolol, timolol), sulfites in food, air pollution (ozone, nitrogen dioxide), and respiratory infections.

APPROACH TO PATIENT **History** Symptoms: wheezing, dyspnea, cough, fever, sputum production, other allergic disorders. Possible precipitating factors (allergens, infection, etc.); asthma attacks often occur at night. Response to medications. Course of previous attacks (e.g., need for hospitalization, steroid treatment).

Physical Exam General: tachypnea, tachycardia, use of accessory respiratory muscles, cyanosis, pulsus paradoxus (accessory muscle use and pulsus paradoxus correlate with severity of obstruction). Lungs: adequacy of aeration, symmetry of breath sounds, wheezing, prolongation of expiratory phase, hyperinflation. Heart: evidence for CHF. ENT/skin: evidence of allergic nasal, sinus, or skin disease.

Laboratory While pulmonary function test (PFT) findings are not diagnostic, they are very helpful in judging severity of airway obstruction and in following response to therapy in both chronic and acute situations. FVC, FEV_1, MMEFR, PEFR, FEV_1/FVC are decreased; RV and TLC increased during episodes of obstruction; $D_{L_{CO}}$ usually normal or slightly increased. Reduction of FEV_1 to <25% predicted or <0.75 L after administration of a bronchodilator indicates severe disease. CBC may show eosinophilia. IgE may show mild elevations; marked elevations may suggest evidence of allergic bronchopulmonary aspergillosis (ABPA). Sputum examination: eosinophilia, Curschmann's spirals (casts of small airways), Charcot-Leyden crystals; presence of large numbers of neutrophils suggests bronchial infection. Arterial blood gases: uniformly show hypoxemia during attacks; usually hypocarbia and respiratory alkalosis present; normal or elevated P_{CO_2} worrisome as may suggest severe respiratory muscle fatigue and airways obstruction. CXR not always necessary: may show hyperinflation, patchy infiltrates due to atelectasis behind plugged airways; important when complicating infection is a consideration.

DIFFERENTIAL DIAGNOSIS "All that wheezes is not asthma": CHF; chronic bronchitis/emphysema; upper airway obstruction due to foreign body, tumor, laryngeal edema; carcinoid tumors (usually associated with stridor, not wheezing); recurrent pulmonary emboli; eosinophilic pneumonia; vocal cord dysfunction; systemic vasculitis with pulmonary involvement.

TREATMENT Five major categories of pharmacologic therapy after removal, if possible, of inciting agent:

1. Beta-adrenergic agonists: inhaled route provides most rapid effect and best therapeutic index; isotharine, albuterol, terbutaline, metaproterenol, fenoterol, or isoproterenol may be given by nebulizer or metered-dose inhaler. Epinephrine

0.3 mL of 1:1000 solution SC (for use in acute situations in absence of cardiac history).

2. *Methylxanthines:* theophylline and various salts; adjust dose to maintain blood level between 10 and 20 μg/mL; may be given PO or IV (as aminophylline). Theophylline clearance varies widely and is reduced with age, hepatic dysfunction, cardiac decompensation, cor pulmonale, febrile illness. Many drugs also alter theophylline clearance (decrease half-life: cigarettes, phenobarbitol, phenytoin; increase half-life: erythromycin, allopurinol, cimetidine, propranolol).

3. *Glucocorticoids:* prednisone 40–60 mg PO daily followed by tapering schedule of 50% reduction every 3–5 d; hydrocortisone 4 mg/kg IV loading dose followed by 3 mg/kg q 6 h; methylprednisolone 50–100 mg IV q 6 h. Evidence is accumulating that very large doses of glucocorticoids have no advantage over more conventional doses. Steroids in acute asthma require 6 h or more to have an effect. Inhaled glucocorticoid preparations are important adjuncts to chronic therapy; not useful in acute attacks.

4. *Cromolyn sodium:* not a bronchodilator; useful in chronic therapy for prevention, not useful during acute attacks; administered as metered-dose inhaler or nebulized powder.

5. *Anticholinergics:* aerosolized atropine and related compounds, such as ipratropium, a nonabsorbable quaternary ammonium. May enhance the bronchodilation achieved by sympathomimetics but is slow acting (30–60 min). Ipratropium may be given by metered-dose inhaler, 2 puffs up to every 6 h. Expectorants and mucolytic agents add little to the management of acute or chronic asthma.

HYPERSENSITIVITY PNEUMONITIS

DEFINITION   Hypersensitivity pneumonitis (HP) or extrinsic allergic alveolitis is an immunologically mediated inflammation of lung parenchyma involving alveolar walls and terminal airways secondary to repeated inhalation of a variety of organic dusts by a susceptible host.

ETIOLOGY   A variety of inhaled substances have been implicated (see Table 205-1, p. 1054, in HPIM-12). These substances are usually organic antigens, particularly thermophilic actinomycetes, but may include inorganic compounds such as isocyanates.

CLINICAL MANIFESTATIONS   Symptoms may be acute, subacute, or chronic depending on the frequency and intensity of exposure to the causative agent; in acute form, cough, fever, chills, dyspnea appear 6–8 h after exposure to antigen; in subacute and chronic forms, temporal relationship to antigenic exposure may be lost and insidiously increasing dyspnea may be predominant symptom.

DIAGNOSIS   History   Occupational history and history of possible exposures and relationship to symptoms are very important.

Physical Exam   Nonspecific; may reveal rales in lung fields, cyanosis in advanced cases.

Laboratory   Serum precipitins to offending antigen may be present but are not specific; eosinophilia is not a feature. CXR: nonspecific changes in interstitial structures; pleural changes or hilar adenopathy rare. PFTs and ABGs: restrictive pattern possibly associated with airway obstruction; diffusing capacity decreased; hypoxemia at rest or with exercise. Bronchoalveolar lavage may show increased lymphocytes of suppressor-cytotoxic phenotype. Lung biopsy may be necessary in some patients who do not have sufficient other criteria; transbronchial biopsy may suffice, but open lung biopsy is frequently necessary.

DIFFERENTIAL DIAGNOSIS   Other interstitial lung diseases, including sarcoidosis, idiopathic pulmonary fibrosis, lung disease associated with collagen-vascular diseases, drug-induced lung disease; eosinophilic pneumonia; allergic bronchopulmonary aspergillosis; silo-fillers' disease; "pulmonary mycotoxicosis" or "atypical" farmer's lung; infection.

TREATMENT   Avoidance of offending antigen is essential. Chronic form may be partially irreversible at the time of diagnosis. Prednisone 1 (mg/kg)/d for 7–14 d, followed by tapering schedule over 2–6 weeks to lowest possible dose.

For a more detailed discussion, see McFadden ER Jr: Asthma, Chap. 204, p. 1047, and Hunninghake GW, Richerson HB: Hypersensitivity Pneumonitis, Chap. 205, p. 1053, in HPIM-12

82 ENVIRONMENTAL LUNG DISEASES

APPROACH TO PATIENT

Ask about workplace and work history in detail: Specific contaminants? Availability and use of protective devices? Ventilation? Do coworkers have similar complaints? Ask about every job; short-term exposures may be significant. CXR may over- or underestimate functional impact of pneumoconioses. PFTs may both quantify impairment and suggest the nature of exposure.

An individual's dose of an environmental agent is influenced by intensity as well as by physiologic factors (ventilation rate and depth).

OCCUPATIONAL EXPOSURES AND PULMONARY DISEASE

INORGANIC DUSTS   Asbestosis   Exposures may occur in mining, milling, and manufacture of asbestos products, construction trades (pipefitting, boilermaking), and manufacture of safety garments, filler for plastic material, and friction materials (brake and clutch linings). Major health effects of asbestos include pulmonary fibrosis (asbestosis) and cancers of the respiratory tract, pleura, and peritoneum.

Asbestosis is a diffuse interstitial fibrosing disease of the lung that is directly related to intensity and duration of exposure, usually requiring ≥10 years of moderate to severe exposure. PFTs show a restrictive pattern. CXR reveals irregular or linear opacities, greatest in lower lung fields. *Pleural plaques* indicate past exposure. Excess frequency of *lung cancer* occurs 15 to 20 years after first asbestos exposure. Smoking substantially increases risk of lung cancer after asbestos exposure but does not alter risk of *mesotheliomas*, which peaks 30 to 35 years after initial exposure.

Silicosis   Exposure to free silica (crystalline quartz) occurs in mining, stone cutting, abrasive industries, blasting, quarrying, farming. Short-term, high-intensity exposures (as brief as 10 months) may produce acute silicosis—rapidly fatal pulmonary fibrosis with radiographic picture of profuse miliary infiltration or consolidation. Longer-term, less-intense exposures are associated with upper lobe fibrosis and hilar adenopathy ≥15 years after exposure. Fibrosis is nod-ular and may lead to pulmonary restriction and airflow obstruction. Pts with silicosis are at higher than normal risk for tuberculosis, and pts with chronic silicosis and a positive PPD warrant antituberculous treatment.

Coal worker's pneumoconiosis (CWP) Symptoms of simple CWP are additive to the effects of cigarette smoking on chronic bronchitis and obstructive lung disease. X-ray signs of simple CWP are small, irregular opacities (reticular pattern) that may progress to small, rounded opacities (nod-ular pattern). Complicated CWP is indicated by roentgeno-graphic appearance of nodules >1 cm in diameter in upper lung fields; $D_{L_{CO}}$ is reduced.

Berylliosis Beryllium exposure may produce acute pneu-monitis or chronic interstitial pneumonitis. Histology is indistinguishable from sarcoidosis.

ORGANIC DUSTS **Cotton dust (byssinosis)** Exposures occur in production of yarns for cotton, linen, and rope making. (Flax, hemp, and jute produce a similar syndrome.) Chest tightness occurs typically on first day of work week. After 10 years, recurrent symptoms are associated with airflow obstruction. Therapy includes bronchodilators, anti-histamines, and elimination of exposure.

Grain dust Farmers and grain elevator operators are at risk. Symptoms are those of cigarette smokers—cough, mucus production, wheezing, and airflow obstruction.

Farmer's lung Persons exposed to moldy hay with spores of thermophilic actinomycetes may develop a hypersensitiv-ity pneumonitis. Acute farmer's lung causes fever, chills, malaise, cough, and dyspnea 4 to 8 h after exposure. Chronic low-intensity exposure causes interstitial fibrosis.

TOXIC CHEMICALS Many toxic chemicals can affect the lung in the form of vapor and gases.

Smoke inhalation Kills more fire victims than does thermal injury. Severe cases may develop pulmonary edema. CO poisoning causing O_2 desaturation may be fatal.

Agents used in the manufacture of synthetic materials may produce sensitization to isocyanates, aromatic amines, and aldehydes. Repeated exposure causes some workers to de-velop productive cough, asthma, or low-grade fever and malaise.

Fluorocarbons, transmitted from a worker's hands to cigarettes, may be volatilized. The inhaled agent causes fever, chills, malaise, and sometimes wheezing. Occurring in plastics workers, the syndrome is termed *polymer fume fever*.

GENERAL ENVIRONMENTAL EXPOSURES

Air pollution   Difficult to relate specific health effects to any single pollutant. Symptoms and diseases of air pollution are also the nononcogenic conditions associated with cigarette smoking (respiratory infections, airway irritation).

Passive cigarette smoking   Increased respiratory illness and reduced lung function have been found in children of smoking parents. Lung cancer risk is elevated in adults exposed to passive smoke.

Radon   Risk factor for lung cancer, exacerbated by cigarette smoke.

PRINCIPLES OF MANAGEMENT

With many environmental agents, lung disease occurs years after exposure. If exposure continues, inciting agent must be eliminated, usually by removing pt from workplace. Pulmonary fibrosis (e.g., asbestosis, CWP) is not responsive to glucocorticoids. Therapy of occupational asthma follows usual guidelines (see Chap. 81). Lung cancer screening has not yet proven effective, even in high-risk occupations.

For a more detailed discussion, see Speizer FE: Environmental Lung Disease, Chap. 206, in HPIM-12, p. 1056

83 CHRONIC BRONCHITIS, EMPHYSEMA, AND AIRWAYS OBSTRUCTION

DEFINITIONS **Chronic bronchitis** Excessive tracheobronchial mucus secretion sufficient to cause cough with expectoration for at least 3 months of the year for 2 consecutive years.

Simple chronic bronchitis Characterized by mucoid sputum production.

Chronic mucopurulent bronchitis Characterized by recurrent purulent sputum in the absence of localized suppurative disease (e.g., bronchiectasis).

Chronic asthmatic bronchitis Cough and mucus hypersecretion associated with dyspnea and wheezing with acute respiratory infections or exposure to inhaled irritants.

Emphysema Distention of air spaces distal to the terminal bronchioles with destruction of alveolar septa.

Chronic obstructive lung disease (COLD) Condition with chronic expiratory airflow obstruction due to chronic bronchitis and/or emphysema. Obstruction is assessed by the expiratory FVC maneuver (see Fig. 80-1). Severity of obstruction may fluctuate in COLD, but some degree of obstruction is always present.

PATHOLOGY Chronic bronchitis is associated with hyperplasia and hypertrophy of submucosal mucus glands. There is Goblet-cell hyperplasia, mucosal edema and inflammation, and increased smooth muscle in small airways. Emphysema may be panacinar (affecting both central and peripheral portions of the acinus) or centriacinar (primary involvement of respiratory bronchioles and alveolar ducts and little involvement of peripheral acina). Panacinar and centriacinar emphysema may exist in the same lung, and both produce similar physiologic changes, primarily increased wasted ventilation.

PATHOGENESIS

1. Cigarette smoking: Responsible for most cases of chronic bronchitis and emphysema; also causes obstruction of small airways in young, asymptomatic persons. Nonsmokers who remain in the presence of cigarette smokers (passive smokers) are significantly exposed to tobacco products. Children of smoking parents may experience more frequent and severe respiratory infections and have a higher prevalence of respiratory symptoms. However, a causal connection between passive smoking and chronic obstructive lung diseases has not been established.

2. Occupational exposures: Dust or gases such as cotton dust and toluene diisocyanate accelerate decline of pulmonary function in COLD.

3. Acute infections: May contribute to exacerbations of COLD and lead to chronic obstruction.

4. Familial aggregation of emphysema: Occurs with deficiency of α_1-antitrypsin, a protease inhibitor.

5. Air pollution: Although exacerbations of chronic bronchitis and mortality rates from emphysema and bronchitis are associated with air pollution, the role of pollutants in the pathogenesis of COLD is unclear.

CLINICAL MANIFESTATIONS   COLD is a progressive disorder even when contributing factors are eliminated and aggressive therapy is instituted. Although most patients demonstrate features of both bronchitis and emphysema, two distinct syndromes exist (see Table 83-1).

Predominant emphysema ("pink puffer")   Scant sputum production but prominent exertional dyspnea; asthenic body build, tachypnea, prolonged expiration, hyperresonant chest, diminished breath sounds. Gas exchange is impaired with mildly reduced arterial P_{O_2} and low or normal P_{CO_2}. PFTs show reduced maximal flow rates and diffusing capacity and evidence of gas trapping. Cor pulmonale and hypercapneic respiratory failure occur late in the course.

Predominant bronchitis ("blue bloater")   Chronic cough and mucus production; dyspnea is less prominent. Pts are often cyanotic and overweight; auscultation reveals coarse rhonchi and wheezes. RV heave, RV S_3, and edema are present. Arterial blood gases are severely deranged, both arterial P_{O_2} and P_{CO_2} (in mmHg) may be in high 40s to low 50s. Maximal expiratory flow rates are reduced, residual volume is moderately elevated, and diffusing capacity normal or slightly $\downarrow$. Episodes of respiratory failure are frequent, but recovery usually occurs with therapy.

PRINCIPLES OF MANAGEMENT   Because emphysema is untreatable, therapeutic efforts are directed at prevention and management of reversible airways obstruction.

Assessment   In addition to Hx and physical exam, pts should receive a CXR as well as PFTs (spirometry, lung volumes, $D_{L_{CO}}$, arterial blood gases). Effects of inhaled bronchodilator should be assessed after acute administration and PFTs should be repeated regularly with and between exacerbations.

Prevention   COLD is progressive; however, the decline is accelerated by smoking, and all pts should be urged to

TABLE 83-1 Chronic obstructive lung disease: Salient features of the two types

	Predominant emphysema	Predominant bronchitis
Age at time of diagnosis, yrs	60 ±	50 ±
Dyspnea	Severe	Mild
Cough	After dyspnea starts	Before dyspnea starts
Sputum	Scanty, mucoid	Copious, purulent
Bronchial infections	Less frequent	More frequent
Respiratory insufficiency episodes	Often terminal	Repeated
Chest film	"Hyperinflation" ± bullous changes, small heart	Increased bronchovascular markings at bases, large heart
Chronic Pa_{CO_2}	35–40 mmHg	50–60 mmHg
Chronic Pa_{O_2}	65–75 mmHg	45–60 mmHg
Hematocrit	35–45%	50–55%
Pulmonary hypertension:		
Rest	None to mild	Moderate to severe
Exercise	Moderate	Worsens
Cor pulmonale	Rare, except terminally	Common
Elastic recoil	Severely decreased	Normal
Resistance	Normal to slight increase	High
Diffusing capacity	Decreased	Normal to slight decrease

From Ingram RH Jr.: HPIM-12, p. 1077.

Improvement c̄ bronchodilⁱⁿ   no   *yes*

quit. Eliminate aerosol sprays and occupational factors that may accelerate disease. Administer yearly influenza vaccinations.

Infections Increases in sputum purulence, volume, and viscosity suggest infection. Nonbacterial infections precipitate most exacerbations, but antibiotics lower intensity and duration of symptoms.

Bronchodilators Methylxanthines (theophylline), sympathomimetics, and anticholinergics may alleviate symptoms by reducing bronchial tone. Selective β_2-stimulating drugs (albuterol and metoproterenol, 2 puffs q 4–6 h metered-dose inhaler) are most effective and are associated with fewest side effects. Ipratropium, an anticholinergic agent, is also available in metered-dose inhaler (2 puffs q 6–8 h) as an alternative or supplement to sympathomimetic agents. Glucocorticoids should be employed when other measures are insufficient and only with objective documentation of improvement. Oral prednisone should be started at 30 mg/d, with serial PFTs to assess response. The dose should be tapered to the lowest effective level and should be stopped if there is no objective improvement.

Other   Bronchopulmonary drainage is important in pts with mucus hypersecretion. Continuous O_2 should be given when severe hypoxia is present (P_{O_2} <55 mmHg) and/or there is evidence of cor pulmonale. Exercise programs do not improve lung function but may increase task-specific exercise tolerance.

ACUTE RESPIRATORY FAILURE Diagnosis   Made on the basis of arterial blood gas from baseline (P_{O_2} drop ≥10–15 mmHg and/or increase in P_{CO_2} associated with pH ≤7.30).

Precipitating factors   Infection, exacerbation of bronchospasm, pneumothorax, pulmonary thromboembolism, and sedative administration all may precipitate respiratory failure.

Treatment   (1) Maintain oxygenation with low-flow O_2 therapy (1–2 L/min by nasal prongs or 24% by Venturi mask). If O_2 results in a large increase in arterial P_{CO_2} with acidosis, mechanical ventilation is required; do not stop O_2 administration abruptly. (2) Treat infection (antibiotics), remove secretions (postural drainage), reverse bronchoconstriction (aminophylline, inhaled sympathomimetics at intervals of 1–2 h, oral or IV glucocorticoids equivalent to 30 mg prednisone each day).

Complications   Arrhythmias, heart failure, pulmonary thromboembolism, GI hemorrhage.

For a more detailed discussion, see Ingram RH Jr.: Chronic Bronchitis, Emphysema, and Airways Obstruction, Chap. 210, in HPIM-12, p. 1074

84 PNEUMONIA AND LUNG ABSCESS

PNEUMONIA

Clinical manifestations ± Cough, fever, chest pain, dyspnea, sputum. Physical exam: ↓ respiratory excursion, high-pitched end-inspiratory crackles from fluid-filled alveoli; bronchial breath sounds (↑ inspiratory and expiratory phases) from consolidation with patent bronchus.

X-rays Alveolar: nonsegmental consolidation with air bronchograms (pneumococcal pneumonia). Bronchopneumonia: segmental involvement without bronchograms (staphylococcal). Interstitial: reticular pattern (*Mycoplasma*).

Diagnosis Gram's stain of sputum with >25 WBC per low-power field. Expectorated sputum (not for anaerobic cultures), transtracheal aspiration, bronchoscopy with bronchoalveolar lavage or brush biopsy, transthoracic needle aspiration, lung biopsy. Cultures of blood, skin lesions, joint effusions, CSF.

Community-acquired pneumonias Pneumococcal (see Chap. 42). Streptococcal (see Chap. 44). *S. aureus* (see Chap. 43). *H. influenzae* (see Chap. 48). *Klebsiella pneumoniae:* middle-aged or elderly pts with underlying alcoholism or diabetes; abrupt fever, rigors, productive cough (± bloody sputum); CXR—usually upper-lobe air space pneumonia with abscess and pleural effusion ± bulging of interlobar fissure. Anaerobic (see Chap. 45). Legionnaire's disease (see Chap. 64). *Mycoplasma pneumoniae* (see Chap. 60). Viral pneumonia (see Chap. 51).

Hospital-acquired pneumonia Most often gram-negative bacilli; diagnosis in intubated pt requires purulent sputum plus fever, leukocytosis, new or progressive infiltrate, and increase in alveolar-arterial P_{O_2} gradient.

Treatment Outpatient without sputum: erythromycin 500 mg qid × 7–14 d; follow-up CXR in 6 weeks. Hospitalize with: hypoxia, empyema, extrapulmonary focus, severe systemic manifestations. Pneumococcal most common—2.4 million U penicillin IV or IM. Aspiration: penicillin 10–12 million U IV qd; clindamycin 300 mg IV q 6 h. Postviral (pneumococcal or staphylococcal)—nafcillin 9 g qd. Chronic bronchitis with pneumonia (pneumococcus, *H. influenzae*): ampicillin 2–6 g qd or cefuroxime 750 mg IV tid. Hospital-acquired pneumonia: good sputum cultures and blood cultures critical; predominant gram-negative rods on Gram's stain—ticarcillin or mezlocillin 16–18 g qd + gentamicin 1.5 mg/kg then 1 mg/kg tid, or third-generation cephalosporin; gram-positive cocci—vancomycin 500 mg IV tid or nafcillin. Compromised hosts: see Chap. 36 for associated organisms and individual chapters for treatment.

LUNG ABSCESS

Symptoms Cough productive of moderate to large amounts of purulent, sometimes foul sputum, fever, chest pain, dyspnea, anorexia, weight loss. *clubbing*

Laboratory findings   ↑ WBC ± anemia, hypoalbuminemia; CXR—consolidation with radiolucency and surrounding wall or border.

Treatment Anaerobic abscess—penicillin 10–12 million U IV, then penicillin V 750 mg–1 g qid or clindamycin 600 mg q 8 h IV, then oral 300 mg qid × 6 weeks.

For a more detailed discussion, see Reynolds HY: Pneumonia and Lung Abscess, Chap. 207, in HPIM-12, p. 1064

85 PULMONARY THROMBOEMBOLISM AND PRIMARY PULMONARY HYPERTENSION

PULMONARY EMBOLISM (PE) (see Fig. 85-1)

NATURAL HISTORY Immediate result is obstruction of pulmonary blood flow to the distal lung. Respiratory consequences include: (1) wasted ventilation (lung ventilated but not perfused), (2) atelectasis that occurs 2–24 h following PE; and (3) widened alveolar-arterial P_{O_2} gradient, usually with arterial hypoxemia. Hemodynamic consequences may include: (1) pulmonary hypertension, (2) acute RV failure, and (3) decline in cardiac output. These occur only when significant fraction of pulmonary vasculature is obstructed. Infarction of lung tissue is uncommon, occurring only with underlying cardiac or pulmonary disease.

SYMPTOMS Sudden onset of dyspnea most common; chest pain, hemoptysis accompany infarction; syncope may indicate massive embolism.

PHYSICAL EXAM Tachypnea and tachycardia common; RV gallop; loud P_2 and prominent jugular *a* waves suggest RV failure; temperature >39°C uncommon. Hypotension suggests massive PE.

LABORATORY FINDINGS Routine studies contribute little to diagnosis; normal CXR does not exclude PE, but normal perfusion scintiscan is not seen with a clinically significant embolism. Detection of venous thrombosis with impedance plethysmography, femoral ultrasound, or venography should prompt therapy for venous thromboembolism in a pt with a suspicion of embolism. A segmental or larger perfusion defect with normal ventilation ("mismatch") is highly suggestive of PE; pulmonary angiography remains definitive test.

TREATMENT IV heparin (approximately 1000 U/h) by continuous infusion is therapy of choice for most pts; usual goal is to maintain activated PTT 1.5–2.0 × control; heparin is continued 7 to 10 days for deep venous thrombosis (DVT) and 10 days for thromboembolism. Most patients receive minimum of 3 months of oral coumadin therapy after PE. Thrombolytic therapy hastens resolution of venous thrombi and is probably indicated for pts with massive embolism and

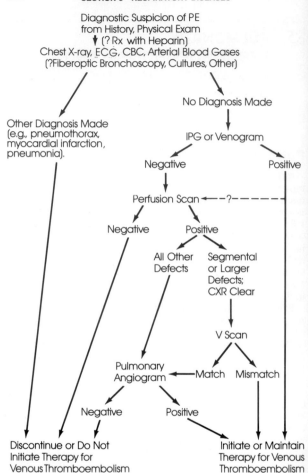

* **FIGURE 85-1** Flow chart used in diagnosis of pulmonary embolism (PE). IPG, impedance plethysmogram; V scan, ventilation scan. (*Reproduced from Moser KM: HPIM-12, p. 1093.*)

systemic hypotension. Surgical therapy is rarely employed for DVT or acute PE. IVC interruption (clip or filter) is used in pts with recurrent PE despite anticoagulants and in those who cannot tolerate anticoagulants. Surgical extraction of old emboli may be helpful in pts with chronic pulmonary hypertension due to repeated PE without spontaneous resolution.

PRIMARY PULMONARY HYPERTENSION (PPH)

HISTORY   Uncommon condition. Typical pt is female of 20–40. At presentation, symptoms are usually of recent onset and natural history is ordinarily less than 5 years. Early symptoms are nonspecific—hyperventilation, chest discomfort, anxiety, weakness, fatigue. Later, dyspnea develops and precordial pain on exertion occurs in 25–50%. Effort syncope occurs very late and signifies ominous prognosis.

PHYSICAL EXAM   Prominent a wave in jugular venous pulse, right ventricular heave, narrowly split S_2 with accentuated P_2. Terminal course is characterized by signs of right-sided heart failure. *CXR:* RV and central pulmonary arterial prominence. Pulmonary arteries taper sharply. *ECG:* RV enlargement, right axis deviation, and RV hypertrophy. *Echocardiogram:* RA and RV enlargement and tricuspid regurgitation.

DIFFERENTIAL DIAGNOSIS   Other disorders of heart, lungs, and pulmonary vasculature must be excluded. Lung function studies will identify chronic pulmonary disease causing pulmonary hypertension and cor pulmonale. Interstitial diseases and hypoxic pulmonary hypertension should be excluded. Perfusion lung scan should be performed to exclude chronic PE. Pulmonary arteriogram and even open lung biopsy may be required to distinguish PE from PPH. Rarely, pulmonary hypertension is due to parasitic disease (schistosomiasis, filariasis). Cardiac disorders to be excluded include pulmonary artery and pulmonic valve stenosis. Pulmonary artery and ventricular and atrial shunts with pulmonary vascular disease (Eisenmenger reaction) should be sought. Silent mitral stenosis should be excluded by echocardiography.

THERAPY   Course is usually one of progressive deterioration despite treatment; therapy is palliative. If begun within 12 months of diagnosis, anticoagulants may improve survival but do not cause regression of disease. In some pts, other pharmacologic therapy may produce clinical and hemodynamic improvement. Categories of drugs used include (1) direct vascular smooth muscle relaxants (nitroglycerin, diazoxide, hydralazine), (2) beta agonists (isoproterenol, terbutaline), (3) alpha-adrenergic blocking agents (phentolamine, phenoxybenzamine), (4) calcium antagonists (nifedipine, verapamil), and (5) ACE inhibitors. Careful drug testing is required to assess efficacy and detect unfavorable effects. Heart-lung transplantation is a potential therapy in selected patients.

For a more detailed discussion, see Rich S: Primary Pulmonary Hypertension, Chap. 212, p. 1087, and Moser KM: Pulmonary Thromboembolism, Chap. 213, p. 1090, in HPIM-12

**INTERSTITIAL LUNG
DISEASE (ILD)**

Chronic, nonmalignant, noninfectious diseases of the lower
respiratory tract characterized by inflammation and derange-
ment of the alveolar walls; >180 separate diseases that may
be grouped into those of known cause and unknown cause.
Each group can be divided into subgroups according to the
presence or absence of histologic evidence of granulomas in
interstitial or vascular areas (Table 86-1).

CLINICAL FEATURES **History** First symptoms are usually
exertional—fatigue, malaise, dyspnea in everyday activities.
Systemic symptoms are infrequent.

**TABLE 86-1 Major categories of alveolar and interstitial
inflammatory lung diseases (ILDs)**

Known cause	Unknown cause
LUNG RESPONSE: ALVEOLITIS, INTERSTITIAL INFLAMMATION, AND FIBROSIS	
Asbestos	Idiopathic pulmonary fibrosis
Fumes, gases	Collagen vascular diseases
Drugs (antibiotics) and chemo-	Pulmonary hemorrhage syn-
therapy drugs	dromes:
Radiation	Goodpasture's syndrome, idio-
Aspiration pneumonia	pathic pulmonary hemoside-
Residual of adult respiratory dis-	rosis
ress syndrome	Pulmonary alveolar proteinosis
	Lymphocytic infiltrative disorders
	Eosinophilic pneumonias
	Lymphangioleiomyomatosis
	Amyloidosis
	Graft vs. host disease (bone mar-
	row transplantation)
LUNG RESPONSE: AS ABOVE BUT WITH GRANULOMA	
Hypersensitivity pneumonitis (or-	Sarcoidosis
ganic dusts)	Langerhans cell granulomatosis
Inorganic dusts: beryllium silica	(eosinophilic granuloma)
	Granulomatous vasculitides:
	Wegener's granulomatosis, al-
	lergic granulomatosis of Churg-
	Strauss, lymphomatoid granu-
	lomatosis
	Bronchocentric granulomatosis

Source: Modified from Reynolds HY: HPIM-12, p. 1083.

Physical exam   Late inspiratory crackles at posterior lung bases. Signs of pulmonary hypertension and clubbing occur late in course.

Laboratory findings   ESR may be elevated. Hypoxemia is common, but polycythemia is rare. Abnormalities of lung parenchyma on CXR in 90%. However, a normal CXR does *not* exclude the possibility of significant infiltrative lung disease.

Scintigraphic findings   Gallium lung scanning is usually positive with diffuse inflammation.

PFTs   Typically restrictive pattern (see Fig. 80-1) with reduced total lung capacity. D_{LCO} often decreased; mild hypoxemia, which worsens with exercise.

Bronchoalveolar lavage   Cells recovered (alveolar macrophages, lymphocytes, neutrophils, eosinophils) may reflect the type of alveolar inflammation in specific disorders.

DIAGNOSTIC EVALUATION   Rarely, clinical syndrome can be related to causative agent, but histologic exam is usually necessary. With exception of sarcoidosis, which can often be diagnosed by transbronchial biopsy, most infiltrative diseases require open lung biopsy for diagnosis. Gallium scans and bronchoalveolar lavage do not yield a specific diagnosis but help to document the extent and character of inflammation.

INDIVIDUAL ILDs   Idiopathic pulmonary fibrosis   Also known as cryptogenic fibrosing alveolitis. Chronic, usually progressive disorder affecting only the lower respiratory tract. Males and females equally affected. One-third date onset of symptoms (dyspnea) to aftermath of viral respiration infection. Usually fatal within 5 years after onset of symptoms.

ILD associated with collagen-vascular disorders   Usually follows development of collagen-vascular disorder; typically mild but occasionally fatal.

Rheumatoid arthritis (RA)   50% of pts with RA have abnormal lung function, 25% have abnormal CXR. Rarely causes symptoms.

Progressive systemic sclerosis   Fibrosis with little inflammation; poor prognosis. Must be distinguished from pulmonary vascular disease.

SLE   Uncommon complication. When it occurs, it is most often an acute, inflammatory patchy process.

Langerhans cell granulomatosis (eosinophilic granuloma or hystiocytosis X)   Disorder of the dendritic cell system, related to Letterer-Siwe and Hand-Schüller-Christian diseases. Develops between 20 and 40 years of age; 90% are present or former smokers. Complicated frequently by pneu-mothoraces. No therapy available.

Chronic eosinophilic pneumonia   Affects females more than males. Often have history of chronic asthma. Symptoms include weight loss, fever, chills, fatigue, dyspnea. CXR shows "photonegative pulmonary edema" pattern with central sparing. Very responsive to glucocorticoids.

Idiopathic pulmonary hemosiderosis   Characterized by recurrent pulmonary hemorrhage; may be life-threatening. Not associated with renal disease.

Goodpasture's syndrome   Relapsing pulmonary hem-orrhage, anemia, and renal failure. Adult males most com-monly affected. Circulating anti-basement membrane anti-bodies.

Inherited disorders   ILD may be associated with tuber-ous sclerosis, neurofibromatosis, Gaucher's disease, Her-mansky-Pudlak syndrome, and Niemann-Pick disease.

TREATMENT   Most important is removal of causative agent. With exception of pneumoconioses, which are generally not treated, and some other specific disorders, therapy is directed toward suppressing the inflammatory process, usually with glucocorticoids. After diagnosis, pts given oral prednisone, 1 mg/kg/d, for 8–12 weeks. Response is assessed by symptoms and PFTs. For idiopathic pulmonary fibrosis and some other disorders, if pt fails to respond to prednisone, consider immunosuppressive therapy with cyclophosphamide (1.0 mg/kg/d) added to prednisone (0.25 mg/kg/d). Smoking cessation, supplemental oxygen (when P_{O_2} <55 mmHg), and therapy for right heart failure and bronchospasm may all improve symptoms.

For a more detailed discussion, see Reynolds HY: Interstitial Lung Diseases, Chap. 211, in HPIM-12, p. 1082

87 CARCINOMA OF THE LUNG

CLASSIFICATION AND CLINICAL CHARACTERISTICS Four major types account for 95% of primary lung cancers: epidermoid (squamous), adenocarcinoma (including bronchioloalveolar), large cell, small cell (including oat cell). Major treatment decisions are made on basis of whether tumor is classified histologically as small cell or non-small cell. Small cell is usually widely disseminated at presentation, while non-small cell may be localized. Epidermoid most common type in males; adenocarcinoma most common type in females. Epidermoid and small cell typically present as central masses, while adenocarcinomas and large cell usually present as peripheral nodules or masses. Epidermoid and large cell cavitate in 20 to 30% of pts.

CLINICAL MANIFESTATIONS Most pts have signs or symptoms of disease at presentation. Central endobronchial tumors cause cough, hemoptysis, wheeze, stridor, dyspnea, pneumonitis. Peripheral lesions cause pain, cough, dyspnea, symptoms of lung abscess resulting from cavitation. Metastatic spread of primary lung cancer may cause tracheal obstruction, dysphagia, hoarseness, Horner's syndrome. Other problems of regional spread include superior vena cava syndrome, pleural effusion, respiratory failure. Extrathoracic metastatic disease affects 50% of pts with epidermoid cancer, 80% with adenocarcinoma and large cell, over 95% with small cell. Clinical problems result from brain metastases, pathologic fractures, liver invasion, and spinal cord compression. Paraneoplastic syndromes may be a presenting finding of lung cancer or first sign of recurrence. Systemic symptoms include weight loss, anorexia, fever. Endocrine syndromes include hypercalcemia (epidermoid), syndrome of inappropriate antidiuretic hormone secretion (small cell), gynecomastia (large cell). Skeletal connective tissue syndromes include clubbing in 30% (most often non-small cell) and hypertrophic pulmonary osteoarthropathy in 1–10% (most often adenocarcinomas), with clubbing, pain, and swelling.

STAGING (Table 87-1) Two parts to staging: (1) determination of location (anatomic staging); (2) assessment of pt's ability to withstand antitumor treatment (physiologic staging). Non-small cell tumors are staged by the TNM/International Staging System (ISS). The T (tumor), N (regional node involvement), and M (presence or absence of distant metastasis) factors are taken together to define different stage

TABLE 87-1   TNM classification of lung cancer using the new International Staging System

PRIMARY TUMOR (T)

T1	Tumor ≤3 cm in greatest dimension, surrounded by lung or visceral pleura, and without evidence of invasion proximal to a lobar bronchus at bronchoscopy
T2	Tumor >3 cm in greatest dimension *or* a tumor of any size that either invades the visceral pleura or has associated atelectasis-obstructive pneumonitis extending to the hilar region
T3	A tumor of any size with direct extension into the chest wall (including superior sulcus tumors), diaphragm, mediastinal pleura, or pericardium
T4	A tumor of any size with invasion of the mediastinum or involving heart, great vessels, trachea, esophagus, vertebral body, or carina *or* the presence of a malignant pleural effusion

REGIONAL LYMPH NODES (N)

N0	No demonstrable metastasis to regional lymph nodes
N1	Metastasis to lymph nodes in the peribronchial and/or ipsilateral hilar region
N2	Metastasis to ipsilateral mediastinal or subcarinal lymph nodes
N3	Metastasis to contralateral mediastinal, contralateral hilar, ipsilateral or contralateral scalene, or supraclavicular lymph nodes

DISTANT METASTASIS (M)

M0	No known distant metastasis
M1	Distant metastasis present with site specified (e.g., brain)

Source: Modified from Minna J, HPIM-12, p. 1105.

groups. Small cell tumors are staged by two-stage system: limited stage disease—confined to one hemithorax and regional lymph nodes; extensive disease—involvement beyond this. General staging procedures include careful ENT exam, CXR, and chest CT scanning. CT scans may suggest mediastinal lymph node involvement and pleural extension in non-small cell lung cancer, but definitive evaluation of mediastinal spread requires histologic exam. Routine radionuclide scans are not obtained in asymptomatic pts. If mass lesion on CXR and no obvious contraindications to curative surgical approach, mediastinum should be investigated. Major contraindications to curative surgery include extrathoracic metastases, superior vena cava syndrome, vocal cord and phrenic nerve paralysis, malignant pleural effusions, metastases to contralateral lung, and histologic diagnosis of small cell cancer.

TREATMENT (Table 87-2)

1. Surgery in pts with localized disease and non-small cell cancer; however, majority initially thought to have "curative" resection ultimately succumb to metastatic disease.

2. Solitary pulmonary nodule: risk factors favoring resection include cigarette smoking, age ≥35, relatively large (>2 cm) lesion, lack of calcification, chest symptoms, and growth of lesion compared to old CXR.

3. For unresectable non-small cell cancer, metastatic disease, or refusal of surgery: consider for radiation therapy; there is no consensus for "debulking" surgery or adjuvant chemotherapy.

4. Small cell cancer: combination chemotherapy is standard mode of therapy; response after 6 to 12 weeks predicts median- and long-term survival.

TABLE 87-2   Summary of treatment approach to lung cancer patients

NON-SMALL CELL LUNG CANCER

Resectable (stages I, II, IIIa, and selected T3, N2 lesions)
  Surgery
  Radiotherapy for "nonoperable" patients
  Postoperative radiotherapy for N2 disease
Nonresectable (N2 and M1)
  Confined to chest: high-dose chest radiotherapy (RT) if possible
  Extrathoracic: RT to symptomatic local sites; chemotherapy (CT) (for
  good-performance-status patients, with evaluable lesions)

SMALL CELL LUNG CANCER

Limited stage (good performance status)
  Combination chemotherapy + chest RT
Extensive stage (good performance status)
  Combination chemotherapy
Complete tumor responders (all stages)
  Prophylactic cranial RT
Poor-performance-status patients (all stages)
  Modified dose combination chemotherapy
  Palliative RT

ALL PATIENTS

Radiotherapy for brain metastases, spinal cord compression, weight-bearing lytic bony lesions, symptomatic local lesions (never paralyses, obstructed airway, hemoptysis in non-small cell lung cancer and in small cell cancer not responding to chemotherapy)
Appropriate diagnosis and treatment of other medical problems and supportive care during chemotherapy
Encouragement to stop smoking

Source: Minna J: HPIM-12, p. 1107.

5. Laser obliteration of tumor through bronchoscopy in presence of bronchial obstruction.

PROGNOSIS At time of diagnosis, only 20% of pts have localized disease. Even in those with apparent localized disease, overall 5-year survival is 30% for males and 50% for females; rates—unchanged over past 20 years.

For a more detailed discussion, see Minna JD: Neoplasms of the Lung, Chap. 215, in HPIM-12, p. 1102

PLEURAL DISEASE

PLEURITIS Inflammation of pleura may occur with pneumonia, tuberculosis, pulmonary infarction, and neoplasm. Pleuritic pain without physical and x-ray findings suggests epidemic pleurodynia (viral inflammation of intercostal muscles); hemoptysis and parenchymal involvement on CXR suggest infection or infarction. Pleural effusion without parenchymal disease suggests postprimary tuberculosis, subdiaphragmatic abscess, mesothelioma, connective tissue disease, or primary bacterial infection of pleural space.

PLEURAL EFFUSION May or may not be associated with pleuritis. In general, effusions due to pleural disease resemble plasma (exudates); effusions with normal pleura are ultrafiltrates of plasma (transudates). Exudates have high protein content (>30 g/L) [or high total fluid/serum protein ratio

TABLE 88-1 Evaluation of pleural fluid

	Transudate	Exudate
Typical appearance	Clear	Clear, cloudy, or bloody
Protein		
Absolute value	<3.0 g/dL	>3.0 g/dL*
Pleural fluid/serum ratio	<0.5	>0.5
Lactic dehydrogenase		
Absolute value	<200 IU/L	>200 IU/L
Pleural fluid/serum ratio	<0.6	>0.6
Glucose	>60 mg/dL (usually same as in blood)	Variable; often <60 mg/dL
Leukocytes	<1000/mL	>1000/mL
Polymorphonuclear	<50%	Usually >50% in acute inflammation
Erythrocytes	<5000/mL†	Variable
pH	↑	↓
Pleural biopsy indicated?	No	Parapneumonic/other acute inflammation
	Yes	Chronic/subacute or undiagnosed effusion

* Less in hypoproteinemic states.
† Assuming atraumatic tap.

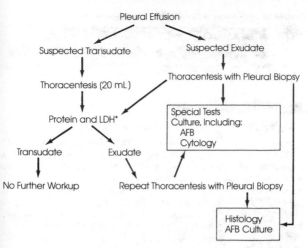

*Draw Blood Sample Simultaneously to Compare with Pleural Fluid Values

FIGURE 88-1   Approach to the diagnosis of pleural effusions. The special tests are summarized in Table 88-2. *(Reproduced from Ingram RH, Jr.: HPIM-11, p. 1125.)*

(>0.5)] and/or pleural/serum LDH activity ratio >0.6. With empyema, pH <7.2, WBCs ↑ (>1000/mL), and glucose ↓. If neoplasm or tuberculosis is considered, closed pleural biopsy should be performed (see Table 88-1, Fig. 88-1). Despite full evaluation, no cause for effusion will be found in 25% of pts.

POSTPRIMARY TUBERCULOSIS EFFUSIONS   Fluid is exudative with predominant lymphocytosis; bacilli are rarely seen on smear and fluid culture is positive in fewer than 20%; closed biopsy required for diagnosis.

NEOPLASTIC EFFUSIONS   Most often lung cancer, breast cancer, or lymphoma. Fluid is exudative; fluid cytology and pleural biopsy will confirm diagnosis in 60%; pleural sclerosis with tetracycline or cytotoxic agents may be required for management.

RHEUMATOID ARTHRITIS (RA)   Exudative effusions may precede articular symptoms; very low glucose and pH; usually males.

PANCREATITIS   Typically left-sided; up to 15% of pts with pancreatitis; high pleural fluid amylase is suggestive but also may occur with effusions due to neoplasms, infection, and esophageal rupture.

TABLE 88-2 Special tests for pleural effusions

	Transudate	Exudate
RBC	<10,000/mL	>100,000/mL suggests neoplasm, infarction, trauma; >10,000 to <100,000/mL is indeterminate
WBC	<100/mL	Usually >1000/mL
Differential WBC	Usually >50% lymphocytes or mononuclear cells	>50% lymphocyts (tuberculosis, neoplasm)
		>50% polymorphonuclear (acute inflammation)
pH	>7.3	<7.3 (inflammatory)
Glucose	Same as blood ($\pm$)	Low (infection)
		Extremely low (rheumatoid arthritis, occasionally neoplasm)
Amylase		>500 units/mL (pancreatitis; occasionally neoplasm, infection)
Specific proteins		Low C3, C4 components of complement (SLE, rheumatoid arthritis)
		Rheumatoid factor
		Antinuclear factor

From Ingram RH, Jr, HPIM-11, p. 1125.

EOSINOPHILIC EFFUSION Defined as more than 10% eosinophils; nonspecific finding may occur with viral, bacterial, traumatic, and pancreatic effusions and may follow prior thoracentesis.

HEMOTHORAX Most commonly follows blunt or penetrating trauma. Pts with bleeding disorders may develop hemothorax following trauma or invasive procedures on pleura. Adequate drainage mandatory to avoid fibrothorax and "trapped" lung.

EMPYEMA An infected pleural effusion or frank pus in pleural space. Usually results from spread of infection from contiguous space. Chest pain, fever, night sweats, cough, and weight loss are common. Thick liquid with loculations, high leukocyte count, and low pH suggest that drainage is required in addition to antibiotics. If closed drainage does not result in marked symptomatic improvement in several days, limited thoracotomy and open drainage are indicated.

PNEUMOTHORAX (PNTX) Spontaneous PNTX most commonly occurs between 20 and 40 years of age; causes sudden, sharp chest pain and dyspnea. Treatment depends on size— if small, observation is sufficient; if large, closed drainage with chest tube is necessary. 50% suffer recurrence, and application of irritants either by surgery or through chest tube may be required so that surfaces become adherent (pleurodesis). Complications include hemothorax, cardiovascular compromise secondary to tension PNTX, and bronchopleural fistula. Many interstitial and obstructive lung diseases may predispose to PNTX.

MEDIASTINAL DISEASE

MEDIASTINITIS   Usually infections. Routes of infection include esophageal perforation or tracheal disruption (trauma, instrumentation, eroding carcinoma). Radiographic hallmarks include mediastinal widening, air in mediastinum, pneumo- or hydropneumothorax. Therapy usually involves surgical drainage and antibiotics.

TUMORS AND CYSTS   Most common mediastinal masses in adults are metastatic carcinomas and lymphomas. Sarcoidosis, infectious mononucleosis, and AIDS may produce mediastinal lymphadenopathy. Neurogenic tumors, teratodermoids, thymomas, and bronchogenic cysts account for two-thirds of remaining mediastinal masses. Specific locations for specific etiologies (see Table 88-3). Evaluation includes CXR, CT scan, and when diagnosis remains in doubt, mediastinoscopy and biopsy.

NEUROGENIC TUMORS   Most common primary mediastinal neoplasms; majority are benign; vague chest pain and cough.

TERATODERMOIDS   Anterior mediastinum; 10–20% undergo malignant transformation.

THYMOMAS   10% primary mediastinal neoplasms; one-quarter are malignant; myasthenia gravis occurs in half.

SUPERIOR VENA CAVA SYNDROME   Dilation of veins of upper thorax and neck, plethora, facial and conjuctival edema, headache, visual disturbances, and reduced state of consciousness; most often due to malignant disease—75% bronchogenic carcinoma, most others lymphoma.

TABLE 88-3   Nature of masses in various locations in mediastinum

Superior	Anterior and middle	Posterior
Lymphoma	Lymphoma	Neurogenic tumors
Thymoma	Metastatic carcinoma	Lymphoma
Retrosternal thyroid	Teratodermoid	Hernia (Bochdalek)
Metastatic carcinoma	Bronchogenic cyst	Aortic aneurysm
Parathyroid tumors	Aortic aneurysm	
Zenker's diverticulum	Pericardial cyst	
Aortic aneurysm		

DISORDERS OF DIAPHRAGM

DIAPHRAGMATIC PARALYSIS   Unilateral paralysis   Usually caused by phrenic nerve injury due to trauma or mediastinal tumor, but nearly half are unexplained; usually asymptomatic; suggested by CXR, confirmed by fluoroscopy.

Bilateral paralysis   May be due to high cervical cord injury, motor neuron disease, poliomyelitis, polyneuropathies, bilateral phrenic involvement by mediastinal lesions, after cardiac surgery, dyspnea; paradoxical abdominal motion should be sought in supine pts.

For a more detailed discussion, see Pierson DJ: Diseases of the Pleura, Mediastinum, and Diaphragm, Chap. 216, in HPIM-12, p. 1111

ALVEOLAR HYPOVENTILATION Exists when arterial P_{CO_2} increases above the normal 37–43 mmHG. In most clinically important chronic hypoventilation syndromes Pa_{CO_2} is 50–80 mmHg.

CAUSE Underlying alveolar hypoventilation always is (1) a defect in the metabolic respiratory control system; (2) a defect in the respiratory neuromuscular system; or (3) a defect in the ventilatory apparatus (Table 89-1).

TABLE 89-1 Chronic hypoventilation syndromes

Mechanism	Site of defect	Disorder
Impaired respiratory drive	Peripheral and central chemoreceptors	Carotid body dysfunction, trauma
		Prolonged hypoxia
		Metabolic alkalosis
	Brainstem respiratory neurons	Bulbar poliomyelitis, encephalitis
		Brainstem infarction, hemorrhage, trauma
		Brainstem demyclination, degeneration
		Chronic drug administration
		Primary alveolar hypoventilation syndrome
Defective respiratory neuromuscular system	Spinal cord and peripheral nerves	High cervical trauma
		Poliomyelitis
		Motor neuron disease
		Peripheral neuropathy
	Respiratory muscles	Myasthenia gravis
		Muscular dystrophy
		Chronic myopathy
Impaired ventilatory apparatus	Chest wall	Kyphoscoliosis
		Fibrothorax
		Thoracoplasty
		Ankylosing spondylitis
		Obesity-hypoventilation
	Airways and lungs	Laryngeal and tracheal stenosis
		Obstructive sleep apnea
		Cystic fibrosis
		Chronic obstructive pulmonary disease

Source: Phillipson EA: HPIM-12, p. 1116.

Disorders associated with impaired respiratory drive, defects in respiratory neuromuscular system, and upper airway obstruction produce an increase in Pa_{CO_2}, despite normal lungs, because of a decrease in overall minute ventilation.

Disorders of chest wall, lower airways, and lungs produce an increase in Pa_{CO_2}, despite a normal or increased minute ventilation.

Increased Pa_{CO_2} leads to respiratory acidosis, compensatory increase in HCO_3^-, and decrease in Pa_{O_2}.

Hypoxemia may induce secondary polycythemia, pulmonary hypertension, right heart failure. Gas exchange worsens during sleep, resulting in morning headache, impaired sleep quality, fatigue, daytime somnolence, mental confusion (Fig. 89-1).

HYPOVENTILATION SYNDROMES

PRIMARY ALVEOLAR HYPOVENTILATION   Cause unknown; rare; thought to arise from defect in metabolic respiratory control

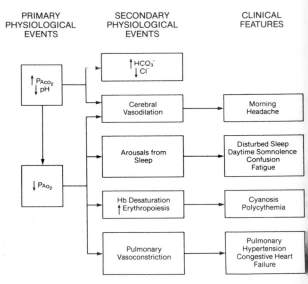

FIGURE 89-1   Physiologic and clinical features of alveolar hypoventilation. *(After Phillipson EA: HPIM-12, p. 1117.)*

system; key diagnostic finding is chronic respiratory acidosis without respiratory muscle weakness or impaired ventilatory mechanics. Some pts respond to respiratory stimulants and supplemental O_2.

RESPIRATORY NEUROMUSCULAR DISORDERS   Several primary neuromuscular disorders produce chronic hypoventilation (see Table 89-1). Hypoventilation usually develops gradually but acute, superimposed respiratory loads (e.g., viral bronchitis with airways obstruction) may precipitate respiratory failure. Diaphragm weakness is a common feature, with orthopnea and paradoxical abdominal movement in supine posture. Testing reveals low maximum voluntary ventilation and reduced maximal inspiratory and expiratory pressures. Therapy involves treatment of underlying condition. Many pts benefit from mechanical ventilatory assistance at night or the entire day.

OBESITY-HYPOVENTILATION SYNDROME   Massive obesity imposes a mechanical load on the respiratory system. Small percentage of morbidly obese pts develop hypercapnia, hypoxemia, and ultimately polycythemia, pulmonary hypertension, and right heart failure. Obstructive sleep apnea may contribute in many pts. Most pts have mild to moderate airflow obstruction. Treatment includes weight loss, smoking cessation, and pharmacologic respiratory stimulants such as progesterone.

SLEEP APNEA   By convention, apnea is defined as cessation of airflow for >10 s. Minimum number of events per night for diagnosis is uncertain but most pts have at least 10–15/h of sleep. Some patients have *central apnea* with transient loss of neural drive to respiratory muscles during sleep. Vast majority have primarily *obstructive apnea* with occlusion in the upper airway. Sleep plays a permissive role in collapse of upper airway. Alcohol and sedatives exacerbate the condition. Most pts have structural narrowing of upper airway. Symptoms include snoring, excessive daytime sleepiness, memory loss, and impotence. Nocturnal hypoxia, a consequence of apnea, may contribute to arrhythmias, pulmonary hypertension, and right heart failure.

Diagnosis   This requires overnight polysomnography. Therapy is directed at increasing upper airway size, increasing upper airway tone, and minimizing upper airway collapsing pressures. Some pts benefit from protriptyline (20–30 mg at bedtime) or surgery (uvulopalatopharyngoplasty). Weight loss often reduces disease severity. Majority of pts with severe sleep apnea require nasal continuous positive airway pressure (nasal C-PAP).

HYPERVENTILATION

Increased ventilation, causing Pa_{CO_2} <37 mmHg. Causes include lesions of the CNS, metabolic acidosis, anxiety, drugs (e.g., salicylates), hypoxemia, hypoglycemia, hepatic coma, and sepsis. Hyperventilation also may occur with some types of lung disease, particularly interstitial disease and pulmonary edema.

For a more detailed discussion, see Phillipson EA: Disorders of Ventilation, Chap. 217, in HPIM-12, p. 1116

---

90 DISEASES OF THE UPPER RESPIRATORY TRACT

NOSE

ANOSMIA (LOSS OF OLFACTORY SENSE) When *transient,* it is usually due to acute infections of the upper respiratory tract. When *chronic,* it is usually due to congenital defects, tumors, trauma, nasal polyps, or chronic nasal obstruction.

RHINITIS (NASAL DISCHARGE) May be caused by hay fever, vasomotor rhinitis, acute coryza, chronic use of vasoconstrictor drugs, atrophy of mucosal tissue, and upper respiratory manifestations of measles, syphilis, tuberculosis. Less commonly, rhinitis and nasal obstruction may be caused by neoplasms and granulomatous disorders (Wegener's granulomatosis, sarcoidosis, midline granuloma).

NASAL OBSTRUCTION When *acute,* it is usually due to viral infection, whereas *chronic* obstruction may be due to allergic reactions or deviated septum. Treatment depends on cause.

EPISTAXIS Most commonly due to trauma, especially "nose picking," with bleeding from Kiesselbach's plexus on the nasal septum. Also occurs with viral infections, typhoid fever, malaria. Noninfectious causes include bleeding diatheses, polycythemia vera, acute sinusitis, tumors.

NASAL FURUNCULOSIS Most common organism is *Staphylococcus aureus.* Potentially life-threatening because of threat of spread to cavernous sinus. Treatment consists of antistaphylococcal antibiotics. Lesions *must* not be squeezed; incision and drainage discouraged except for large or painful lesions.

PHARYNX

ACUTE PHARYNGITIS Symptoms range from "scratchy throat" to severe pain with difficulty swallowing. Lingual tonsillitis associated with streptococcal pharyngitis may cause pain on moving tongue. Findings may range from simple erythema to vascular congestion, exudate, and lymphoid hypertrophy. Presence of exudate does not establish a specific etiology. Single throat culture yields *Streptococcus pyogenes* in only 70% of pts with pharyngitis due to this organism. Following culture, initial treatment may be based on clinical diagnosis, with modifications based on results of culture.

PERITONSILLAR CELLULITIS AND ABSCESS A complication of acute pharyngitis. First sign is tonsillar enlargement, which

371

may progress to occlusion of upper airway. May progress from cellulitis to abscess; diagnosis based on PE. Initial treatment consists of antibiotics, with incision and drainage if large abscess persists.

PARAPHARYNGEAL ABSCESS   Also a complication of acute pharyngitis. Bacterial invasion of tonsil leads to intratonsillar abscess and inflammation of parapharyngeal space; usually unilateral. May spread to jugular vein causing septic thrombophlebitis. If large abscess persists, treatment with antibiotics is followed by incision and drainage.

RETROPHARYNGEAL ABSCESS   Most common under age 4. In adults, may follow acute otitis, dental disease, regional trauma. May complicate cervical or cervicodorsal vertebral osteomyelitis. Diabetes mellitus, immunosuppression are predisposing factors. Treatment as for parapharyngeal abscess.

CHRONIC SORE THROAT   May be symptom of upper airway neoplasm. Also caused by mouth breathing (often with sleep apnea), cigarette smoking, subacute thyroiditis.

SINUSES

ACUTE SINUSITIS   Most common organisms are *S. pneumoniae*, *S. pyogenes*, and *H. influenzae*. Most common predisposing factor is viral URI. *Diagnosis* is made clinically; localized pain and tenderness, nasal obstruction, recurrent headaches, fever, and chills. *Therapy* includes antibiotics, intranasal vasoconstrictors, and in some cases, surgical drainage. Failure to respond to therapy or relapse should prompt a search for a complicating condition such as fracture, tumor, Wegener's granulomatosis. *Complications* include osteomyelitis, meningitis, as well as infection and thrombosis of cavernous and sagittal veins.

CHRONIC SINUSITIS   A difficult diagnosis to establish. Symptoms include headaches, nasal obstruction, and tenderness. X-ray exams of paranasal sinuses reveal thickening of mucus membranes. Allergic background frequent.

LARYNX

Principal symptom of laryngeal disease is hoarseness, which may be due to inflammatory lesions, functional disturbances (hysterical aphonia), and local or generalized neurologic disease (see Table 90-1); cough is common. Stridor and dyspnea are uncommon and suggest obstruction.

EPIGLOTTITIS   Uncommon in adults; men are affected more than women. Immunosuppression predisposes to epiglottitis. Organisms include *H. influenzae, S. pneumoniae, S. py-*

TABLE 90-1   Differential diagnosis of hoarseness and other manifestations of laryngeal dysfunction

INTRALARYNGEAL DISEASE

Infectious:
  Common cold, viral laryngitis, herpes simplex, *Haemophilus influenzae*, membranous laryngitis *(Streptococcus pyogenes, Pseudomonas, Fusobacterium)*
Noninfectious:
  Trauma (edema or hematoma); vocal cord nodules, papillomas and leukoplakia of vocal cords
  Inhalation of smoke, fire, irritating gases, tobacco smoke
  Tumors (benign or malignant), foreign bodies

EXTRALARYNGEAL DISEASE

Lesions in neck:
  Hemorrhages and/or edema due to trauma, severe traction of neck, thyroidectomy, tracheostomy, and biopsy of scalene node
  Tumors of hypopharynx
Local and systemic disorders outside the neck (produce hoarseness by pressure on laryngeal nerves anywhere along the course outside the neck, or paresis or paralysis of the vocal cords as a manifestation of generalized neurologic dysfunction):
  Local lesions: infectious mononucleosis (enlarged mediastinal nodes), angioedema
  Aneurysms of arch of aorta, carotid or innominate arteries
  Tumors of mediastinal structure
  Tumors of parotid gland, relapsing polychondritis
  Systemic disorders: infectious mononucleosis (nervous system involvement), herpes zoster, mucoviscidosis

Source: Modified from Weinstein L: HPIM-11, p. 1114.

ogenes, E. coli, and anaerobes. Bacteremia occurs in 50%. Sore throat is always present. Fever, dyspnea, dysphagia, and hoarseness also occur. Antibiotics are mandatory. Fiberoptic exam best way to confirm diagnosis. Tracheostomy may be necessary.

TUBERCULOSIS LARYNGITIS   Usually in older men. Hoarseness nearly always present. Pulmonary tuberculosis may be absent. Hyperemia and edema may be only signs on exam. Highly contagious.

CANCER OF LARYNX   Develops at average age of 60; 10 times more common in men. Therapy includes radiation or surgery.

For a more detailed discussion, see Lebovics R: Diseases of the Upper Respiratory Tract, Chap. 214, in HPIM-12, p. 1096

91 PULMONARY INSUFFICIENCY AND ADULT RESPIRATORY DISTRESS SYNDROME (ARDS)

ARDS is a descriptive term applied to many acute, diffuse infiltrative lung lesions of diverse etiologies (see Table 91-1) with severe arterial hypoxemia.

CLINICAL CHARACTERISTICS AND PATHOPHYSIOLOGY Earliest sign is often tachypnea followed by dyspnea. Arterial blood gas shows reduction of P_{O_2} and P_{CO_2} with widened alveolar-arterial O_2 difference. Physical exam and CXR may be normal initially. With progression, pt becomes cyanotic, dyspneic, and increasingly tachypneic. Crackles become audible diffusely and chest radiograph shows diffuse, bilateral, interstitial and alveolar infiltrates.

ARDS increases lung water without increasing hydrostatic forces. Toxic gases (chlorine, NO_2, smoke) and gastric acid aspiration damage the alveolar-capillary membrane directly, whereas sepsis increases alveolar-capillary permeability by producing activation and aggregation of formed blood elements. Though radiologically diffuse, regional lung dysfunction is nonhomogeneous with severe ventilation-perfusion imbalance and actual shunting of blood through collapsed alveoli.

TABLE 91-1 Conditions that may lead to the adult respiratory distress syndrome

1. Diffuse pulmonary infections (e.g., viral, bacterial, fungal, *Pneumocystis*)
2. Aspiration (e.g., gastric contents with Mendelson's syndrome, water with near drowning)
3. Inhalation of toxins and irritants (e.g., chlorine gas, NO_2, smoke, ozone, high concentrations of oxygen)
4. Narcotic overdose pulmonary edema (e.g., heroin, methadone, morphine, dextropropoxyphene)
5. Nonnarcotic drug effects (e.g., nitrofurantoin)
6. Immunologic response to host antigens (e.g., Goodpasture's syndrome, systemic lupus erythematosus)
7. Effects of nonthoracic trauma with hypotension
8. In association with systemic reactions to processes initiated outside the lung (e.g., gram-negative septicemia, hemorrhagic pancreatitis, amniotic fluid embolism, fat embolism)
9. Postcardiopulmonary bypass ("pump lung," "postperfusion lung")

Source: Ingram RH Jr.: HPIM-12, p. 1122.

MANAGEMENT Early in illness supplemental O_2 may be sufficient to correct hypoxemia, but with progression mechanical ventilatory support is necessary. Goal of therapy is to provide adequate tissue O_2 delivery—determined by arterial oxygen saturation (Sa_{O_2}), hemoglobin (Hb), cardiac output, and blood flow distribution. Reasonable objective is to achieve 90% saturation (Pa_{O_2} 8 kPa or 60 mmHg) with the lowest inspired O_2 concentration practical to avoid O_2 toxicity. Hb should be $\geq$100 g/L ($\geq$10 g/dL). Cardiac output is supported as necessary with IV fluids and inotropic agents. Pulmonary artery catheter insertion may be necessary for accurate assessment of ventricular filling pressures, hemodynamics, and O_2 transport. Mechanical ventilation is delivered to improve oxygenation by increasing mean lung volume. This is accomplished using large tidal volumes (12–15 mL/kg lean body weight). If Pa_{O_2} cannot be increased to or above 8 kPa (60 mmHg) with large tidal breaths and high inspired fraction of O_2, then positive end expiratory pressure (PEEP) should be added, beginning generally at 5 cmH_2O and increasing in 2.5-cmH_2O increments while monitoring O_2 delivery.

COMPLICATIONS

1. LV failure is a common, easily missed complication, particularly in pts receiving mechanical ventilation.

2. Secondary bacterial infection may be obscured by the diffuse roentgenographic changes.

3. Bronchial obstruction may be caused by endotracheal or tracheostomy tubes.

4. Pneumothorax and pneumomediastinum may cause abrupt deterioration in pts receiving mechanical ventilation.

PROGNOSIS Overall mortality rate is 50% and varies with the intrinsic mortality of the underlying condition. If ARDS occurs as a result of extrapulmonic sepsis, multiple organ failure often supervenes.

For a more detailed discussion, see Ingram RH Jr.: Adult Respiratory Distress Syndrome, Chap. 218, in HPIM-12, p. 1122

SECTION 6   RENAL DISEASES

92   APPROACH TO PATIENT WITH RENAL DISEASE

Despite the complexity of renal function, diseases of the kidney and urinary tract give rise to a finite number of clinical syndromes (see Table 92-1). The approach to renal disease begins with recognition of a particular syndrome based on findings such as presence or absence of azotemia, proteinuria, hypertension, edema, abnormal UA, electrolyte disorders, abnormal urine volumes, or infection.

ACUTE RENAL FAILURE (Chap. 93)   Clinical syndrome due to diverse causes characterized by a rapid, severe decrease in GFR (rise in serum creatinine and BUN), usually with reduced urine output. Extracellular fluid expansion leads to edema, hypertension, and CHF. Hyperkalemia, hyponatremia, and acidosis are common. Etiologies include ischemia, nephrotoxic injury due to drugs or endogenous pigments, sepsis, severe renovascular disease, or conditions related to pregnancy. Prerenal and postrenal failure are potentially reversible causes.

Rapidly progressive glomerulonephritis (RPGMN)   Loss of renal function occurs over weeks to months. Early, pts are nonoliguric and may have recent flulike symptoms; later, oliguric renal failure with uremic symptoms supervenes. Pulmonary manifestations range from asymptomatic infiltrates to life-threatening hemoptysis. UA shows hematuria, proteinuria, and RBC casts.

Acute glomerulonephritis (Chap. 96)   An acute illness with sudden onset of hematuria, edema, hypertension, oliguria, and elevated BUN and creatinine. Mild pulmonary congestion may be present. An antecedent or concurrent infection or multisystem disease may be causative, or glomerular disease may exist alone. Hematuria, proteinuria, and pyuria are present in the majority, and RBC casts confirm the diagnosis. Serum complement may be decreased.

CHRONIC RENAL FAILURE (Chap. 94)   Progressive permanent loss of renal function over months to years. Because of adaptive mechanisms, symptoms of uremia do not appear

TABLE 92-1   Initial clinical and laboratory data base for defining major syndromes in nephrology

Syndromes	Important clues to diagnosis	Common findings that are not diagnostic
Acute or rapidly progressive renal failure	Anuria, oliguria. Recent decline in GFR.	Hypertension, hematuria, proteinuria, pyuria casts, edema.
Acute nephritis	Hematuria, RBC casts. Azotemia, oliguria. Edema, hypertension.	Proteinuria, pyuria, circulatory congestion.
Chronic renal failure	Azotemia for >3 months. Symptoms or signs of uremia. Symptoms or signs of renal osteodystrophy. Kidneys reduced in size bilaterally. Broad casts in urinary sediment.	Hematuria, proteinuria. Casts, oliguria. Polyuria, nocturia. Edema, hypertension. Electrolyte disorders.
Nephrotic syndrome	Proteinuria >3.5 g/1.73 m²/d. Hypoalbuminemia, hyperlipidemia, lipiduria.	Casts, edema.
Asymptomatic urinary abnormalities	Hematuria, proteinuria (below nephrotic range), sterile pyuria, casts.	
UTI	Bacteriuria >10⁵ colonies/mL. Infectious agent documented in urine. Pyuria, WBC casts. Frequency, urgency. Bladder tenderness, flank tenderness.	Hematuria, mild azotemia, mild proteinuria, fever.
Renal tubule defects	Electrolyte disorders. Polyuria, nocturia. Symptoms or signs of renal osteodystrophy. Large kidneys. Renal transport defects.	Hematuria, "tubular" proteinuria, enuresis.
Hypertension	Systolic/diastolic hypertension.	Proteinuria, casts, azotemia.
Nephrolithiasis	Previous history of stone passage or removal. Previous history of stone seen by x-ray. Renal colic.	Hematuria, pyuria, frequency, urgency.

TABLE 92-1 Initial clinical and laboratory data base for defining major syndromes in nephrology *(Continued)*

Syndromes	Important clues to diagnosis	Common findings that are not of diagnostic value
Urinary tract obstruction	Azotemia, oliguria, anuria. Polyuria, nocturia, urinary retention. Slowing of urinary stream. Large prostate, large kidneys. Flank tenderness, large residual volume.	Hematuria, pyuria, enuresis, dysuria.

Source: Modified from Coe FL, Brenner BM: HPIM-12, p. 1134.

until GFR is reduced to about 25% of normal. Hypertension may occur early. Later, signs and symptoms include anorexia, nausea, vomiting, insomnia, weight loss, weakness, paresthesias, bleeding, serositis, anemia, acidosis, and hyperkalemia. Evidence for a *specific* cause may be present (diabetes mellitus, hypertension, urinary tract obstruction, interstitial nephritis). Indications of chronicity include long-standing azotemia, anemia, hyperphosphatemia, hypocalcemia, shrunken kidneys, renal osteodystrophy by x-ray, or findings on renal biopsy.

NEPHROTIC SYNDROME (Chap. 96) Defined as heavy albuminuria (>3.5 g/day in the adult); may be accompanied by edema, hypoalbuminemia, hyperlipidemia, and varying degrees of renal insufficiency. Can be idiopathic or due to drugs, infections, neoplasms, multisystem or hereditary diseases. Complications include severe edema, thromboembolic events, infection, and protein malnutrition.

ASYMPTOMATIC URINARY ABNORMALITIES May include isolated hematuria, proteinuria, or pyuria. Hematuria may be due to neoplasms, stones, or infection at any level of the urinary tract, sickle cell disease, or analgesic abuse. Renal parenchymal causes are suggested by RBC casts, proteinuria, or dysmorphic RBCs in urine. Pattern of gross hematuria may be helpful in localizing site. Hematuria with low-grade proteinuria may be due to benign recurrent hematuria or IgA nephropathy. Modest proteinuria may be an isolated finding due to fever, exertion, CHF, or upright posture. Renal causes include diabetes mellitus, amyloidosis, or other mild forms of glomerular disease. Pyuria can be caused by UTI, interstitial nephritis, SLE, or renal transplant rejection. "Sterile" pyuria is associated with UTI treated with antibiotics, glucocorticoid therapy, acute febrile episodes, cyclophosphamide therapy, pregnancy, renal transplant rejection, genitourinary trauma, prostatitis, cystourethritis, tuberculosis and other mycobacterial infections, fungal infection, *Haemophilus influenzae*, anaerobic infection, fastidious bacteria, and bacterial L forms.

UTI (Chap. 98)   Generally defined as bacteriuria greater than 10^5 bacteria/mL of urine. Levels between 10^2 and 10^5/mL may indicate infection in some pts but are commonly due to poor sample collection, especially if mixed flora are present. Adults at risk are sexually active women or anyone with urinary tract obstruction, reflux, catheterization, or neurogenic bladder. Prostatitis, urethritis, and vaginitis may be distinguished by quantitative urine culture. Flank pain, nausea, vomiting, fever, and chills indicate renal infection. UTI is a common cause of sepsis.

RENAL TUBULAR DEFECTS (Chap. 97)   Generally inherited, they include anatomic defects (polycystic kidneys, medullary cystic disease, medullary sponge kidney) detected in the evaluation of hematuria, flank pain, infection, or renal failure of unknown cause; as well as disorders of tubular transport that cause glucosuria, aminoaciduria, stones, or rickets. Fanconi syndrome is a generalized tubular defect that can be hereditary or acquired from drugs, heavy metals, multiple myeloma, amyloidosis, or renal transplantation. Nephrogenic diabetes insipidus (polyuria, polydypsia, hypernatremia, hypernatremic dehydration) and renal tubular acidosis are additional tubular disorders.

HYPERTENSION (Chap. 69)   Blood pressure >140/90 mmHg may affect 20% of the U.S. adult population and when inadequately controlled is an important contributor to cerebrovascular accident, MI, CHF, and renal failure. Hypertension is usually asymptomatic until cardiac, renal, or neurologic symptoms appear. Most cases are idiopathic, and occur between the ages of 25 and 45 years.

NEPHROLITHIASIS (Chap. 100)   Patients with colicky pain, UTI, hematuria, dysuria, or unexplained pyuria. Unsuspected stones may be found on routine x-ray. Most are radiopaque Ca stones, commonly with a high level of urinary Ca excretion as underlying cause. Staghorn calculi are large, branching radiopaque stones within the renal pelvis due to recurrent infection. Uric acid stones are radiolucent. UA may reveal hematuria, pyuria, or pathologic crystals.

URINARY TRACT OBSTRUCTION (Chap. 101)   Causes variable symptoms depending on whether it is acute or chronic, unilateral or bilateral, complete or partial, and on underlying etiology. It is an important reversible cause of unexplained renal failure. Upper tract obstruction may be silent or produce flank pain, hematuria, and renal infection. Bladder symptoms may be present in lower tract obstruction. Functional consequences include polyuria, anuria, nocturia, acidosis, hyperkalemia, and hypertension. A flank or suprapubic mass may be found on physical exam.

For a more detailed discussion, see Coe FL, Brenner BM: Approach to the Patient with Diseases of the Kidneys and Urinary Tract, Chap. 221, in HPIM-12, p. 1134

93 ACUTE RENAL FAILURE (ARF)

CAUSES (see Table 93-1)   These are categorized as prerenal, intrinsic renal, or postrenal. Only about half of pts with ARF have anuria-oliguria; those with preserved urine output usually have a mild disorder and a better prognosis.

Prerenal failure, the most common cause of acute azotemia, results from inadequate perfusion of kidneys. This may be due to severe hemorrhage, volume contraction, extracellular fluid sequestration, low cardiac output, vascular pooling, or renal artery obstruction. NSAIDs may also cause functional prerenal azotemia, especially in pts with chronic renal failure (CRF), nephrotic syndrome, CHF, cirrhosis, those on diuretics, and the elderly. Prolonged renal hypoperfusion is a risk factor for ARF due to acute tubular necrosis (ATN).

Intrinsic renal causes include renovascular disease (Chap. 99), glomerulonephritis (Chap. 96), and interstitial nephritis (Chap. 97). Some are amenable to specific treatment.

Postrenal causes of ARF are those producing urinary obstruction at any level from the kidneys to the urethra (Chap. 101). ARF due to urinary obstruction above the

TABLE 93-1   Causes of ARF

Disorder	Causes
PRERENAL FAILURE	
Hypovolemia	Diarrhea, vomiting, hemorrhage, overdiuresis, pancreatitis, peritonitis
Vasodilatation	Sepsis, drugs, anaphylaxis, *liver → varices*
Cardiovascular ↓ *output*	CHF, MI, tamponade
Renal hypoperfusion	Renal artery obstruction, NSAIDs
INTRARENAL FAILURE (INTRINSIC RENAL DISEASE)	
	Hypotension, sustained prerenal failure, postoperative, rhabdomyolysis, aminoglycosides, contrast dye, NSAIDs, glomerulonephritis, vasculitis, interstitial nephritis
POSTRENAL FAILURE	
Intrarenal	Crystals, calculi, papillary necrosis
Extrarenal	Prostate, pelvic, bladder neoplasm, retroperitoneal neoplasm or fibrosis, urethral or bladder neck obstruction

bladder requires simultaneous bilateral involvement or unilateral disease with an absent or impaired contralateral kidney.

ATN This is due to ischemic or toxic injury acting on renal vessels, glomeruli, and/or tubules causing ↓ GFR and ↑ intratubular pressure.

Ischemic ATN may follow abrupt hypoperfusion or evolve from any condition causing severe prerenal failure, particularly in elderly pts or when nephrotoxins are present.

Nephrotoxic ATN can result from exogenous or endogenous causes. Common exogenous nephrotoxins are (1) aminoglycoside antibiotics (dose-related in elderly dehydrated pts or those with prior renal impairment), and (2) contrast dye (in the elderly, diabetics, pts with prior renal impairment, dehydration, myeloma; can be prevented by volume expansion and use of minimal dose). Endogenous nephrotoxins causing ATN include myoglobin released after muscle trauma or with coma or heat stroke. Intravascular hemolysis may cause ARF in the setting of hypotension or sepsis.

Pathophysiologic theories of ATN include obstruction or backleak through damaged tubules and diminished glomerular perfusion secondary to afferent arteriolar vasoconstriction. Histopathologic features are variable. Specific evidence of glomerulonephritis, vasculitis, or interstitial nephritis may be present. Tubular necrosis may coexist with normal glomeruli and blood vessels.

CLINICAL FEATURES Pts with *prerenal failure* have clinical features of volume contraction, hypotension, or impaired cardiac function. Dx is confirmed only when renal perfusion improves, as with volume repletion or improvement in cardiac function.

Postrenal failure may be evident from a distended bladder, large prostate, pelvic mass, or hydronephrosis. The pattern of urinary flow may indicate total (anuria) or partial (polyuria) obstruction. Crystals or urinary infection may be present in urinary sediment. Early (hours) obstruction causes urinary indices identical to those of prerenal failure; later, the indices of obstruction resemble those of ATN (Table 20-1).

ARF due to *intrinsic renal diseases* may require a renal biopsy for diagnosis. RBC casts and heavy proteinuria suggest glomerulonephritis (GN) or vascular inflammatory disease. Interstitial nephritis may also cause fever, skin eruption, and pyuria with eosinophils on Wright's stain of urinary sediment.

With ATN, brown cellular casts and renal tubular epithelial cells may be present in urine sediment. ATN with a low U_{Na} may be due to contrast dye, acute GN, burns, or myoglobinuria. Toxic ATN due to rhabdomyolysis is suggested by a heme-positive dipstick in the absence of microscopic hematuria and a markedly elevated serum CK.

Clinical course ATN begins with diminished urine output within a day of the insult and may cause anuria; oliguria lasts for 10–14 days. If oliguria persists >2–3 weeks, other diagnoses should be considered. The daily increments in BUN and creatinine average 3.6–7.1 mmol/L (10–20 mg/dL) and 45–90 μmol/L (0.5–1.0 mg/dL), respectively, but will be greater in catabolic states.

Complications Include salt and water overload, hypertension, and CHF. Hyperkalemia results from impaired K excretion. Retention of acid causes an anion gap metabolic acidosis. Other complications include hyperphosphatemia, hypocalcemia, hypermagnesemia, mild hyperuricemia, anemia, infection, GI bleeding, ileus, pericarditis, and neurologic abnormalities.

During the recovery phase of ARF, urine volume increases progressively; BUN and creatinine level off and then begin to fall. However, major complications of ARF may first appear during this stage. Fluid and electrolyte depletion may complicate postobstructive diuresis and post ATN.

Principles of *management* of acute renal failure are listed in Table 93-2.

TABLE 93-2 Management of ARF

1. Search for and correct prerenal and postrenal causes.
2. Search for evidence of ischemic or nephrotoxic injury or renal parenchymal disease.
3. Attempt to establish a urine output with volume challenge or furosemide.
4. Conservative therapy:
   Discontinue indwelling catheter
   Measure intake and output
   Daily weights
   Limit fluids to 400 mL + previous day's losses
   Alter medication doses as indicated
   Add phosphate binders
   Treat hyperkalemia and acidosis
5. Dialysis for volume overload, pericarditis, GI bleeding, symptomatic uremia, severe hyperkalemia or acidosis.

For a more detailed discussion, see Anderson RJ, Schrier RW: Acute Renal Failure, Chap. 223, in HPIM-12, p. 1144

CRF refers to the permanent loss of renal function, which, when advanced, results in the signs and symptoms termed *uremia*. Unlike ARF, from which recovery is frequent, CRF is not reversible and may lead to a vicious cycle with progressive loss of remaining nephrons.

CAUSES The common causes of CRF are <u>diabetic nephropathy</u> (28%), <u>hypertension</u> (24%), <u>glomerulonephritis</u> (21%), and <u>polycystic kidney disease</u>.

The specific causes of the <u>uremic syndrome</u> are unknown. In addition to failure of renal excretion of solutes and products of metabolism, CRF causes loss of metabolic and endocrine function of the healthy kidney. The most likely retained toxins causing this syndrome are breakdown products of proteins and amino acids. <u>Urea</u> itself is the most abundant and may account, in part, for <u>malaise, anorexia, and vomiting</u>. Another nitrogenous compound, <u>guanidinosuccinic acid</u>, contributes to <u>platelet dysfunction</u>. Larger compounds ("<u>middle molecules</u>") are implicated in <u>uremic neuropathy</u>. A variety of <u>polypeptide hormones, including parathyroid hormone</u> (PTH), circulate at high levels in CRF and contribute to the uremic syndrome.

CONSEQUENCES CRF and uremia cause deleterious effects on cellular functions and metabolism and on volume and composition of body fluids. Defective membrane transport can cause dysfunction of RBCs and skeletal muscle. Protein malnutrition and inadequate energy intake are common. Hypertriglyceridemia is common, although cholesterol levels are usually normal.

With progressive nephron loss, the ability of the diseased kidney to concentrate urine is impaired, resulting in isosthenuria and leading to polyuria and nocturia. Thus, fluid restriction is potentially hazardous; impaired diluting capacity may result in hyponatremia due to water retention.

In early CRF external Na balance is maintained by an increase in fractional Na excretion, due to altered peritubular factors and osmotic diuresis due to retained solutes. Late in CRF the remaining nephrons cannot excrete normal amounts of Na so that dietary salt is retained, resulting in hypertension and volume overload. However, severe Na restriction may cause Na depletion, with worsening of renal function due to superimposed prerenal azotemia.

Little or no change in blood pH, HCO_3, or P_{CO_2} occur until GFR falls below 50% of normal. <u>Metabolic acidosi</u> results, in part, from diminished NH_3 production. However positive H balance causes only mild nonprogressive metaboli acidosis, probably because of bone buffering. In moderat renal failure, chloride retention leads to hyperchloremi acidosis (normal anion gap acidosis). Retention of sulfate phosphate, and other unmeasured anions in severe CR results in an anion gap acidosis.

With advancing renal disease, phosphate balance is achieve by reduced fractional phosphate reabsorption, mediated b enhanced PTH secretion; the latter is due to ↓ in serum Ca^{2+}, associated with retention of phosphate, as GFR falls Elevated PTH levels cause many of the bone changes o renal osteodystrophy. Other abnormalities include skeleta resistance to PTH and <u>reduced circulating 1,25(OH)₂D</u>.

Clinical spectrum of abnormalities in uremia are listed i Table 94-1. Signs and symptoms typically appear late in th course of CRF, when GFR <25% of normal.

TABLE 94-1 Consequences of CRF

VOL/COMPOSITION BODY FLUIDS	NEUROMUSCULAR
	confusion somnolence
Na retention or depletion	*seizures coma*
Hyponatremia	Encephalopathy
Hyperkalemia	Peripheral neuropathy *flapping tre*
Metabolic acidosis	Dialysis dementia *– Al* *tocking -g*
Hyperphosphatemia	Dialysis disequilibrium *– sensory convulsion*
Hypocalcemia	
Hypermagnesemia	GASTROINTESTINAL
Hyperuricemia	
	Anorexia, nausea, vomiting
CARDIOPULMONARY	Gastroenteritis
	Peptic ulcer *(↓ gastrin catabolism)*
CHF	Ascites
Hypertension *– volume overload (↓ GFR)*	Diverticulosis
Pericarditis	Viral hepatitis
Accelerated atherosclerosis *– angina*	
Pneumonitis	ENDOCRINE
Pleuritis	
	Secondary hyperparathyroidism
HEMATOLOGIC	Vitamin D disorders
	Glucose intolerance *(↓ insulin catabol*
Anemia *pallor, fatigue dyspnea, tachycardia*	Amenorrhea *+ high spontaneous abor*
Poor hemostasis *hemic murmur (pulm)*	Impaired testicular function
Leukocyte abnormalities	Impotence
BONE	SKIN
Osteodystrophy – PTH : Ca++ resorption + remodeling	Pruritus *– metastatic calcification*
Rickets . osteomalacia – Vit. D.	Ecchymosis
Osteoporosis – met- acidosis – Ht accum. in bone	Hyperpigmentation

hypercalcemia – metastatic calcification in skin – pruritus
*   – gastritis*
*   – band keratopathy ← deposition around cornea*

Excessive salt ingestion leads to CHF, hypertension, and edema; extrarenal fluid losses may cause extracellular volume depletion. Excessive water ingestion results in hyponatremia. Hyperkalemia results from excessive K intake, antikaliuretic drugs, acidosis, or oliguria. Hyperphosphatemia and hypocalcemia develop when GRF falls to <25% of normal. Hypermagnesemia is a hazard in pts given Mg-containing antacids or cathartics.

In addition to CHF, pulmonary edema may be due to ↑ capillary permeability in the absence of volume overload. Both forms respond to dialysis. Pericarditis can be due to uremia itself or to a systemic disease. There is a high incidence of accelerated atherosclerosis in dialysis pts. Normochromic normocytic anemia results from diminished erythropoiesis, shortened RBC survival, and, in some cases, blood loss. Abnormalities in hemostasis, characterized by prolonged bleeding time, lower platelet factor III activity, and platelet function abnormalities, may produce hemorrhagic complications; GI bleeding is common. Mild thrombocytopenia may be present. The hemostatic defect responds to effective dialysis. Cryoprecipitate may be useful. A variety of WBC functions may be impaired.

Encephalopathy and peripheral neuropathy are common in advanced CRF and improve with dialysis. GI symptoms of uremia include anorexia, nausea, and vomiting, especially in the morning. Shallow mucosal ulcers, peptic ulcers, and diverticulitis may be sites of GI bleeding. Overproduction of PTH contributes to bone changes of osteitis fibrosa cystica. Abnormal vitamin D metabolism may induce rickets and osteomalacia. Glucose intolerance results largely from resistance to insulin. Amenorrhea, impaired testicular function, and impotence are common.

Uremic pruritus, ecchymosis, a yellow hyperpigmentation due to retention of urochromes, and discoloration due to hemachromatosis are cutaneous manifestations of CRF.

metallic taste, muscle cramps, restless legs.

For a more detailed discussion, see Brenner BM, Lazarus JM: Chronic Renal Failure: Pathophysiologic and Clinical Considerations, Chap. 224, in HPIM-12, p. 1151

Kidney normally degrades insulin + gastrin ∴ glucose intolerance + gastritis
↓ wbc. fxn - ↓ chemotactic factors → infection

95 DIALYSIS AND TRANSPLANTATION

CHRONIC HEMODIALYSIS

The usual therapy for end-stage renal disease (ESRD) and many forms of poisoning is perfusion of pt's blood and a dialysate solution on opposite sides of a membrane. Solutes such as urea diffuse out, and salt and water are attracted by hyperfiltration. Efficiency of dialysis depends on solute size, blood and dialysate flow rates, and characteristics of dialysis membrane.

INDICATIONS These include ARF (Chap. 93), CRF in pts due for early transplantation, and other pts with CRF in whom the quality of life has deteriorated. Most pts are dialyzed for 4 h three times per week and are maintained on a 40–60 g protein diet with Na and K restriction. Phosphate-binding antacids, folate, and multivitamins are added.

ACCESS Commonly achieved by creation of a subcutaneous AV fistula or shunt. Alternatives include prosthetic fistulas and percutaneous subclavian or femoral catheters. In pts with CRF, access surgery should be performed when the serum creatinine level has reached 600–800 μmol/L (7–9 mg/dL), since the native fistula cannot be used for several weeks. Shunts and catheters are temporary devices. Prosthetic fistulas are more likely to cause infection, thrombosis, and aneurysm. Other complications of access sites and of dialysis are shown in Table 95-1. Access infections are usually staphylococcal and may lead to sepsis and/or endocarditis.

Many manifestations of uremia persist in pts on chronic hemodialysis, although they are less severe. Anemia may be

TABLE 95-1 Complications of dialysis

Access	Dialysis procedure
Infection	Hemorrhage
Thrombosis	Hypotension
Vascular compromise	Cardiac ischemia
High-output CHF	Cramps, nausea, vomiting
Carpal tunnel syndrome	Seizures
Recirculation of blood flow	Hypoventilation, hypoxemia
	Anticoagulation
	Air embolism
	Hemolysis

aggravated by blood loss and folate deficiency. Accelerated atherosclerosis is common in pts on chronic hemodialysis. Pericarditis, diverticulosis, hepatitis (most frequently non-A, non-B), impotence, and acquired renal cysts are other complications. Dialysis dementia, a syndrome of speech dyspraxia, seizures, and myoclonus, linked to aluminum intoxication is usually fatal. *Disequilibrium* refers to CNS symptoms ranging from nausea to seizures related to volume depletion and osmolar shifts, usually occuring with early treatments. Renal osteodystrophy may progress or appear in the form of osteomalacia with bone pain and fractures.

PERITONEAL DIALYSIS This alternative to chronic hemodialysis has the advantage of safety, lack of need for blood access, lack of blood loss, less cardiovascular stress, and pt independence. The major complication is peritonitis, most commonly staphylococcal. Malnutrition due to protein loss, hypertriglyceridemia, hypernatremia, hyperglycemia, obesity, and cardiopulmonary compromise are other complications.

RENAL TRANSPLANTATION

Now a commonplace therapy for ESRD. Immunologic rejection is the major hazard in graft survival, but recent advances have improved transplant success and lessened recipient risk.

Graft acceptance is determined by genetic compatibility of donor and recipient, based on matching of antigens (Ag) of *HLA* genes. Class I Ag are detected by a lymphocyte assay; class II Ag ("DR") by the mixed lymphocyte culture (MLC). HLA genes are inherited as a haplotype from each parent. Graft survival in living related transplants improves with matching of class I Ag. Class II Ag matching is more important to success of cadaveric transplants. Presensitization (the presence of antibody against donor ABO or class I Ag), is detected by a positive cross-match and is a contraindication to transplantation. Pretransplant blood transfusion enhances graft survival, although it risks sensitization in some pts.

Contraindications to transplantation include presensitization; major extrarenal diseases (such as coronary artery or cerebrovascular disease, respiratory failure, or malignancy), active infection, advanced age, active glomerulonephritis, and treatable renal disease (see Table 95-2).

REJECTION May be (1) hyperacute (immediate graft failure due to presensitization); (2) acute (within weeks to months with a rise in creatinine, hypertension, fever, graft tenderness, volume overload, and low urine output, treated by intense

TABLE 95-2   **Contraindications to kidney transplantation**

Absolute contraindications	Relative contraindications
Reversible renal involvement	Age
Ability of conservative measures to maintain useful life	Severe bladder or urethral abnormalities
Advanced forms of major extrarenal complications (cerebrovascular or coronary disease, neoplasia)	Iliofemoral occlusive disease
	Diabetes mellitus
	Severe psychiatric disease
	Oxalosis
Active infection	
Active glomerulonephritis	
Previous sensitization to donor tissue	

Reproduced from Carpenter CB, Lazarus JM: HPIM-12, p. 1157.

immunosuppression); or (3) chronic (months to years with ongoing loss of function and hypertension).

IMMUNOSUPPRESSIVE THERAPY   Used to prevent or impede allograft rejection (see Table 95-3). Azathioprine inhibits synthesis of DNA, RNA, or both and is the keystone of immunosuppressive therapy. It is begun at transplantation and continued throughout and is useful in preventing acute rejection. CBC must be monitored. If renal function worsens, smaller doses may be required. Toxicity is indicated by low WBC, occasional thrombocytopenia, jaundice, and alopecia. Glucocorticoids are used for maintenance and are given in higher doses to reverse acute rejection; chronic rejection is often steroid-resistant. Cyclosporine blocks formation of interleukin 2 by helper-inducer (CD4+) T lymphocytes; it has improved survival rates, decreased severity of acute rejection episodes, and allowed lower doses of prednisone. The most important limiting factor is dose-dependent nephrotoxicity that does not correlate well with blood levels. Manifestations of cyclosporin-induced nephrotoxicity include posttransplant oliguria, an insidious rise in serum creatinine, hypertension, hyperkalemia, and renal tubular acidosis. Other complications are hepatotoxicity, tremor, gingival hypertrophy, and hirsutism.

Efficacies of antithrombocyte globulin and monoclonal antibodies are being studied.

In addition to acute rejection, other causes of early posttransplant oliguria include volume depletion, ureteral obstruction or leak, and renal artery stenosis. Workup includes renal ultrasound and radioisotope scan. Acute rejection may begin several days after transplant. Urinary Na may be low. A renal transplant biopsy may be preferable to empiric therapy of suspected rejection.

ABLE 95-3   Complications of immunosuppressive therapy

ZATHIOPRINE	GLUCOCORTICOIDS
Sone marow suppression	Infection
Hepatitis	Diabetes mellitus
Malignancy	Adrenal suppression
	Euphoria, psychosis
CYCLOSPORINE	Peptic ulcer disease
	Hypertension
Nephrotoxicity	Osteoporosis
Hepatotoxicity	Myopathy
Tremor	
Gingival hypertrophy	
Hirsutism	
Lymphoma	

Glomerular diseases in transplants include recurrent glomerulonephritis, chronic rejection, and CMV glomerulopathy with nephrotic syndrome.

For a more detailed discussion, see Carpenter CB, Lazarus M: Dialysis and Transplantation in the Treatment of Renal Failure, Chap. 225, in HPIM-12, p. 1157

96 GLOMERULAR DISEASES

ACUTE GLOMERULONEPHRITIS (AGN)

Characterized by development, over days, of azotemia, hypertension, edema, hematuria, proteinuria, and sometimes oliguria. Salt and water retention are due to reduced GFR and may result in circulatory congestion. RBC casts on UA confirm Dx. Proteinuria usually <3 g/d. Most forms of AGN are mediated by humoral immune mechanisms. Clinical course depends on underlying lesion (see Table 96-1).

ACUTE POSTSTREPTOCOCCAL GN The prototype and most common cause in childhood. Nephritis develops 1–3 weeks after pharyngeal or cutaneous infection with nephritogenic strains of group A β-hemolytic streptococci. Dx depends on a positive pharyngeal or skin culture, rising antibody titers, and hypocomplementemia. Renal biopsy reveals diffuse proliferative GN. Treatment consists of correction of fluid and electrolyte imbalance. In most cases the disease is self-limited, although the prognosis in adults is less favorable and urinary abnormalities more likely to persist.

POSTINFECTIOUS GN May follow other bacterial, viral, and parasitic infections. Examples are bacterial endocarditis, sepsis, hepatitis B, and pneumococcal pneumonia. Feature

TABLE 96-1 Causes of acute glomerulonephritis

I. Infectious diseases
   A. Poststreptococcal glomerulonephritis*
   B. Nonstreptococcal postinfectious glomerulonephritis
      1. Bacterial: infective endocarditis,* "shunt nephritis," sepsis, pneumococcal pneumonia, typhoid fever, secondary syphilis, meningococcemia
      2. Viral: hepatitis B, infectious mononucleosis, mumps, measles, varicella, vaccinia, echovirus, and coxsackievirus
      3. Parasitic: malaria, toxoplasmosis
II. Multisystem diseases: systemic lupus erythematosus,* vasculitis, Henoch-Schönlein purpura,* Goodpasture's syndrome
III. Primary glomerular diseases: mesangiocapillary glomerulonephritis, Berger's disease (IgA nephropathy),* "pure" mesangial proliferative glomerulonephritis
IV. Miscellaneous: Guillain-Barré syndrome, irradiation of Wilm's tumor, self-administered diphtheria-pertusis-tetanus vaccine, serum sickness

* Most common causes.
From Glassock RJ, Brenner BM: HPIM-12, p. 1170.

are milder than with poststreptococcal GN. Control of primary infection usually produces resolution of GN.

AGN may occur in several *multisystemic diseases*. In SLE, renal involvement is due to deposition of circulating immune complexes. Clinical features include arthralgias, skin rash, serositis, hair loss, and CNS disease. Renal biopsy reveals mesangial, focal, or diffuse GN and membranous nephropathy; nephrotic syndrome with renal insufficiency is typical. Clinical and biopsy findings may not correlate. Diffuse GN, the most common finding, is characterized by an active sediment, severe proteinuria, and progressive renal insufficiency and may have an ominous prognosis. Pts have a positive ANA, anti-dsDNA, and ↓ complement. Treatment includes oral and/or IV glucocorticoids and cytotoxic agents.

GOODPASTURE'S SYNDROME   Characterized by lung hemorrhage, GN, and circulating antibody to basement membrane, usually in young men. Hemoptysis may precede nephritis. Rapidly progressive renal failure is typical. Circulating anti-GBM antibody and linear immunofluorescence on renal biopsy establish Dx. Linear IgG is also present on lung biopsy. Plasma exchange may produce remission. Severe lung hemorrhage is treated with IV glucocorticoids.

HENOCH-SCHÖNLEIN PURPURA   A generalized vasculitis causing GN, purpura, arthralgias, and abdominal pain; occurs mainly in children. Renal involvement is manifested by hematuria and proteinuria. Serum IgA is increased in half of pts. Renal biopsy is useful for prognosis. Treatment is symptomatic.

VASCULITIS   Several distinct syndromes cause GN. *Polyarteritis nodosa* causes hypertension, arthralgias, neuropathy, and renal failure. Similar features plus palpable purpura and asthma are common in *hypersensitivity angiitis*. *Wegener's granulomatosis* involves upper respiratory tract and kidney and responds to cyclophosphamide.

RAPIDLY PROGRESSIVE GLOMERULONEPHRITIS

Characterized by gradual onset of hematuria, proteinuria, and renal failure, which progresses over a period of weeks to months. Crescentic GN is usually found on renal biopsy. The causes are outlined in Table 96-2. Prognosis for preservation of renal function is poor. Fifty percent of pts refuse dialysis within 6 months of diagnosis. Glucocorticoids in pulsed doses, cytotoxic agents (azathioprine, cyclophosphamide), and intensive plasma exchange in combination have produced encouraging preliminary results.

TABLE 96-2   Causes of rapidly progressive glomerulonephritis

I. Infectious diseases
    A. Post streptococcal glomerulonephritis*
    B. Infective endocarditis*
    C. Occult visceral sepsis
    D. Hepatitis B infection (with vasculitis and/or cryoimmunoglobulinemia)
    E. Human immunodeficiency virus infection(?)
II. Multisystem diseases
    A. Systemic lupus erythematosus*
    B. Henoch-Schönlein purpura*
    C. Systemic necrotizing vasculitis (including Wegener's granulomatosis)*
    D. Goodpasture's syndrome*
    E. Essential mixed (IgG/IgM) cryoimmunoglobulinemia
    F. Malignancy
    G. Relapsing polychondritis
    H. Rheumatoid arthritis (with vasculitis)
III. Drugs
    A. Penicillamine*
    B. Hydralazine
    C. Allopurinol (with vasculitis)
    D. Rifampin
IV. Idiopathic or primary glomerular disease
    A. Idiopathic crescentic glomerulonephritis*
        1. Type I—with linear deposits of Ig (anti-glomerular basement membrane antibody–mediated)
        2. Type II—with granular deposits of Ig (immune-complex–mediated)
        3. Type III—with few or no immune deposits of Ig ("pauci-immune")
        4. Anti-neutrophil cytoplasmic antibody–induced, *? forme fruste* of vasculitis
    B. Superimposed on another primary glomerular disease
        1. Mesangiocapillary (membranoproliferative glomerulonephritis)* (especially type II)
        2. Membranous glomerulonephritis*
        Berger's disease (IgA nephropathy)*

* Most common causes.
From Glassock RJ, Brenner BM: HPIM-12, p. 1172.

NEPHROTIC SYNDROME (NS)

Characterized by albuminuria (>3.5 g/d) and hypoalbuminemia (<30 g/L) and accompanied by edema, hyperlipidemia, and lipiduria. Complications include renal vein thrombosis and other thromboembolic events, infection, vitamin D deficiency, protein malnutrition, and drug toxicities due to decreased protein binding.

In adults, a minority of cases are secondary to diabetes mellitus, SLE, amyloidosis, drugs, neoplasia, or other disorders (see Table 96-3). By exclusion, the remainder are idiopathic. Renal biopsy is required to make the diagnosis and determine therapy in idiopathic NS.

MINIMAL CHANGE DISEASE   Causes about 15% of idiopathic NS in adults. Blood pressure is normal; GFR is normal or slightly reduced; urinary sediment is benign or may show few RBCs. Protein selectivity is variable in adults. Recent URI, allergies, or immunizations are present in some cases. ARF may rarely occur. Renal biopsy shows only foot process fusion on electron microscopy. Remission of proteinuria with glucocorticoids carries a good prognosis; cytotoxic therapy may be required for relapse. Progression to renal failure is uncommon. Later focal sclerosis has been suspected in some cases.

MEMBRANOUS GN   Characterized by subepithelial IgG deposits; accounts for 45% of adult NS. Pts present with edema, nephrotic proteinuria, and normal BP, GFR, and urine sediment, and hypertension, mild renal insufficiency, and abnormal urine sediment develop later. Renal vein thrombosis is common. Underlying diseases such as SLE, hepatitis B, and solid tumors and exposure to such drugs as captopril or penicillamine should be sought. Glucocorticoids may reduce the decline in renal function if given prior to renal insufficiency, but they do not induce full remission of proteinuria. Some pts progress to end-stage renal disease.

FOCAL GLOMERULOSCLEROSIS   Involves fibrosis of portions of some (primarily juxtamedullary) glomeruli and is found in 15% of pts. Hypertension, reduced GFR, and hematuria are typical. Some cases may be a late stage of minimal change disease or be due to heroin abuse, vesicoureteral reflux, or AIDS. Fewer than half undergo remission with glucocorti-

TABLE 96-3   Causes of nephrotic syndrome (NS)

Systemic causes (25%)	Glomerular disease (75%)
Diabetes mellitus, SLE, amyloidosis	Membranous (40%)
Drugs: gold, penicillamine, probenecid, street heroin, captopril, NSAIDs	Minimal change disease (15%)
	Focal glomerulosclerosis (15%)
	Membranoproliferative GN (7%)
Infections: bacterial endocarditis, hepatitis B, shunt infections, syphilis, malaria	Mesangioproliferative GN (5%)
Malignancy: Hodgkin's and other lymphomas, leukemia, carcinoma of breast, GI tract	
Allergic reactions	

Modified from Glassock RJ, Brenner BM: HPIM-12, p. 1175.

coids. Half progress to renal failure in 10 years; may recur in a renal transplant. Pressure of azotemia or hypertension reflects poor prognosis. Role of dietary protein restriction is unclear.

MEMBRANOPROLIFERATIVE   GLOMERULONEPHRITIS   (MPGN) Mesangial expansion and proliferation extends into the capillary loop. Two ultrastructural variants exist. In MPGN I, subendothelial electron-dense deposits are present, C3 is deposited in a granular pattern indicative of immune-complex pathogenesis, and IgG and the early components of complement may or may not be present. In MPGN II, the lamina densa of the glomerular basement membrane (GBM) is transformed into an electron-dense character, as is the basement membrane in Bowman's capsule and tubules. C3 is found irregularly in the GBM. Small amounts of Ig (usually IgM) are present, but early components of complement are absent. Decreased serum complement levels are characteristic. MPGN affects young adults; blood pressure and GFR are abnormal, and the urine sediment is active. Some present with acute nephritis or hematuria. Similar lesions occur in SLE and hemolytic-uremic syndrome. Renal function declines over several years. Glucocorticoids may delay progression. ASA plus dipyridamole appears beneficial in some pts. May recur in allografts.

DIABETIC NEPHROPATHY Common cause of NS. Pathologic changes include diffuse and/or nodular glomerulosclerosis, nephrosclerosis, chronic pyelonephritis, and papillary necrosis. *Clinical features* include proteinuria, hypertension, azotemia, and bacteriuria. Duration of diabetes mellitus is variable, but proteinuria may develop 10–15 years after onset, progress to NS, and then eventuate in renal failure over 3–5 years. Retinopathy is nearly universal. Treatment with ACE inhibitors may delay the onset of nephropathy. Aggressive management of hypertension and restriction of dietary protein may retard decline of renal failure. Mortality rates on dialysis are high, and successful transplantation is somewhat less frequent than in nondiabetics.

Evaluation of NS is shown in Table 96-4.

ASYMPTOMATIC URINARY ABNORMALITIES

Proteinuria in the nonnephrotic range and/or hematuria unaccompanied by edema, reduced GFR, or hypertension can be due to multiple causes (see Table 96-5).

IDIOPATHIC RENAL HEMATURIA (Berger's disease, IgA nephropathy) The most common cause of recurrent hematuria of glomerular origin. It is most common in young adults, mostly men. Episodes of macroscropic hematuria are present

TABLE 96-4   Evaluation of nephrotic syndrome

24-h urine for protein; creatinine clearance
Serum albumin, cholesterol, complement
Urine protein electrophoresis
Rule out SLE, diabetes mellitus
Review drug exposure
Renal biopsy
Consider malignancy (in elderly pt with membranous GN or minimal change disease)
Consider renal vein thrombosis (if membranous GN or symptoms of pulmonary embolism are present)

TABLE 96-5   Glomerular causes of asymptomatic urinary abnormalities

I. Hematuria with or without proteinuria
  A. Primary glomerular diseases
    1. Berger's disease (IgA nephropathy)*
    2. Mesangiocapillary glomerulonephritis
    3. Other primary glomerular hematurias accompanied by "pure" mesangial proliferation, focal and segmental proliferative glomerulonephritis, or other lesions
    4. "Thin basement membrane" disease (? *forme fruste* of Alport's syndrome)
  B. Associated with multisystem or heredofamilial diseases
    1. Alport's syndrome and other "benign" familial hematurias*
    2. Fabry's disease
    3. Sickle cell disease
  C. Associated with infections
    1. Resolving poststreptococcal glomerulonephritis*
    2. Other postinfectious glomerulonephritides*
II. Isolated nonnephrotic proteinuria
  A. Primary glomerular diseases
    1. "Orthostatic" proteinuria*
    2. Focal and segmental glomerulosclerosis*
    3. Membranous glomerulonephritis*
  B. Associated with multisystem or heredofamilial diseases
    1. Diabetes mellitus*
    2. Amyloidosis*
    3. Nail-patella syndrome

* Most common.
From Glassock RJ, Brenner BM: HPIM-12, p. 1179.

with flu-like symptoms, without skin rash, abdominal pain, or arthritis. Renal biopsy shows diffuse mesangial deposition of IgA, often with lesser amounts of IgG, nearly always by C3 and properdin but not by C1q or C4. Prognosis is variable; 50% develop ESRD within 25 years. Therapy does not influence natural history.

TABLE 96-6 Serologic findings in selected multisystem diseases

Disease	C3	Ig	FANA	Anti-dsDNA	Anti-GBM	Cryo-Ig	CIC	ANCA
Systemic lupus erythematosus	↓↓	↑ IgG	+++	++	-	++	+++	±
Goodpasture's syndrome	-	-	-	-	+++	-	±	-
Henoch-Schönlein purpura	-	↑ IgA	-	-	-	±	++	-
Polyarteritis	↓←	↑ IgG	+	±	-	++	+++	+++
Wegener's granulomatosis	←	↑ IgA, IgE	-	-	-	±	++	+++
Cryoimmunoglobulinemia	↓→	± → ↑ IgG, IgA, IgD, IgE	-	-	-	+++	++	-
Multiple myeloma	-	→ ↑ IgG	-	-	-	+	-	-
Waldenström's macroglobulinemia	-	↑ IgM	-	-	-	-	-	-
Amyloidosis	-	± Ig	-	-	-	-	-	-

NOTE: C3 = C3 component; Ig = immunoglobulin levels; FANA = fluorescent antinuclear antibody assay; anti-dsDNA = antibody to double-stranded (native) DNA; anti-GBM = antibody to glomerular basement membrane antigens; cryo-Ig = cryoimmunoglobulin; CIC = circulating immune complexes; ANCA = anti-neutrophil cytoplasmic antibody; − = normal; + = occasionally slightly abnormal; + + = often abnormal; + + + = severely abnormal.
From Glassock RJ, Brenner BM: HPIM-12, p. 1181.

CHRONIC GLOMERULONEPHRITIS

This syndrome is characterized by persistent urinary abnormalities and slow progressive impairment of renal function; symmetrically contracted kidneys, moderate to heavy proteinuria; abnormal urinary sediment, especially RBC (casts), and x-ray evidence of normal pyelocalyceal systems. The time to progression to ESRD is variable, hastened by uncontrolled hypertension and infections.

GLOMERULOPATHIES ASSOCIATED WITH MULTISYSTEM DISEASE (Table 96-6)

For a more detailed discussion, see Glassock RJ, Brenner BM: Immunopathogenic Mechanisms of Renal Injury, Chap. 226, p. 1166; Glassock RJ, Brenner BM: The Major Glomerulopathies, Chap. 227, p. 1170; and Glassock RJ, Brenner BM: Glomerulopathies Associated with Multisystem Diseases, Chap. 228, p. 1180, HPIM-12

97 RENAL TUBULAR DISEASES

Tubulointerstitial diseases form a diverse group of acute and chronic hereditary and acquired disorders involving renal tubules and supporting structures (Table 97-1). Functionally, they may result in nephrogenic DI with polyuria, nocturia, non-anion gap acidosis, saltwasting, and hypo- or hyperkalemia. Azotemia is frequently present, owing to associated glomerulofibrosis or ischemia. Compared to glomerulopathies, proteinuria is modest, hypertension less common, but anemia more severe.

ACUTE INTERSTITIAL NEPHRITIS (IN) Drugs are a leading cause of this type of renal failure (RF), identifiable by acute oliguria and sometimes an allergic reaction with fever, rash, and arthralgias. In addition to azotemia, tubular dysfunction may be present. Common causes are methicillin and other penicillins, sulfonamides, diuretics, rifampin, cimetidine, cephalosporin, and allopurinol; NSAIDs cause IN with nephrotic syndrome associated with minimal change disease that may lack allergic manifestations.

Eosinophilia is common; UA shows RBCs, pyuria, and eosinophiluria on Wright's stain. On renal biopsy, interstitial edema with WBC infiltration is present. RF commonly responds to withdrawal of offending drug, and most pts have good recovery. Uncontrolled studies support more rapid and complete renal recovery with glucocorticoids, which may outweigh their risk.

Acute bacterial pyelonephritis may cause acute IN but does not generally cause RF unless complicated by dehydration, sepsis, or urinary obstruction.

CHRONIC INTERSTITIAL NEPHRITIS Analgesic nephropathy is an important cause of RF and results from prolonged consumption of combination analgesics (5–10 tablets/d for 3 years), usually of phenacetin and aspirin. Nephropathy may be manifested as chronic IN, uremia, acute papillary necrosis in nondiabetics, sterile pyuria, or renal calculi. Pts are often women with headaches, anemia, and GI symptoms. Renal function stabilizes with total cessation of drugs.

Other drugs causing chronic IN include lithium (polyuria is common but RF due to chronic IN is unusual in the absence of toxic levels), cisplatin (nephrotoxicity reduced by saline diuresis), and semustine. Metabolic causes of chronic IN include (1) chronic hypercalcemia (fibrosis with tubular Ca deposits; initially causes nephrogenic diabetes

TABLE 97-1   Principal causes of tubulointerstitial disease of the kidney

---

I. Toxins
    A. Exogenous toxins
        1. Analgesic nephropathy
        2. Lead nephropathy
        3. Miscellaneous nephrotoxins (e.g., antibiotics, cyclosporine, radiographic contrast media, heavy metals)
    B. Metabolic toxins
        1. Acute uric acid nephropathy
        2. Gouty nephropathy
        3. Hypercalcemic nephropathy
        4. Hypokalemic nephropathy
        5. Miscellaneous metabolic toxins (e.g., hyperoxaluria, cystinosis, Fabry's disease)
II. Neoplasia
    A. Lymphoma
    B. Leukemia
    C. Multiple myeloma
III. Immune disorders
    A. Hypersensitivity nephropathy
    B. Sjögren's syndrome
    C. Amyloidosis
    D. Transplant rejection
    E. Tubulointerstitial abnormalities associated with glomerulonephritis
    F. AIDS
IV. Vascular disorders
    A. Arteriolar nephrosclerosis
    B. Atheroembolic disease
    C. Sickle cell nephropathy
    D. Acute tubular necrosis
V. Hereditary renal diseases
    A. Hereditary nephritis (Alport's syndrome)
    B. Medullary cystic disease
    C. Medullary sponge kidney
    D. Polycystic kidney disease
VI. Infectious injury
    A. Acute pyelonephritis
    B. Chronic pyelonephritis
VII. Miscellaneous disorders
    A. Chronic urinary tract obstruction
    B. Vesicoureteral reflux
    C. Radiation nephritis

From Brenner BM, Hostetter TH: HPIM-12, p. 1187.

insipidus (DI) and late causes chronic RF); (2) hypokalemia (may cause fibrosis after many years); and (3) uric acid nephropathy (acute RF due to acute hyperuricemia or chronic RF due to chronic hyperuricemia, hypertension, and uric acid stones).

Chronic IN also may be due to multiple myeloma, in which progressive RF follows precipitation of immunoglobulin light chains in tubules and fibrosis (''myeloma kidney'') and correlates with Bence Jones proteinuria. Other renal manifestations of myeloma include ARF, proteinuria, amyloidosis, tubular defects, and hypercalcemic nephropathy. Chronic IN is also caused by Sjögren's syndrome, sarcoidosis, tuberculosis, and radiation nephritis.

Medullary sponge kidney is a disorder, usually sporadic, of ectatic collecting ducts that presents as hematuria, urinary infection, distal renal tubular acidosis (RTA), and/or nephrolithiasis in the fourth and fifth decades. Dx is made by IVP. RF is rare.

In *amyloidosis of the kidney*, glomerular pathology usually predominates leading to heavy proteinuria and azotemia. Tubular function may also be deranged, resulting in nephrogenic DI and distal (type I) RTA.

In *AIDS kidney disease*, proteinuria and renal insufficiency are due to tubulointerstitial and glomerular pathology. Glomerular sclerosis has been reported as a complication of AIDS without apparent other cause.

Several *inherited* disorders affect the renal tubules and interstitium. *Polycystic kidney disease* is a frequent cause of CRF; inheritance is autosomal dominant, and men and women are equally affected. Symptoms of flank pain, nocturia, hematuria, and urinary infection appear in the third or fourth decade. Kidneys are palpable. Hepatic cysts and intracranial aneurysms also may be present. Progressive azotemia occurs in most pts. Dx is by IVP or ultrasound. Dialysis and transplantation are routinely used in treatment. In *medullary cystic disease*, polyuria, acidosis, and salt wasting precede slowly progressive RF. Genetics is variable. Dx may be made by IVP, arteriography, or renal biopsy.

Congenital disorders of tubular transport include

1. Bartter's syndrome: Hypokalemia due to renal K wasting, weakness, polyuria, beginning in childhood; autosomal recessive; high renin and aldosterone, often responsive to indomethacin.

2. Renal tubular acidosis:

Distal (type I) RTA: Patients are unable to lower urine pH normally despite acidosis; autosomal dominant but frequently sporadic due to autoimmune disease, obstruction, or amphotericin; associated with hypokalemia, hypercalciuria, and osteomalacia.

Proximal (type II) RTA: A defect in HCO_3 reabsorption, usually associated with glucosuria, aminoaciduria, phosphaturia; may also be due to myeloma, drugs, or renal transplant; requires large amounts of HCO_3, which aggravates hypokalemia.

Type IV RTA: Occurs with hyperkalemia and usually low renin and aldosterone levels and is generally associated with diabetes, advanced age, chronic IN, or nephrosclerosis.

TABLE 97-2 Comparison of three types of renal tubular acidosis*

Finding	Type 1	Type 2	Type 4
Non-anion gap acidosis	Yes	Yes	Yes
Minimum urine pH	>5.5	<5.5	<5.5
% filtered HCO_3 excreted	<10	>15	<10
Serum potassium	Low	Low	High
Fanconi syndrome	No	Yes	No
Stones/nephrocalcinosis	Yes	No	No
Daily acid excretion	Low	Normal	Low
Ammonium excretion	High for pH	Normal	Low for pH
Daily HCO_3 replacement needs	<4 mmol/kg	>4 mmol/kg	<4 mmol/kg

* HCO_3, bicarbonate. Type 3 renal tubular acidosis is a rare form of a mixture of types 1 and 2.
From Coe FL, Kathpalia S: HPIM-12, p. 1199.

For a more detailed discussion, see Brenner BM, Hostetter TH: Tubulointerstitial Diseases of the Kidney, Chap. 229, and Coe FL, Kathpalia S: Hereditary Tubular Disorders, Chap. 331, p. 1196, in HPIM-12

98 URINARY TRACT INFECTIONS (UTI)

ETIOLOGY

• 80% *E. coli;* increased with calculi—*Proteus* (positive urease) and *Klebsiella.* • *Staphylococcus saprophyticus* 10–15% in young women. • A third of women with dysuria have $<10^5$ organisms/mL of urine, three-quarters have pyuria, most have usual pathogens; others have *Chlamydia, Neisseria gonorrhoeae,* herpes simplex.

Increased risk Sexually active women, prostatitis, prostatic hypertrophy, pregnancy (20–30% with asymptomatic bacteriuria develop pyelonephritis), obstruction, neurogenic bladder dysfunction, vesicoureteral reflux.

CLINICAL PRESENTATION

• Cystitis: dysuria, frequency, urgency, suprapubic pain, 30% bloody urine; usually *E. coli.*
• Acute pyelonephritis: fever, chills, nausea, vomiting, costovertebral angle tenderness; usually *E. coli.*
• Urethritis: dysuria, frequency but no or insignificant bacterial growth; frequently sexually transmitted infection.
• Catheter-associated infections: risk of infection 5% per day of catheterization; usually *E. coli, Proteus, Pseudomonas, Klebsiella, Serratia.*

TREATMENT Treat specific organism whenever possible.

1. Cystitis: Single-dose therapy (reliable nonpregnant pts with uncomplicated cystitis): trimethoprim-sulfamethoxazole (TMP/SMX) 2–3 double-strength tablets, TMP 400 mg, or SMX 2 g; amoxicillin (3 g) less effective since 20–30% of *E. coli* are resistant. 7–10-d therapy (children, pregnant women, catheter-associated): TMP/SMX* 1 double-strength tablet PO bid, TMP 100 mg PO bid, cephalexin or cephradine 250–500 mg PO qid, tetracycline* 250–500 mg PO qid, amoxicillin 500 mg PO tid, nitrofurantoin 100 mg PO qid, indanyl carbenicillin 1–2 tablets PO qid, quinolone* for resistant organisms. (*avoid if pt pregnant)

2. Acute pyelonephritis: Treat with IV aminoglycoside, first-generation cephalosporin, or TMP/SMX for several days, then PO for a total of 10–14 d. May treat entirely PO if pt is not pregnant, only mildly ill, and reliable for follow-up.

3. Asymptomatic bacteriuria: Document twice before treatment orally × 7 days; if it persists, follow without further treatment unless neutropenic, renal transplant, or previous pyelonephritis → 6 weeks oral therapy.

   4. Catheter-associated UTI: Cure unlikely unless catheter removed; if asymptomatic, do not treat unless at risk for sepsis (1–2%) with old age, underlying disease, diabetes, pregnancy.

Urologic evaluation   IVP and cystoscopy only for women with relapsing infection, history of childhood infections, stones, recurrent pyelonephritis; investigate all men or any pt with symptoms suggestive of obstruction or stones.

Prophylaxis   >2 infections in 6 months; single-dose TMP/ SMX or nitrofurantoin 50 mg qd after urine sterilized.

CHRONIC PYELONEPHRITIS

Chronic interstitial nephritis attributed to chronic renal infection in pts with normal or abnormal urinary tracts. No pathognomonic features. Diagnosis: recurrent UTIs, impaired renal function, pyuria with WBC casts, bacteriuria, IVP with irregularly outlined renal pelvis with caliectasis and cortical scars; symptoms often minimal; may have hypertension; progression to uremia.

PAPILLARY NECROSIS

Increased risk with gout, diabetes, phenacetin-containing analgesics, sickle cell anemia, alcoholism, vascular disease. *Symptoms:* hematuria, flank pain, chills, fever. *Treatment:* antibiotics for severe pyelonephritis; with overwhelming infection, if unilateral, may require nephrectomy.

PROSTATITIS

ACUTE BACTERIAL PROSTATITIS   Usually young males or indwelling catheter; physical exam: fever, chills, dysuria, boggy or tender prostate; diagnose by urine gram stain and culture (prostatic massage may cause bacteremia); usually gram-negative rods or *S. aureus;* treat with IV cephalosporin, TMP/SMX, or aminoglycoside.
CHRONIC BACTERIAL PROSTATITIS   Usually no symptoms, normal prostate, pyuria; treat with prolonged courses (e.g., 12 weeks) of TMP/SMX, a quinolone, or nitrofurantoin.

For a more detailed discussion, see Stamm WE, Turck M: Urinary Tract Infections and Pyelonephritis, Chap. 95, in HPIM-12, p. 538

---

99 RENOVASCULAR DISEASE

Vascular occlusion of the large and small renal arteries produces ischemic injury whose expression depends on the rate, site, severity, and duration of vascular compromise. Signs and symptoms range from painful infarction to acute renal failure (ARF), impaired GFR, hematuria, or tubular dysfunction. Renal ischemia of any etiology may cause renin-mediated hypertension.

ACUTE OCCLUSION OF A RENAL ARTERY May be due to thrombosis or embolism (from valvular disease, endocarditis, mural thrombi, or atrial arrhythmias). Large renal infarcts cause pain, vomiting, nausea, hypertension, fever, proteinuria, hematuria, and elevated LDH and SGOT. Renal functional loss depends on contralateral function. IVP or radionuclide scan shows unilateral hypofunction; ultrasound is normal. Renal arteriography establishes diagnosis. With occlusions of large arteries, surgery may be the initial therapy; with occlusions of small arteries, anticoagulation should be used.

RENAL ATHEROEMBOLISM Usually arises when aortic angiography or surgery causes cholesterol embolization of small renal vessels. Renal insufficiency may develop suddenly or gradually. Other findings are GI or retinal ischemia with cholesterol emboli visible on fundoscopic examination, neurologic deficits, livedo reticularis, toe gangrene, and hypertension. UA is negative, and U_{Na} may be low. Skin or renal biopsy may be necessary for diagnosis. Heparin is contraindicated.

RENAL VEIN THROMBOSIS This occurs in a variety of settings including pregnancy, oral contraceptive use, trauma, nephrotic syndrome, dehydration (in infants), extrinsic compression of the renal vein (lymph nodes, aortic aneurysm, tumor), and invasion of the renal vein by renal cell carcinoma. Definitive Dx is established by selective renal renography. Streptokinase may be effective.

RENAL ARTERY STENOSIS Main cause of renovascular hypertension; due to (1) atherosclerosis (two-thirds of cases, usually men >60 years, advanced retinopathy) or (2) fibromuscular dysplasia (a third of cases, white women <45 years, brief history of hypertension). Renal hypoperfusion activates renin-angiotensin-aldosterone axis. Suggestive clinical features include onset of hypertension <30 or >50 years, bruits, hypokalemic alkalosis, acute onset of hypertension or malignant hypertension, and hypertension resistant to medical therapy.

The gold standard in diagnosis of renal artery stenosis is arteriography. Digital subtraction angiography is useful in some settings. The least invasive and most reliable screening test in pts with normal renal function is the captopril renogram when combined with: (1) post-captopril plasma renin activity measurement of ≥ 12 μg/L/h, (2) an absolute increase of plasma renin activity of ≥ 10 μg/L/h, and (3) increase in plasma renin of $\geq 150\%$ or $\geq 400\%$ if baseline plasma renin activity is ≤ 3 μg/L/h. Measurement of renal vein renin may be necessary to demonstrate functional significance of a lesion.

Surgical revascularization Achieves best results in fibromuscular disease. Those with localized atherosclerosis do well, but mortality is higher; surgery in patients with diffuse or bilateral lesions is best reserved for urgent cases who have failed medical management.

Angioplasty Also most successful with fibromuscular disease and nonoccluded, nonostial atherosclerotic lesions; has a low complication rate and cost. In many pts (the elderly, those with impaired renal function, or those with high surgical risk), pharmacotherapy is employed. Converting-enzyme inhibitors are ideal drugs except in pts with bilateral stenosis or disease in solitary kidney.

Malignant hypertension (Chap. 69) also may be caused by renal vascular occlusion with severe hypertension, papilledema, headache, malaise, encephalopathy, and renal impairment. Nitroprusside or calcium antagonists are generally effective in lowering BP.

In some pts with previously stable scleroderma (Chap. 118), sudden oliguric renal failure and severe hypertension occur due to small vessel occlusion. Aggressive control of BP with converting-enzyme inhibitors and dialysis improves survival and may restore renal function.

Sludging of blood in the renal medulla causes hematuria in pts with sickle cell anemia or trait. It may cause nephrogenic diabetes insipidus (DI), papillary necrosis, proteinuria, and mild renal insufficiency.

HEMOLYTIC-UREMIC SYNDROME Characterized by ARF, microangiopathic hemolytic anemia, and thrombocytopenia; increasingly recognized in adults; may be preceded by a prodrome of bloody diarrhea and abdominal pain. Fibrin deposition leads to small vessel occlusion. Lack of fever or CNS involvement helps to distinguish it from thrombotic thrombocytopenic purpura. Treatment is symptomatic; prognosis for recovery of renal function is poor.

TOXEMIAS OF PREGNANCY   *Preeclampsia* is characterized by hypertension, proteinuria, edema, consumptive coagulopathy, sodium retention, and hyperreflexia; *eclampsia* is the further development of seizures. Glomerular swelling causes renal insufficiency. Coagulation abnormalities and ARF may occur. Treatment consists of bed rest, sedation, control of neurologic manifestations with magnesium sulfate, control of hypertension with vasodilators, and delivery of the infant.

VASCULITIS   Renal complications are frequent and severe in polyarteritis nodosa, hypersensitivity angiitis, Wegener's granulomatosis, and other forms of vasculitis (see Chap. 119). Therapy is directed toward the underlying disease.

SICKLE CELL NEPHROPATHY   The hypertonic and relatively hypoxic renal medulla coupled with slow blood flow in the vasa recta favors sickling. Papillary necrosis, cortical infarcts, functional tubule abnormalities (nephrogenic DI), glomerulopathy, nephrotic syndrome, and, rarely, end-stage renal disease may be complications.

For a more detailed discussion, see Badr KF, Brenner BM: Vascular Injury to the Kidney, Chap. 230, in HPIM-12, p. 1192

Renal stones are common (1% of population) and recurrent (50–85%) disorders that are usually preventable. Stone formation begins when urine becomes supersaturated with insoluble component(s) due to excessive excretion or factors that diminish solubility. Stones are 75% Ca, 15% struvite (magnesium-ammonium-phosphate), 5% uric acid, and 1% cystine. Composition reflects the metabolic disorders from which they arise.

SYMPTOMS Similar for most types of stones. Those in the renal pelvis may be asymptomatic or cause hematuria, and obstruction may occur at any site. On passage, severe colicky migrating pain and hematuria are typical. Symptoms of UTI or obstruction can occur. Staghorn calculi cause recurrent infection.

STONE COMPOSITION Most stones are composed of *Ca oxalate;* 30% are associated with hypercalciuria, whereas hyperoxaluria is rare. Hypercalciuria without hypercalcemia is usually idiopathic, i.e., without specific etiology (sarcoidosis, immobilization, furosemide, renal tubular acidosis, Cushing's syndrome). The abnormality in idiopathic hypercalciuria ranges from excessive GI Ca absorption to increased renal Ca excretion and appears to be familial. Standard treatment of both GI and renal forms is high fluid intake and thiazide diuretics.

Other causes of Ca oxalate stones include (1) hyperuricosuria due to dietary purine excess (uric acid initiates Ca oxalate crystal formation); treatment is low purine diet and allopurinol; (2) primary hyperparathyroidism (hypercalcemic hypercalciuria with high parathyroid hormone); parathyroidectomy prevents stones; (3) distal renal tubule acidosis (renal acidosis causes hypercalciuria; with alkaline urine and low urine citrate, Ca phosphate stones form, along with nephrocalcinosis); treat with alkali; (4) hyperoxaluria (usually due to excess GI absorption associated with steatorrhea); therapy is correction of fat malabsorption, oral Ca lactate and/or cholestyramine; and (5) idiopathic (normocalciuric); treat with hydration and dietary Ca restriction.

Struvite stones form in the collecting system when infection with urea-splitting organisms (usually *Proteus*) is present. High urine pH (8–9), magnesium, ammonium, and carbonate levels result, producing struvite ($MgNH_4PO_4$) stones. It is the most common cause of staghorn calculi and obstruction. Risk factors include urinary catheters, neurogenic bladder, and repeated instrumentation. Mandelamine and antibiotics are useful for lowering urine pH, suppressing infection, and preventing stone growth and/or recurrence. Cure requires lithotripsy or surgical removal. Partial dissolution may occur with chronic antibacterial therapy. Irrigation of renal pelvis with renacidin, which dissolves struvite, is possible in some centers.

Uric acid stones occur when urine is saturated with uric acid in the presence of an acid urine pH and dehydration. Occur in pts with (1) gout, where they may precede arthritis; (2) myeloproliferative disorders, particularly when chemotherapy increases uricosuria; (3) diarrhea, inflammatory bowel disease, or ileostomy; or (4) idiopathic. Treatment is with fluids, alkalinization of urine, and allopurinol. When hyperuricosuria (>1 g/d) is present, reduced purine intake is indicated.

CYSTINURIA A rare inherited disorder of defective renal (and intestinal) transport resulting in overexcretion of cystine. Stones begin to form in childhood and are a rare cause of staghorn calculi. Hexagonal cystine crystals identified in urine should be further assessed by measurement of urine cystine excretion. Treatment is with high urine volume, alkali therapy (urine pH >7.5). Penicillamine, which binds cystine, is reserved for refractory cases. Mercaptopropinylglycine has been used to dissolve renal calculi by perfusion of the renal pelvis and can be given orally as prophylaxis.

EVALUATION Yields an identifiable cause in many and should be offered to all stone formers. History may reveal prior episodes or positive family history of dietary excess or low fluid intake, UTI, gout, bowel disease, or a specific cause of hypercalciuria. Serum Ca, HCO_3, and creatinine should be measured. Cystine, struvite, or other crystals may be found in urine; a culture should be done if infection is suggested. Abdominal film (KUB) and IVP will reveal stone location, quantity, size, and opacity, as well as presence of obstruction. Obtained stones should always be analyzed. No matter what the composition, urine volume should be increased by high fluid intake.

All patients with infection, uric acid, or cystine stones should be evaluated and specific therapy instituted. For Ca stone formers, hypercalcemia and hyperparathyroidism should be ruled out. 24-h urines should be obtained to detect hypercalciuria (>300 mg in men, >250 mg in women); urine pH and excretion of uric acid and oxalate may guide specific therapy.

Management of stones already present in kidney and urinary tract depends on the location and whether they are obstructing or causing infection or impairing renal function.

Stone migration and risk of removal should be assessed. Lithotripsy, if available, is a useful alternative to surgical lithotomy.

For a more detailed discussion, see Coe FL, Favus MJ: Nephrolithiasis, Chap. 232, in HPIM-12, p. 1202

UTO is a potentially reversible cause of renal failure; should be considered in all cases of acute renal failure (ARF) or when chronic renal failure (CRF) worsens abruptly. Consequences depend on duration and severity and whether obstruction is unilateral or bilateral.

UTO may occur at any level from collecting tubule to urethra. In adults, UTO is preponderant in women (pelvic tumors), elderly men (prostatic disease), diabetics (papillary necrosis, neurogenic bladder), and pts with retroperitoneal disease, vesicoureteral reflux, stones, or functional urinary retention.

The initial effect of renal function is a prompt increase in renal blood flow (RBF) in an attempt to preserve GFR. Later RBF and GFR $\downarrow$ and tubular pressures $\uparrow$. As a result, oliguria with low U_{Na} and high osmolality (similar to prerenal azotemia) develop followed by indices similar to ARF (Chap. 93). Complete and bilateral obstruction causes anuria. The effects of chronic UTO on renal function resemble other forms of CRF; Na wasting and impaired K secretion are prominent.

CLINICAL MANIFESTATIONS Pain due to distention of upper urinary tract or bladder, renal colic, prostatic symptoms, nocturia, and diminished urine output. UTO should be considered in pts with UTI (Chap. 98) and stones (Chap. 100) and in all pts with unexplained azotemia.

PHYSICAL EXAM May reveal large bladder, palpable kidneys, prostatic or pelvic disease, rectal mass, or abnormal sphincter tone. Suspected lower tract obstruction may be confirmed by large residual urine on bladder catheterization.

On UA, pyuria, hematuria, bacteriuria, or crystalluria may be found without heavy proteinuria. Opaque stones should be sought on x-ray. Abdominal ultrasound should be performed to assess bladder and kidney size, the presence of hydronephrosis, and degree of preservation of renal parenchyma. Dilatation may be absent in UTO due to tubular obstruction, upper tract encasement by tumors or retroperitoneal fibrosis, staghorn calculus, very early ARF, or antecedent CRF with small kidneys. Unilateral hydronephrosis may be responsible for azotemia when contralateral kidney is diseased or absent.

IVP may be employed to determine level of obstruction and its cause. IVP should not be attempted in severe renal failure. To examine the renal pelvis and ureter in patient with RF, either retrograde or antegrade pyelography should be performed. CT scan is helpful in elucidating etiology, particularly in pts with retroperitoneal disease causing UTO without hydronephrosis.

ARF due to UTO requires rapid intervention, since return of renal function depends in part on duration of obstruction. Bladder catheterization and nephrostomy relieve obstruction in lower and upper tracts, respectively. Infection should be treated aggressively. Dialysis is indicated in severe RF due to reversible UTO.

Relief of severe bilateral obstruction is typically followed by physiologic *diuresis* lasting several days, with excretion of large quantities of water and electrolytes. Volume depletion, hypokalemia, hyponatremia, and hypomagnesemia may result. IV fluids (one-half normal saline with added K and Mg prn) should be used to replace urinary losses. Close monitoring of fluid balance is mandatory.

For a more detailed discussion, see Brenner BM, Milford EL, Seifter JL: Urinary Tract Obstruction, Chap. 233, in HPIM-12, p. 1206

RENAL CELL CARCINOMA Of renal tumors, 85% are *renal cell carcinomas;* the remainder arise in the renal pelvis. Occur typically in men in sixth decade; cigarette smoking is a risk factor. Rare forms are inherited (in von Hippel–Lindau disease) and some are due to chromosomal translocations. Renal cysts in hemodialysis patients may become malignant.

Clinical manifestations Include hematuria (gross or microscopic), flank pain, abdominal mass (and systemic symptoms), fever, fatigue, weight loss, cachexia, anemia. Paraneoplastic syndromes include fever of unknown origin, hypercalcemia, galactorrhea, Cushing's syndrome, erythrocytosis, or hypertension. LFTs may be abnormal.

Diagnosis Usually begins with discovery of a flank mass by IVP (space-occupying lesion, distorted collecting system), often in pt with systemic symptoms or manifestations of metastases. When renal mass is detected, CT and ultrasound can differentiate benign cysts from tumor. Percutaneous needle aspiration for cytology is frequently helpful. CT may reveal solid mass, occasionally with extension into renal vein. Renal arteriography may show hypervascular tumor. *Staging* begins with search for metastatic disease (CXR, bone and liver scans). If negative, radical nephrectomy is indicated. Five-year survival rates range from about 70% (tumor confined to kidney) to under 5% (distant spread). Metastatic disease is resistant to hormonal and/or chemotherapy. Cure is occasionally achieved by excision of solitary metastasis.

TUMORS OF THE URINARY COLLECTION SYSTEM Tumors of *renal pelvis* are usually *transitional cell carcinomas.* Risk factors include smoking, chemical exposure, and analgesic abuse; present with painless gross hematuria; IVP and urine cytology are positive. Treatment of advanced disease is radical nephroureterectomy. Survival is 10–50% after 5 years. Close follow-up is required.

Bladder (transitional cell) carcinoma is most common in men over age 40. Risk factors are smoking and chemical exposure. Bladder cancer also may follow cyclophosphamide therapy or chronic *Schistosoma haematobium* infection. Hematuria or other bladder symptoms are usually present. Dx is by urine cytology and cystoscopy with biopsy. Prognosis depends on depth of invasion of bladder and systemic involvement. Superficial disease is treated by endoscopic resection with frequent follow-up; recurrences may require intravesical chemotherapy. Metastatic disease may remit with surgery and combination chemotherapy.

Tumors metastatic to kidney (principally liver cancer and lymphoma) are rarely evident clinically. Leukemic infiltration is common.

For a more detailed discussion, see Garnick MB, Brenner BM: Tumors of the Urinary Tract, Chap. 234, in HPIM-12, p. 1209

SECTION 7 GASTROINTESTINAL DISEASES

103 ESOPHAGEAL DISEASES

DYSPHAGIA

OROPHARYNGEAL Difficulty initiating swallowing; food sticks at level of suprasternal notch; nasopharyngeal regurgitation; aspiration. Not to be confused with globus hystericus, the sensation of a constant lump in the throat.

Solids only Carcinoma, aberrant vessel, congenital web (Plummer-Vinson syndrome), web, cervical osteophyte.

Solids and liquids Cricopharyngeal achalasia, hypertensive or hypotensive upper esophageal sphincter, Zenker's diverticulum, myasthenia gravis, steroid myopathy, hyperthyroidism, hypothyroidism, myotonic dystrophy, amyotrophic lateral sclerosis, multiple sclerosis, parkinsonism, stroke, and bulbar and pseudobulbar palsy.

ESOPHAGEAL Food sticks in mid or lower sternal area; odynophagia (pain on swallowing); regurgitation; aspiration.

Solids only initially *Intermittent:* lower esophageal (Schatski) ring; *progressive:* peptic stricture (with heartburn), carcinoma (no heartburn), lye stricture.

Solids and liquids *Intermittent:* diffuse esophageal spasm (with chest pain); *progressive:* scleroderma (with heartburn), achalasia (no heartburn).

ESOPHAGEAL MOTOR DISORDERS

Patients with esophageal motility disturbances may have a spectrum of manometric findings ranging from nonspecific abnormalities to defined clinical entities.

ACHALASIA (1) Hypertensive lower esophageal sphincter (LES); (2) inadequate relaxation of LES; (3) loss of peristalsis in smooth-muscle portion of esophageal body.

Causes Primary (idiopathic) or secondary: Chagas' disease, lymphoma, carcinoma, chronic idiopathic intestinal pseudoobstruction, ischemia, neurotropic viruses, drugs, toxins, radiation, postvagotomy.

Diagnosis CXR: absence of gastric air bubble; barium swallow: dilated esophagus with distal beaklike narrowing and air-fluid level; endoscopy: exclude tumor; manometry: normal or elevated LES pressure, decreased LES relaxation, absent peristalsis.

Treatment Trial of calcium antagonists (e.g., nifedipine 10–20 mg or isosorbide dinitrate 5–10 mg SL ac) in pts at high risk for dilatation or surgery; pneumatic (forceful) balloon dilatation—effective in 85%, small risk of perforation, bleeding; Heller's extramucosal myotomy of LES—equally effective, risk of reflux esophagitis.

DIFFUSE ESOPHAGEAL SPASM Multiple spontaneous and swallow-induced contractions of the esophageal body that are of simultaneous onset, high amplitude, long duration, and repetitive occurrence.

Causes Primary (idiopathic) or secondary: reflux esophagitis, emotional stress, diabetes, alcoholism, neuropathy, radiation, ischemia, collagen-vascular disease, aging (presbyesophagus).

Variants Example, nutcracker esophagus—high-amplitude peristaltic contractions; may be associated with pain or dysphagia.

Diagnosis Barium swallow: corkscrew esophagus, pseudodiverticula; manometry: contractions in esophageal body that are of simultaneous onset, high amplitude, long duration, and repetitive occurrence (in nutcracker esophagus, contractions are peristaltic and of high amplitude); possible provocation with edrophonium, ergonovine, bethanecol, etc. (first exclude CAD).

Treatment Trials of anticholinergics (usually of limited value), nitrates (isosorbide dinitrate 5–10 mg SL ac), Ca antagonists (nifedipine 10–20 mg SL ac); balloon dilatation may be attempted in some cases refractory to medical therapy; longitudinal myotomy of esophageal circular muscle in severe, resistant cases.

SCLERODERMA (1) Aperistalsis due to atrophy of esophageal smooth muscle ± fibrosis; (2) incompetent LES leading to reflux esophagitis, stricture. Treat as for reflux (see below).

GASTROESOPHAGEAL REFLUX

PATHOPHYSIOLOGY Reflux episode (1) Increased gastric volume (after meal, gastric stasis, acid hypersecretion); (2) contents near gastroesophageal junction (bending, recumbency); (3) increased gastric pressure (obesity, tight clothes, pregnancy, ascites); (4) loss of LES-gastric pressure gradient:

LES pressure decreased by smoking, anticholinergics, Ca antagonists, pregnancy, scleroderma; role of hiatal hernia unclear.

Heartburn Occurrence may depend on amount refluxed and frequency; decreased esophageal clearance by gravity and peristalsis; decreased neutralization by salivary secretion.

Esophagitis Results when refluxed acid (or bile) overwhelms esophageal mucosal defenses.

CLINICAL FEATURES Heartburn, dysphagia due to stricture, aspiration; complications: esophageal ulcer, bleeding, Barrett's esophagus (replacement of squamous with columnar epithelium, premalignant), adenocarcinoma.

DIAGNOSIS History often suffices; further testing in atypical or refractory cases.

- Barium swallow: frequent false-negatives for reflux or esophagitis; detects strictures.
- Endoscopy and mucosal biopsy: may be normal in gastroesophageal reflux, detects esophagitis, Barrett's esophagus.
- Bernstein test: reproduction of symptoms with 0.1 N HCl but not normal saline infused by tube into esophagus; less sensitive than 24-h esophageal luminal pH recording.
- ^{99m}Tc sulfur colloid scintiscan: to document and quantitate reflux.
- 24-h esophageal luminal pH recording: most sensitive test for reflux.

TREATMENT General Weight reduction; sleeping with elevated head of bed; avoidance of smoking, large meals, caffeine, alcohol, chocolate, fatty foods, citrus juices.

Medical therapy Antacids, H-2-receptor blockers, or sucralfate (initial doses as for peptic ulcer; Chap. 104); in unresponsive cases, higher than standard doses of H-2-receptor blockers may be effective (e.g., cimetidine 800 mg PO bid, ranitidine 300 mg PO bid, famotidine 40 mg PO bid) or consider adding an agent to increase LES pressure and enhance gastric emptying—metoclopramide 10–20 mg PO ac + hs (side effects: tremor, spasms, parkinsonism, elevated prolactin) or bethanechol 25 mg PO ac + hs (side effects: dry mouth, urinary retention; avoid in glaucoma, prostatism). Long-term therapy often necessary. Omeprazole 20–40 mg PO qAM, a substituted benzimidazole and H^+,K^+-ATPase inhibitor, is very effective, even in resistant cases; recommended for no longer than 8 weeks' duration because of uncertain risks of prolonged gastric antacidity. Dilate strictures. Surgical therapy (Belsey repair, Nissen fundoplication, Hill repair) in severe and refractory cases.

OTHER FORMS OF ESOPHAGITIS

HERPES ESOPHAGITIS Cause Herpesvirus I or II, varicella-zoster, cytomegalovirus. In immunocompromised persons (e.g., those with AIDS), may present with odynophagia, dysphagia, fever, bleeding; diagnosis by endoscopy with biopsy, brush cytology, culture. Treatment: May be self-limited in immunocompetent person; viscous lidocaine for pain; in prolonged cases and in immunocompromised hosts, herpes and varicella esophagitis are treated with acyclovir 250 mg/m^2 IV q 8 h, then 200–400 mg PO 5 times daily; CMV is treated with ganciclovir 5 mg/kg IV q 12 h until healing, which may take weeks to months.

CANDIDA **ESOPHAGITIS** In immunocompromised hosts (e.g., AIDS), malignancy, diabetes, hypoparathyroidism, hemoglobinopathy, SLE, corrosive esophageal injury; may present with odynophagia, dysphagia, oral thrush (in 50%); diagnosis by barium swallow (large filling defects), endoscopy with brushings (KOH stain), biopsy, culture. Treatment—oral nystatin (100,000 U/mL) 5 mL q 6 h or clotrimazole 10 mg tablet sucked q 6 h; in immunocompromised host, ketoconazole 200–400 mg PO qd for 7–10 days, often followed by long-term maintenance therapy; poorly responsive pts can be treated with amphotericin 10–15 mg IV q 6 h for a total dose of 300–500 mg.

PILL-RELATED ESOPHAGITIS Doxycycline, tetracycline, aspirin, NSAIDs, KCl, quinidine, ferrous sulfate, clindamycin, alprenolol. Predisposing factors: recumbency after swallowing pills with small sips of water; anatomic factors (e.g., enlarged left atrium or ectatic aorta impinging on esophagus).

Treatment Withdraw offending drug, antacids; dilate any resulting stricture.

ESOPHAGEAL CANCER (see Chap. 107)

For a more detailed discussion, see Goyal RK: Dysphagia, Chap. 42, and Diseases of the Esophagus, Chap. 237, in HPIM-12, pp. 249 and 1222

PEPTIC ULCER DISEASE, GASTRITIS, AND ZOLLINGER-ELLISON SYNDROME

PEPTIC ULCER DISEASE

Most commonly in duodenal bulb (duodenal ulcer—DU) and stomach (gastric ulcer—GU). May also occur in esophagus, pyloric channel, duodenal loop, jejunum, Meckel's diverticulum. Results from imbalance between "aggressive" factors (gastric acid, pepsin) and "defensive" factors involved in mucosal resistance (gastric mucus, bicarbonate, microcirculation, prostaglandins, *Helicobacter pylori*, mucosal "barrier").

RISK FACTORS AND ASSOCIATIONS **General** Heredity, smoking, gastrinoma (Zollinger-Ellison syndrome), hypercalcemia, mastocytosis. *H. pylori:* spiral urease-producing organism that colonizes gastric antral mucosa in up to 100% of persons with DU and 70% with GU (those not due to NSAIDs). Also found in normals (increasing prevalence with age). Invariably associated with histologic evidence of active chronic gastritis. Role in ulcer pathogenesis unclear, but may be prequisite and act by rendering mucosa more susceptible to acid-pepsin injury. (*Unproven:* Stress, coffee, alcohol.)

DU Relative gastric acid hypersecretion in one-third of pts. Elevated serum pepsinogen I in 50% (autosomal dominant trait). Glucocorticoids, chronic renal failure, renal transplantation, cirrhosis, chronic lung disease.

GU Gastric acid secretory rates usually normal or reduced. Gastritis, reflux of duodenal contents (including bile) frequently found. Chronic salicylate or NSAID use may account for up to 30% of GUs and increase risk of bleeding, perforation.

CLINICAL FEATURES **DU** Burning epigastric pain 90 min to 3 h after meals, often nocturnal, relieved by food.

GU Burning epigastric pain made worse by or unrelated to food; anorexia, food aversion, weight loss (in 40%). Great individual variation. Similar symptoms may occur in persons without demonstrated peptic ulcers ("nonulcer dyspepsia"); less responsive to standard therapy.

COMPLICATIONS Bleeding, obstruction, penetration causing acute pancreatitis, perforation, intractability, frequent recurrences.

DIAGNOSIS **DU** Upper endoscopy or upper GI barium radiography.

GU   Upper endoscopy often preferable to exclude possibility that ulcer is malignant (brush cytology, $\geq$6 pinch biopsies of ulcer margin). Radiographic features suggesting malignancy: ulcer within a mass, folds that do not radiate from ulcer margin, a large ulcer (>2.5–3 cm); however, 1% of radiographically benign-appearing ulcers prove to be malignant.

TREATMENT   **Medical**   Objectives: pain relief, healing, prevention of complications, prevention of recurrences. For GU, exclude malignancy (follow endoscopically to healing). Dietary restriction unnecessary with contemporary drugs; smoking prevents healing and should be stopped. Available drugs (in U.S.A.) equally effective (80–90% healing of DUs and 60% healing of GUs in 6 weeks; larger ulcers heal more slowly than smaller ones) (see Table 104-1). Only regimens that eradicate *H. pylori* from stomach (see below) appear to decrease the subsequent ulcer relapse rate.

Maintenance therapy   After healing (cimetidine 300 mg hs, ranitidine or nizatidine 150 mg hs, famotidine 20 mg hs, sucralfate 1 g bid), lowers 1-year relapse rate from 60–70% to 20%; reserved for pts with frequent recurrences or following a complication.

Surgery   For complications (persistent or recurrent bleeding, obstruction, perforation) or intractability (check serum gastrin to exclude gastrinoma). For *DU* see Table 104-2. For *GU* perform subtotal gastrectomy.

Complications of surgery   (1) Obstructed afferent loop (Billroth II), (2) bile reflux gastritis, (3) dumping syndrome (rapid gastric emptying with abdominal distress + postprandial vasomotor symptoms), (4) postvagotomy diarrhea, (5) bezoar, (6) anemia (iron, B_{12}, folate malabsorption), (7) malabsorption (poor mixing of gastric contents, pancreatic juices, bile; bacterial overgrowth), (8) osteomalacia and osteoporosis (vitamin D and Ca malabsorption), (9) gastric remnant carcinoma.

GASTRITIS

EROSIVE GASTRITIS   (Hemorrhagic gastritis, multiple gastric erosions)   Caused by aspirin, NSAIDs, alcohol, severe stress (burns, sepsis, trauma, surgery, shock, or respiratory, renal, or liver failure). May be asymptomatic or associated with epigastric discomfort, nausea, hematemesis, or melena. Diagnosis by upper endoscopy.

Treatment   Removal of offending agent and maintenance of O_2 and blood volume as required. For prevention of stress ulcers in critically ill pts, hourly oral administration of liquid antacids (e.g., Maalox 30 mL), IV H-2-receptor antagonist (e.g., cimetidine 300-mg bolus + 37.5–50 mg/h IV), or both is recommended to maintain gastric pH $\geq$4. Alternatively, su

TABLE 104-1   Drug treatment of peptic ulcer disease

Drug	Mechanism	Dose	Side effects
Antacids	Acid neutralization	140 mmol 1 h + 3 h pc + hs (e.g., 30 mL Maalox); lower doses (15 mL pc + hs) appear to be as effective	Diarrhea (Mg), constipation (Al), osteomalacia, milk-alkali syndrome (elevated serum Ca, P, BUN, creatinine, HCO_3; due to Ca carbonate)
Cimetidine	H-2-receptor blockade	300 mg qid or 400 mg bid or 800 mg hs	Uncommon: antiandrogen (high doses), confusion, ↑ creatinine, ↓ hepatic drug metabolism, ↑ serum aminotransferase levels, rare blood dyscrasias
Ranitidine	H-2-receptor blockade	150 mg bid or 300 mg hs	As for cimetidine but antiandrogen, mental status and drug metabolism effects are less frequent; rare cases of hepatitis
Famotidine	H-2-receptor blockade	40 mg hs	Probably as for ranitidine
Nizatidine	H-2-receptor blockade	300 mg hs	Probably as for ranitidine
Sucralfate	Ulcer coating, pepsin binding	1 g 1 h ac + hs or 2 g bid	Constipation, binding to coadministered drugs
Misoprostol	Prostaglandin (enhance mucosal defense, reduce gastric acid secretion)	200 μg qid for prevention of NSAID-induced ulcers	Diarrhea, uterine contraction (do not use in women of child-bearing age)
Omeprazole	Inhibits H^+,K^+-ATPase (proton pump) on gastric parietal cell	20 mg qAM	↓ Hepatic drug metabolism; approved only for short-term (8-week) treatment of refractory ulcers and for hypersecretory states (Zollinger-Ellison syndrome) because of concern that drug-induced antacidity and consequent hypergastrinemia may lead to increased cancer risk.

TABLE 104-2   Surgical treatment of duodenal ulcer

Operation	Recurrence rate	Complication rate
Vagotomy + antrectomy (Billroth I or II)*	1%	Highest
Vagotomy and pyloroplasty	10%	Intermediate
Parietal cell (proximal gastric, superselective) vagotomy	$\geq$10%	Lowest

* Billroth I = gastroduodenostomy; Billroth II = gastrojejunostomy.

cralfate slurry 1 g PO q 6 h can be given; does not raise gastric pH and may thus avoid increased risk of aspiration pneumonia. As above (Table 104-1), misoprostol 200 μg PO qid can be used with NSAIDs to prevent NSAID-induced ulcers.

NONEROSIVE GASTRITIS   Fundal gland (type A) gastritis Three patterns: superficial gastritis, atrophic gastritis, gastric atrophy. Generally asymptomatic, common in elderly; atrophic types may be associated with achlorhydria, pernicious anemia, and increased risk of gastric cancer (value of screening endoscopy uncertain).

Superficial (type B) gastritis   Usually antral and caused by *H. pylori* (see above). Diagnosis of *H. pylori* gastritis can be made by histology, rapid urease test of gastric biopsy material, urea breath testing, and detection in serum of antibodies to *H. pylori*. Often asymptomatic but may be associated with dyspepsia. May also lead to atrophic gastritis and gastric atrophy. Eradication of *H. pylori* is associated with resolution of gastritis but usually requires cumbersome, multidrug regimen (e.g., bismuth subsalicylate 30 mL PO qid, amoxicillin 50 mg PO tid, and metronidazole 500 mg PO tid for 3–4 weeks), is of uncertain clinical benefit, and may be followed by recolonization of stomach by *H. pylori*.

Pyloric gland gastritis   May result from regurgitation of duodenal contents. Generally asymptomatic, but may be associated with gastric ulcers.

SPECIFIC TYPES OF GASTRITIS   Ménétrier's disease (hypertrophic gastropathy), eosinophilic gastritis, granulomatous gastritis, Crohn's disease, sarcoidosis, infections (tuberculosis, syphilis, fungi, viruses, parasites), pseudolymphoma, radiation, corrosive gastritis.

ZOLLINGER-ELLISON (Z-E) SYNDROME (GASTRINOMA)

Consider when ulcer disease is severe, refractory to therapy, associated with ulcers in atypical locations, or associated with diarrhea. Tumors usually pancreatic, often multiple, slowly growing; >60% malignant; 20–25% associated with multiple endocrine neoplasia type I (gastrinoma, hyperparathyroidism, pituitary neoplasm).

DIAGNOSIS   Suggestive   Basal acid output >15 mmol/h; basal/maximal acid output >60%; upper GI radiograph: large mucosal folds.

Confirmatory   Serum gastrin >1000 ng/L or rise in gastrin of 200 ng/L following IV secretin (see Table 104-3).

DIFFERENTIAL DIAGNOSIS   Increased gastric acid secretion Z-E syndrome, antral G-cell hyperplasia, postgastrectomy retained antrum, renal failure, massive small bowel resection, chronic gastric outlet obstruction.

Normal or decreased gastric acid secretion   Pernicious anemia, chronic gastritis, gastric cancer, vagotomy, pheochromocytoma.

TREATMENT   Omeprazole, beginning at 40 mg PO qAM and increasing until maximal gastric acid output is <10 mmol/h before next dose, is drug of choice during evaluation and in pts who are not surgical candidates. Tumor localization can be attempted with ultrasound, CT, selective angiography, and, in selected cases, venous sampling for gastrin. Exploratory laparotomy with resection of primary tumor and solitary metastases when possible; in pts with MEN I, tumor is often multifocal and unresectable. For unresectable tumors, parietal cell vagotomy may enhance control of ulcer disease by drugs. Occasional gastrinomas are located in duodenum or other extrapancreatic sites. Chemotherapy for metastatic tumor (e.g., streptozocin and 5-fluorouracil); 40% partial response rate.

TABLE 104-3   Differential diagnostic tests

Condition	Fasting gastrin	Gastrin response to	
		IV Secretin	Food
DU	N* (≤150 ng/L)	NC†	Slight ↑
Z-E	↑ ↑ ↑	↑ ↑ ↑	NC
Antral G (gastrin) cell hyperplasia	↑	↑ , NC	↑ ↑ ↑

* N = normal.
† NC = no change.

For a more detailed discussion, see McGuigan JE: Peptic Ulcer and Gastritis, Chap. 238, and Mayer RJ: Neoplasms of the Esophagus and Stomach, Chap. 239, in HPIM-12, pp. 1229 and 1248

ACUTE PANCREATITIS

The differentiation between acute and chronic pancreatitis is based on clinical criteria. In acute pancreatitis, there is restoration of normal pancreatic function; in the chronic form there is permanent loss of function and pain may predominate. There are two pathologic types of acute pancreatitis: edematous and necrotizing.

ETIOLOGY Most common causes in the U.S. are alcohol and cholelithiasis. Others include abdominal trauma; postoperative, postendoscopic retrograde cholangiopancreatography (ERCP); metabolic (e.g., hypertriglyceridemia, hypercalcemia, renal failure); hereditary pancreatitis; infection (e.g., mumps, viral hepatitis, coxsackievirus, ascariasis *Mycoplasma*); medications (e.g., azathioprine, sulfonamides, thiazides, furosemide, estrogens, tetracycline, valproic acid, pentamidine); vasculitis (e.g., lupus, necrotizing angiitis, thrombotic thrombocytopenic purpura); penetrating peptic ulcer; obstruction of the ampulla of Vater (e.g., regional enteritis); pancreas divisum.

SYMPTOMS AND SIGNS Can vary from mild abdominal pain to shock. *Common symptoms:* (1) Steady, boring midepigastric pain radiating to the back; (2) nausea, vomiting. *Physical exam:* (1) Low-grade fever, tachycardia, hypotension; (2) erythematous skin nodules due to subcutaneous fat necrosis; (3) basilar rales, pleural effusion (often on the left); (4) abdominal tenderness and rigidity, diminished bowel sounds, palpable upper abdominal mass; (5) Cullen's sign—blue discoloration in the periumbilical area due to hemoperitoneum; (6) Turner's sign—blue-red-purple or green-brown discoloration of the flanks due to tissue catabolism of hemoglobin.

LABORATORY

1. Serum amylase: Large elevations ($>3 \times$ normal) virtually assure the diagnosis if salivary gland disease and intestinal perforation/infarction are excluded. However, normal serum amylase does *not* exclude the diagnosis of acute pancreatitis, and the degree of elevation does not predict severity of pancreatitis. Amylase levels typically return to normal in 48–72 h.

2. Urinary amylase-creatinine clearance ratio may be helpful in distinguishing between pancreatitis and other causes of hyperamylasemia (e.g., macroamylasemia) but is invalid in the presence of renal failure. Simultaneous serum and urine amylase values are used. $C_{am}/C_{Cr} = (am_{urine} \times CR_{serum}) / (am_{serum} \times Cr_{urine})$. Normal value is less than 4%.

3. Serum lipase level is more specific for pancreatic disease and remains elevated for 7–14 d.

4. Other tests: Hypocalcemia occurs in approximately 25% of patients. *Leukocytosis* (15,000–20,000/μL) occurs frequently. *Hypertriglyceridemia* occurs in 15% of cases and can cause a spuriously normal serum amylase level. *Hyperglycemia* is common. *Serum bilirubin, alkaline phosphatase,* and *aspartate aminotransferase* can be transiently elevated. *Hypoalbuminemia* and marked elevations of serum lactic dehydrogenase (LDH) are associated with an increased mortality rate. *Hypoxemia* is present in 25% of pts. The ECG may demonstrate ST-segment and T-wave abnormalities.

IMAGING

1. Abdominal radiographs are abnormal in 50% of pts but are not specific for pancreatitis. Common findings include total or partial ileus ("sentinel loop") and spasm of transverse colon. Useful for excluding other diagnoses such as intestinal perforation.

2. Ultrasound often fails to visualize the pancreas because of overlying intestinal gas but may detect gallstones or edema or enlargement of the pancreas.

3. CT can confirm diagnosis of pancreatitis (edematous pancreas) and is useful for predicting and identifying late complications.

DIFFERENTIAL DIAGNOSIS   Intestinal perforation (especially peptic ulcer), cholecystitis, acute intestinal obstruction, mesenteric ischemia, renal colic, myocardial ischemia, aortic dissection, connective tissue disorders, pneumonia, and diabetic ketoacidosis.

TREATMENT   Most (90%) cases subside over a period of 3–7 d. Conventional measures: (1) analgesics, such as meperidine; (2) IV fluids and colloids; (3) no oral alimentation; (4) treatment of hypocalcemia, if symptomatic; (5) antibiotics only if there is established infection. Cimetidine (or related agents), nasogastric suction, glucagon, peritoneal lavage, and anticholinergic medications have not been shown effective. In mild or moderate pancreatitis, a clear liquid diet can usually be started after 3–6 d. Fulminant pancreatitis usually requires aggressive fluid support and meticulous management of cardiovascular collapse, respiratory insufficiency, and pancreatic infection. Laparotomy with removal of necrotic material and adequate drainage should be considered if pt continues to deteriorate despite conventional therapy. Pts with severe gallstone-induced pancreatitis often benefit from early (<3 d) papillotomy.

COMPLICATIONS   Increased mortality with respiratory failure, shock, massive colloid requirements, hypocalcemia, or hemorrhagic peritoneal fluid. _Early:_ Shock, GI bleeding, common duct obstruction, ileus, splenic infarction or rupture, DIC, subcutaneous fat necrosis, ARDS, pleural effusion, hematuria, acute renal failure. _Late:_ (1) _Pancreatic phlegmon_ is a solid mass of swollen, inflamed pancreas and should be suspected if abdominal pain, fever, and hyperamylasemia persist for more than 5 d. Phlegmons may become secondarily infected resulting in abscess formation (see below). (2) _Pancreatic pseudocysts_ develop over 1–4 weeks. Abdominal pain is the usual complaint and a tender upper abdominal mass may be present. Can be detected by abdominal ultrasound or CT. In pts who are stable and uncomplicated treatment is supportive; if there is no resolution within 6 weeks, consider CT-guided needle aspiration/drainage, surgical drainage, or resection. In pts with an expanding pseudocyst or complicated by hemorrhage, rupture, or abscess surgery should be performed. (3) _Pancreatic abscess_ (signalled by fever, leukocytosis, ileus, and rapid deterioration in a pt recovering from pancreatitis) is most often due to _E coli_. The diagnosis of pancreatic infection can be established by CT-guided needle aspiration of phlegmons and pseudocysts. Treatment consists of antibiotic therapy and surgical drainage. (4) _Pancreatic ascites and pleural effusions_ are usually due to disruption of the main pancreatic duct. Treatment involves nasogastric suction and parenteral alimentation for 2–3 weeks. If medical management fails, pancreatography followed by surgery should be performed.

CHRONIC PANCREATITIS

Chronic pancreatitis may occur as recurrent episodes of acute inflammation superimposed upon a damaged pancreas or as chronic damage with pain and malabsorption. The causes of relapsing pancreatitis are similar to acute pancreatitis.

ETIOLOGY   Chronic alcoholism most frequent in U.S.; also hypertriglyceridemia, hypercalcemia, hereditary pancreatitis, hemochromatosis, and cystic fibrosis. In 25% of adults etiology is unknown.

SYMPTOMS AND SIGNS   _Pain_ is cardinal symptom. Weight loss, steatorrhea, and other signs and symptoms of malabsorption common. Physical exam often unremarkable.

LABORATORY   No specific laboratory test for chronic pancreatitis. Serum amylase and lipase levels are often normal.

Serum bilirubin and alkaline phosphatase may be elevated. Steatorrhea (fecal fat concentration ≥9.5%) late in the course. The bentiromide test, a simple, effective test of pancreatic exocrine function may be helpful. D-Xylose urinary excretion test is usually normal. Impaired glucose tolerance is present in over 50% of pts. Secretin stimulation test is a relatively sensitive test for pancreatic exocrine deficiency.

IMAGING *Plain films of the abdomen* reveal pancreatic calcifications in 30–60%. *Ultrasound* and *CT scans* may show pseudocysts or dilation of the pancreatic duct. *ERCP* often reveals irregular dilation of the main pancreatic duct and pruning of the branches.

DIFFERENTIAL DIAGNOSIS Important to distinguish from pancreatic carcinoma; may require radiographically guided biopsy.

TREATMENT Aimed at controlling pain and malabsorption. Intermittent attacks treated like acute pancreatitis. Alcohol and large, fatty meals must be avoided. Narcotics for severe pain but subsequent addiction is common. Surgery may control pain if there is a ductal stricture. Subtotal pancreatectomy may also control pain but at the cost of exocrine insufficiency and diabetes. Malabsorption is managed with a low-fat diet and pancreatic enzyme replacement (8 conventional tablets or 3 enteric-coated tablets with meals). Because pancreatic enzymes are inactivated by acid, agents that reduce acid production (e.g., omeprazole or sodium bicarbonate) may improve their efficacy (but bicarbonate should not be given with enteric-coated preparations). Insulin may be necessary to control serum glucose.

COMPLICATIONS Vitamin B_{12} malabsorption in 40% of alcohol-induced and all cystic fibrosis cases. Impaired glucose tolerance. Nondiabetic retinopathy due to vitamin A and/or zinc deficiency. GI bleeding, icterus, effusions, subcutaneous fat necrosis, and bone pain occasionally occur. Increased risk for pancreatic carcinoma. Narcotic addiction common.

For a more detailed discussion, see Greenberger NJ, Toskes, PP, Isselbacher KJ: Acute and Chronic Pancreatitis, Chap. 260, in HPIM-12, p. 1372

106 INFLAMMATORY BOWEL DISEASES

Chronic inflammatory disorders of unknown etiology involving the GI tract. Peak occurrence between ages 15 and 35, but onset may occur at any age.

ULCERATIVE COLITIS (UC)

Pathology   Colonic *mucosal* inflammation; rectum almost always involved, with inflammation extending continuously (no skip areas), proximally for a variable extent; histologic features include epithelial damage, inflammation, crypt abscesses, loss of goblet cells.

Clinical manifestations   Bloody diarrhea, mucus, fever, abdominal pain, tenesmus, weight loss; spectrum of severity (majority of cases are mild, limited to rectosigmoid). In severe cases dehydration, anemia, hypokalemia, hypoalbuminemia.

Complications   Toxic megacolon, colonic perforation; cancer risk related to extent and duration of colitis; preceded by dysplasia (precancer), which may be detected on surveillance colonoscopic biopsies.

Diagnosis   Sigmoidoscopy/colonoscopy: mucosal erythema, granularity, friability, exudate, hemorrhage, ulcers, pseudopolyps (regenerating mucosa). Barium enema: loss of haustrations, mucosal irregularity, ulcerations.

CROHN'S DISEASE (CD)

Pathology   Any part of GI tract, usually terminal ileum and/or colon; *transmural* inflammation, bowel wall thickening, linear ulcerations, and submucosal thickening leading to cobblestone pattern; discontinuous involvement (skip areas); histologic features include transmural inflammation, granulomas, fissures, fistulas.

Clinical manifestations   Fever, abdominal pain, diarrhea (often without blood), fatigue, weight loss, growth retardation in children; acute ileitis mimicking appendicitis; anorectal fissures, fistulas, abscesses.

Complications   Intestinal obstruction (edema vs. fibrosis); rarely toxic megacolon or perforation; intestinal fistulas to bowel, bladder, vagina, skin, soft tissue, often with abscess formation; bile salt malabsorption leading to cholesterol gallstones and/or oxalate kidney stones; intestinal malignancy; amyloidosis.

Diagnosis Sigmoidoscopy/colonoscopy, barium enema, upper GI and small bowel series: nodularity, rigidity, ulcers that may be deep or longitudinal, cobblestoning, skip areas, strictures, fistulas. CT may show thickened, matted bowel loops or an abscess.

DIFFERENTIAL DIAGNOSIS

Infectious enterocolitis *Shigella, Salmonella, Campylobacter, Yersinia* (acute ileitis), *Gonorrhea, Lymphogranuloma venereum, Clostridium difficile* toxin, tuberculosis, amebiasis.

Others Ischemic bowel disease, diverticulitis, radiation enterocolitis, bleeding colonic lesion (e.g., neoplasm), irritable bowel syndrome (no bleeding).

EXTRAINTESTINAL MANIFESTATIONS (UC AND CD)

1. *Joint:* Peripheral arthritis—parallels activity of bowel disease; ankylosing spondylitis and sacroiliitis (associated with HLA-B27)—activity independent of bowel disease.
2. *Skin:* Erythema nodosum, aphthous ulcers, pyoderma gangrenosum, cutaneous Crohn's disease.
3. *Eye:* Episcleritis, iritis, uveitis.
4. *Liver:* Fatty liver, pericholangitis (intrahepatic sclerosing cholangitis), sclerosing cholangitis, cholangiocarcinoma, chronic hepatitis.
5. *Others:* Autoimmune hemolytic anemia, phlebitis, pulmonary embolus.

TREATMENT

Supportive Antidiarrheal agents (diphenoxylate and atropine, loperamide) in mild disease; IV hydration and blood transfusions in severe disease; parenteral nutrition or defined enteral formulas (effective as primary therapy in CD, although high relapse rate when oral feeding is resumed; should not replace drug therapy; important role in preoperative preparation of malnourished pt); emotional support.

Sulfasalazine Active component is 5-aminosalicylic acid (5-ASA) linked to sulfapyridine carrier; useful in colonic disease of mild to moderate severity (1–1.5 g PO qid); efficacy in maintaining remission demonstrated only for UC (500 mg PO qid). Toxicity (generally due to sulfapyridine component):

dose-related—nausea, headache, rarely hemolytic anemia—may resolve when drug dose is lowered; idiosyncratic—fever, rash, neutropenia, pancreatitis, hepatitis, etc.; miscellaneous—oligospermia. For fever and some rashes, desensitization can be attempted—after 2 weeks reintroduce drug in very low dose (0.125 g qd) and increase by 0.125 g weekly; for more severe side effects, do not restart the drug. New alternative drugs: 5-ASA (mesalamine) linked to other carriers, in slow release form, or as enema: e.g., 4-g 5-ASA enemas in distal UC, 1 PR retained qhs until remission, then q 2 hs or q 3 hs.

Glucocorticoids   Useful in severe disease and ileal or ileocolonic CD. Prednisone 40–60 mg PO qd, then taper; IV hydrocortisone 100 mg tid or equivalent in hospitalized pts; IV ACTH drip (120 U per day) may be preferable in first attacks of UC. Nightly hydrocortisone retention enemas in proctosigmoiditis.

Immunosuppressive agents (Azathioprine, 6-mercaptopurine 50 mg PO qd up to 1.5 mg/kg qd)   Useful as steroid-sparing agents and in intractable CD (may require 4- to 8-month trial period). Toxicity—immunosuppression, pancreatitis, ? carcinogenicity.

Metronidazole   Appears <u>effective in colonic CD</u> (500 mg PO bid) and <u>refractory perineal CD</u> (10–20 mg/kg PO qd). Toxicity—peripheral neuropathy, metallic taste, ? carcinogenicity.

Experimental   Cyclosporine, methotrexate, chloroquine, fish oil, others.

Surgery   *UC:* Colectomy (curative) for intractability, toxic megacolon (if no improvement with aggressive medical therapy in 24–48 h), cancer, severe dysplasia. Alternatives to conventional ileostomy—continent ileostomy (Koch pouch), ileal pouch–anal anastomosis. *CD:* Resection for fixed obstruction (or stricturoplasty), abscesses, persistent symptomatic fistulas, intractability.

For a more detailed discussion, see Glickman RM: Inflammatory Bowel Disease, Chap. 241, in HPIM-12, p. 1268

107 TUMORS OF THE GASTROINTESTINAL TRACT

ESOPHAGEAL CARCINOMA

Fifth most common cancer in men; less frequent in women. Highest incidence in focal regions of China, Iran, Soviet Union. In U.S. blacks more frequently affected than whites; 5-year survival <5%.

Pathology 85% squamous cell carcinoma, most commonly in upper two-thirds; <15% adenocarcinoma, usually in distal third, arising in region of columnar metaplasia (Barrett's esophagus), glandular tissue, or as direct extension of proximal gastric adenocarcinoma; lymphoma and melanoma rare.

Etiology and risk factors Cause unknown; major risk factors for squamous cell carcinoma: ethanol abuse, smoking (combination is synergistic); other risks: lye ingestion and esophageal stricture, radiation exposure, head and neck cancer, achalasia, smoked opiates, Plummer-Vinson syndrome, tylosis, chronic ingestion of extremely hot tea, deficiency of vitamin A, zinc, molybdenum.

Clinical features Progressive dysphagia (first with solids, then liquids), rapid weight loss common, chest pain (from mediastinal spread), pulmonary aspiration (obstruction, tracheoesophageal fistula), hoarseness (laryngeal nerve palsy), hypercalcemia (parathyroid hormone–related peptide hypersecretion by squamous carcinomas); bleeding infrequent, occasionally severe; examination often unremarkable.

Diagnosis Double-contrast barium swallow useful for screening; flexible esophagogastroscopy most sensitive and specific test; pathologic confirmation by combination of endoscopic biopsy and cytologic examination of mucosal brushings (neither alone sufficiently sensitive); CT valuable to assess local and nodal spread.

Therapy *Squamous cell carcinoma:* Surgical resection after chemotherapy [5-fluorouracil (5-FU), cisplatin] prolongs survival and provides somewhat improved chance of cure. *Adenocarcinoma:* Curative resection rarely possible. Overall, 40% resectable with less than one-fifth of these surviving 5 years. Palliative measures include laser ablation, mechanical dilatation, radiotherapy, luminal prosthesis to bypass tumor, and bypass surgery. Gastrostomy or jejunostomy frequently required for nutritional support.

GASTRIC CARCINOMA

Common worldwide, with highest incidence in Japan, China, Chile, Ireland; although incidence decreasing worldwide, dramatically in U.S.; twice as common as esophageal carcinoma. Male:female = 2:1; peak incidence sixth and seventh decades; overall 5-year survival less than 15%.

Etiology and risk factors   Cause unknown; environmental component of focal tumors, suggested by studies of migrants and their offspring. Several dietary factors correlated with increased incidence: nitrates, smoked foods, heavily salted foods; genetic component suggested by increased incidence in first-degree relatives of affected pts; other risk factors: atrophic gastritis, Billroth II gastrectomy, gastrojejunostomy, adenomatous gastric polyps, pernicious anemia, hyperplastic gastric polyps (latter two associated with atrophic gastritis). Ménétrier's disease; slight increased risk with blood group A.

Pathology   Adenocarcinoma in ~90%; usually focal (polypoid, ulcerative), two-thirds arising in antrum or lesser curvature, less commonly diffuse infiltrative (linitis plastica) or superficial spreading (diffuse lesions more prevalent in younger pts with significant geographic variation); spreads primarily to local nodes, liver, peritoneum; systemic spread uncommon; lymphoma accounts for ~7% (most frequent extranodal site in immunocompetent pts) and leiomyosarcoma less than 3% of gastric malignancies.

Clinical features   Most commonly presents with progressive upper abdominal discomfort, frequently with weight loss, anorexia, nausea; acute or chronic GI bleeding (mucosal ulceration) common; dysphagia (location in cardia); vomiting (pyloric and widespread disease); early satiety; examination often unrevealing early in course; later, abdominal tenderness, pallor, and cachexia most common signs; palpable mass uncommon; metastatic spread may be manifest by hepatomegaly, ascites, left supraclavicular or scalene adenopathy, periumbilical, ovarian, or prerectal mass (Blummer's shelf), low-grade fever, skin abnormalities (nodules, dermatomyositis, acanthosis nigricans, or multiple seborrheic keratoses). *Laboratory findings*: iron deficiency anemia in two-thirds of pts; fecal occult blood in 80%; rarely associated with pancytopenia or microangiopathic hemolytic anemia (from marrow infiltration), or leukemoid reaction, or migratory thrombophlebitis.

Diagnosis   Double-contrast barium swallow useful for screening; gastroscopy most sensitive and specific test; pathologic confirmation by biopsy and cytologic examination of mucosal brushings; superficial biopsies less sensitive for lymphomas (frequently submucosal); important to differentiate benign from malignant gastric ulcers with multiple biopsies and follow-up examinations to demonstrate ulcer healing.

Treatment *Adenocarcinoma*: Gastrectomy offers only chance of cure; the rare tumors limited to mucosa are resectable for cure in 80%; deeper invasion, nodal metastases decrease 5-year survival to 20% of pts with resectable tumors in absence of obvious metastatic spread, CT may aid in determining tumor resectability. Palliative therapy for pain, obstruction, and bleeding includes surgery, endoscopic dilatation, radiation, chemotherapy. *Lymphoma*: Resectable in two-thirds of pts leading to 50% 5-year survival; unresectable gastric lymphoma treated with radiation and chemotherapy, with occasional long-term survival. *Leiomyosarcoma:* Surgical resection curative in most pts.

BENIGN GASTRIC TUMORS

Much less common than malignant gastric tumors; hyperplastic polyps most common, with adenomas, hamartomas, and leiomyomas rare; 30% of adenomas and occasional hyperplastic polyps are associated with gastric malignancy; polyposis syndromes include Peutz-Jeghers and familial polyposis (hamartomas and adenomas), Gardner's (adenomas), and Cronkhite-Canada (cystic polyps). See section on Colonic Polyps below.

Clinical features Usually asymptomatic; occasionally present with bleeding or vague epigastric discomfort.

Treatment Endoscopic or surgical excision.

SMALL BOWEL TUMORS

Clinical features Uncommon tumors (~5% of all GI neoplasms); usually present with bleeding, abdominal pain, weight loss, or intestinal obstruction (intermittent or fixed); increased incidence of lymphomas in pts with gluten-sensitive enteropathy, Crohn's disease involving small bowel deficiency states.

Pathology Usually benign; adenomas (usually duodenal), leiomyomas (intramural), and lipomas (usually ileal) most common; 50% of *malignant* tumors are adenocarcinoma, usually in duodenum (at or near ampulla of Vater) or jejunum, commonly coexisting with benign adenomas; lymphomas account for 25%; occur as focal mass (western type) or diffuse infiltration (Mediterranean type); immunoproliferative small intestinal disease (IPSID) can present as intestinal malabsorption; carcinoid tumors; diffuse tumors usually asymptomatic; carcinoid syndrome limited to pts with metastic spread to liver; leiomyosarcomas rare, frequently large at diagnosis.

Diagnosis Barium x-ray examination best diagnostic test; direct small bowel instillation of contrast (enteroclysis) occasionally reveals tumors not seen with routine small bowel radiography; angiography (to detect plexus of tumor vessels) or laparotomy often required for diagnosis; CT useful to evaluate extent of tumor (esp. lymphomas).

Treatment Surgical excision; adjuvant chemotherapy for focal lymphoma, no proven role for chemotherapy or radiation therapy for other small bowel tumors; no current therapy alters variable course of IPSID.

COLONIC POLYPS

TUBULAR ADENOMAS Present in ~15% of adults; pedunculated or sessile; usually asymptomatic; may cause bleeding or, rarely, obstruction; risk of malignant degeneration correlates with size and is higher in sessile polyps; 65% found in rectosigmoid colon; diagnosis by barium enema, sigmoidoscopy, or colonoscopy. *Treatment:* Full colonoscopy to detect synchronous lesions (present in 30%); endoscopic resection (surgery if polyp large or inaccessible by colonoscopy); follow-up surveillance by colonoscopy every 2–3 years.

VILLOUS ADENOMAS Generally larger than tubular adenomas at diagnosis; often sessile; high risk of malignancy (up to 50% when greater than 2 cm); more prevalent in left colon; occasionally associated with potassium-rich secretory diarrhea. *Treatment:* As for tubular adenomas.

HYPERPLASTIC POLYPS Asymptomatic; usually incidental finding at colonoscopy; rarely greater than 5 mm; no malignant potential. *No treatment* required.

HEREDITARY POLYPOSIS SYNDROMES

1. Familial polyposis coli (FPC): Diffuse pancolonic adenomatous polyposis (up to several thousand polyps); autosomal dominant inheritance associated with deletion in chromosome 5; colon carcinoma from malignant degeneration of polyp in 100% by age 40. *Treatment:* Prophylactic total colectomy or subtotal colectomy with ileoproctostomy before age 30; subtotal resection avoids ileostomy but necessitates *frequent* proctoscopic surveillance; periodic colonoscopic or radiologic screening of siblings and offspring of patients with FPC until age 35.

2. Gardner's syndrome: Variant of FPC with associated soft tissue tumors (sebaceous cysts, osteomas, lipomas, desmoids); higher incidence of gastroduodenal polyps, ampullary adenocarcinoma. *Treatment:* As for FPC; surveillance for small bowel disease with fecal occult blood testing after colectomy.

3. Turcot's syndrome: Rare variant of FPC with associated malignant brain tumors. *Treatment:* As for FPC.

4. Juvenile polyposis: Multiple benign colonic and small bowel hamartomas; intestinal bleeding common; other symptoms: abdominal pain, diarrhea; occasional intussusception; rarely recur after excision; diffuse polyposis associated with somewhat increased incidence of colon cancer from malignant degeneration of interspersed *adenomatous* polyps. Prophylactic colectomy controversial.

5. Peutz-Jeghers syndrome: Numerous hamartomatous polyps of entire GI tract; polyps more prevalent in small bowel than colon; GI bleeding common; increased risk for the development of cancer at gastrointestinal and non-gastrointestinal sites. Prophylactic surgery *not* recommended.

COLON CANCER

Second most common internal cancer in humans; accounts for 20% of cancer-related deaths in U.S., incidence increases dramatically above age 50, equal in men and women.

Etiology and risk factors Cause unknown; increased prevalence in developed countries; increased risk in pts with hypercholesterolemia, coronary artery disease; environmental factors suggested by studies of migrants, correlation of risk with low-fiber, high animal fat diets, although direct effect of diet remains unproven; possible decreased risk with long-term dietary calcium supplementation; risk increased in first-degree relatives of pts, families with increased prevalence of cancer, and pts with history of breast or gynecologic cancer, familial polyposis syndromes, >10-year history of ulcerative colitis, Crohn's colitis, >15-year history of ureterosigmoidostomy, asbestosis; tumors in pts with strong family history of malignancy, frequently in right colon, and commonly present before age 50; high prevalence in pts with *Streptococcus bovis* bacteremia.

Pathology Nearly always adenocarcinoma; 75% located distal to the splenic flexure (except in association with polyposis or hereditary cancer syndromes); may be polypoid, sessile, fungating, or constricting; subtype and degree of differentiation do not correlate with course; degree of invasiveness at surgery (Dukes' classification) single best predictor of prognosis: >90% 5-year survival for cancer confined to mucosa and submucosa (stage A); 70–85% with extension to muscularis or serosa; (stage B; survival in this group worse with tumor penetration of pericolic fat); 30–60% with regional lymph node involvement (stage C; survival in this group better with involvement of <5 lymph nodes); 5% with distant metastasis (e.g., liver, lung, bone; stage D); rectosigmoid tumors may spread to lungs early because of systemic paravertebral venous drainage of this area; other predictors of poor prognosis: preoperative serum carcinoembryonic antigen (CEA) >5 ng/mL (>5 μg/L), poorly differentiated histology, bowel perforation, venous invasion, adherence to adjacent organs, aneuploidy, specific deletions in chromosomes 5, 17, 18.

Clinical features   Left-sided colon cancers present most commonly with rectal bleeding, altered bowel habits (narrowing, constipation, intermittent diarrhea, tenesmus), and abdominal or back pain; cecal and ascending colon cancers more frequently present with symptoms of anemia, occult blood in stool, or weight loss; other complications: perforation, fistula, volvulus, inguinal hernia; laboratory findings: anemia in 50% of right-sided lesions.

Diagnosis   Early diagnosis aided by screening asymptomatic persons with fecal occult blood testing (see below); more than half of all colon cancers are within reach of a 60-cm flexible sigmoidoscope; air-contrast barium enema will diagnose approximately 85% of colon cancers not within reach of sigmoidoscope; colonoscopy most sensitive and specific, permits tumor biopsy and removal of synchronous polyps, but incurs somewhat greater expense.

Treatment   *Local disease:* Surgical resection of colonic segment containing tumor; preoperative evaluation to assess prognosis and surgical approach includes chest films, biochemical liver tests, plasma CEA level, and possible abdominal CT; resection of isolated hepatic metastases possible in selected cases; adjuvant radiation therapy to pelvis (with or without concomitant chemotherapy) to decrease local recurrence rate of *rectal* carcinoma (no apparent effect on survival); radiotherapy without benefit on more proximal tumors; adjuvant chemotherapy (5-FU and levamisole) to decrease recurrence rate of stage C tumors (may also improve survival); periodic determination of serum CEA level useful to follow therapy and assess recurrence. *Follow-up after curative resection:* Yearly liver tests, CBC, follow-up radiologic or colonoscopic evaluation at 1 year, if normal repeat every 3 years, with routine screening interim (see below); if polyps detected, repeat 1 year after resection. *Advanced tumor* (locally unresectable or metastatic): Systemic chemotherapy (5-FU and folinic acid), intraarterial chemotherapy [floxuridine (FUDR)] and/or radiotherapy may palliate symptoms.

Prevention Early detection of colon carcinoma may be facilitated by routine screening of stool for occult blood (Hemoccult II, Colo-Test, etc.); false positives: ingestion of red meat, iron, aspirin; upper GI bleeding; false negatives: vitamin C ingestion, intermittent bleeding; annual testing recommended for pts over age 40, earlier in pts with increased risk (see above); *screening* flexible sigmoidoscopy recommended every 3 years; careful evaluation of all pts with positive fecal occult blood tests (flexible sigmoidoscopy *and* air-contrast barium enema or colonoscopy alone) reveals polyps in 20–40% and carcinoma in approximately 5%; screening of asymptomatic persons allows earlier detection of colon cancer (i.e., earlier Dukes' stage), greater resectability rate; however, routine fecal occult blood testing has not been shown to affect overall mortality from colon carcinoma. More intensive evaluation of first degree relatives of pts with colon carcinoma frequently includes *screening* air-contrast barium enema or colonoscopy after age 40.

For a more detailed discussion, see Mayer RJ: Neoplasms of the Esophagus and Stomach, Chap. 239, p. 1248; Mayer RJ: Tumors of the Large and Small Intestine, Chap. 243, p. 1289; and Richter JM, Isselbacher KJ: Gastrointestinal Bleeding, Chap. 46, p. 261, in HPIM-12

IRRITABLE BOWEL SYNDROME

A motor disorder characterized by altered bowel habits, abdominal pain, and absence of detectable organic pathology. Most common GI disease in clinical practice. Three variants: (1) spastic colon (chronic abdominal pain and constipation), (2) alternating constipation and diarrhea, and (3) chronic, painless diarrhea.

Pathophysiology Alteration in colonic motility (increased resting colonic motility in spastic colon; decreased motility in diarrhea); motility increases in response to stress, cholinergic drugs, cholecystokinin; psychologic disturbances in some patients—depression, hysteria, obsessive-compulsive traits; specific food intolerances in a few cases.

Clinical manifestations Onset often before age 30; females/males = 2:1; pasty stools, ribbony or pencil-thin stools, mucus in stools (no blood), heartburn, bloating, back pain, weakness, faintness, palpitations, urinary frequency.

Diagnosis Often by history; consider sigmoidoscopy and barium radiographs to exclude inflammatory bowel disease or malignancy; consider excluding giardiasis, intestinal lactase deficiency, hyperthyroidism.

Treatment Reassurance, avoidance of stress or precipitating factors, dietary bulk (fiber, psyllium extract, e.g., Metamucil 1 tbsp bid-tid); occasional trials of loperamide (2 PO qA.M. then 1 PO after each loose stool to a maximum of 8/d, then titrate), diphenoxylate (Lomotil)(up to 2 PO qid), or cholestyramine (up to 1 packet mixed in water PO qid), for diarrhea or, for pain, anticholinergics (e.g., dicyclomine HCl 10–40 mg PO qid).

DIVERTICULAR DISEASE

Herniations or saclike protrusions of the mucosa through the muscularis at points of nutrient artery penetration; possibly due to increased intraluminal pressure, low-fiber diet; most common in sigmoid colon.

Clinical presentations and treatment

1. Asymptomatic

2. Pain: Recurrent left lower quadrant pain relieved by defecation; alternating constipation and diarrhea. Diagnosis by barium enema. *Treatment:* high-fiber diet, psyllium extract (e.g., Metamucil 1 tbsp PO bid-tid), anticholinergics (e.g., dicyclomine hydrochloride 10–40 mg PO qid).

3. Diverticulitis: Pain, fever, altered bowel habits, tender colon, leukocytosis. *Treatment:* nothing by mouth, IV fluids, antibiotics (e.g., cefoxitin 2g IV q 6 h or imipenem 500 mg IV q 6–8 h); for ambulatory patients ampicillin or tetracycline 500 mg PO qid (clear liquid diet); surgical resection in refractory or frequently recurrent cases. *Complications:* pericolic abscess, perforation, fistula (to bladder, vagina, skin, soft tissue), liver abscess, stricture.

4. Hemorrhage: Usually in absence of diverticulitis, often from ascending colon and self-limited. If persistent, manage with mesenteric arteriography and intraarterial infusion of vasopressin or surgery (see Chap. 17).

INTESTINAL PSEUDOOBSTRUCTION

Recurrent attacks of nausea, vomiting, and abdominal pain and distention mimicking mechanical obstruction; may be complicated by steatorrhea due to bacterial overgrowth.

Causes *Primary:* Familial visceral neuropathy, familial visceral myopathy, idiopathic. *Secondary:* Scleroderma, amyloidosis, diabetes, celiac disease, parkinsonism, muscular dystrophy, drugs, electrolyte imbalance, postsurgical.

Treatment Acute attacks—intestinal decompression with long tube. Oral antibiotics for bacterial overgrowth (e.g., tetracycline 500 mg PO qid 1 week out of each month). Avoid surgery. In refractory cases, consider long-term parenteral hyperalimentation.

VASCULAR DISORDERS (SMALL AND LARGE INTESTINES)

MECHANISMS OF MESENTERIC ISCHEMIA (1) *Occlusive:* arterial thrombus (atherosclerosis); embolus (atrial fibrillation, valvular heart disease); venous thrombosis (trauma, neoplasm, infection, cirrhosis, oral contraceptives, antithrombin-III deficiency, protein S or C deficiency, lupus anticoagulant, idiopathic); vasculitis (SLE, polyarteritis, rheumatoid arthritis, Henoch-Schönlein purpura); (2) *nonocclusive:* hypotension, heart failure, arrhythmia.

ACUTE MESENTERIC ISCHEMIA Periumbilical pain out of proportion to tenderness; nausea, vomiting, distention, GI bleeding, altered bowel habits. Abdominal x-ray shows bowel distention, air-fluid levels, thumbprinting (submucosal edema). Peritoneal signs indicate infarcted bowel requiring surgical resection. In suspected arterial embolus, consider early celiac and mesenteric arteriography and surgical embolectomy.

CHRONIC MESENTERIC INSUFFICIENCY   "Abdominal angina"—dull, crampy periumbilical pain 15–30 min after a meal and lasting for several hours; weight loss. Evaluate with mesenteric arteriography for possible bypass graft surgery.

ISCHEMIC COLITIS   Usually due to nonocclusive disease in patient with atherosclerosis. Severe lower abdominal pain, rectal bleeding, hypotension. Abdominal x-ray shows colonic dilatation, thumbprinting. Sigmoidoscopy shows submucosal hemorrhage, friability, ulcerations; rectum often spared. Conservative management (NPO, IV fluids); surgical resection for infarction or postischemic stricture.

COLONIC ANGIODYSPLASIA

Vascular ectasias usually in right colon in persons over age 60. Account for up to 40% of cases of chronic or recurrent lower GI bleeding in elderly. May be associated with aortic stenosis. Diagnosis by arteriography (clusters of small vessels, early and prolonged opacification of draining vein) or colonoscopy (flat, bright red, fernlike lesions). For bleeding, treat by colonscopic electro- or laser coagulation, arteriographic embolization, or if necessary, right hemicolectomy (see Chap. 17).

COLONIC POLYPS AND COLON CANCER

(See Chap. 107)

ANORECTAL DISEASES

HEMORRHOIDS   Due to increased hydrostatic pressure in hemorrhoidal venous plexus (straining at stool, pregnancy, portal hypertension). May be external, internal, thrombosed, acute (prolapsed or strangulated), or bleeding. Treat pain with bulk laxative and stool softeners (psyllium extract, dioctyl sodium sulfosuccinate 100–900 mg/d), sitz baths 1–4/d, witch hazel compresses, analgesics as needed. Bleeding may require rubber band ligation or injection sclerotherapy. Operative hemorrhoidectomy in severe or refractory cases.

ANAL FISSURES   Medical therapy as for hemorrhoids. Internal anal sphincterotomy in refractory cases.

PRURITUS ANI   Often of unclear cause; may be due to poor hygiene, fungal or parasitic infection. Treat with thorough cleansing after bowel movement, topical glucocorticoid, antifungal agent if indicated.

For a more detailed discussion, see LaMont JT, Isselbacher KJ: Diseases of the Small and Large Intestine, Chap. 242, in HPIM-12, p. 1281

CHOLELITHIASIS

There are three major types of gallstones: cholesterol, pigment, and mixed stones. In the U.S., 80% of stones are cholesterol or mixed, 20% pigment.

Epidemiology One million new cases of cholelithiasis per year in the U.S. Increased incidence in American Indians and with obesity, diabetes, ileal disease, pregnancy, estrogen or oral contraceptive use, type IV hyperlipidemia, and cirrhosis. Females/males = 4:1.

Symptoms and signs Many gallstones are "silent," i.e., present in asymptomatic pts. Symptoms occur when stones produce inflammation or obstruction of the cystic or common bile ducts. Major symptoms: (1) biliary colic which is usually constant, RUQ or epigastric pain that occurs 30–90 min after meals, lasts for several hours, and occasionally radiates to the right scapula or back; and, (2) nausea, vomiting. Physical exam may be normal or show epigastric or RUQ tenderness.

Laboratory Occasionally, mild and transient elevations in bilirubin [<85 μmol/L (<5 mg/dL)] accompany biliary colic.

Imaging Only 10% of gallstones are radioopaque. Ultrasonography is best diagnostic test. The oral cholecystogram (OCG) requires a functioning gallbladder and serum bilirubin <51 μmol/L (<3 mg/dL).

Differential diagnosis Includes peptic ulcer disease, gastroesophageal reflux, irritable bowel syndrome, and hepatitis.

Treatment Since risk of developing complications requiring surgery is small in asymptomatic pts, elective cholecystectomy should be reserved for: (1) *symptomatic* pts [i.e., biliary colic despite dietary restriction (low-fat diet)]; (2) persons with previous complications of cholelithiasis (see below); and, (3) asymptomatic pts with an increased risk of complications (calcified or nonfunctioning gallbladder, cholesterolosis, adenomyomatosis). Patients with large (>2 cm) gallstones or with an anomalous gallbladder containing gallstones should also be considered for surgery. Oral dissolution agents (chenodeoxycholic acid, ursodeoxycholic acid) partially or completely dissolve radiolucent stones in 50% of pts but are ineffective in dissolving large, radioopaque or pigment stones and those within a poorly opacified gallbladder following oral cholecystography. Recurrence is likely if the medication is stopped. Extracorporeal shockwave lithotripsy followed by medical litholytic therapy is effective therapy in selected pts with radiolucent gallstones. Direct dissolution of gallstones using solvents such as methyl-*tert*-butyl ether instilled through a percutaneously placed biliary catheter appears promising.

Complications   See Acute Cholecystitis below.

ACUTE CHOLECYSTITIS

Acute inflammation of the gallbladder usually caused by cystic duct obstruction by an impacted stone.

Etiology   90% calculous; 10% acalculous; latter caused by prolonged acute illness, fasting, hyperalimentation leading to gallbladder stasis, vasculitis, carcinoma of gallbladder or common bile duct.

Symptoms and signs   (1) RUQ or epigastric pain; (2) nausea, vomiting, anorexia; and (3) fever. Examination typically reveals RUQ tenderness; palpable RUQ mass found in 20% of pts.

Laboratory   Mild leukocytosis; serum bilirubin, alkaline phosphatase, and SGOT may be mildly elevated.

Imaging   Ultrasonography is useful for demonstrating gallstones and occasionally a phlegmonous mass surrounding the gallbladder. Radionuclide scans (HIDA, DISIDA, etc.) may identify cystic duct obstruction.

Differential diagnosis   Includes acute pancreatitis, appendicitis, pyelonephritis, peptic ulcer disease, hepatitis, and hepatic abscess.

Treatment   Bowel rest, nasogastric suction, IV fluids and electrolytes, analgesia (meperidine or pentazocine), and antibiotics (ampicillin, cephalosporins, or aminoglycosides) are the mainstays of treatment. Diabetic, septic, or debilitated pts should receive combination antibiotic therapy. Surgery is definitive and should be performed as soon as feasible (within 24–48 h of admission). Delayed surgery reserved for pts with high risk of emergent surgery and where the diagnosis is in doubt.

Complications   Empyema, hydrops, gangrene, perforation, fistulization, gallstone ileus.

CHRONIC CHOLECYSTITIS

Etiology   Chronic cholecystitis usually caused by gallstones.

Symptoms and signs   Often non-specific; include dyspepsia, fatty food intolerance, and abdominal pain.

Laboratory   Tests are usually normal.

Imaging   Ultrasonography preferred; usually shows gallstones within a contracted gallbladder.

Differential diagnosis   Peptic ulcer disease, esophagitis, irritable bowel syndrome.

Treatment   Surgery is treatment of choice if symptomatic.

CHOLEDOCHOLITHIASIS/CHOLANGITIS

Symptoms and signs   Choledocholithiasis may present as an incidental finding, biliary colic, obstructive jaundice, cholangitis, or pancreatitis. Cholangitis usually presents as fever, RUQ pain, and jaundice (Charcot's triad).

Laboratory   Elevations in serum bilirubin, alkaline phosphatase, and aminotransferases.

Imaging   Ultrasonography may reveal dilated bile ducts but is not sensitive for detecting common duct stones. Endoscopic retrograde cholangiopancreatography or transhepatic cholangiography will confirm the diagnosis.

Differential diagnosis   Acute cholecystitis, renal colic, perforated viscus, pancreatitis.

Treatment   Cholecystectomy with choledocholithotomy and T-tube drainage of the bile ducts is the treatment of choice for most pts. If retained calculi are evident on a follow-up T-tube cholangiogram, percutaneous basket extraction should be performed. In elderly or poor surgical-risk pts, endoscopic papillotomy with stone extraction is possible. Cholangitis treated like acute cholecystitis; bowel rest, hydration, and analgesia are the mainstays; stones should be removed surgically or endoscopically.

Complications   Cholangitis, obstructive jaundice, and gallstone-induced pancreatitis.

PRIMARY SCLEROSING CHOLANGITIS (PSC)

PSC is a sclerosing inflammatory process involving the biliary tree.

Etiology   Males outnumber females and most patients are 25–45 years old. Associations: ulcerative colitis (60% of cases of PSC), AIDS, rarely Crohn's disease and retroperitoneal fibrosis.

Symptoms and signs Pruritus, RUQ pain, jaundice, fever, weight loss, and malaise. May progress to cirrhosis with portal hypertension.

Laboratory Evidence of cholestasis (elevated bilirubin and alkaline phosphatase) common.

Radiology/endoscopy Transhepatic or endoscopic cholangiograms reveal stenosis and dilation of the intra- and extrahepatic bile ducts.

Differential diagnosis Cholangiocarcinoma, Caroli's disease (cystic dilation of bile ducts), Fasciola hepatica, echinococcosis, and ascariasis.

Treatment No satisfactory therapy. Cholangitis should be treated as outlined above. Cholestyramine may control pruritus. Supplemental vitamin D and Ca may retard bone loss. Surgical relief of biliary obstruction may be appropriate but has a high complication rate. The efficacy of colectomy for pts with ulcerative colitis is uncertain. Liver transplantation should be considered in patients with endstage cirrhosis.

For a more detailed discussion, see Greenberger NJ, Isselbacher KJ: Diseases of the Gallbladder and Bile Ducts, Chap. 258, in HPIM-12, p. 1358

PANCREATIC CARCINOMA

Fifth most common cause of cancer death in the U.S., accounts for 10% of GI tumors; peak incidence in seventh decade; male:female = 1.5:1; somewhat more common in blacks.

Etiology and risk factors Cause unknown; three-fold increased incidence in smokers; proposed relationships to diabetes mellitus, chronic pancreatitis, cholelithiasis, ethanol, coffee, or caffeine ingestion not substantiated; may be associated with diet high in grilled meats.

Pathology 70% in head, 30% in body and tail; almost always ductal adenocarcinoma; 85% already locally invasive or metastatic at time of initial diagnosis.

Clinical features Weight loss, anorexia, abdominal pain, back pain, depression common; pain may be relieved by leaning forward; painless jaundice (with dark urine, clay-colored stools, occasional pruritus) frequent presenting feature of tumors in pancreatic head. Examination commonly reveals jaundice, hepatomegaly, abdominal mass, or abdominal tenderness, but may be unremarkable; enlarged, palpable gallbladder (Courvoisier's) in about 25% with tumors in pancreatic head. Complications include portal vein thrombosis (leading to splenomegaly, gastric varices, GI bleeding) and duodenal invasion (causing GI bleeding, obstruction); occasionally, hyperglycemia due to new-onset diabetes mellitus, and elevated amylase and lipase levels from associated pancreatitis.

Diagnosis Ultrasound useful screening test; shows abnormalities in about 75% of pts; most sensitive for lesions over 2 cm in head and body; CT most accurate noninvasive test (80% sensitivity; frequently able to detect lesions in tail); ERCP is most sensitive test for pts with carcinoma in pancreatic head (bile duct deformity); pancreatic duct abnormalities seen in >50% of pts regardless of location. Pathologic confirmation by aspiration of biliary secretions during cholangiography or percutaneous needle biopsy of mass under sonographic or CT guidance; serum tumor markers (e.g., carcinoembryonic antigen, CA19-9) insensitive, still too nonspecific for population screening; utility of MRI undefined.

Treatment Surgical resection by partial pancreatectomy or pancreaticoduodenectomy (Whipple procedure) potentially curative; however, tumor resectable in only 15% of pts and curable in less than 3%; preoperative screening for resectability includes chest films, CT scan, and celiac angiography; utility of laparoscopy unproven. Intraoperative irradiation may improve survival from unresectable local disease. Median survival with unresectable tumor 5 months. Palliative relief of biliary obstruction provided by surgical bypass or endoscopic or transhepatic stent placement; stenting preferable in elderly pts with multiple medical problems and those with advanced disease and short life expectancy; radiotherapy (RT) may reduce pain; 5-fluorouracil (5 FU) enhances palliative effect of RT: combination of RT and 5-FU may prolong survival of pts with both resectable and unresectable tumors; benefit of chemotherapy alone unproven.

OTHER PANCREATIC TUMORS

ISLET CELL TUMORS   Second most common class of pancreatic neoplasms; often suspected because of clinical effects of the hormones secreted. Table 110-1 lists the most common islet cell tumors. "Nonsecreting" islet cell tumors produce no discernible endocrine abnormalities. Most often located in body and tail of pancreas, can grow to 10 cm or more before causing pain, palpable mass, weight loss, or splenomegaly (from splenic vein compression).
   Treatment   Surgical resection, pharmacologic inhibition of hormonal effects; chemotherapy (streptozotocin, 5-FU) for unresectable tumor.
   CYSTADENOCARCINOMA   Rare, slow-growing, cystic neoplasms; symptoms caused by mass effect. Two pathologic

---

TABLE 110-1   Clinical features of most common islet cell tumors

Gastrinoma: Zollinger-Ellison syndrome; serum gastrin >200 ng/L, frequently increasing after IV secretion, basal acid output >4.2 μmol/s (>15 mmol/h); peptic ulcers, diarrhea; 25–50% associated with MEN I. *Treatment options*: H-2 blockers of omeprazole [goal: BAO <2.8 μmol/s (<10 mmol/h)], subtotal gastrectomy, tumor resection occasionally possible.

Insulinoma: Fasting hypoglycemia; rarely malignant. *Treatment*: partial pancreatectomy, diazoxide, octreotide, chemotherapy for metastases.

VIP-oma: Verner-Morrison syndrome, pancreatic cholera, or WDHA syndrome (*w*atery *d*iarrhea, *h*ypokalemia, *a*chlorhydria); mass effect. *Treatment*: tumor resection, octreotide.

Nonfunctioning: No detectable endocrine abnormality; abdominal or back pain, mass, effect from tumor that is frequently large, occasional splenic vein compression. *Treatment*: tumor resection, poor response to chemotherapy.

forms: mucinous (malignant) and serous (benign); differentiation by CT and chemical analysis of cyst fluid.

Treatment Surgical resection.

BENIGN PANCREATIC MASSES Pseudocysts complicating pancreatitis, true cysts (isolated or in association with polycystic kidney and liver disease; usually asymptomatic), and abscesses (which usually present with fever or signs of sepsis; see Chap. 105).

BILIARY TRACT CANCERS

Courvoisier's law - a non-palpable gall bladder in jaundiced pt. suggests malignant obstruction of

Less common than pancreatic carcinoma; usually present with obstructive jaundice, pruritus, RUQ pain, nausea, vomiting, anorexia, weight loss.

CHOLANGIOCARCINOMA Adenocarcinoma of bile duct epithelium; highest incidence in fifth to seventh decades; male/female = 1.5:1. Predisposing factors: choledochal (biliary) cysts, primary sclerosing cholangitis, ulcerative colitis, chronic *Clonorchis sinensis* infestation, but *not* gallstones. Usually presents with obstructive jaundice, occasionally with GI bleeding from hematobilia; usually unresectable at time of diagnosis.

Diagnosis Ultrasonography, CT scan, ERCP; ERCP appearance may mimic primary sclerosing cholangitis; CT-guided biopsy for tissue diagnosis.

Treatment Similar to carcinoma of head of pancreas; 5-year survival approximately 5%.

AMPULLARY CARCINOMA Tumor of papilla of Vater or ampullary involvement of duodenal adenocarcinoma. Usual presentation is obstructive jaundice and GI bleeding; stools occasionally silver (combination of acholic and melenic).

Diagnosis Ultrasonography, upper GI series, duodenal endoscopy and biopsy. Papillary tumors are rare but slow-growing and commonly resectable (Whipple procedure); duodenal carcinoma less often resectable.

GALLBLADDER CARCINOMA Rare complication of chronic cholelithiasis; male/female = 1:4. May be found incidentally at laparotomy (usually cholecystectomy) or autopsy (1% prevalence). Advanced tumor usually presents in seventh to eighth decades with RUQ pain, mass, jaundice, and weight loss; preoperative diagnosis occasionally made by ultrasound or CT.

Treatment Surgical resection or palliation; cure rate of advanced or symptomatic tumors less than 5%.

HEPATOCELLULAR CARCINOMA

Most common form of internal cancer worldwide; highest incidence in areas where hepatitis B virus infection endemic (esp. Southeast Asia, sub-Saharan Africa); far less common in U.S. (1–2% of malignant tumors). Peak incidence fifth and sixth decades in U.S., fourth and fifth in endemic areas; male/female = 2:1–4:1.

Etiology and risk factors Strong correlation with chronic hepatitis B infection suggests causative role of this virus in majority of cases. Neonatal infection carries highest risk of subsequent carcinoma. Hepatitis C virus infection also increases risk. Other risk factors: cirrhosis (esp. alcohol-induced), hemochromatosis, α_1-antitrypsin deficiency, tyrosinosis, ingested fungal metabolites (e.g., aflatoxin), use of anabolic steroids, administration of Thorotrast (radiologic contrast agent used in 1940s and 1950s).

Clinical features In cirrhotic pts, often presents as decompensation of underlying liver disease; weight loss, RUQ pain (occasionally acute due to tumor hemorrhage or rupture); jaundice rare except in terminal stages. Examination commonly reveals tender hepatomegaly; palpable liver mass, ascites (often blood-tinged) present in about 25% at time of diagnosis; occasional bruit or hepatic friction rub. Laboratory studies: elevated alkaline phosphatase and 5′-nucleotidase, often out of proportion to other liver tests; elevated serum α-fetoprotein [(AFP) often >400 µg/L (>400 ng/mL)] in 80% of pts worldwide (~50% in U.S.). Other causes of elevated AFP include cirrhosis, acute or chronic hepatitis, liver metastases (all with mild elevations), normal pregnancy, malignant teratomas.

Diagnosis CT, MRI most sensitive for detection of liver mass; radionuclide scanning (e.g., gallium, ethiotol) may suggest primary hepatocellular carcinoma; angiography often reveals typical vascularity of lesions and may detect small tumors. Pathologic confirmation by radiologically guided percutaneous liver biopsy, laparoscopy, or laparotomy.

Treatment Curative resection possible in fewer than 5% of pts; liver transplantation may benefit selected pts with small tumors confined to the liver; preoperative MRI angiography to assess resectability; radiation therapy or selective arterial embolization for palliation of pain only; systemic and intraarterial chemotherapy of no proven benefit. Prevention may ultimately be achieved by effective global immunization against hepatitis B infection.

OTHER LIVER TUMORS

Most common liver tumors in U.S. population are metastases from other primary cancers; liver is second most common site of metastases after lymph nodes; most common primaries are tumors of GI tract (colon, pancreas, stomach), lung, breast, lymphoma, and melanoma.

Clinical features   Metastatic liver tumors usually asymptomatic or associated with nonspecific symptoms (weight loss, fever, weakness, etc.); abdominal pain, hepatomegaly less common; ascites, jaundice, liver dysfunction rare. Laboratory findings: elevated alkaline phosphatase and 5'-nucleotidase, anemia, hypoalbuminemia.

Diagnosis   As for hepatocellular carcinoma; CT-guided biopsy most sensitive means of tissue diagnosis short of laparotomy; MRI may detect lesions not visualized on CT.

Treatment   On rare occasions, resection of isolated hepatic metastases and primary tumor can be curative; usual therapy is palliative, either by surgery, radiation, or chemotherapy. Direct hepatic artery floxuridine administration for hepatic metastases of primary colon carcinoma or carcinoma of unknown primary may improve survival slightly; overall, prognosis poor unless primary tumor sensitive to chemotherapy.

BENIGN LIVER TUMORS

1. Hemangiomas: Most common benign hepatic tumors; usually single and small, but may present as large mass. Diagnosis by MRI, CT with intravenous contrast, angiography. *Treatment:* surgical resection for symptomatic tumors only.

2. Adenomas: Increased incidence in women taking oral contraceptives; lesions often regress after stopping these agents; biopsy required to exclude malignancy. Major complications include bleeding, rupture. *Treatment:* curative therapy by surgical excision.

3. Focal nodular hyperplasia: Usually asymptomatic, incidental finding at laparotomy; not caused by oral contraceptives, but may enlarge and become hypervascular under influence of estrogen; rarely bleed or rupture. Surgical resection required only to exclude adenoma or carcinoma or to treat hemorrhagic complications.

For a more detailed discussion, see Isselbacher KJ, Wands JR: Neoplasms of the Liver, Chap. 255, p. 1350; Greenberger NJ, Isselbacher KJ: Diseases of the Gallbladder and Bile Ducts, Chap. 258, p. 1358; Mayer RJ: Pancreatic Cancer, Chap. 261, p. 1383; Kaplan LM: Endocrine Tumors of the Gastrointestinal Tract and Pancreas, Chap. 262, p. 1388, in HPIM-12

VIRAL HEPATITIS

Clinically characterized by malaise, nausea, vomiting, diarrhea, and low-grade fever followed by dark urine, jaundice, and tender hepatomegaly; may be subclinical and detected on basis of elevated aspartate and alanine aminotransferase (AST and ALT) levels. Hepatitis B may be associated with immune complex phenomena, including arthritis, glomerulonephritis, and polyarteritis nodosa. Hepatitis-like illnesses may be caused not only by hepatotropic viruses (A, B, C, D, E), but also by other viruses (Epstein-Barr, cytomegalovirus, coxsackievirus, etc.), alcohol, drugs, hypotension and ischemia, and biliary tract disease.

HEPATITIS A (HAV)   27-nm enterovirus (picornavirus) with single-stranded RNA genome. Course: See Fig. 111-1.

Outcome   Recovery within 6–12 months, occasionally after one or two apparent clinical and serologic relapses; in some cases pronounced cholestasis suggesting biliary obstruction may occur; rare fatalities (fulminant hepatitis), no chronic carrier state.

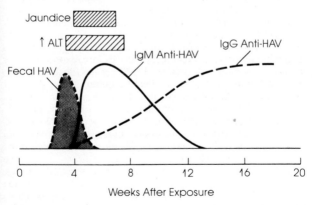

FIGURE 111-1 Scheme of typical clinical and laboratory features of HAV. (Reproduced from Dienstag JL, Wands JR, Isselbacher KJ, HPIM-12, p. 1323.)

Diagnosis IgM anti-HAV in acute or early convalescent serum sample.

Epidemiology Fecal-oral transmission; endemic in underdeveloped countries; food-borne and waterborne epidemics; outbreaks in day-care centers, residential institutions.

Prevention After exposure—immune globulin 0.02 mL/kg IM within 2 weeks to household and institutional contacts (not casual contacts at work). Before exposure (e.g., travelers to endemic areas)—immune globulin, 0.02 mL/kg IM for travel <3 months, 0.06 mL/kg IM q 4–6 months for longer travel or residence. Vaccines under development.

HEPATITIS B (HBV) 42-nm hepadnavirus with outer surface coat (HBsAg), inner nucleocapsid core (HBcAg), DNA polymerase, and partially double-stranded DNA genome of 3200 nucleotides. Circulating form of HBcAg is HBeAg, a marker of viral replication and infectivity. Course: see Fig. 111-2.

Outcome Recovery 90%, fulminant hepatitis (<1%), chronic hepatitis or carrier state (up to 10%), cirrhosis and hepatocellular carcinoma (especially following chronic infection beginning in infancy or early childhood) (Chap. 113).

Diagnosis HBsAg in serum (acute or chronic infection); IgM anti-HBc (early anti-HBc indicative of acute or recent infection).

Epidemiology Percutaneous (needlestick), sexual, or perinatal transmission. Endemic in sub-Saharan Africa and Southeast Asia, where up to 20% of population acquire infection, usually early in life.

Prevention After exposure—hepatitis B immune globulin (HBIG) 0.06 mL/kg IM immediately after needlestick, within 14 days of sexual exposure, or at birth (HBsAg+ mother) in combination with vaccine series. Before exposure—recombinant hepatitis B vaccine 10–20 μg IM (dose depends on formulation); half dose to young children, 40-μg dose to immunocompromised adults; at 0, 1, and 6 months; deltoid, not gluteal injection. Recommended for high-risk groups (e.g., health workers, gay men, IV drug users, hemodialysis patients, hemophiliacs, household and sexual contacts of HBsAg carriers, all neonates in endemic areas, or high-risk neonates in lower-risk areas).

HEPATITIS C (HCV) Formerly transfusion-associated non-A, non-B hepatitis. Caused by flavi-like virus with RNA genome of over 9000 nucleotides (similar to yellow fever virus, dengue virus). Incubation period 7–8 weeks. Course often marked by fluctuating elevations of serum aminotransferase levels; >50% likelihood of chronicity, leading to cirrhosis in 20%.

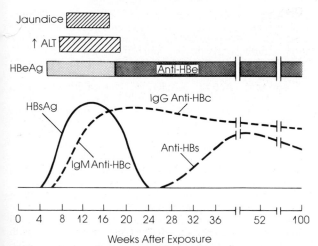

Jaundice

↑ ALT

HBeAg ▭ Anti-HBe

IgG Anti-HBc

HBsAg

IgM Anti-HBc

Anti-HBs

| | | | | | | | | | | |
|0|4|8|12|16|20|24|28|32|36|52|100|

Weeks After Exposure

FIGURE 111-2 Scheme of typical clinical and laboratory features of HBV. (Reproduced from Dienstag JL, Wands JR, Isselbacher KJ, HPIM-12, p. 1324.)

Diagnosis Anti-HCV in serum; often appears after acute illness but generally present by 6 months after exposure.

Epidemiology Percutaneous transmission; non-A, non-B hepatitis accounts for over 90% of transfusion-associated hepatitis cases, of which at least 85% are due to HCV. Little evidence for widespread sexual or perinatal transmission.

Prevention Exclusion of paid blood donors, testing of donated blood for anti-HCV and for surrogate markers of hepatitis (raised ALT levels, anti-HBc).

HEPATITIS D (HDV, DELTA AGENT) Defective 37-nm RNA virus that requires HBV for its replication; either *coinfects* with HBV or *superinfects* a chronic HBV carrier. Enhances severity of HBV infection (acceleration of chronic hepatitis to cirrhosis, occasionally fulminant acute hepatitis).

Diagnosis Anti-HD in serum (acute hepatitis D—often in low titer, transient; chronic hepatitis D—in higher titer, sustained).

Epidemiology Endemic among HBV carriers in Mediterranean basin, areas of South America, etc. Otherwise spread percutaneously among HBsAg+ IV drug users or by transfusion in hemophiliacs and to a lesser extent among HBsAg+ gay men.

Prevention Hepatitis B vaccine (noncarriers only).

HEPATITIS E (HEV)   Formerly enterically transmitted non-A, non-B hepatitis. Caused by 29–32-nm agent thought to be a calicivirus. Responsible for waterborne epidemics of hepatitis in India, parts of Asia and Africa, and Mexico. Self-limited illness with high (10–20%) mortality rate in pregnant women.

Treatment   Activity as tolerated, high-calorie diet (often tolerated best in morning), IV hydration for severe vomiting, cholestyramine up to 4 g PO qid for severe pruritus, avoiding hepatically metabolized drugs; no role for glucocorticoids.

TOXIC AND DRUG-INDUCED HEPATITIS

DOSE-DEPENDENT (DIRECT HEPATOTOXINS)   Onset within 48 h, predictable, necrosis around terminal hepatic venule—e.g., carbon tetrachloride, benzene derivatives, mushroom poisoning, acetaminophen.

IDIOSYNCRATIC   Variable dose and time of onset, small number of exposed persons affected, may be associated with fever, rash, arthralgias, eosinophilia. In some cases mechanism may involve toxic metabolite determined on genetic basis—e.g., isoniazid, halothane, phenytoin, methyldopa.

TREATMENT   Supportive as for viral hepatitis; withdraw suspected agent.

ACUTE HEPATIC FAILURE

Massive hepatic necrosis with impaired consciousness occurring within 8 weeks of the onset of illness.

Causes   Infections (viral, including HAV, HBV, HCV, HDV, bacterial, rickettsial, parasitic), drugs and toxins, ischemia (shock), Budd-Chiari syndrome, idiopathic chronic active hepatitis, acute Wilson's disease, microvesicular fat syndromes (Reye's syndrome, acute fatty liver of pregnancy).

Clinical manifestations   Neuropsychiatric changes—delirium, personality change, stupor, coma, decerebrate rigidity (due to cerebral edema), deep jaundice, coagulopathy, bleeding, renal failure, hypoglycemia, acute pancreatitis, cardiorespiratory failure.

Adverse prognostic indicators   Older age, certain causes (e.g., halothane, non-A, non-B hepatitis), coma (survival <20%), rapid reduction in liver size, respiratory failure, marked prolongation of PT, factor V level <20%.

Treatment   Endotracheal intubation often required. Monitor serum glucose—IV D10 or D20 as necessary. Prevent gastrointestinal bleeding with H-2 receptor antagonists and antacids (maintain gastric pH $\geq$ 3.5). Value of intracranial pressure monitoring and dexamethasone for cerebral edema unclear; IV mannitol may be beneficial. Liver transplantation should be considered in pts with grade III–IV encephalopathy and other adverse prognostic indicators.

For a more detailed discussion, see Dienstag JL, Wands JR, Isselbacher KJ: Acute Hepatitis, Chap. 252, in HPIM-12, p 1322

---

112 CHRONIC HEPATITIS

A group of disorders characterized by a chronic inflammatory reaction in the liver for at least 6 months.

CLASSIFICATION (Table 112-1)

Etiology   Hepatitis B virus (HBV), hepatitis C virus (HCV), hepatitis D virus (HDV, delta agent), drugs (methyldopa, nitrofurantoin, isoniazid), Wilson's disease, alpha$_1$ antitrypsin deficiency, idiopathic (autoimmune, "lupoid").

Presentation   Wide clinical spectrum ranging from asymptomatic serum aminotransferase elevations to acute, even fulminant, hepatitis-like illness. Common symptoms include fatigue, malaise, anorexia, low-grade fever; jaundice is frequent in severe disease. Some pts may present with complications of cirrhosis; ascites, variceal bleeding, encephalopathy, coagulopathy, hypersplenism. In chronic hepatitis B or idiopathic CAH, extrahepatic features may predominate.

TABLE 112-1

Histology	Chronic persistent (CPH)	Chronic active (CAH)
Portal zone infiltrate of lymphocytes and plasma cells	+ +	+ + +
Piecemeal necrosis (extension of portal infiltrate into hepatic lobule with erosion of limiting plate of hepatocytes surrounding portal zones)	–	+ + +
Bridging necrosis (from portal zone to portal zone or portal zone to central vein)	–	±
Multilobular necrosis (extensive inflammation and hepatocyte necrosis)	–	±
Cirrhosis	–	±
Symptoms	Mild or absent	Common
Prognosis	Good	Depends on severity, cause, treatment

CHRONIC HEPATITIS B

Follows up to 10% of cases of acute hepatitis B. Spectrum of severity: asymptomatic antigenemia, CPH, and CAH; *early phase* often associated with continued symptoms of hepatitis, elevated aminotransferase levels, presence in serum of HBeAg and HBV DNA, and presence in liver of replicative form of HBV; *later phase* in some patients may be associated with clinical and biochemical improvement, disappearance of HBeAg and HBV DNA and appearance of anti-HBe in serum, and integration of HBV DNA into host hepatocyte genome. In Mediterranean area, a frequent variant is characterized by a severe and rapidly progressive course and HBV DNA with anti-HBe in serum, due to a mutation in the pre-C region of the HBV genome that prevents HBeAg synthesis. May lead to cirrhosis (particularly in patients with HDV superinfection or the pre-C mutation) and hepatocellular carcinoma (particularly when chronic infection is acquired early in life).

Extrahepatic manifestations (immune-complex–mediated)   Rash, urticaria, arthritis, polyarteritis, polyneuropathy, glomerulonephritis, cryoglobulinemia.

Treatment   Most promising is α-interferon 5 million units qd × 4 months for serum HBeAg/HBV-DNA-positive pts with symptoms, aminotransferase levels over 3 times normal, and biopsy evidence of chronic active hepatitis. Results in HBeAg anti-HBe seroconversion with clinical, biochemical, and histologic improvement in up to 40% of cases. Common side effects—febrile reactions, bone marrow depression, autoimmune thyroid disease, CNS symptoms, anorexia, sleep disturbance. In pts with lower aminotransferase levels, efficacy of interferon may be enhanced by a priming prednisone course, 60 mg PO qd, tapering over 6 weeks.

CHRONIC HEPATITIS C

Follows at least 50% of cases of transfusion-associated and sporadic hepatitis C. Clinically mild, often waxing and waning aminotransferase elevations; mild CAH on liver biopsy. Diagnosis confirmed by detecting anti-HCV in serum. May lead to cirrhosis in 20% of cases. Therapy with α-interferon 2–3 million units 3 times per week for 6 months shows promise for pts with symptoms, aminotransferase elevations, and biopsy evidence of chronic hepatitis; 50% achieve clinical and biochemical remission or improvement after 6 months. However, 50% of pts relapse 6 months after end of treatment.

IDIOPATHIC CAH

Clinical manifestations   80% women, third to fifth decades. Abrupt onset (acute hepatitis) in a third. Insidious onset in two-thirds: progressive jaundice, anorexia, hepatomegaly, abdominal pain, epistaxis, fever, fatigue, amenorrhea. Leads to cirrhosis; >50% 5-year mortality if untreated.

Extrahepatic manifestations   Rash, arthralgias, keratoconjunctivitis sicca, thyroiditis, hemolytic anemia, nephritis.

Serologic abnormalities   Hypergammaglobulinemia, smooth-muscle antibody (40–80%), ANA (20–50%), LE prep (10–20%), antimitochondrial antibody (10–20%).

Treatment   Indicated for symptomatic disease with biopsy evidence of severe CAH (bridging necrosis) and marked aminotransferase elevations (5–10-fold). Prednisone or prednisolone 30 mg PO qd tapered to 10–15 mg qd over several weeks; often azathioprine 50 mg PO qd is also administered to permit lower glucocorticoid doses and avoid steroid side effects. Monitor LFTs monthly. Symptoms may improve rapidly, but biochemical improvement may take weeks or months and subsequent histologic improvement (to lesion of CPH or normal biopsy) up to 18–24 months. Withdrawal of glucocorticoids can be attempted following clinical, biochemical, and histologic remission; relapse occurs in 50–90% of cases (re-treat).

For a more detailed discussion, see Wands JR, Isselbacher KJ: Chronic Hepatitis, Chap. 253, in HPIM-12, p. 1337

113 CIRRHOSIS AND ALCOHOLIC LIVER DISEASE

Chronic disease of the liver characterized by fibrosis, disorganization of the lobular and vascular architecture, and regenerating nodules of hepatocytes.

CAUSES Alcohol, viral hepatitis [B, C, D (delta); see Chap. 111], primary or secondary biliary cirrhosis, hemochromatosis (Chap. 153), Wilson's disease (Chap. 153), alpha$_1$ antitrypsin deficiency, chronic active hepatitis (Chap. 111), Budd-Chiari syndrome, chronic CHF (cardiac cirrhosis), drugs and toxins, schistosomiasis, cryptogenic.

CLINICAL MANIFESTATIONS May be absent.

Symptoms Anorexia, nausea, vomiting, diarrhea, fatigue, weakness, fever, jaundice, amenorrhea, impotence, infertility.

Signs Spider telangiectases, palmar erythema, parotid and lacrimal gland enlargement, nail changes (Muehrcke lines, Terry's nails), clubbing, Dupuytren's contracture, gynecomastia, testicular atrophy, hepatosplenomegaly, ascites, gastrointestinal bleeding (e.g., varices), hepatic encephalopathy.

Laboratory findings Anemia (microcytic due to blood loss, macrocytic due to folate deficiency), pancytopenia (hypersplenism), prolonged PT, rarely DIC; hyponatremia, hypokalemic alkalosis, glucose disturbances, hypoalbuminemia.

Other associations Gastritis; duodenal ulcer; gallstones. Altered drug metabolism because of decreased drug clearance, metabolism (e.g, by cytochrome P_{450}), and elimination; hypoalbuminemia; and portosystemic shunting.

DIAGNOSTIC STUDIES Choices depend on clinical setting. Serum: HBsAg, anti-HBc, anti-HBs, anti-HCV, anti-HD, Fe, total iron binding capacity, ferritin, antimitochondrial antibody (AMA), smooth-muscle antibodies (SMA), ANA, ceruloplasmin, alpha$_1$ antitrypsin (and pi typing); abdominal ultrasound with doppler study, liver scan, portal venography, and wedged hepatic vein pressure measurement. Definitive diagnosis often depends on liver biopsy (percutaneous or open); may be precluded by coagulopathy.

ALCOHOLIC LIVER DISEASE

Three forms: fatty liver, alcoholic hepatitis, cirrhosis; may coexist. History of excessive alcohol use often denied. Severe forms (hepatitis, cirrhosis) associated with ingestion of 80–160 g/d for >5–10 years. Malnutrition may contribute to development of cirrhosis.

FATTY LIVER   May follow even brief periods of ethanol use. Often presents as asymptomatic hepatomegaly and mild elevations in biochemical liver tests. Reverses on withdrawal of ethanol; does not lead to cirrhosis.

ALCOHOLIC HEPATITIS   Clinical presentation ranges from asymptomatic to severe liver failure with jaundice, ascites, GI bleeding, and encephalopathy. Typically anorexia, nausea, vomiting, fever, jaundice, tender hepatomegaly. Occasional cholestatic picture mimicking biliary obstruction. Aspartate aminotransferase (AST) usually less than 300 U and >twofold higher than alanine aminotransferase (ALT). Bilirubin may be >170 μmol/L (>10 mg/dL). WBC may be as high as 20,000/μL. Diagnosis defined by liver biopsy findings: hepatocyte swelling, alcoholic hyaline (Mallory bodies), infiltration of PMNs, necrosis of hepatocytes, pericentral venular fibrosis.

Other metabolic consequences of alcoholism   (increased NADH/NAD ratio)   Lacticacidemia, ketoacidosis, hyperuricemia, hypoglycemia.; also hypomagnesemia, hypophosphatemia.

Adverse prognostic factors   *Short-term:* PT >5 s above control despite vitamin K, bilirubin >170 μmol/L (>10 mg/dL), encephalopathy, hypoalbuminemia, azotemia. *Long-term:* severe hepatic necrosis and fibrosis, portal hypertension, continued alcohol consumption.

Treatment   Abstinence is essential; 8500–12,500 kJ (2000–3000 kcal) diet with 1 g/kg protein (less if encephalopathy). Daily multivitamin, thiamine 100 mg, folic acid 1 mg. Correct potassium, magnesium, and phosphate deficiencies. Transfusions of packed red cells, plasma as necessary. Monitor glucose (hypoglycemia in severe liver disease). Prednisone 40 mg or prednisolone 32 mg PO qd × 1 month may be beneficial in severe alcoholic hepatitis with encephalopathy. Colchicine 0.6 mg PO bid may slow progression of alcoholic liver disease.

PRIMARY BILIARY CIRRHOSIS

Progressive nonsuppurative destructive intrahepatic cholangitis. Affects middle-aged women. Presents as asymptomatic elevation in alkaline phosphatase (better prognosis) or with pruritus, progressive jaundice, consequences of impaired bile excretion, and ultimately cirrhosis and liver failure.

CLINICAL MANIFESTATIONS   Pruritus, jaundice, xanthelasma, xanthomata, osteoporosis, steatorrhea, skin pigmentation, hepatosplenomegaly, portal hypertension, elevations in serum alkaline phosphatase, bilirubin, cholesterol, and IgM levels.

ASSOCIATED DISEASES Sjögren's syndrome, collagen-vascular diseases, thyroiditis, glomerulonephritis, pernicious anemia, renal tubular acidosis.

DIAGNOSIS AMA in >90–95% (directed against the E_2 component of pyruvate dehydrogenase and other mitochondrial enzymes). Liver biopsy: stage 1—destruction of interlobular bile ducts, granulomas; stage 2—ductular proliferation; stage 3—fibrosis; stage 4—cirrhosis.

TREATMENT Cholestyramine 4 g PO with meals for pruritus. Vitamin K 10 mg IM qd × 3 (then once a month) for elevated PT due to intestinal bile salt deficiency. Vitamin D 100,000 U IM q 4 weeks plus oral calcium 1 g qd for osteoporosis (often unresponsive). Vitamin A 25,000–50,000 U PO qd or 100,000 U IM q 4 weeks and zinc 220 mg PO qd may help night blindness. Vitamin E 10 mg IM or PO qd. Substituting dietary fat with medium-chain triglycerides (MCTs) may reduce steatorrhea. Experimental: azathioprine, colchicine, chlorambucil, cyclosporine, ursodeoxycholic acid, methotrexate.

LIVER TRANSPLANTATION

Consider for chronic, irreversible, progressive liver disease or fulminant hepatic failure when no alternative therapy is available. (Also indicated to correct certain congenital enzyme deficiencies and inborn errors of metabolism.)

CONTRAINDICATIONS Absolute: Extrahepatobiliary sepsis or malignancy, cardiopulmonary disease, portal and superior mesenteric vein thrombosis, AIDS.

Relative: Age > 60, HBsAg and HIV, extensive previous abdominal surgery, portal vein thrombosis, active alcoholism or drug abuse, lack of pt understanding.

INDICATIONS Guidelines: expected death in 1 year; preferably in anticipation of major complication (variceal bleeding, irreversible encephalopathy, severe malnutrition and incapacitating weakness, hepatorenal syndrome); refractory ascites, progressive bone disease, recurrent bacterial cholangitis, intractable coagulopathy; bilirubin > 170–340 μmol/L (> 10–20 mg/dL), albumin < 20 g/L (< 2 g/dL), worsening coagulopathy; poor quality of life. In fulminant hepatic failure consider for grade III–IV coma.

SELECTION OF DONOR Matched for ABO blood group compatibility and liver size (reduced-size grafts may be used, esp. in children).

IMMUNOSUPPRESSION   Various combinations of cyclosporine, glucocorticoids, azathioprine, OKT3 (monoclonal antithymocyte globulin).

MEDICAL COMPLICATIONS AFTER TRANSPLANTATION   Liver graft dysfunction (rejection, ischemia, hepatic artery thrombosis, biliary obstruction or leak, recurrent viral infection); infections (bacterial, viral, fungal, opportunistic); renal dysfunction; neuropsychiatric disorders.

SUCCESS RATE   60–80% long-term survival.

For a more detailed discussion, see Podolsky DK, Isselbacher KJ: Cirrhosis of the Liver, Chap. 254, p. 1340; Schmid R: Liver Transplantation, Chap. 257, p. 1355, in HPIM-12

114 PORTAL HYPERTENSION

Any increase in portal vein pressure due to anatomic or functional obstruction to blood flow in the portal venous system.

Normal portal vein pressure is 7–10 mmHg. Indicators of portal hypertension are:

- Intraoperative portal vein pressure · · · · >30 cm saline
- Intrasplenic pressure · · · · >17 mmHg
- Wedged hepatic vein pressure · · · · >4 mmHg above IVC pressure

CLASSIFICATION (Table 114-1)

CONSEQUENCES (1) Increased collateral circulation between high-pressure portal venous system and low-pressure systemic venous system: lower esophagus/upper stomach (varices), rectum (hemorrhoids), anterior abdominal wall (caput Medusae; flow away from umbilicus), parietal peritoneum, splenorenal; (2) increased lymphatic flow; (3) increased plasma volume; (4) ascites (Chap. 19); (5) splenomegaly, possible hypersplenism; (6) portosystemic shunting (including hepatic encephalopathy).

ESOPHAGOGASTRIC VARICES

Bleeding is major life-threatening complication; risk correlates with variceal size above minimal portal venous pressure

TABLE 114-1

Site of obstruction	Pressure		Examples
	Portal	Corrected wedged hepatic vein*	
Presinusoidal	↑	Normal	Splenic AV fistula, portal or splenic vein thrombosis, schistosomiasis
Sinusoidal	↑	↑	Cirrhosis, hepatitis
Postsinusoidal	↑	↑ (May be unmeasurable due to hepatic vein occlusion)	Budd-Chiari syndrome, veno-occlusive disease

* Wedged hepatic vein minus inferior vena cava pressure.

>12 mmHg and presence on varices of red wales. Mortality correlates with severity of underlying liver disease (hepatic reserve).

DIAGNOSIS *Upper GI series:* tortuous, beaded filling defects in lower esophagus. *Esophagogastroscopy:* procedure of choice for acute bleeding. *Celiac and mesenteric arteriography:* when massive bleeding precludes endoscopy and to evaluate portal vein patency (portal vein also may be studied by ultrasound with dopplers).

TREATMENT See Chapter 17 for general measures to treat GI bleeding.

Control of acute bleeding (1) Intravenous vasopressin up to 0.4–0.9 U/min until bleeding is controlled for 12–24 h (50–60% success rate, but no effect on mortality), then discontinue or taper (0.1 U/min q 6–12 h); add nitroglycerin up to 0.6 mg SL q 30 min, 40–400 µg/min IV, or by transdermal patch 10 mg/24 h to prevent coronary and renal vasoconstriction. Maintain systolic BP >90 mmHg. Somatostatin 50–250 µg bolus + 250 µg/h IV infusion as effective as vasopressin with no serious complications. (2) Blakemore-Sengstaken balloon tamponade: can be inflated for up to 24–48 h; complications—obstruction of pharynx, asphyxiation, esophageal ulceration. (3) Endoscopic sclerotherapy—may be procedure of choice (not suitable for gastric varices); variety of techniques, sclerosants; >90% success rate; complications—esophageal ulceration and stricture, fever, chest pain, mediastinitis, pleural effusions, aspiration.

Prevention of recurrent bleeding (1) Repeated endoscopic sclerotherapy (e.g., q 2–4 weeks) until obliteration. Long-term efficacy unclear; decreases but does not eliminate recurrent bleeding; effect on overall survival uncertain but compares favorably to shunt surgery. (2) Propranolol—portal venous antihypertensive; most effective in well-compensated cirrhotics; generally given bid in dose that reduces heart rate by 25%. May be effective in preventing bleeding in pts with large "high-risk" varices that have not previously bled. (3) Splenectomy (for splenic vein thrombosis). (4) Portosystemic shunt surgery: portacaval (total decompression) or distal splenorenal (Warren) (selective; contraindicated in ascites; ? lower incidence of hepatic encephalopathy). Alternative procedure—devascularization of lower esophagus and upper stomach (Sugiura). Surgery is now generally reserved for pts who fail nonsurgical therapy (e.g., sclerotherapy). Liver transplantation should be considered in appropriate candidates. (A prior distal splenorenal shunt does not preclude subsequent liver transplantation.)

PROGNOSIS (AND SURGICAL RISK) Correlated with classification of Child and Turcotte; see Table 114-2.

TABLE 114-2

	Class		
	A	B	C
Serum bilirubin, μmol/L (mg/dL)	<34 (<2)	34–51 (2–3)	>51 (>3)
Serum albumin, g/L (g/dL)	>35 (>3.5)	30–35 (3.0–3.5)	<30 (<3.0)
Ascites	None	Easily controlled	Poorly controlled
Encephalopathy	None	Mild	Advanced
Nutrition	Excellent	Good	Poor
Prognosis	Good	Fair	Poor

HEPATIC ENCEPHALOPATHY

A state of disordered CNS function associated with severe acute or chronic liver disease; may be acute and reversible or chronic and progressive.

CLINICAL FEATURES Mild—day-night reversal of sleep cycle, somnolence, confusion, personality change, asterixis (flapping tremor). More severe—stupor, coma, dementia, occasionally extrapyramidal signs. Fetor hepaticus (odor of breath and urine caused by mercaptans). Characteristic EEG abnormalities.

PATHOPHYSIOLOGY Failure of liver to detoxify agents noxious to CNS [ammonia, mercaptans, fatty acids, γ-aminobutyric acid (GABA)] due to decreased hepatic function and portosystemic shunting. False neurotransmitters also may enter CNS due to increased aromatic and decreased branched-chain amino acid levels in blood. Role of endogenous benzodiazepine agonist uncertain. Blood ammonia most readily measured marker, although may not always correlate with clinical status.

PRECIPITANTS GI bleeding (100 mL = 14–20 g protein), azotemia, constipation, high-protein meal, hypokalemic alkalosis, CNS depressant drugs (e.g., benzodiazepines), hypoxia, hypercarbia, sepsis.

TREATMENT Remove precipitants; reduce blood ammonia by decreasing protein intake (20–30 g/day, vegetable sources); enemas/cathartics to clear gut. Lactulose (converts NH_3 to unabsorbed NH_4^+, produces diarrhea, alters bowel flora) 30–50 mL PO qh until diarrhea, then 15–30 mL tid-qid prn 2–3 loose stools/day. In coma, give as enema (300 mL in 700 mL H_2O). In refractory cases, add neomycin 1 g PO bid. *Unproven*: IV branched-chain amino acids, levodopa, bromocriptine, keto-analogues of essential amino acids. *Experimental*: flumazenil, a GABA-benzodiazepine receptor antagonist; lactilol, a second-generation disaccharide that is less sweet than lactulose and can be dispensed as a powder.

For a more detailed discussion, see Podolsky DK, Isselbacher KJ: Cirrhosis of the Liver, Chap. 254, in HPIM-12, p. 1340

115 DISEASES OF IMMEDIATE TYPE HYPERSENSITIVITY

DEFINITION   Diseases of immediate type hypersensitivity result from IgE-dependent release of mediators from sensitized basophils and mast cells on contact with appropriate antigen (allergen). Associated disorders include anaphylaxis, allergic rhinitis, urticaria, asthma, and eczematous (atopic) dermatitis. *Atopic allergy* implies a familial tendency to the development of these disorders singly or in combination.

PATHOPHYSIOLOGY   IgE binds to surface of mast cells and basophils through a high-affinity receptor. Cross-linking of this IgE by antigen causes cellular activation with the subsequent release of preformed and newly synthesized mediators. These include histamine, prostaglandins, leukotrienes (including leukotrienes C_4, D_4, and E_4, collectively known as slow-reacting substance of anaphylaxis, SRS-A), acid hydrolases, neutral proteases, and proteoglycans. These mediators have been implicated in many pathophysiologic events associated with immediate-type hypersensitivity, such as vasodilatation, increased vasopermeability, smooth-muscle contraction, and chemotactic attraction of neutrophils and other inflammatory cells. The clinical manifestations of each allergic reaction depend largely on the anatomic site(s) and time course of this mediator release.

URTICARIA AND ANGIOEDEMA

DEFINITION   May occur together or separately. *Urticaria* involves superficial dermis and presents as circumscribed wheals with raised serpiginous borders and blanched centers; wheals may coalesce. *Angioedema* involves deeper layers of skin and may include subcutaneous tissue. These disorders may be classified as (1) IgE-dependent, including atopic, secondary to specific allergens, and physical stimuli, especially cold, (2) complement-mediated (including hereditary angioedema and hives related to serum sickness or vasculitis), (3) nonimmunologic due to direct mast cell-releasing agents or drugs that influence mediator release, and (4) idiopathic.

PATHOPHYSIOLOGY Characterized by massive edema formation in the dermis (and subcutaneous tissue in angioedema). Presumably the edema is due to increased vasopermeability caused by mediator release from mast cells or other cell populations.

DIAGNOSIS
• *History:* special attention to possible offending exposures and/or ingestion. • Skin testing to food and/or inhalant antigens. • Physical provocation, e.g., challenge with vibratory or cold stimuli. • *Laboratory examination:* complement levels, ESR; Cl-esterase inhibitor levels if history suggests hereditary angioedema; cryoglobulins, hepatitis B antigen and antibody studies; autoantibody screen. • Skin biopsy may be necessary.

DIFFERENTIAL DIAGNOSIS Atopic dermatitis, cutaneous mastocytosis (urticaria pigmentosa), systemic mastocytosis.

PREVENTION AND TREATMENT

• Identification and avoidance of offending agent(s), if possible.
• H1 and H2 antihistamines may be helpful; e.g., ranitidine 150 mg PO bid; diphenhydramine 25–50 mg PO qid; hydroxyzine 25–50 mg PO qid.
• Cyproheptadine 4 mg PO tid may be helpful.
• Sympathomimetic agents may occasionally be useful.

ALLERGIC RHINITIS

DEFINITION An inflammatory condition of the nose characterized by sneezing, rhinorrhea, and obstruction of nasal passages; may be associated with conjunctival and pharyngeal itching, lacrimation, and sinusitis. *Seasonal* allergic rhinitis is commonly caused by exposure to pollens, especially from grasses, trees, weeds, and molds. *Perennial* allergic rhinitis is frequently due to contact with house dust (containing dust mite antigens) and animal danders.

PATHOPHYSIOLOGY Impingement of pollens and other allergens on nasal mucosa of sensitized individual results in IgE-dependent triggering of mast cells with subsequent release of mediators that cause development of mucosal hyperemia, swelling, and fluid transudation. Inflammation of nasal mucosal surface probably allows penetration of allergens deeper into tissue, where they contact perivenular mast cells. Obstruction of sinus ostia may result in development of secondary sinusitis, with or without bacterial infection.

DIAGNOSIS

- Accurate *history* of symptoms correlated with time of pollination of plants in a given locale; special attention must be paid to other potentially sensitizing antigens such as pet danders.
- *Physical examination:* nasal mucosa may be boggy or erythematous; nasal polyps may be present; sinuses may demonstrate decreased transillumination; conjunctivae may be inflamed or edematous; manifestations of other allergic conditions (e.g., asthma, eczema) may be present.
- Skin tests to inhalant and/or food antigens.
- Nasal smear may reveal large numbers of eosinophils; presence of neutrophils may suggest infection.
- Total and specific serum IgE may be elevated.

DIFFERENTIAL DIAGNOSIS Vasomotor rhinitis, URI, irritant exposure, pregnancy with nasal mucosal edema, rhinitis medicamentosa, nonallergic rhinitis with eosinophilia.

PREVENTION AND THERAPY

- Identification and avoidance of offending antigen(s).
- Antihistamines, e.g., sustained-release chlorpheniramine 12 mg PO bid or terfenadine 60 mg PO bid; utility of these agents may be limited by side effects, chiefly drowsiness.
- Oral sympathomimetics, e.g., pseudoephedrine 30–60 mg PO qid; may aggravate hypertension; combination antihistamine/decongestant preparations may balance side effects and provide improved pt convenience.
- Topical vasoconstrictors—should be used sparingly due to rebound congestion and chronic rhinitis associated with prolonged use.
- Topical nasal steroids, e.g., beclomethasone 2 sprays in each nostril bid–tid.
- Topical nasal cromolyn sodium 1–2 sprays in each nostril qid.
- Hyposensitization therapy if more conservative therapy is unsuccessful.

For a more detailed discussion, see Austen KF: Diseases of Immediate Type Hypersensitivity, Chap. 267 in HPIM-12, p. 1422

116 **PRIMARY IMMUNODEFICIENCY DISEASE**

DEFINITION Disorders involving the cell-mediated (T-cell) or antibody-mediated (B-cell) arm of immune system; some disorders may manifest abnormalities of both pathways. Pts are prone to development of recurrent infections and, in certain disorders, lymphoproliferative neoplasms. *Primary disorders* may be congenital or acquired; some are familial in nature. *Secondary disorders* are not caused by intrinsic abnormalities of immune cells but may be due to infection (such as in AIDS; see HPIM-12, Chap. 264), treatment with cytotoxic drugs, radiation therapy, or lymphoreticular malignancies. Pts with disorders of antibody formation are chiefly prone to infection with encapsulated bacterial pathogens (e.g., streptococci, *Haemophilus,* meningococcus) and *Giardia*. Individuals with T-cell defects are generally susceptible to infections with viruses, fungi, and protozoa.

CLASSIFICATION **Severe combined immunodeficiency (SCID)** Congenital (autosomal recessive or X-linked); affected infants rarely survive beyond 1 year. Dysfunction of both cellular and humoral immunity:

- Swiss-type: autosomal recessive; severe lymphopenia involving B and T cells.
- Adenosine deaminase deficiency: autosomal recessive.
- X-linked patterns: some pts have normal numbers of B cells but few or no circulating T cells.

Bone marrow transplantation is useful in some pts.

Other well-defined immunodeficiency syndromes

1. DiGeorge syndrome: Maldevelopment of organs derived embryologically from third and fourth pharyngeal pouches (including thymus); associated with congenital cardiac defects, parathyroid hypoplasia with hypocalcemic tetany, abnormal facies, thymic aplasia; serum Ig levels may be normal, but specific antibody responses are impaired.

2. Ataxia-telangiectasia: Autosomal recessive; cerebellar ataxia, oculocutaneous telangiectasia, immunodeficiency; not all pts have immunodeficiency; lymphomas common; IgG subclasses may be abnormal.

3. Wiskott-Aldrich syndrome: X-linked genetic disorder characterized by eczema, thrombocytopenia, and infections.

Predominantly antibody deficiencies

1. X-linked agammaglobulinemia: Marked deficiency of circulating lymphocytes; all Ig classes low; arthritis associated with *Mycoplasma* and chronic echovirus encephalitis are common complications.

2. Transient hypogammaglobulinemia of infancy: This occurs between 3 and 6 months of age as maternally derived IgG levels decline.

3. Isolated IgA deficiency: Most common immunodeficiency; many affected pts do not have increased infections; antibodies against IgA may lead to anaphylaxis during transfusion of blood or plasma; may be associated with deficiencies of IgG subclasses.

4. X-linked immunodeficiency with increased IgM.

5. Isolated deficiency of IgM.

6. Common variable immunodeficiency: Heterogeneous group of syndromes characterized by panhypogammaglobulinemia, deficiency of IgG and IgA, or selective IgG deficiency; associated conditions include lymphoreticular neoplasms, arthritis, ulcerative colitis.

7. Immunodeficiency with thymoma.

8. Selective deficiency of IgG subclasses (with or without IgA deficiency).

Miscellaneous immunodeficiency syndromes

• Mucocutaneous candidiasis. • Immunodeficiency associated with serum lymphocytotoxins. • X-linked lymphoproliferative syndrome.

PRELIMINARY EVALUATION

• CBC with differential. • Quantitative immunoglobulin levels. • Isoagglutinins, diphtheria and tetanus antibody titers. • Complement levels (C3, C4, and CH_{50}). • Skin tests for T-cell function (PPD, *Candida, Trichophyton, tetanus toxoid*).

TREATMENT Treatment of T-cell disorders is complex and largely investigational. Therapy of humoral immunodeficiencies with intravenous IgG preparations should aim to keep IgG levels near low-normal range.

For a more detailed discussion, see Cooper MD, Lawton AR III: Primary Immune Deficiency Diseases, Chap. 263, in HPIM-12, p. 1395

117 **ACQUIRED IMMUNODEFICIENCY SYNDROME (AIDS)**

DEFINITION AIDS was originally defined empirically by the Centers for Disease Control (CDC) as "the presence of a reliably diagnosed disease that is at least moderately indicative of an underlying defect in cell-mediated immunity." Examples of such diseases are Kaposi's sarcoma in an individual under 60 or a life-threatening opportunistic infection such as *Pneumocystis carinii* pneumonia. Following the recognition of the causative virus HIV, formerly called HTLV-III/LAV, the diagnosis of AIDS is now excluded if tests for the presence of the virus or its antibodies are negative and the number of T helper lymphocytes is normal.

AIDS is now best considered as a part of the *spectrum of HIV infection*. Stages of the infection are:

Group I   Acute infection
Group II   Asymptomatic infection
Group III Persistent generalized adenopathy
Group IV   Other disease:
    Subgroup A   Constitutional disease (e.g., fever, weight loss, diarrhea)
    Subgroup B   Neurologic disease
    Subgroup C   Secondary infectious diseases
    Subgroup D   Secondary neoplasms
    Subgroup E   Other conditions

ETIOLOGY AIDS is caused by infection with the human retroviruses HIV-1 or HIV-2. HIV-1 is most common cause worldwide; HIV-2 has about 40% sequence homology, is more closely related to simian immunodeficiency viruses, and has been identified predominantly in western Africa. The virus is passed through sexual contact; through contact with blood, blood products, or other bodily fluids (as in drug users who share contaminated IV needles); or perinatally from mother to infant. There is no evidence that the virus can be passed through casual or family contact.

EPIDEMIOLOGY AIDS first appeared in the U.S. in the late 1970s and was first recognized in 1981, when the CDC announced the unexplained occurrence of *P. carinii* pneumonia and Kaposi's sarcoma in previously healthy homosexual men from New York City and Los Angeles. Since that time there has been a geometric increase in the number of cases, and it is anticipated that there will be over 365,000 cases in the U.S. by 1992. The disease is also occurring with increased frequency in virtually all countries, particularly those of Europe, central Africa, and South America.

Among adult U.S. cases, approximately 60% are in homosexual or bisexual men who do not use IV drugs; 20% are in heterosexual male and female IV drug users; 7% are in homosexual or bisexual men who also use IV drugs; approximately 1% are in hemophiliacs with no history of other risk factors, exposed to HIV in large quantities of blood products; 2% are in nonhemophiliacs who have received transfusions of blood or blood products; 5% of cases have had sexual contact with an infected individual or one in a known risk group, frequently a user of IV drugs. Importantly, rate of new infections among homosexual and bisexual men is decreasing, leading to a higher proportion of cases among drug users, with consequent increase in number of heterosexually transmitted, perinatally transmitted, and pediatric cases.

PATHOPHYSIOLOGY AND IMMUNOPATHOGENESIS The characteristic immunologic feature of AIDS is a profound defect in cell-mediated immunity, leading to the development of opportunistic infections and neoplasms. The main cause of the immune defect is a quantitative and qualitative deficiency in CD4+ thymus-derived helper/inducer lymphocytes (termed T4 cells). The CD4 molecule, present on T4 lymphocytes and other cells, including the monocyte/macrophage lineage, is the cell surface receptor with which the HIV virion interacts during the process of cellular infection.

Because of the central role of the helper/inducer T-cell subset in inducing and coordinating many varied components of the immune response, there are global defects of immune function present in AIDS. These include defects in natural killer cells, monocytes, virus-specific cytotoxic T cells, and B cells. B cells are polyclonally activated, resulting in hypergammaglobulinemia with elevated levels of IgG, IgM, and IgA.

In addition to its effects on the immune system, HIV may directly infect other organ systems such as the brain and cause pathology there. This may be especially important in explaining the neuropsychiatric abnormalities frequently observed in HIV-infected pts.

CLINICAL MANIFESTATIONS Group I: acute infection Majority of infected individuals recall no recognizable symptoms or signs at time of initial infection. Acute syndrome follows acute infection by 3–6 weeks. Characterized by fevers, rigors, arthralgias, myalgias, maculopapular rash, urticaria, abdominal cramps, diarrhea, and aseptic meningitis; lasts 2–3 weeks and resolves spontaneously.

Group II: asymptomatic infection Length of time between infection and development of disease varies greatly, but mean is estimated to be 8–10 years.

Group III: persistent generalized lymphadenopathy Palpable adenopathy at two or more extrainguinal sites that persists for >3 months without explanation other than HIV infection. Many pts will go on to disease progression.

Group IV: other disease *Subgroup A: constitutional symptoms* Fever persisting for more than 1 month, involuntary weight loss of more than 10% of baseline, diarrhea for >1 month in absence of explainable cause.

Subgroup B: neurologic disease Most common is HIV encephalopathy (AIDS dementia complex); other neurologic complications include opportunistic infections or primary CNS lymphoma.

Subgroup C: secondary infectious diseases (For complete list, see Table 264-2, p. 1406 in HPIM-12.) *P. carinii* pneumonia is most common opportunistic infection, occurring in approximately 80% of pts during the course of their illness. Other common pathogens include CMV (chorioretinitis, colitis, pneumonitis, adrenalitis), *Candida albicans* (oral thrush, esophagitis), *Mycobacterium avium-intracellulare* (localized or disseminated infection), *M. tuberculosis, Cryptococcus neoformans* (meningitis, disseminated disease), *Toxoplasma gondii* (encephalitis, intracerebral mass lesion), herpes simplex virus (severe mucocutaneous lesions, esophagitis), diarrhea due to *Cryptosporidium* or *Isospora belli,* bacterial pathogens (especially in pediatric cases).

Subgroup D: secondary neoplasms Kaposi's sarcoma (cutaneous and visceral, more fulminant course than in non-HIV infected pts), lymphoid neoplasms (especially B-cell lymphomas of brain, marrow, GI tract).

Subgroup E: other diseases Thrombocytopenia, nonspecific interstitial pneumonitis.

DIAGNOSIS AIDS is diagnosed in an HIV-infected individual with group IV disease (see above).

Documentation of HIV infection by detection of antibodies against virus using ELISA confirmed by western blot. 95% of infected pts will develop detectable antibodies within 5 months of infection.

TREATMENT AND PROGNOSIS Prognosis is variable. Mean incubation period in infected adults estimated to be 8–10 years. Current evidence suggests that all infected individuals will eventually develop progressive disease. Treatment strategy is: (1) treatment of HIV infection with antiretroviral drugs, (2) prophylactic treatment of certain infections, and (3) treatment of opportunistic infections and neoplasms as they occur.

Antiretroviral therapy Pts with AIDS or AIDS-related complex (group III) should be treated with zidovudine (3'-azido-3'-deoxythymidine, AZT), 200 mg PO q 4 h (reduced to 100 mg q 4 h if higher dose not tolerated). Complications include bone marrow suppression with anemia and neutropenia, and GI intolerance. Asymptomatic infected individuals with CD4+ T-cell counts less than 500/μL may benefit from 100 mg q 4 h while awake (total daily dose 500 mg). Studies have demonstrated improvement in HIV-related symptoms and slowing of disease progression.

Prophylaxis of infections Aerosolized pentamidine isethionate 300 mg once a month or trimethoprim/sulfamethoxazole 320/1600 mg bid may help prevent *P. carinii* pneumonia in pts with history of previous episode or T4 lymphocytes ≤200/μL.

Treatment of infections and neoplasms Treatment of opportunistic infections is outlined in HPIM-12, Table 264-2. Kaposi's sarcoma should be treated when it is cosmetically unacceptable, causes symptoms, or interferes with function. Radiation therapy, interferon-α, and single- and multiagent chemotherapy are useful. Lymphoid neoplasms are treated in same fashion as for non-AIDS pts.

EDUCATION AND PREVENTION Education of individuals in risk groups regarding modification of behavior is of prime importance in attempting to halt spread of virus. Screening of blood supplies and use of universal precautions by health care workers are other important efforts. Vaccine development is currently underway and would mark a major advance in control of this disorder.

For a more detailed discussion, see Fauci AS, Lane HC: The Acquired Immunodeficiency Syndrome (AIDS), Chap. 264, in HPIM-12, p. 1402

DEFINITION Heterogeneous disorders that share certain common features, including inflammation of skin, joints, and other structures rich in connective tissue, as well as altered patterns of immunoregulation, including production of auto-antibodies and abnormalities of cell-mediated immunity. While certain distinct clinical entities may be defined, manifestations may vary considerably from one pt to the next and overlap of clinical features between and among specific diseases is common.

SYSTEMIC LUPUS ERYTHEMATOSUS (SLE)

Definition and pathogenesis Disease of unknown etiology in which tissues and cells are damaged by deposition of pathogenic antibodies and immune complexes. Genetic, environmental, and sex hormonal factors are likely of pathogenetic importance. B-cell hyperactivity, production of auto-antibodies with specificity for nuclear antigenic determinants, and abnormalities of T-cell function occur.

Clinical manifestations May involve virtually any organ system. Course of disease is one of periods of exacerbation and remission. *Common features* include fatigue, fever, malaise, weight loss, skin rashes (especially malar "butterfly" rash), photosensitivity, arthritis, myositis, oral ulcers, vasculitis, alopecia, anemia (may be hemolytic), neutropenia, thrombocytopenia, lymphadenopathy, splenomegaly, organic brain syndromes, seizures, psychosis, pleuritis, pericarditis, myocarditis, pneumonitis, nephritis, venous or arterial thrombosis, mesenteric vasculitis, sicca syndrome. Antinuclear antibodies are usually present. Syndrome may be *drug-induced* (especially by procainamide, hydralazine, isoniazid).

Evaluation Hx and physical exam, appropriate radiographic studies, ECG, UA, CBC, ESR, serum immunoglobulins, antinuclear antibodies and subtypes (dsDNA, ssDNA, anti-Sm, anti-Ro, anti-La, antihistone), complement levels (C3, C4, CH_{50}), VDRL, PT, PTT.

Treatment No cure; treatment is directed at controlling inflammation. Useful drugs include salicylates (especially enteric-coated aspirin, 2–4 g/d in divided doses), NSAIDs (e.g., ibuprofen 400–800 mg tid–qid), and hydroxychloroquine, 400 mg/d; glucocorticoids [1–2 (mg/kg)/d prednisone or equivalent] may be necessary for life-threatening or severely disabling manifestations; cytotoxic agents [cyclophosphamide 1.5–2.5 (mg/kg)/d or azathioprine 2–3 (mg/kg)/d] may be required for manifestations not successfully controlled by acceptable doses of steroids; IV pulse cyclophosphamide (10–15 mg/kg every 4 weeks) is an alternative regimen to daily cytotoxic therapy.

RHEUMATOID ARTHRITIS (RA)

Definition and pathogenesis A chronic multisystem disease of unknown etiology characterized chiefly by persistent inflammatory synovitis, usually involving peripheral joints in a symmetrical fashion. Cartilaginous destruction, bony erosions, and joint deformation are hallmarks of persistent synovial inflammation. Pathogenesis is not well understood; synovial hyperplasia and hypertrophy, lymphocytic infiltration of synovial tissue, joint infiltration by neutrophils, protease release, and chondrocyte activation occur.

Clinical manifestations Hallmark is symmetrical polyarthritis of peripheral joints with pain, tenderness, and swelling of affected joints; morning stiffness is common; PIP and MCP joints frequently involved; joint deformities may develop after persistent inflammation. *Extraarticular manifestations* include rheumatoid nodules, rheumatoid vasculitis, pleuropulmonary inflammation, scleritis, sicca syndrome, Felty's syndrome (splenomegaly and neutropenia), osteoporosis.

Evaluation Hx and physical exam with careful examination of all joints; CBC, ESR, rheumatoid factor, complement levels, synovial fluid analysis, chest and joint radiographs.

Treatment (1) Aspirin (2–4 g/d in divided doses) and NSAIDs (e.g., ibuprofen 400–800 mg tid–qid) are mainstays of therapy; (2) disease-modifying drugs, e.g., oral gold salts (auranofin 6 mg/d), hydroxychloroquine 400 mg/d, D-penicillamine 500 mg/d, sulfasalazine 500 mg/d; (3) low-dose prednisone (e.g., 7.5 mg/d); (4) methotrexate 7.5–15 mg/week; (5) surgery.

SYSTEMIC SCLEROSIS (scleroderma, SSc)

Definition and pathogenesis Multisystem disorder characterized by inflammatory, vascular, and fibrotic changes of skin and various internal organ systems (chiefly GI tract, lungs, heart, and kidney). Pathogenesis not clear; primary event may be endothelial cell injury with eventual intimal proliferation, fibrosis, and vessel obliteration.

Clinical manifestations Raynaud's phenomenon, fibrosis of the skin (scleroderma), telangiectasis, calcinosis, esophageal hypomotility, arthralgias and/or arthritis, intestinal hypofunction, pulmonary fibrosis, hypertension, renal failure (leading cause of death).

Evaluation Hx and physical exam, ESR, CXR, barium swallow, ANA [specific antibodies may include antibodies to nucleolar antigens, ribonucleoprotein, centromere, and antitopoisomerase I (Scl-70)], ECG, UA, skin biopsy.

Treatment SSc cannot be cured but appropriate treatment can relieve symptoms and improve function. D-penicillamine 250 mg/d starting dose may reduce skin thickening and prevent organ involvement. Glucocorticoids (prednisone 40–60 mg/d with subsequent taper) are indicated for inflammatory myositis or pericarditis. Calcium channel blockers (e.g., nifedipine 10–20 mg PO tid) are useful for Raynaud's phenomenon, as adjuncts to warm clothing, smoking cessation, etc. Antacids, H-2 antagonists (e.g., ranitidine 150 mg PO bid), and metoclopramide 10 mg PO ac and hs may be useful for esophageal reflux. ACE inhibitors (e.g., captopril 25 mg PO tid) may be particularly useful for controlling hypertension and limiting progression of renal disease.

MIXED CONNECTIVE TISSUE DISEASE (MCTD)

Definition and pathogenesis Syndrome characterized by a combination of clinical features similar to those of SLE, SSc, polymyositis, and RA; unusually high titers of circulating antibodies to a nuclear ribonucleoprotein (RNP) are found. Pathogenic mechanisms are unknown, but evidence exists for abnormal immunoregulation and proliferative intimal and/or medial vascular lesions resulting in narrowing of vessel lumens.

Clinical manifestations Raynaud's phenomenon, polyarthritis, swollen hands or sclerodactyly, esophageal dysfunction, pulmonary fibrosis, inflammatory myopathy. Renal involvement is less common than in SSc. Laboratory abnormalities include high-titer ANAs, positive rheumatoid factor in >50% of pts, very high titers of antibody to RNP component of extractable nuclear antigen.

Evaluation Similar to that for SLE and SSc.

Treatment Similar to that for SLE; directed at controlling inflammatory manifestations of disease.

SJÖGREN'S SYNDROME

Definition and pathogenesis An immunologic disorder characterized by progressive destruction of exocrine glands leading to mucosal and conjunctival dryness (sicca syndrome); may be primary or in association with other autoimmune diseases; affected tissues demonstrate lymphocytic infiltration and immune-complex deposition.

Clinical manifestations   Xerostomia and keratoconjunctivitis sicca, nephritis, vasculitis (usually cutaneous), polyneuropathy, interstitial pneumonitis, pseudolymphoma, autoimmune thyroid disease, congenital cardiac conduction defects in children born to women with anti-Ro (SSA) antibodies.

Evaluation   Hx and physical exam, with special attention to determining extent of disease and presence of other autoimmune disorders; CBC, UA, CXR, ECG, thyroid function tests, Schirmer's test, ESR, cryoglobulins.

Treatment   Symptomatic relief of dryness with artificial tears, ophthalmic lubricating ointments, nasal saline sprays, frequent sips of water, moisturizing skin lotions; treatment of associated autoimmune phenomena.

For a more detailed discussion, see Hahn BH: Systemic Lupus Erythematosus, Chap. 269, p. 1432; Lipsky PE: Rheumatoid Arthritis, Chap. 270, p. 1437; Gilliland BC: Systemic Sclerosis (Scleroderma), Chap. 271, p. 1443; Sharp GC: Mixed Connective Tissue Disease, Chap. 272, p. 1448; and Lanc HC, Fauci AS: Sjögren's Syndrome, Chap. 273, p. 1449, in HPIM-12

---

119 VASCULITIS

DEFINITION AND PATHOGENESIS A clinicopathologic process characterized by inflammation of and damage to blood vessels, compromise of vessel lumen, and resulting ischemia. Clinical manifestations of ischemic damage depend on size and location of vessel. May be primary or sole manifestation of a disease or secondary to another disease process.

Most vasculitic syndromes appear to be mediated in whole or in part by immune mechanisms, particularly deposition of immune complexes in vessel walls.

CLASSIFICATION Systemic necrotizing vasculitis

1. Classic polyarteritis nodosa (PAN): Small and medium-sized muscular arteries involved, esp. branch points; commonly involves kidney, heart, liver, GI tract, peripheral nerves, skin; lungs usually spared.

2. Allergic angiitis and granulomatosis (Churg-Strauss disease): Granulomatous vasculitis of multiple organ systems, particularly the lung; similar to PAN but with higher frequency of involvement of lungs and vessels of multiple sizes and types; eosinophilic tissue infiltration, peripheral eosinophilia, and association with severe asthma.

3. Polyangiitis overlap syndrome: Overlap of PAN, allergic angiitis and granulomatosis, and manifestations of small-vessel hypersensitivity vasculitis.

Hypersensitivity vasculitis Heterogeneous group of disorders; common feature is small-vessel involvement; skin disease usually predominates.

Exogenous stimuli proved or suspected

• Henoch-Schönlein purpura. • Serum sickness and serum sickness-like reactions. • Drug-induced vasculitis. • Vasculitis associated with infectious diseases.

Endogenous antigens likely involved

• Vasculitis associated with neoplasms. • Vasculitis associated with connective tissue disorders. • Vasculitis associated with other underlying diseases. • Vasculitis associated with congenital deficiencies of complement system.

Wegener's granulomatosis Granulomatous vasculitis of upper and lower respiratory tracts together with glomerulonephritis; paranasal sinus congestion and pain, drainage, purulent or bloody nasal discharge. Mucosal ulceration, septal perforation, and cartilaginous destruction (saddle nose deformity) may result. Lung involvement may be asymptomatic or cause cough, hemoptysis, or dyspnea; eye involvement may occur; renal involvement accounts for most deaths.

Giant cell arteritis

1. Temporal arteritis: Inflammation of medium- and large-sized arteries; temporal artery usually involved, but systemic involvement may occur; fever, high ESR, anemia, musculoskeletal symptoms (polymyalgia rheumatica), sudden blindness are major manifestations; glucocorticoid therapy necessary to prevent ocular complications.

2. Takayasu's arteritis: Vasculitis of medium- and large-sized arteries with strong predilection for aortic arch and its branches; most common in young women; presents with inflammatory or ischemic symptoms in arms and neck, systemic inflammatory symptoms, aortic regurgitation.

Miscellaneous vasculitic syndromes

• Mucocutaneous lymph node syndrome (Kawasaki's disease).   • Isolated vasculitis of the central nervous system.
• Thromboangiitis obliterans (Buerger's disease).

EVALUATION

• Thorough Hx and physical exam, with special reference to ischemic manifestations and systemic inflammatory signs/symptoms.
• CBC, ESR, serum chemistries, UA, ECG.
• Quantitative serum immunoglobulins.
• ANA, rheumatoid factor, VDRL, hepatitis B antigen and antibody, immune complexes, complement levels.
• Antineutrophil cytoplasmic autoantibodies may be positive in pts with Wegener's granulomatosis.
• Radiographic studies, including angiography of affected organs when necessary.
• Biopsy of affected organ system(s) necessary to establish diagnosis.

THERAPY   Once diagnosis is established, therapy may be necessary with glucocorticoids and/or cytotoxic agents. Cytotoxic agents are particularly important in syndromes with life-threatening organ system involvement, including Wegener's granulomatosis, PAN, allergic angiitis and granulomatosis, and isolated CNS vasculitis. Glucocorticoids alone may control temporal arteritis and Takayasu's arteritis. Some of the small-vessel syndromes may be particularly resistant to therapy. *Useful medications:*

• Prednisone 1 (mg/kg)/d initially, then tapered.
• Cyclophosphamide 2 (mg/kg)/d, adjusted to avoid severe leukopenia. Pulse administration of cyclophosphamide (1 g/m^2 per month) may be useful in selected pts who cannot tolerate chronic administration of the drug.

- Azathioprine 2 (mg/kg)/d, adjusted to avoid severe leuko-penia; used when side effects of cyclophosphamide are prohibitive.
- Plasmapheresis may have an adjunctive role in management if manifestations not controlled by above measures.

For a more detailed discussion, see Fauci AS: The Vasculitis Syndromes, Chap. 276, in HPIM-12, p. 1456

120 SARCOIDOSIS

DEFINITION A systemic granulomatous disease of unknown etiology. Affected organs are characterized by an accumulation of T lymphocytes and mononuclear phagocytes, non-caseating epithelioid granulomas, and derangements of normal tissue architecture.

PATHOPHYSIOLOGY Mononuclear cells, mostly T helper lymphocytes and mononuclear phagocytes, accumulate in affected organs followed by formation of granulomas. No evidence that this process by itself permanently injures parenchyma of organ system; however, distortion of organ architecture from accumulation of these inflammatory components occurs. Granulomatous inflammation is maintained by secretion of mediators (including interleukin 2 and γ-interferon) by the activated T helper lymphocytes. Severe damage of parenchyma can lead to irreversible fibrosis, which can alter further the structural integrity of organ and in advanced cases lead to serious organ dysfunction.

CLINICAL MANIFESTATIONS

- May be asymptomatic and discovered on routine CXR as hilar adenopathy and slight infiltrative disease of lung parenchyma.
- Constitutional symptoms: fever, weight loss, anorexia, fatigue.
- Lung: hilar adenopathy, alveolitis, interstitial pneumonitis, cough, dyspnea; pleural disease and hemoptysis rare; airways may be involved and cause obstruction to airflow; lung most commonly involved organ—90% with sarcoidosis will have abnormal CXR some time during course.
- Lymph nodes: intrathoracic and peripheral lymph nodes may be enlarged.
- Skin: 25% will have skin involvement; lesions include erythema nodosum, plaques, maculopapular eruptions, subcutaneous nodules, and lupus pernio (indurated blue-purple shiny lesions on face, fingers, and knees).
- Eye: uveitis in approximately 25%; may progress to blindness.
- Bone marrow and spleen: mild anemia and thrombocytopenia may occur.
- Liver: involved on biopsy in 60–90%; rarely important clinically.
- Kidney: may have parenchymal disease or more commonly nephrolithiasis secondary to abnormalities of calcium metabolism.

- Nervous system: may involve CNS, cranial nerves, peripheral nerves.
- Heart: may involve left ventricular wall or conduction system, causing disturbances of rhythm and/or contractility.

COMPLICATIONS Major morbidity and mortality related to progressive respiratory dysfunction in association with severe interstitial lung disease; eye involvement (including blindness) is most common extrapulmonary complication, but is manageable with glucocorticoid treatment.

EVALUATION

- Hx and physical exam to rule out exposures and other evidence of interstitial lung disease.
- CBC, Ca^{++}, angiotensin converting enzyme, PPD and control skin tests, LFTs.
- CXR, ECG, PFTs.
- Biopsy of lung or other affected organ is mandatory to establish diagnosis before starting therapy. Transbronchial lung biopsy usually adequate to make diagnosis.
- Bronchoalveolar lavage and gallium scan of lungs may help decide when treatment is indicated and to follow therapy.

TREATMENT Many cases remit spontaneously; therefore, deciding when treatment is necessary is difficult and controversial. Progressive lung involvement, eye disease, and cardiac disease are unequivocal indications for treatment. Bronchoalveolar lavage and gallium scanning may help to identify individuals with high risk of progression to end-stage lung disease; however, these are not uniformly accepted. Glucocorticoids are mainstay of therapy. Usual therapy is prednisone 1 (mg/kg)/d for 4–6 weeks followed by taper over 2–3 months. Anecdotal reports suggest that cyclosporine may be useful in extrathoracic sarcoid not responding to glucocorticoids.

For a more detailed discussion, see Crystal RG: Sarcoidosis, Chap. 277, in HPIM-12, p. 1463

---

121 APPROACH TO PATIENT WITH MUSCULOSKELETAL DISEASE

Musculoskeletal complaints are extremely common among pts seen in outpatient medical practice and are among the leading causes of disability and absenteeism from work. Musculoskeletal complaints must be evaluated in a uniform, thorough, and logical fashion to ensure the best chance of accurate diagnosis and to plan appropriate follow-up testing and therapy.

HISTORIC FEATURES

- Age, sex, race, family history.
- Mode of onset: characteristically acute in infection or gout, more chronic in osteoarthritis, rheumatoid arthritis.
- Duration of symptoms.
- Precipitating events: e.g., trauma, drug administration, associated illnesses.
- Number and pattern of involved structures: symmetrical? one joint or more than one? migratory? intermittent or continuous?
- Associated features: fever, rash, morning stiffness, involvement of other organ systems.

PHYSICAL EXAMINATION

- Complete examination with special attention to eyes, skin, mucous membranes, heart, lungs, nails (may reveal characteristic pitting in psoriasis), nervous system.
- Careful and thorough examination of involved and uninvolved joints and periarticular structures; this should proceed in an organized fashion from head to foot or from extremities inward toward axial skeleton; special attention should be paid to identifying the presence or absence of (1) warmth, erythema, swelling; (2) joint or bursal effusions; (3) subluxation, dislocation, joint deformity; (4) synovial thickening; (5) joint instability; (6) limitations to active and passive range of motion; (7) crepitus.

ADDITIONAL INVESTIGATIONS

- CBC, ESR, serum uric acid.
- Joint radiographs.
- ANA, rheumatoid factor, antistreptolysin O titer, complement levels.
- Synovial fluid aspiration and analysis; especially important in acute monarthritis or when crystal-induced or septic

arthritis is suspected. Should be examined for (1) appearance, viscosity; (2) cell count; (3) glucose, protein; (4) crystals using polarizing microscope; (5) Gram's stain, cultures.

For a more detailed discussion, see Cush JJ, Lipsky PE: Approach to Articular and Musculoskeletal Disorders, Chap. 280, in HPIM-12, p. 1472

---

122 ANKYLOSING SPONDYLITIS

DEFINITION   Also known as rheumatoid spondylitis and Marie-Strümpell disease, this is a chronic and progressive inflammatory disease of spinal joints, sacroiliac joints, hips, shoulders, and occasionally peripheral joints. Most frequently presents in young men in third decade; strong association with histocompatibility antigen HLA-B27.

PATHOLOGY   Earliest changes found in sacroiliac joints. Synovitis resembles that seen in rheumatoid arthritis (RA) with synovial hyperplasia, lymphoid cell accumulation, bony erosions, cartilage destruction followed by fibrosis and bony ankylosis (fusion). Ossification of the annulus fibrosis of intervertebral disks and anterior longitudinal ligament causes "bamboo spine" appearance on spine radiographs. Inflammation at insertion of tendons, ligaments, and capsules into bone is called "enthesitis." Focal medial necrosis at root of aorta may be seen.

CLINICAL MANIFESTATIONS

- Morning back pain and stiffness; peripheral joint pain (esp. hip).
- Chest pain from involvement of thoracic skeleton and muscular insertions.
- Aortic valve incompetence and regurgitation in 3%.
- Cardiac conduction defects.
- Acute anterior uveitis in 20–30%; may be recurrent.
- Constitutional symptoms may be severe: fever, anemia, fatigue, weight loss.
- Rare: amyloidosis, bilateral upper lobe lung fibrosis.
- Cauda equina syndrome: buttock or leg pain; leg weakness; loss of bladder or rectal sphincter control.
- Physical findings: tenderness over involved joints, diminished chest expansion, diminished anterior flexion of lumbar spine (Schober test).

LABORATORY FINDINGS

- ESR elevated in majority; normal in 20% of pts with mild disease; rheumatoid factor negative; mild anemia.
- Radiographs: early may be normal but will soon show progressive sclerosis of sacroiliac joints; spinal x-rays show straightening of lumbar spine, squaring of vertebrae, syndesmophytes ("bamboo spine").

DIFFERENTIAL DIAGNOSIS   RA; juvenile RA; spondylitis associated with Reiter's syndrome, psoriatic arthritis, inflammatory bowel disease; diffuse idiopathic skeletal hyperostosis.

TREATMENT Exercise program designed to maintain posture and mobility is key to management. NSAIDs (e.g., indomethacin 75 mg slow-release qd or bid) useful in most pts. Sulfasalazine 2–3 g/d may be useful. Adjunctive therapy includes intraarticular glucocorticoids for persistent enthesopathy or synovitis; ocular glucocorticoids for uveitis; surgery for severely affected or deformed joints.

For a more detailed discussion, see Taurog JD, Lipsky PE: Ankylosing Spondylitis and Reactive Arthritis, Chap. 274, in HPIM-12, p. 1451

DEFINITION Osteoarthritis (OA) is a disorder characterized by progressive deterioration and loss of articular cartilage accompanied by proliferation of new bone and soft tissue in and around involved joint. Most common form of arthritis, OA affects almost all joints, especially weight-bearing and frequently used joints. In *primary* (idiopathic) OA no underlying cause is apparent. In *secondary* OA, a predisposing factor such as trauma, congenital abnormality, or metabolic disorder is present.

PATHOGENESIS Earliest physicochemical change is increased water content in cartilage, due to disruption of collagen network. Leads to softened cartilage. Increased synthesis of matrix-degrading enzymes by chondrocytes, possibly due to cytokines or mechanical factors. Subchondral bone is metabolically active and becomes sclerotic. Geometry of joint is altered, with subsequent pain, stiffness, and swelling.

CLINICAL MANIFESTATIONS

- Pain usually limited to one or a few joints, but may be generalized.
- Stiffness in morning or after rest may occur but usually brief.
- Pain at night or with weather changes may occur; pts may note crepitus.
- With progressive disease, joint motion becomes limited; subluxation and deformity may occur.
- Heberden's or Bouchard's nodes may occur at interphalangeal joints.
- Hip involvement more common in men than women; may be unilateral at first; internal rotation most limited in early stages.
- OA of knee may involve medial, lateral, or patellofemoral compartments; pain may be diffuse or localized to one compartment.
- Spine involvement may affect intervertebral disks, apophyseal joints, and paraspinal ligaments.
- Lumbar stenosis may cause cord compression due to posterior vertebral osteophytes; symptoms provoked by hyperextension of lumbar spine, relieved by flexion; laminectomy may be required if symptoms progress.
- Secondary OA due to traumatic, systemic, or congenital disorders may be unilateral, appear at early age, or involve joints not usually seen in OA.

LABORATORY FINDINGS

- Routine lab work usually normal.
- ESR usually normal but may be elevated in pts with primary generalized or erosive OA.
- Joint fluid is straw-colored with good viscosity; fluid WBCs < 2000; calcium pyrophosphate or hydroxyapatite crystals may be found in some fluids.
- Radiographs may be normal at first but as disease progresses may show joint space narrowing, subchondral bone sclerosis, osteophytes, joint surface erosions, subchondral cysts.
- Rheumatoid factor, ANA studies normal.

DIAGNOSIS   Usually established on basis of pattern of joint involvement, normal laboratory tests, synovial fluid findings, and radiographic features. Differential diagnosis includes rheumatoid arthritis and crystal-induced arthritides.

TREATMENT   Pt education, weight reduction, appropriate use of cane and other supports, isometric exercises to strengthen muscles around affected joints. Medical treatment includes salicylates or NSAIDs (e.g., ibuprofen 400–800 mg tid or qid), intraarticular glucocorticoid injections; surgery and/or splinting may be necessary.

For a more detailed discussion, see Brandt KD, Kovalov-St. John K: Osteoarthritis, Chap. 281, in HPIM-12, p. 1475

124 GOUT, PSEUDOGOUT, AND RELATED DISEASES

GOUT

The term *gout* is applied to a spectrum of disorders that may encompass (in their fully developed states) five cardinal features, which may occur singly or in combination:

1. Increased serum urate concentration
2. Recurrent arthritic attacks with urate crystals demonstrable in synovial fluid leukocytes
3. Appearance of tophi, aggregated deposits of monosodium urate monohydrate
4. Renal disease involving interstitial tissues and blood vessels
5. Uric acid nephrolithiasis

Pathogenesis *Hyperuricemia* May arise from the overproduction or reduced excretion of uric acid or a combination of the two. Uric acid represents the end product of degradation of purine nucleotides; thus uric acid production is closely linked to pathways of purine metabolism, with the intracellular concentration of 5-phosphoribosyl-1-pyrophosphate (PRPP) being the major determinant of the rate of uric acid biosynthesis.

Primary hyperuricemia may occur from undefined metabolic defects or as the result of two inborn metabolic errors, partial hypoxanthine-guanine phosphoribosyltransferase (HGPRT) deficiency or PRPP synthetase superactivity.

Secondary hyperuricemia may be due to an increased rate of purine biosynthesis, type I glycogen storage disease, certain myeloproliferative and lymphoproliferative disorders, hemolytic anemias, thalassemia, certain hemoglobinopathies, pernicious anemia, infectious mononucleosis, and some carcinomas. Reduced excretion of uric acid may arise from renal causes, diuretic therapy, treatment with certain drugs, volume depletion, and competition by certain organic acids (e.g., in starvation ketosis, diabetic ketoacidosis, and lactic acidosis).

Acute gouty arthritis Results from release of monosodium urate crystals into joint space, phagocytosis of these crystals by leukocytes, recruitment of additional phagocytes into joint space, and inflammation of joint induced by activation of kallikrein and complement systems and release of lysosomal products and other toxins into synovial fluid.

Clinical manifestations

1. Asymptomatic hyperuricemia: Nearly all pts with gout are hyperuricemic; however, only about 5% of hyperuricemic pts develop gout.

2. Acute gouty arthritis: Usually an exquisitely painful monarthritis but may be polyarticular and accompanied by fever; podagra (attack in the great toe) may occur eventually in 90% and may be site of first attack in half; attack will generally subside spontaneously after days to weeks; during the subsequent intercritical period, pt is asymptomatic; diagnosis of acute gouty arthritis made by demonstration of characteristic monosodium urate crystals in joint fluid by polarizing microscopy.

3. Tophi and chronic gouty arthritis: Nodular (tophaceous) deposits of monosodium urate may develop after long periods of untreated hyperuricemia; commonly involve helix and antihelix of ears, ulnar surface of forearm, Achilles tendon; incidence has fallen due to effective antihyperuricemic therapy.

4. Nephropathy: May be due to deposition of monosodium urate crystals in renal interstitium or to obstruction of collecting system and ureter by urate crystals.

5. Nephrolithiasis.

Evaluation

• Quantitation of urine uric acid.   • Abdominal flat plate, possibly IVP.   • Chemical analysis of renal stones.   • Joint x-rays and synovial fluid analysis.   • If overproduction is suspected, measurement of erythrocyte HGPRT and PRPP levels may be indicated.

Treatment

- Necessity for treatment of asymptomatic hyperuricemia is controversial; probably not indicated unless pt becomes symptomatic; has strong family history of gout, renal disease, or stones; or excretes >1100 mg uric acid per day.
- Treatment of acute gouty attack: colchicine 0.6 mg PO every hour until pt improves, GI side effects develop, or maximal dose of 6 mg is reached; or indomethacin 75 mg PO then 50 mg PO q 6 h.
- Prophylaxis with chronic colchicine (1–2 mg/d) or indomethacin (25 mg PO bid or tid); avoidance of precipitating factors (e.g., alcohol, purine-rich foods); antihyperuricemic therapy.

- Uricosuric agents: probenicid (250–1500 mg PO bid) or sulfinpyrazone (50 mg PO bid, may be increased up to 800 mg/d in divided doses).
- Allopurinol (300 mg PO qd): decreases uric acid synthesis by inhibiting xanthine oxidase.

PSEUDOGOUT

Definition and pathogenesis   Calcium pyrophosphate deposition disease (CPDD) characterized by acute and chronic inflammatory joint disease, usually affecting older individuals. The knee and other large joints most commonly affected. Calcium deposits in articular cartilage (chondrocalcinosis) may be seen radiographically.

CPDD may be classified into three categories: (1) a hereditary type; (2) a form associated with metabolic disorders, including hyperparathyroidism, hemochromatosis, hypophosphatasia, hypomagnesemia, hypothyroidism, gout, ochronosis, and Wilson's disease; and (3) an idiopathic form.

Crystals are not thought to form in synovial fluid but probably are shed from articular cartilage into joint space, where similar to gout they are phagocytosed by neutrophils and incite the characteristic inflammatory response.

Clinical manifestations   Acute *pseudogout* occurs in approximately 25% of pts with CPDD; knee is most frequently involved, but other joints may be affected; involved joint is erythematous, swollen, warm, and painful; most pts have evidence of chondrocalcinosis.

A minority will have involvement of multiple joints (*pseudorheumatoid disease*). Approximately half of pts with CPDD will have *chronic disease* with progressive degenerative changes in multiple joints. These pts may also have intermittent acute attacks.

Diagnosis   Made by demonstration of calcium pyrophosphate dihydrate crystals (appearing as short blunt rods, rhomboids, and cuboids with weak positive birefringence) in synovial fluid and finding of chondrocalcinosis in joint radiographs.

Treatment   Indomethacin or other NSAIDs (see above); intraarticular injection of glucocorticoids; colchicine is variably effective.

HYDROXYAPATITE ARTHROPATHY

Crystal-induced arthritis may be observed due to calcium hydroxyapatite crystals; described mainly in knee and shoulder. Hydroxyapatite crystals may coexist with pyrophosphate crystals and must be identified using electromagnetic or x-ray diffraction studies. Radiographic appearance resembles CPDD. Treatment involves NSAIDs, repeated joint aspiration, and rest of affected joint.

For a more detailed discussion, see Kelley WN, Palella TD: Gout and Other Disorders of Purine Metabolism, Chap. 329, p. 1834; and Hoffman GS: Arthritis Due to Deposition of Calcium Crystals, Chap. 282, p. 1479, in HPIM-12

---

125 PSORIATIC ARTHRITIS

Approximately 5% of pts with psoriasis develop arthritis related to their skin disease. Some 50% of pts with psoriasis and spondylitis have the HLA-B27 histocompatibility antigen; however, there is no apparent relation between HLA-B27 and psoriatic peripheral arthritis. Onset of psoriasis usually precedes development of joint disease; approximately 15% of pts develop arthritis prior to onset of skin disease.

PATTERNS OF JOINT INVOLVEMENT

- Approximately 16–70% (mean 47%) of pts have asymmetric oligoarticular arthritis affecting two or three joints simultaneously; proximal joints of hands and feet are frequently affected; "sausage digits" may be present reflecting involvement of interphalangeal joints.
- Some 25% of pts have symmetrical polyarthritis resembling rheumatoid arthritis; rheumatoid factor is negative.
- Approximately 10% have predominantly distal interphalangeal joint involvement with psoriatic changes of adjacent nail. _pitting. onycholysis_
- Rare pts have aggressive, destructive form of arthritis known as "arthritis mutilans" with severe joint deformities and bony dissolution.
- Approximately 20% of pts with psoriatic arthritis have spondylitis and/or sacroiliitis; spondylitis may occur in absence of peripheral arthritis.

LABORATORY FINDINGS

• Hypoproliferative anemia, elevated ESR. • Negative tests for rheumatoid factor. • Hyperuricemia. • Inflammatory synovial fluid and biopsy without specific findings. • Radiographic features include severe joint destruction with bony ankylosis, osteolysis, whittling of tufts of terminal phalanges, "pencil-in-cup" deformity.

DIAGNOSIS Suggested by presence of inflammatory arthritis in pt with skin and nail changes of psoriasis and in absence of findings characteristic of other chronic inflammatory arthritides.

TREATMENT

- Aspirin 2–4 g/d or NSAIDs (especially indomethacin 25–50 mg PO tid).
- Intraarticular steroid injections for acute inflammation.
- Gold salts (e.g., auranofin 6 mg PO qd) may be helpful in some pts.

- Methotrexate (7.5–15 mg PO weekly) in advanced cases, especially with severe skin involvement.

For a more detailed discussion, see Schur PH: Psoriatric Arthritis and Arthritis Associated with Gastrointestinal Diseases, Chap. 283, in HPIM-12, p. 1482

---

126 REITER'S SYNDROME AND REACTIVE ARTHRITIDES

DEFINITION Reiter's syndrome is a disorder characterized by seronegative, oligoarticular, asymmetric arthritis with urethritis and/or cervicitis. The term *reactive arthritis* refers to acute nonpurulent arthritis complicating an infection elsewhere in the body.

PATHOGENESIS Two clinical forms of syndrome are recognized: postvenereal and postdysenteric (see also Chap. 127). Reiter's syndrome is most common cause of arthritis in young men. Up to 90% of pts carry the HLA-B27 alloantigen.

Syndrome is thought to be triggered in individuals with appropriate genetic background by an infection of urogenital or GI tracts with organisms such as *Chlamydia trachomatis*, *Ureoplasma urealyticum*, *Shigella dysenteriae*, *S. flexneri*, *Salmonella enteritidis*, *Yersinia enterocolitica*, or *Campylobacter jejuni*.

CLINICAL MANIFESTATIONS

- Usually begins with urethritis followed by conjunctivitis and arthritis; urethral discharge intermittent and may be asymptomatic; conjunctivitis, usually minimal; uveitis, keratitis, and optic neuritis rarely present.
- Arthritis usually acute, asymmetric, oligoarticular, involving predominantly lower extremities; plantar fasciitis and Achilles tendonitis common; sacroiliitis may occur.
- Mucocutaneous lesions: painless lesions on glans penis and oral mucosa in approximately a third of pts; keratoderma blenorrhagica (crusted scaling papules) may occur in postvenereal form but not in postdysenteric variety.
- Uncommon manifestations: pleuropericarditis, aortic regurgitation, neurologic manifestations, secondary amyloidosis.
- Prognosis is variable; a third will have recurrent or sustained disease, with 15–25% developing permanent disability.

LABORATORY FINDINGS Nonspecific; rheumatoid factor and ANA negative; mild anemia, leukocytosis, elevated ESR may be seen; synovial fluid analysis nondiagnostic.

DIAGNOSIS Presence of asymmetric seronegative oligoarthritis for >1 month with nonspecific urethritis or cervicitis allows diagnosis with approximately 80% specificity; differential diagnosis includes gonococcal arthritis and psoriatic arthritis.

TREATMENT NSAIDs (e.g., indomethacin 25–50 mg PO tid) benefit most pts; debilitating manifestations refractory to NSAIDs may require cytotoxic therapy, such as azathioprine [1–2 (mg/kg)/d] or methotrexate (7.5–15 mg/week); sulfasalazine up to 3 g/d in divided doses may help some pts with persistent arthritis. Uveitis may require aggressive therapy with ocular or systemic glucocorticoids. Intralesional steroid injections may help tendinitis. Zidovudine (AZT) may help reactive arthritis associated with HIV infection.

For a more detailed discussion, see Taurog JD, Lipsky PE: *Ankylosing Spondylitis and Reactive Arthritis*, Chap. 274, in HPIM-12, p. 1451

---

127 OTHER ARTHRITIDES

ARTHRITIS ASSOCIATED WITH BOWEL DISEASE Both peripheral arthritis and spondylitis may be associated with *ulcerative colitis* or *regional enteritis*. Spondylitis associated with inflammatory bowel disease (IBD) is indistinguishable from ankylosing spondylitis. Peripheral arthritis is episodic, asymmetric, and most frequently affects knee and ankle. Attacks usually subside within several weeks and characteristically resolve completely without residual joint damage.

Laboratory findings are nonspecific; rheumatoid factors absent; radiographs of peripheral joints usually normal; spine films resemble ankylosing spondylitis.

Treatment is directed at underlying IBD; aspirin and NSAIDs may alleviate joint symptoms.

Some pts will develop arthritis and/or vasculitis following *intestinal bypass* surgery. Treatment involves reconnection of bowel, if possible, or suppression of bacterial overgrowth with tetracycline or other antibiotics. Aspirin and NSAIDs may be of benefit.

Whipple's disease Characterized by arthritis in approximately two-thirds of pts and usually precedes appearance of intestinal symptoms. GI and joint manifestations respond to antibiotic therapy.

NEUROPATHIC JOINT DISEASE Also known as Charcot's joint, this is a severe form of osteoarthritis that occurs in joints deprived of pain and position sense; may occur in tabes dorsalis, diabetic neuropathy, meningomyelocele, amyloidosis, or leprosy. Usually begins in a single joint but may spread to involve other joints. *Treatment* involves stabilization of joint; surgical fusion may improve function.

RELAPSING POLYCHONDRITIS An idiopathic disorder characterized by recurrent inflammation of cartilaginous structures, eyes, ears, and cardiovascular system. Cardinal manifestations include ear and nose involvement with floppy ear and saddle nose deformities, scleritis, conjunctivitis, iritis, oral and/or genital ulcerations, episodic nondeforming polyarthritis, collapse of tracheal and bronchial cartilage rings, aortic regurgitation, and vasculitis of medium or large vessels.

Diagnosis is made clinically and may be confirmed by biopsy of affected cartilage. *Treatment* is glucocorticoids (prednisone 40–60 mg/d with subsequent taper), with addition of cytotoxic agents if disease progresses.

HYPERTROPHIC OSTEOARTHROPATHY Syndrome consisting of periosteal new bone formation, digital clubbing, and arthritis. Most commonly seen in association with lung carcinoma, but also occurs with chronic lung or liver disease; congenital heart, lung, or liver disease in children; and idiopathic and familial forms. *Symptoms* include burning and aching pain most pronounced in distal extremities. Radiographs show periosteal thickening with new bone formation of distal ends of long bones. *Treatment* is that of associated disorder. Vagotomy or percutaneous nerve block, aspirin, NSAIDs, and other analgesics may help to relieve symptoms.

FIBROSITIS A common disorder characterized by pain, aching, and stiffness of trunk and extremities, and presence of a number of specific tender sites (trigger points). More common in women than men. Frequently associated with sleep disorders. *Diagnosis* is made clinically; there are no laboratory or radiographic abnormalities. *Treatment* is supportive care, salicylates, NSAIDs, benzodiazepines or tricyclics for sleep disorder, and local measures (heat, massage, injection of trigger points).

REFLEX SYMPATHETIC DYSTROPHY SYNDROME (RSDS) A syndrome of pain and tenderness, usually of a hand or foot, associated with vasomotor instability, trophic skin changes, and rapid development of bony demineralization. Frequently, development will follow a precipitating event (local trauma, myocardial infarction, stroke, or peripheral nerve injury). Early recognition and treatment can be effective in preventing disability. *Therapeutic options* include pain control, application of heat or cold, exercise, sympathetic nerve block, and short courses of high-dose prednisone in conjunction with physical therapy.

PERIARTICULAR DISORDERS **Bursitis** Inflammation of the thin-walled bursal sac surrounding tendons and muscles over bony prominences. The subacromial and greater trochanteric bursae are most commonly involved. *Treatment* involves prevention of aggravating conditions, rest, NSAIDs, and local glucocorticoid injections.

Tendonitis May involve virtually any tendon but frequently affects tendons of the rotator cuff around shoulder, especially the supraspinatus. Pain is dull and aching but becomes acute and sharp when tendon is squeezed below acromion. NSAIDs, glucocorticoid injection, and physical therapy may be beneficial. The rotator cuff tendons or biceps tendon may rupture acutely, frequently requiring surgical repair.

Calcific tendonitis Results from deposition of calcium salts in tendon, usually supraspinatus. The resulting pain may be sudden and severe.

Adhesive capsulitis ("frozen shoulder") Results from conditions that enforce prolonged immobility of shoulder joint. Shoulder is painful and tender to palpation, and both active and passive range of motion is restricted. Spontaneous improvement may occur; NSAIDs, local injections of glucocorticoids, and physical therapy may be helpful.

For a more detailed discussion, see Schur PH: Psoriatic Arthritis and Arthritis Associated with Gastrointestinal Diseases, Chap. 283, p. 1482; and Gilliland BC: Relapsing Polychondritis and Miscellaneous Arthritides, Chap. 284, p. 1484, in HPIM-12

DEFINITION A disease characterized by deposition of the fibrous protein amyloid in one or more sites of the body. Clinical manifestations depend on anatomic distribution and intensity of amyloid protein deposition and range from local deposition with little significance to involvement of virtually any organ system with consequent severe pathophysiologic changes.

BIOCHEMISTRY OF AMYLOID FIBRILS Chemical characterization of amyloid fibrils reveals several varieties associated with different clinical situations:

1. *AL:* Associated with primary amyloid and amyloid associated with multiple myeloma; has significant homology to *N*-terminal sequence of immunoglobulin light chains.
2. *AA:* Found in secondary amyloid deposits and pts with familial Mediterranean fever (FMF); formed from serum precursor (SAA); SAA release from hepatocytes induced by interleukin 1.
3. *AF:* Found in familial form; identical to prealbumin (transthyretin) except for single amino acid substitution.
4. *AE:* Associated with medullary thyroid carcinoma (fibril is probably a calcitonin precursor) and focal forms.
5. *AS:* Related to prealbumin (transthyretin), atrial natriuretic peptide, or beta protein of Alzheimer's disease. Associated with senile amyloid of heart and brain.
6. *AP:* P component; found in most systemic forms; distinct from amyloid fibrils.
7. *AH:* Chronic hemodialysis-related amyloid; identical to $beta_2$ microglobulin.

CLASSIFICATION

1. *Primary amyloidosis:* No evidence for preexisting or coexisting disease; AL type deposits.
2. *Amyloidosis associated with myeloma:* AL type.
3. *Secondary (reactive) amyloidosis:* AA type; associated with chronic infectious or inflammatory diseases.
4. *Heredofamilial amyloidosis:* AF type; amyloidosis associated with FMF (AA type), and a variety of other syndromes (AF type).
5. *Local amyloidosis.*
6. *Senile amyloidosis:* Associated with aging; heart and brain especially involved.
7. *Chronic hemodialysis-related amyloidosis.*

CLINICAL MANIFESTATIONS   Major clinical findings may include proteinuria, nephrosis, azotemia, CHF, cardiomegaly, arrhythmias, cutaneous involvement with raised waxy papules, GI obstruction or ulceration, hemorrhage, protein loss, diarrhea, macroglossia, disordered esophageal motility, neuropathy, postural hypotension, arthritis, respiratory obstruction, and selective clotting factor deficiency.

DIAGNOSIS   Requires demonstration of amyloid in a biopsy of affected tissue using appropriate stains (e.g., Congo red). Electrophoresis and immunoelectrophoresis of serum and urine may assist in detecting paraproteins. Aspiration of abdominal fat pad or biopsy of rectal mucosa may demonstrate amyloid fibrils.

PROGNOSIS AND TREATMENT   Prognosis is variable and depends on underlying disorder. Prognosis is poor when associated with myeloma, but when associated with chronic infections and infection is successfully treated, remission is possible. Renal failure is major cause of death in progressive amyloidosis.

Management regimens for amyloidosis are not clearly proven effective. Clearly, the underlying disorder should be treated. Primary amyloidosis may respond to regimens incorporating prednisone and alkylating agents (e.g., melphalan), presumably because of the effects of these agents on synthesis of the AL amyloid protein. Colchicine (1–2 mg/d) may block amyloid deposition.

Adjunctive therapies such as renal transplantation may be effective in selected pts.

For a more detailed discussion, see Cohen AS: Amyloidosis, Chap. 266, in HPIM-12, p. 1417

SECTION 9 HEMATOLOGY AND ONCOLOGY

129 EXAMINATION OF BLOOD SMEARS AND BONE MARROW

BLOOD SMEARS

ERYTHROCYTE (RBC) MORPHOLOGY Normal: 7.5-μm diameter.

- *Reticulocytes* (Wright's stain)—large, grayish-blue, admixed with pink (polychromasia); variation in RBC size (anisocytosis) or abnormal shapes (poikilocytosis) may provide clues to causes of anemia.
- *Acanthocytes* (spur cells)—irregularly spiculated; abetalipoproteinemia, severe liver disease, rarely anorexia nervosa.
- *Echinocytes* (burr cells)—regularly shaped, uniformly distributed spiny projections; uremia, RBC volume loss.
- *Elliptocytes*—elliptical; hereditary elliptocytosis.
- *Schizocytes* (schistocytes)—fragmented cells of varying sizes and shapes; microangiopathic or macroangiopathic hemolytic anemia.
- *Sickled cells*—elongated, crescentic; sickle cell anemias.
- *Spherocytes*—small hyperchromic cells lacking normal central pallor; hereditary spherocytosis, extravascular hemolysis as in autoimmune hemolytic anemia, glucose-6-phosphate dehydrogenase (G6PD) deficiency.
- *Target cells*—central and outer rim staining with intervening ring of pallor; liver disease, thalassemia, hemoglobin C and sickle C diseases.
- *Teardrop cells*—myelofibrosis, other infiltrative processes of marrow (e.g., carcinoma).
- *Rouleaux formation*—alignment of RBCs in stacks; may be artifactual or due to paraproteinemia (e.g., multiple myeloma, macroglobulinemia).

RBC INCLUSIONS

- *Howell-Jolly bodies*—1-μm diameter basophilic cytoplasmic inclusion, usually single; asplenic pts.
- *Basophilic stippling*—multiple, punctate basophilic cytoplasmic inclusions; lead poisoning, thalassemia, myelofibrosis.
- *Pappenheimer (iron) bodies*—resemble basophilic stippling, but also stain with Prussian blue; lead poisoning, other sideroblastic anemias.
- *Heinz bodies*—seen only with supravital stains, such as crystal violet; G6PD deficiency (after oxidant stress such as infection, certain drugs), unstable hemoglobin variants.
- *Parasites*—characteristic intracytoplasmic inclusions; malaria, babesiosis.

LEUKOCYTE INCLUSIONS

- *Toxic granulations*—dark cytoplasmic granules; bacterial infection.
- *Döhle bodies*—1–2 μm blue, oval cytoplasmic inclusions; bacterial infection, Chediak-Higashi anomaly.
- *Auer rods*—eosinophilic, rodlike cytoplasmic inclusions; acute myelogenous leukemia (some cases).

PLATELET ABNORMALITIES

- *Platelet clumping*—an in vitro artifact, often readily detectable on smear; can lead to falsely low platelet count by automated cell counters.

BONE MARROW

Aspiration assesses cell morphology. *Biopsy* assesses overall marrow architecture, including degree of cellularity.

INDICATIONS   Aspiration   Hypoproliferative anemia, unexplained leukopenia or thrombocytopenia, suspected leukemia or myeloma, evaluation of iron stores.

Special tests: Histochemical staining (leukemias), cytogenetic studies (leukemias, lymphomas), microbiology (bacterial, mycobacterial, fungal cultures); Prussian blue (iron) stain (assess iron stores; diagnosis of sideroblastic anemias).

Biopsy   Performed in addition to aspiration for possible pancytopenia (rule out aplastic anemia), metastatic tumor, granulomatous infection (e.g., mycobacteria, brucellosis, histoplasmosis), myelofibrosis, lipid storage disease (e.g., Gaucher's, Niemann-Pick), any case with "dry tap" on aspiration.

Special tests: Histochemical staining (e.g., acid phosphatase for metastatic prostate carcinoma), immunoperoxidase staining (e.g., immunoglobulin detection in multiple myeloma, lysozyme detection in monocytic leukemia), reticulin staining (increased in myelofibrosis), microbiological staining (e.g., acid-fast staining for mycobacteria).

INTERPRETATION **Cellularity** Varies inversely with age; a simple formula is: Normal marrow cellularity (%) = 100 − age of patient. Therefore, 70% cellularity normal for a 30-year-old pt but abnormally hypercellular for a 70-year-old pt.

Myeloid:erythroid (M:E) ratio Normally 3:1 to 4:1. The M:E ratio is *increased* in acute and chronic infection, leukemoid reactions (e.g., chronic inflammation, metastatic tumor), acute and chronic myelogenous leukemia, myelodysplastic disorders ("preleukemia") and pure red cell aplasia; *decreased* in agranulocytosis, anemias with erythroid hyperplasia (megaloblastic, iron-deficiency, thalassemia, hemorrhage, hemolysis, sideroblastic), and erythrocytosis (excessive RBC production); *normal* in aplastic anemia (though marrow hypocellular), myelofibrosis (marrow hypocellular), multiple myeloma, lymphoma, anemia of chronic disease.

For a more detailed discussion, see Bunn HF: Anemia, Chap. 61, p. 344, and Dale D: Leukocytosis, Leukopenia, and Eosinophilia, Chap. 64, p. 359, in HPIM-12

ANEMIA

Blood hemoglobin (Hb) concentration <140 g/L (<14 g/dL) or hematocrit (Hct) <42% in adult males; Hb <120 g/L (<12 g/dL) or Hct <37% in adult females.

Basic evaluations: (1) *reticulocyte index,* (2) review of *blood smear* and *RBC indices* [mean corpuscular volume (MCV), mean corpuscular hemoglobin (MCH), mean corpuscular hemoglobin concentration (MCHC)], and (3) determination of *acuteness* or *chronicity* of anemia (Table 130-1).

The *reticulocyte index* (RI) = [reticulocyte count (%) × observed Hct]/(2 × normal Hct). RI <2% implies inadequate RBC production; RI >2% implies excessive RBC destruction or loss.

ANEMIA DUE TO EXCESSIVE RBC DESTRUCTION OR LOSS Blood Loss Trauma, GI hemorrhage (may be occult); less commonly genitourinary sources (menorrhagia, gross hematuria), internal—retroperitoneal, iliopsoas hemorrhage (e.g., in hip fractures).

Hemolysis (see Table 130-2)

1. Hypersplenism (pancytopenia may be present).

2. Immunohemolytic anemia (positive Coombs' test, spherocytes). Two types: (a) *warm* antibody (usually IgG)—idiopathic, lymphomas, chronic lymphocytic leukemia, SLE, drugs (e.g., methyldopa, penicillins, quinine, quinidine, isoniazid, sulfonamides); and (b) *cold* antibody—cold agglutinin disease (IgM) due to *Mycoplasma* infection, infectious mononucleosis, lymphoma, idiopathic; paroxysmal cold hemoglobinuria (IgG) due to syphilis, viral infections.

3. Mechanical trauma (macro- and microangiopathic hemolytic anemias; schistocytes)—prosthetic heart valves, vas-

TABLE 130-1 Initial evaluation of anemia

Blood loss (common)	Under-production (common)	Hemolysis (uncommon)
Test stool for occult blood	↓ Reticulocyte count; RBC indexes and bone marrow are informative	↑ Reticulocyte count ↑ Bilirubin ↓ Haptoglobin Abnormal RBC morphology

From Bunn HF: HPIM-12, p. 345.

TABLE 130-2   Laboratory evaluation of hemolysis

	Moderate hemolysis (RBC life span 20–40 days)	Severe hemolysis (RBC life span 5–20 days)
HEMATOLOGIC		
Routine blood film	Polychromatophilia	Polychromatophilia
Reticulocyte count	↑	↑ ↑
Bone marrow examination	Erythroid hyperplasia	Erythroid hyperplasia
PLASMA OR SERUM		
Bilirubin	↑ Unconjugated	↑ Unconjugated
Haptoglobin	↓, absent	Absent
Hemopexin	Normal, ↓	↓, absent
Plasma hemoglobin	↑	↑ ↑
Lactate dehydrogenase	↑ (variable)	↑ ↑ (variable)
Methemalbumin	0	+ *
URINE		
Bilirubin	0	0
Urobilinogen	Variable	Variable
Hemosiderin	0, +	+
Hemoglobin	0	+ *

* Intravascular hemolysis.
From Cooper RA, Bunn HF: HPIM-12, p. 1532.

culitis, malignant hypertension, eclampsia, renal graft rejection, giant hemangioma, scleroderma, thrombotic thrombocytopenic purpura, hemolytic-uremic syndrome, DIC, march hemoglobinuria (e.g., marathon runners).

4. Direct toxic effect—infections (e.g., malaria, *Clostridia*, toxoplasmosis).

5. Membrane abnormalities—spur cell anemia (cirrhosis, anorexia nervosa), paroxysmal nocturnal hemoglobinuria, hereditary spherocytosis (increased RBC osmotic fragility, spherocytes).

6. Intracellular RBC abnormalities—enzyme defects [glucose-6-phosphate dehydrogenase deficiency (G6PD) (Table 130-3), pyruvate kinase deficiency (PK)], hemoglobinopathies, sickle cell anemia and variants (Table 130-4), thalassemia, unstable hemoglobin variants.

Laboratory abnormalities   Elevated reticulocyte index, polychromasia and nucleated RBCs on smear; also spherocytes, schistocytes, target, spur, or sickle cells may be present depending on disorder; elevated unconjugated serum bilirubin and lactate dehydrogenase (LDH), elevated plasma

TABLE 130-3 Drugs causing hemolysis in subjects deficient in G6PD

Antimalarials: primaquine, pamaquine, chloroquine, dapsone
Sulfonamides: sulfanilamide, sulfasoxazole, etc.
Nitrofurantoin
Analgesics: phenacetin, acetanilid
Miscellaneous: vitamin K (water-soluble form), probenecid, methylene blue, *p*-aminosalicylic acid, nalidixic acid, quinine,* quinidine,* chloramphenicol*

* Not known to cause hemolysis in blacks with A-type G6PD.
From Cooper RA, Bunn HF: HPIM-12, p. 1542.

hemoglobin, low or absent haptoglobin; look for urine hemosiderin or hemoglobin (latter seen in brisk, *intravascular* hemolysis); Coombs' test (immunohemolytic anemias), osmotic fragility test (hereditary spherocytosis), hemoglobin electrophoresis (sickle cell anemia, thalassemia), G6PD assay (best performed *after resolution* of hemolytic episode to prevent false-negative result).

ANEMIA DUE TO INADEQUATE RBC PRODUCTION (Table 130–5)
Hypochromic anemias (MCHC <32%) (1) *Iron deficiency* (e.g., blood loss, pregnancy, impaired gut absorption); (2) *thalassemia;* (3) *sideroblastic anemias* (e.g., hereditary, 2° to drugs such as alcohol, lead). Anemia of chronic disorders (inflammatory, infectious, neoplastic) is also occasionally hypochromic.

Iron studies may help in the differential diagnosis (see Table 130-6).

Normochromic anemias (MCHC 32–36%) May be *normocytic* (MCV 82–94 fL) or *macrocytic* (MCV >94 fL).

Normocytic anemias—(1) Anemia of chronic disease (Table 130-7); (2) endocrinopathies (e.g., hypothyroidism, adrenal insufficiency, hyperparathyroidism); (3) marrow failure

TABLE 130-4 Clinical manifestations of sickle cell anemia

I. Constitutional
   A. Impaired growth and development
   B. Increased susceptibility to infection
II. Vasoocclusive
   A. Microinfarcts → Painful crisis
   B. Macroinfarcts
          Organ damage
III. Anemia
   A. Severe hemolysis
   B. Aplastic crises ←

From Bunn HF: HPIM-12, p. 1545.

TABLE 130-5   Anemias due to decreased red cell production

RBC Indexes	Marrow	Additional lab tests	Diagnosis
Hypochromic, microcytic ($\downarrow$MCV)	0 Iron	$\downarrow$Fe, $\uparrow$TIBC	Iron deficiency
	+ Iron	$\uparrow$Hb A$_2$, $\uparrow$Hb F	β Thalassemia
	Ring sideroblasts	$\downarrow$Hb A$_2$	Sideroblastic anemia
Macrocytic ($\uparrow$MCV)	Megaloblastic	$\downarrow$Serum B$_{12}$, achlorhydria	Vitamin B$_{12}$ deficiency, pernicious anemia
		$\downarrow$Serum folate	Folic acid deficiency
Normochromic, normocytic	Normal	$\downarrow$Fe, $\downarrow$TIBC	Anemia of chronic inflammation
		$\uparrow$Creatinine	Anemia of uremia
		Abn LFT	Anemia of liver disease
		$\downarrow$T$_4$	Anemia of myxedema
Normoblasts, teardrops	Aplastic	Pancytopenia	Aplastic anemia
	Infiltrated: tumor, lymphoma, etc.		Myelophthisic
	Fibrosis	$\uparrow$LAP	Myeloid metaplasia

NOTE: Fe, iron; TIBC, total iron-binding capacity; Hb, hemoglobin; LAP, leukocyte alkaline phosphatase; LFT, liver function tests; Abn, abnormal; MCV, mean corpuscular volume.
From Bunn HF: HPIM-12, p. 345.

(e.g., irradiation, drugs—chloramphenicol, antineoplastic agents; chemicals—benzene; viral—parvovirus, hepatitis B, human immunodeficiency virus); (4) marrow replacement (e.g., metastatic carcinoma, leukemia, myelofibrosis).

Macrocytic anemias—(1) Chronic hepatic disorders (e.g., cirrhosis, chronic hepatitis); (2) alcoholism; (3) hypothyroidism (anemia may also be normocytic); (4) megaloblastic anemias (e.g., B$_{12}$, folate deficiencies); (5) myelodysplasia (Chap. 135).

BONE MARROW EXAMINATION FOR ANEMIA See Chap. 129.

TREATMENT OF ANEMIA   General approaches The acuteness and severity determine whether *transfusion therapy* with packed RBCs is indicated. Rapid occurrence of severe anemia (e.g., after acute GI hemorrhage resulting in Hct <25, following volume repletion) is a general indication for transfusion. For each unit of packed RBCs, Hct should increase 3–4% [Hb by 10 g/L (1 g/dL)], assuming no ongoing losses. *Chronic* anemia (e.g., B$_{12}$ deficiency secondary to pernicious anemia), even when severe, may not require

TABLE 130-6   Differential diagnosis of microcytic, hypochromic anemia

	Iron-deficiency anemia	β-Thalassemia trait	Anemia of chronic disease	Sideroblastic anemia
Serum iron	↓	N	↓	↑
TIBC	↑	N	↓	N
Serum ferritin	↓	N	↑	↑
Red cell protoporphyrin	↑	N	↑	↑ or N
Hb A₂	↓	↑	N	↓

NOTE: ↑ = increased; ↓ = decreased; N = normal; TIBC = total iron-binding capacity.
From Bridges KR, Bunn HF: HPIM-12, p. 1521.

TABLE 130-7   Anemias secondary to chronic systemic diseases

1. Anemia of chronic inflammation
  a. Infection
  b. Connective tissue disorders, etc.
  c. Malignancy
2. Anemia of uremia
3. Anemia due to endocrine failure
4. Anemia of liver disease

From Bunn HF: HPIM-12, p. 1529.

transfusion therapy if the patient is compensated and specific therapy (e.g. parenteral B₁₂) is instituted.

Specific disorders   (1) *Autoimmune hemolysis:* glucocorticoids, sometimes immunosuppressive agents, danazol, plasmapheresis; (2) *G6PD deficiency:* avoid agents known to precipitate hemolysis (e.g., primaquine, sulfonamides, nitrofurantoin); (3) *aplastic anemia:* antithymocyte globulin, bone marrow transplantation; (4) *iron deficiency:* treat cause of blood loss; oral iron (e.g., FeSO₄ 300 mg tid); (5) *B₁₂ deficiency:* parenteral B₁₂ required in most cases (e.g., pernicious anemia—lack of *intrinsic factor* prevents dietary absorption); vitamin B₁₂ 100 μg IM qd for 7 days, then 100–1000 μg IM per month; (6) *folate deficiency:* common in malnourished, alcoholics; folic acid 1 mg PO qd (5 mg qd for patients with malabsorption); (7) *anemia of chronic disease:* treat underlying disease; in uremia use recombinant human erythropoietin.

ERYTHROCYTOSIS

Also known as polycythemia, this is an increase above the normal range of RBCs in the circulation. *Relative erythro-*

cytosis—due to plasma volume loss (e.g., severe dehydration, burns); does not represent a true increase in total RBC mass. *Absolute erythrocytosis*—increase in total RBC mass.

Causes   Polycythemia vera (Chap. 135), erythropoietin-producing neoplasms (e.g., hypernephroma, cerebellar hemangioma), chronic hypoxemia (e.g., high altitude, pulmonary disease), carboxyhemoglobin excess (e.g. smokers), high-affinity hemoglobin variants, Cushing's syndrome, androgen excess.

Complications   Hyperviscosity (with diminished O_2 delivery) with risk of ischemic organ injury.

Treatment   Phlebotomy recommended for Hct >55%, regardless of cause.

For a more detailed discussion, see Bunn HF: Anemia, Chap. 61, p. 344, and Bunn HF et al: The Anemias, Chaps. 290–298, pp. 1514–1570, in HPIM-12

APPROACH Review *smear* (? abnormal cells present) and obtain *differential* count. The normal values for concentration of blood leukocytes are shown in Table 131-1.

NEUTROPHILIA Absolute neutrophil count (polys and bands) >10,000/μL.

Causes (1) *Exercise, stress;* (2) *infections*—esp. bacterial; smear shows increased numbers of immature neutrophils ("left shift"), toxic granulations, Döhle bodies; (3) *burns;* (4) *tissue necrosis* (e.g., myocardial, pulmonary, renal infarction); (5) *chronic inflammatory disorders* (e.g., gout, vasculitis); (6) *drugs* (e.g., glucocorticoids, epinephrine, lithium); (7) *myeloproliferative disorders* (Chap. 135); (8) *metabolic* (e.g., ketoacidosis, uremia); (9) *other*—malignant neoplasms, acute hemorrhage or hemolysis, after splenectomy.

LEUKEMOID REACTION Extreme elevation of leukocyte count (>50,000/μL) secondary to mature and/or immature neutrophils.

Causes (1) *Infection* (severe, chronic), esp. in children; (2) *hemolysis* (severe); (3) *malignant neoplasms* (esp. carcinoma of the breast, lung, kidney). May be distinguished from chronic myelogenous leukemia (CML) by measurement of the *leukocyte alkaline phosphatase (LAP) level:* elevated in leukemoid reactions, depressed in CML.

LEUKOERYTHROBLASTIC REACTION Similar to leukemoid reaction with addition of <u>nucleated RBCs</u> on blood smear.

Causes (1) *Myelophthisis*—invasion of the bone marrow by tumor, fibrosis, granulomatous processes; smear shows "teardrop" RBCs; (2) *hemorrhage or hemolysis* (rarely, in severe cases).

LYMPHOCYTOSIS Absolute lymphocyte count >5000/μL.

Causes (1) *Infection*—infectious mononucleosis, hepatitis, CMV, rubella, pertussis, tuberculosis, brucellosis, syphilis; (2) *endocrine*—thyrotoxicosis, adrenal insufficiency; (3)

TABLE 131-1

Cell type	Mean (cells/μL)	95% confidence limits (cells/μL)	Percent total WBC
Neutrophil	3650	1830–7250	30–60
Lymphocyte	2500	1500–4000	20–50
Monocyte	430	200–950	2–10
Eosinophil	150	0–700	0.3–5
Basophil	30	0–150	0.6–1.8

neoplastic—chronic lymphocytic leukemia (CLL), most common cause of lymphocyte count >10,000/μL.

MONOCYTOSIS   Absolute monocyte count >800/μL.

Causes   (1) *Infection*—subacute bacterial endocarditis, tuberculosis, brucellosis, rickettsial diseases (e.g., Rocky Mountain spotted fever), malaria, leishmaniasis; (2) *granulomatous diseases*—sarcoidosis, Crohn's disease; (3) *collagen-vascular diseases*—rheumatoid arthritis, SLE, polyarteritis nodosa, polymyositis, temporal arteritis; (4) *hematologic*—leukemias, lymphoma, myeloproliferative and myelodysplastic syndromes, hemolytic anemia, chronic idiopathic neutropenia; (5) *malignant neoplasms*.

EOSINOPHILIA   Absolute eosinophil count >500/μL.

Causes   (1) *Drugs;* (2) *parasitic infections;* (3) *allergic diseases;* (4) *collagen-vascular diseases;* (5) *malignant neoplasms;* (6) *hypereosinophilic syndromes*.

BASOPHILIA   Absolute basophil count >100/μL.

Causes   (1) *Allergic diseases;* (2) *myeloproliferative disorders* (esp. CML); (3) *chronic inflammatory disorders* (rarely).

For a more detailed discussion, see Adamson JW: The Myeloproliferative Diseases, Chap. 297, p. 1561; Champlin R, Golde DW: The Leukemias, Chap. 296, p. 1552, HPIM-12

DEFINITION   Total leukocyte count <4300/μL.
NEUTROPENIA   Absolute neutrophil count <2500/μL (increased risk of bacterial infection with count <1000/μL).
Causes   (1) *Drugs*—phenytoin, carbamazepine, indomethacin, chloramphenicol, penicillins, sulfonamides, cephalosporins, propylthiouracil, phenothiazines, captopril, methyldopa, procainamide, chlorpropamide, thiazides, cimetidine, allopurinol, colchicine, ethanol, penicillamine, chemotherapeutic and immunosuppressive agents; (2) *infections*—viral (e.g., influenza, hepatitis, infectious mononucleosis, human immunodeficiency virus), bacterial (e.g., typhoid fever, miliary tuberculosis, fulminant sepsis), malaria; (3) *nutritional*—B$_{12}$, folate deficiencies; (4) *benign*—mild neutropenia common in blacks, no associated risk of infection; (5) *hematologic*—cyclic neutropenia (q 21 d, with recurrent infections common), leukemia, myelodysplasia (preleukemia), aplastic anemia, bone marrow infiltration (uncommon cause), Chediak-Higashi syndrome; (6) *hypersplenism*—e.g., Felty's syndrome, congestive splenomegaly, Gaucher's disease; (7) *autoimmune*—idiopathic, SLE, lymphoma (may see positive anti-neutrophil antibodies).
Management of the febrile, neutropenic patient   In addition to usual sources of infection, consider *"occult" sites* (e.g., paranasal sinuses, oral cavity, anorectal region); empiric therapy with broad-spectrum antibiotics is usually indicated after blood and other appropriate cultures are obtained. Prolonged neutropenia (>14 d) leads to increased risk of disseminated *fungal* infections; may require addition of antifungal chemotherapy (e.g., amphotericin B). Granulocyte transfusions may be helpful (controversial). The duration of chemotherapy-induced neutropenia can be shortened by treatment with the cytokines GM-CSF or G-CSF (experimental).
LYMPHOPENIA   Absolute lymphocyte count <1000/μL.
Causes   (1) *Acute stressful illness*—e.g., myocardial infarction, pneumonia, sepsis; (2) *glucocorticoid therapy*; (3) *lymphoma* (esp. Hodgkin's disease); (4) *immune deficiency syndromes*—ataxia telangiectasia, Wiskott-Aldrich, DiGeorge's syndromes; (5) *immunosuppressive therapy*—e.g., antilymphocyte globulin, cyclophosphamide; (6) *after radiotherapy* (esp. for lymphoma); (7) *intestinal lymphangiectasia* (increased lymph loss); (8) *chronic illness*—e.g., CHF, uremia, SLE, disseminated malignancies; (9) *bone marrow*

failure/replacement—e.g., aplastic anemia, miliary tuberculosis.

MONOCYTOPENIA Absolute monocyte count <100/µL.

Causes (1) *Acute stressful illness*; (2) *glucocorticoid therapy*; (3) *aplastic anemia;* (4) *leukemia* (certain types, e.g., hairy cell leukemia); (5) *chemotherapeutic* and *immunosuppressive* agents.

EOSINOPENIA Absolute eosinophil count <50/µL.

Causes (1) *Acute stressful illness;* (2) *glucocorticoid therapy*.

For a more detailed discussion, see Masur H, Fauci AS: Infections in the Compromised Host, Chap. 82, p. 464; Rappeport JM, Bunn HF: Bone Marrow Failure: Aplastic Anemia and Other Primary Bone Marrow Disorders, Chap. 298, p 1567, in HPIM-12

BLEEDING DISORDERS

Bleeding may result from abnormalities of (1) platelets, (2) blood vessel walls, or (3) coagulation. *Platelet disorders* characteristically produce *petechial* and *purpuric skin lesions* and bleeding from *mucosal* surfaces. *Defective coagulation* results in *ecchymoses, hematomas,* and *mucosal* and, in some disorders, recurrent *joint bleeding* (hemarthroses).

PLATELET DISORDERS Thrombocytopenia Normal platelet count is 150,000–350,000/μL. Bleeding is rare if platelet count >100,000/μL. *Bleeding time,* a measurement of platelet function, is abnormally increased if platelet count <100,000/μL; injury or surgery may provoke excess bleeding. Spontaneous bleeding unusual unless count is <20,000/μL; platelet count <10,000/μL often is associated with serious hemorrhage. *Bone marrow examination* shows increased number of megakaryocytes in disorders associated with accelerated platelet destruction; decreased number in disorders of platelet production.

Causes: (1) *Production defects* such as marrow injury (e.g., drugs, irradiation), marrow failure (e.g., aplastic anemia), marrow invasion (e.g., carcinoma, leukemia, fibrosis); (2) *sequestration* due to *splenomegaly;* (3) *accelerated destruction*—causes include:

- *Drugs* such as chemotherapeutic agents, thiazides, ethanol, estrogens, sulfonamides, quinidine, quinine, methyldopa. *Treatment* includes discontinuation of possible offending agents; expect recovery in 7–10 days. *Heparin-induced* thrombocytopenia is seen in 5% of pts receiving >5 days of therapy; is due to in vivo platelet aggregation. Arterial and occasionally venous *thromboses* may result. Treatment of heparin-induced thrombocytopenia includes prompt discontinuation of heparin. Warfarin and/or a fibrinolytic agent (see below) should be used for treatment of thromboses.
- *Autoimmune* destruction by an *antibody* mechanism; may be idiopathic or associated with SLE, lymphoma, human immunodeficiency virus. *Idiopathic thrombocytopenic purpura* (ITP) has two forms: an *acute,* self-limited disorder of childhood requiring no specific therapy, and a *chronic* disorder of adults (esp. women 20–40 years of age).

Treatment of chronic ITP—prednisone (initially 1–2 mg/kg per day, then slow taper) to keep the platelet count >60,000/μL. Splenectomy, danazol (androgen), or other agents (e.g., vincristine, cyclophosphamide) indicated for pts requiring >5–10 mg prednisone daily.

- *Disseminated intravascular coagulation* (DIC)—platelet consumption with coagulation factor depletion (prolonged PT, PTT) and stimulation of fibrinolysis (generation of fibrin split products, FSP). Blood smear shows microangiopathic hemolysis (schistocytes). *Causes*—infection (esp. meningococcal, pneumococcal, gram-negative bacteremias), extensive burns, trauma, or thrombosis; giant hemangioma, retained dead fetus, heat stroke, mismatched blood transfusion, metastatic carcinoma, acute promyelocytic leukemia. *Treatment*—control of underlying disease most important; platelets, fresh frozen plasma (FFP) to correct clotting parameters. Heparin may be beneficial in pts with acute promyelocytic leukemia.

- *Thrombotic thrombocytopenic purpura*—rare disorder characterized by microangiopathic hemolytic anemia, fever, thrombocytopenia, renal dysfunction (and/or hematuria), and neurologic dysfunction. *Treatment*—plasmapheresis and FFP infusions; recovery in two-thirds of cases.

- *Hemorrhage* with extensive *transfusion*.

Pseudothrombocytopenia Platelet clumping secondary to collection of blood in EDTA (0.3% of pts). Examination of *blood smear* establishes diagnosis.

Thrombocytosis Platelet count >350,000/μL. Either *primary* (thrombocythemia; Chap. 135) or *secondary* (reactive); latter secondary to severe hemorrhage, iron deficiency, surgery, after splenectomy (transient), malignant neoplasms, chronic inflammatory diseases (e.g., inflammatory bowel disease), recovery from acute infection, drugs (e.g., vincristine, epinephrine). *Rebound thrombocytosis* may occur after marrow recovery from cytotoxic agents, alcohol. *Primary* thrombocytosis may be complicated by bleeding and/or thrombosis; secondary rarely causes hemostatic problems.

Disorders of platelet function Suggested by the finding of prolonged bleeding time with normal platelet count. *Causes:* (1) *Drugs*—aspirin, other NSAIDs, dipyridamole, heparin, penicillins, esp. carbenicillin, ticarcillin; (2) *uremia;* (3) *cirrhosis;* (4) *dysproteinemias;* (5) *myeloproliferative* and *myelodysplastic* disorders; (6) *von Willebrand's disease* (see below). *Treatment:* Remove or reverse underlying cause. Dialysis and/or cryoprecipitate infusions (10 bags/24 h) may be helpful for platelet dysfunction associated with uremia.

Platelet transfusion therapy   See Chap. 134.

HEMOSTATIC DISORDERS DUE TO BLOOD VESSEL WALL DEFECTS
Causes: (1) *Aging;* (2) *drugs*—e.g., glucocorticoids (chronic therapy), penicillins, sulfonamides; (3) *vitamin C deficiency;* (4) *Henoch-Schönlein purpura;* (5) *paraproteinemias;* (6) *hereditary hemorrhagic telangiectasia* (Osler-Rendu-Weber disease).

DISORDERS OF BLOOD COAGULATION   Congenital disorders
1. Hemophilia A—most common hereditary disorder of coagulation (1:10,000); sex-linked recessive deficiency of factor VIII (low plasma factor VIII *coagulant* activity, but normal amount of factor VIII-related antigen–von Willebrand's factor). *Laboratory features*—elevated PTT, normal PT. *Treatment*—factor VIII replacement for bleeding or before surgical procedure; degree and duration of replacement depends on severity of bleeding. *Degree* of replacement: Give factor VIII to obtain a 15% (for mild bleeding) to 50% (for severe bleeding) factor VIII level. *Duration:* Ranges from a single dose of factor VIII to therapy bid for up to 2 weeks.

2. Hemophilia B—also sex-linked recessive, due to factor IX deficiency. Clinical and laboratory features similar to hemophilia A. *Treatment*—FFP of factor IX concentrates (Proplex, Konyne).

3. von Willebrand's disease—relatively common, usually autosomal dominant; primary defect is reduced synthesis or chemically abnormal factor VIII-related antigen, resulting in *abnormal platelet function.* *Treatment*—cryoprecipitate (plasma product rich in factor VIII); up to 10 bags bid for 48–72 h, depending upon the severity of bleeding. Desmopressin (vasopressin analogue) may benefit some pts.

Acquired disorders
1. Vitamin K deficiency—impairs production of factors II (prothrombin), VII, IX, and X; major source of vitamin K is dietary (esp. green vegetables) with minor production by gut bacteria. *Laboratory features*—elevated PT and PTT.

2. Liver disease—results in deficiencies of all clotting factors except VIII. *Laboratory features*—elevated PT, normal or elevated PTT. *Treatment*—FFP.

3. Other disorders—DIC, fibrinogen deficiency (liver disease, DIC, L-asparaginase therapy, rattlesnake bites), other factor deficiencies, circulating anticoagulants (lymphoma, SLE, idiopathic), massive transfusion (dilutional coagulopathy).

THROMBOTIC DISORDERS

HYPERCOAGULABLE STATE Consider in pts with recurrent episodes of venous thrombosis (i.e., deep venous thrombosis, DVT; pulmonary embolism). *Causes:* (1) *Venous stasis* (e.g., pregnancy, immobilization); (2) *vasculitis;* (3) *myeloproliferative disorders;* (4) *oral contraceptives;* (5) *lupus anticoagulant*—antibody to platelet phospholipid, *stimulates* coagulation; (6) *heparin-induced thrombocytopenia;* (7) *deficiencies of endogenous anticoagulant factors*—antithrombin III, protein C, protein S; (8) *other*—paroxysmal nocturnal hemoglobinuria, dysfibrinogenemias (abnormal fibrinogen).

Treatment Correct underlying disorder whenever possible; long-term warfarin therapy is otherwise indicated.

ANTITHROMBOTIC THERAPY Anticoagulant agents

1. Heparin—enhances activity of antithrombin III; parenteral agent of choice. In adults, 25,000–40,000 U continuous IV infusion over 24 h following initial IV bolus of 5000 U; monitor by following PTT, should be maintained between 1.5 and 2 times upper normal limit. *Prophylactic* anticoagulation to lower risk of venous thrombosis recommended in some pts (e.g., postoperative, immobilized); dosage is 5000 U SC q 8–12 h. Major *complication* of heparin therapy is *hemorrhage*—manage by discontinuing heparin; for severe bleeding, administer *protamine* (1 mg/100 U heparin); results in rapid neutralization.

2. Warfarin (Coumadin)—vitamin K antagonist, decreases levels of factors II, VII, IX, X and anticoagulant proteins C and S. Administered over 2–3 days; initial load of 5–10 mg PO qd followed by titration of daily dose to keep PT 1.5–2 times control PT. *Complications*—hemorrhage, warfarin-induced skin necrosis (rare), teratogenic effects. Warfarin effect reversed by administration of vitamin K; FFP infused if urgent reversal necessary. Numerous drugs potentiate or antagonize warfarin effect. *Potentiating agents*—chlorpromazine, chloral hydrate, sulfonamides, chloramphenicol, other broad-spectrum antibiotics, allopurinol, cimetidine, tricyclic antidepressants, disulfiram, laxatives, high-dose salicylates, thyroxine, clofibrate. *Antagonizing agents*—vitamin K, barbiturates, rifampin, cholestyramine, oral contraceptives, thiazides.

In-hospital anticoagulation usually initiated with heparin with subsequent maintenance on warfarin after an *overlap* of 3 days.

Fibrinolytic agents Two agents currently available; *streptokinase* and *urokinase;* mediate *clot lysis* by activating plasmin, which degrades fibrin. *Indications*—treatment of

DVT, with lower incidence of postphlebitic syndrome (chronic venous stasis, skin ulceration) than with heparin therapy; massive pulmonary embolism, arterial embolic occlusion of extremity, treatment of acute MI, unstable angina pectoris. Recombinant tissue plasminogen activator (tPA, alteplase) is also effective for treatment of acute MI. *Dosages* for fibrinolytic agents: (1) *Streptokinase*—for *acute MI*, 1.5 million IU IV over 60 min; or 20,000 IU as a bolus intracoronary (IC) infusion, followed by 2000 IU/min for 60 min IC. For *pulmonary embolism* or *arterial* or *deep venous thrombosis*, 250,000 IU IV over 30 min, then 100,000 IU/h for 24 h (pulmonary embolism) or 72 h (arterial or deep venous thrombosis). (2) *Urokinase*—for *pulmonary embolism*, 4400 IU/kg IV over 10 min, then 4400 IU/kg/h IV for 12 h. (3) *tPA*—for *acute MI* (adult >65 kg), 10 mg IV bolus over 1–2 min, then 50 mg IV over 1 h and 40 mg IV over next 2 h (total dose = 100 mg).

Fibrinolytic therapy is usually followed by period of anticoagulant therapy with heparin. Fibrinolytic agents are *contraindicated* in pts with: (1) active internal bleeding, (2) recent (<2–3 months) cerebrovascular accident, (3) intracranial neoplasm, aneurysm, or recent head trauma.

Antiplatelet agents   Aspirin (160–325 mg/d) with or without dipyridamole (50–100 mg qid) may be beneficial in lowering incidence of arterial thrombotic events (stroke, MI) in high-risk pts.

For a more detailed discussion, see Handin RI: Bleeding and Thrombosis, Chap. 62, p. 348; Handin RI: Inherited Thrombotic Disorders and Antithrombotic Therapy, Chap. 289, p. 1511, in HPIM-12

---

134 BLOOD TRANSFUSION AND PHERESIS THERAPY

In general, individual components, not whole blood, should be used. With hemorrhage, packed RBCs, fresh frozen plasma (FFP), and platelets in an approximate ratio of 3:1:10 units are an adequate replacement for whole blood.

TRANSFUSIONS

RED BLOOD CELL TRANSFUSION Indicated for symptomatic anemia unresponsive to specific therapy or requiring urgent correction. In general, transfusions should be withheld when Hb >90 g/L (>9 g/dL) (Hct >27%); may be indicated when Hb is between 70 and 90 g/L (7 and 9 g/dL), esp. in pts with ischemic cardiovascular disease. Transfusion almost always necessary when Hb <70 g/L (<7 g/dL). One unit of packed RBCs raises the Hb by approximately 10 g/L (1 g/dL).

Other indications (1) *Hypertransfusion therapy*—e.g., thalassemia, sickle cell anemia; (2) *exchange transfusion*—hemolytic disease of newborn; (3) *transplant recipients*—decreases rejection of cadaveric kidney transplants.

Complications (1) *Transfusion reaction*—immediate or delayed; IgA-deficient pts at particular risk for severe reaction; (2) *infection*—bacterial (rare), hepatitis, most commonly non-A, non-B (also hepatitis B, CMV), human immunodeficiency virus (HIV), cause of AIDS (antibody screening of donated blood now routinely performed); (3) *pulmonary leukoagglutinin reaction*—rare; (4) *circulatory overload*; (5) *iron overload*—usually after 100 U of RBCs (less in children), in absence of blood loss; can result in *hemochromatosis*—iron chelation therapy with *deferoxamine* indicated.

AUTOLOGOUS TRANSFUSION Use of pt's own stored blood; avoids hazards of donor blood; also useful in pts with multiple RBC antibodies.

GRANULOCYTE TRANSFUSION May be of benefit in severe neutropenia (<500 granulocytes/μL) with bacterial infection unresponsive to appropriate antibiotics; short (<24 h) life span and potential for severe leukoagglutinin reactions limit utility.

PLATELET TRANSFUSION Prophylactic transfusions usually reserved for platelet count <10,000/μL. One unit elevates the count by about 10,000/μL if no platelet antibodies are present as a result of prior transfusions. Efficacy assessed by 1-h and 24-h posttransfusion platelet counts. HLA-matched single-donor platelets may be required in pts with platelet alloantibodies.

THERAPEUTIC HEMAPHERESIS

DEFINITION   Removal of a cellular or plasma constituent of blood; specific procedure referred to by the blood fraction removed.

LEUKAPHERESIS   Removal of WBCs; most often used in acute leukemia, esp. acute myelogenous leukemia (AML) in cases complicated by marked elevation ($>$50,000/μL) of the peripheral blast count, to lower risk of *leukostasis* (blast-mediated vasoocclusive events resulting in CNS or pulmonary infarction, hemorrhage).

PLATELETPHERESIS   Used in some patients with *thrombocytosis* associated with myeloproliferative disorders with bleeding and/or thrombotic complications; not practical for long-term control (Chap. 133). Also used to enhance platelet yield from blood donors.

PLASMAPHERESIS   Indications   (1) *Hyperviscosity* states (e.g., Waldenström's macroglobulinemia); (2) *thrombotic thrombocytopenic purpura* (Chap. 133); (3) *immune complex and autoantibody disorders*—e.g., Goodpasture's syndrome, rapidly progressive glomerulonephritis, myasthenia gravis; possibly Guillain-Barré, SLE.

For a more detailed discussion, see Giblett ER: Blood Groups and Blood Transfusion, Chap. 286, in HPIM-12, p. 1494

---

135 MYELOPROLIFERATIVE AND MYELODYSPLASTIC DISORDERS

MYELOPROLIFERATIVE DISEASES

Stem cell disorders characterized by autonomous proliferation of one or more hematopoietic cell lines (erythroid, myeloid, megakaryocytic) in the bone marrow; results in excess number of cells in peripheral blood and, in some cases, liver and spleen (extramedullary hematopoiesis). Four basic disorders.

CHRONIC MYELOGENOUS (GRANULOCYTIC) LEUKEMIA Characterized by splenomegaly and leukocytosis (WBC typically 50,000–200,000) with a spectrum of granulocyte precursors and mature granulocytes in blood. Associated with characteristic chromosomal abnormality (Philadelphia chromosome, a 9;22 translocation). Two phases of disease—*chronic phase*, relatively indolent, lasting 2–3 years, followed by *blastic phase*, resembling acute leukemia, usually rapidly fatal.

Treatment During chronic phase, *cytotoxic agents* (busulfan, hydroxyurea) and/or *interferon* can control granulocyte count, but are not curative; *bone marrow transplantation* may be curative in some pts.

POLYCYTHEMIA VERA Characterized by excessive production of erythroid cells, resulting in elevation of the blood hemoglobin and hematocrit. WBC and platelet overproduction also occurs in >50% of pts. Increased RBC mass results in increased blood volume and blood *viscosity*.

Clinical features Pruritus, plethoric facies, retinal vein engorgement, impairment of cerebral circulation (headache, tinnitus, dizziness, visual disturbances, transient ischemic events). Accelerated *atherosclerotic and thrombotic disease* are typical (stroke, myocardial infarction, peripheral vascular disease; uncommonly mesenteric, hepatic vein thrombosis); *hemorrhage* (esp. epistaxis, GI); *splenomegaly* in 75%.

Diagnosis Exclusion of secondary causes of an elevated RBC mass (e.g., chronic hypoxemia, excess carboxyhemoglobin, erythropoietin-producing neoplasm).

Treatment Aimed at reducing the RBC mass toward normal, usually with repeated *phlebotomy*, ^{32}P radiotherapy. About 20% of pts progress to *myelofibrosis*, <5% to leukemia (higher if treated with alkylating agents; no longer recommended).

MYELOFIBROSIS (MYELOID METAPLASIA)   Fibrosis of bone marrow and extramedullary hematopoiesis (myeloid metaplasia) involving spleen and liver (splenomegaly in all cases; hepatomegaly in one-half).

Clinical features   Thromboses increased, hemorrhage uncommon.

Diagnosis   Anemia, with abnormal blood smear: RBC atypia (teardrops, other poikilocytes, nucleated RBCs, basophilic stippling, giant platelet forms); bone marrow *biopsy* the definitive test—marrow fibrosis can be documented by *reticulin staining*. May also see *osteosclerosis* (increased bone density). *Secondary* causes of myelofibrosis in the differential diagnosis: metastatic tumor, tuberculosis, Paget's disease, Gaucher's disease.

Treatment   Supportive, with median survival about 4 years.

ESSENTIAL THROMBOCYTOSIS (THROMBOCYTHEMIA)   Excessive megakaryocytic proliferation leading to platelet excess; platelet count $>800,000/\mu L$. Anemia usually present, often secondary to iron deficiency from blood loss.

Clinical features   Resembles polycythemia vera; recurrent hemorrhage and thrombosis.

Diagnosis   Elevated platelet count and abnormal platelet forms (e.g., giant platelets) on blood smear; exclude secondary causes of an elevated platelet count (Chap. 133).

Treatment   Aimed at lowering the platelet count (alkylating agents, hydroxyurea, ^{32}P). Acute reduction in platelet count by plateletpheresis indicated in occasional pt presenting with severe hemorrhage. Possible benefit of antiplatelet agents (aspirin, dipyridamole) for recurrent thromboses.

MYELODYSPLASTIC SYNDROMES

A *heterogeneous* group of disorders of persons over age 50 characterized by *peripheral cytopenias* (one or more lines) in the presence of a normocellular or hypercellular marrow and *dysplastic maturation* of one or more of the marrow cell lineages; 25–50% of pts progress to *acute myelogenous leukemia* (AML) (Chap. 136); syndromes often referred to as *preleukemia*.

Treatment   Rarely successful after progression to acute leukemia, in contrast to patients with de novo AML.

For a more detailed discussion, see Adamson JW: The Myeloproliferative Diseases, Chap. 297, in HPIM-12, p. 1561

136 THE LEUKEMIAS

DEFINITION A heterogeneous group of malignant neoplasms developing from hematopoietic (blood-forming) cells. The cells of these neoplasms proliferate in bone marrow and lymphoid tissues and eventually involve peripheral blood and infiltrate other organ systems. These disorders are classified on the basis of the cell line involved as either *myeloid* or *lymphoid* and as acute or chronic depending on the course of progression of the illness.

ETIOLOGY In most cases, the etiology is not known. Congenital syndromes, radiation, and chemical exposure are important factors in some cases. The human T-cell leukemia virus (HTLV-I) is associated with adult T-cell leukemia (see HPIM-12, Chap. 296 for additional details).

PATHOPHYSIOLOGY The proliferating cell in acute leukemias is an immature clonal myeloid or lymphoid cell that may demonstrate varying degrees of differentiation. These proliferating cells accumulate in bone marrow primarily because they fail to mature past the myeloblast or promyelocyte level in acute myelogenous leukemia (AML) or the lymphoblast level in acute lymphocytic leukemia (ALL). The neoplastic cells in many forms of acute and chronic leukemia demonstrate characteristic cytogenetic abnormalities. Many pts with leukemia demonstrate pancytopenia, which may result from bone marrow crowding by malignant cells or may be the result of direct effects of the leukemic cells or their interaction with the bone marrow microenvironment. Infiltration of leukemic cells into other organ systems may produce the varied clinical manifestations of advanced leukemia.

ACUTE LEUKEMIA

PATHOLOGY AND CLASSIFICATION Bone marrow in acute leukemia is typically hypercellular and heavily infiltrated with a monomorphic population of leukemic blasts; numbers of normal bone marrow elements are markedly reduced. Prognostic and therapeutic considerations make it crucial to distinguish between AML and ALL. These disorders are classified on the basis of cellular morphology, cytochemical features, immunologic phenotype, and degree of differentiation. A collaborative French-American-British (FAB) group has divided ALL into 3 subtypes (L1, L2, and L3) and AML into 7 subtypes (M1 through M7) based on morphologic features.

Leukemic lymphoblasts in ALL are typically smaller than in AML and have round or convoluted nuclei and small amounts of cytoplasm. In >90% of pts with ALL, these cells contain terminal deoxynucleotidal transferase (TdT), rarely present in AML cells. In approximately 60% of cases, cells express the common ALL antigen (CALLA) but are negative for surface immunoglobulin or T-cell markers. About 20% of ALL cases are of T-cell type, and the cells express T-cell surface markers; some 5% of ALL are of B-cell type and represent the leukemic form of the B-cell neoplasm, Burkitt's lymphoma (L3 in the FAB classification). Approximately 15% of cases are of null cell type.

AML blasts are usually larger than those seen in ALL and have a lower nuclear-cytoplasmic ratio. Cytoplasm of the cells may stain positive for such enzymatic markers as peroxidase or esterase and may contain Auer rods (abnormal primary granules). Clinical differences among the 7 subtypes of AML in the FAB classification are subtle. Pts with acute promyelocytic leukemia (M3) frequently present with DIC.

CLINICAL AND LABORATORY FEATURES

- Initial symptoms of acute leukemia usually present for less than 3 months; a preleukemic syndrome may be present in some 25% of pts with AML.
- WBC may be low, normal, or markedly elevated; circulating blast cells may or may not be present; with WBC >100,000 blasts/μL leukostasis in lungs and brain may occur.
- Thrombocytopenia and spontaneous bleeding, especially when platelet count <20,000/μL.
- Bacterial and fungal infection common; risk is heightened when total neutrophil count <500/μL; breakdown of mucosal and cutaneous barriers aggravates susceptibility; infections may be clinically occult in presence of severe leukopenia, and prompt recognition requires a high degree of clinical suspicion.
- Hepatosplenomegaly and lymphadenopathy are common in ALL, less so in AML; leukemic meningitis may present with headache, nausea, seizures, papilledema, cranial nerve palsies; testicular involvement in males with ALL.
- Metabolic abnormalities may include hyponatremia, hypokalemia, elevated serum LDH, hyperuricemia, and (rarely) lactic acidosis.

TREATMENT OF ACUTE LEUKEMIA General considerations

Leukemic cell mass at time of presentation may be 10^{11}–10^{12} cells; when total leukemic cell numbers fall below approximately 10^9, they are no longer detectable in blood or bone marrow and pt appears to be in complete remission. Thus aggressive therapy must continue past the point when initial cell bulk is reduced if leukemia is to be eradicated. Typical phases of chemotherapy include *remission induction, consolidation, maintenance,* and *late intensification.*

Supportive care with transfusions of red cells, granulocytes, and platelets is very important, as are aggressive prevention, diagnosis, and treatment of infections.

Treatment of ALL

- With current ALL therapy, >50% of children will achieve probable cure; prognosis for adults not as good.
- Remission-induction chemotherapy usually includes vincristine and prednisone plus either L-asparaginase or daunorubicin.
- CNS prophylaxis with radiation or intrathecal chemotherapy is effective in reducing rates of CNS relapse.
- Maintenance chemotherapy for 2–3 years or longer should follow the above measures.

Treatment of AML   60–80% of pts with AML will achieve initial remission when treated with regimens including cytarabine and daunorubicin with or without 6-thioguanine; following intensive consolidation and maintenance therapy, 10–30% of pts may achieve 5-year disease-free survival and probable cure; duration of remissions induced after relapse is short, and prognosis for pts who have relapsed is poor.

Bone marrow transplantation   Bone marrow transplantation from identical twin or HLA-identical sibling is effective treatment for ALL or AML. Typical protocol uses high-dose chemotherapy or total-body irradiation to ablate host marrow, followed by infusion of marrow from donor. Risks are substantial (unless marrow is from identical twin). Complications include graft-versus-host disease, interstitial pneumonitis, opportunistic infections (especially CMV). Some 10–15% of otherwise end-stage pts with refractory leukemia may achieve probable cure; results are better when transplant is performed during remission. Results are best for children and young adults. Unanswered questions about transplantation include: (1) timing of transplant in adults and children with high-risk forms of ALL; (2) use of transplantation vs. postremission chemotherapy for pts with AML in first remission; (3) role of unrelated HLA-identical donors for pts without related donor; and (4) potential usefulness of *autologous marrow transplantation* (pt's marrow is harvested during remission and cryopreserved for later reinfusion following intensive chemoradiotherapy; harvested marrow is frequently treated to kill residual leukemic cells).

CHRONIC LEUKEMIA

CHRONIC LYMPHOCYTIC LEUKEMIA (CLL)

- CLL is a neoplasm characterized by accumulation of mature-appearing lymphocytes in blood and bone marrow; 95% of cases involve B lymphocytes; spleen and lymph nodes may be infiltrated; pts are usually over 50 years old. CLL is frequently an incidental finding on CBC.
- Complications include cytopenia, Coombs-positive hemolytic anemia, hypogammaglobulinemia, infection, evolution into lymphoma (Richter's syndrome).
- Many pts require no therapy; some may need therapy with alkylating agents, glucocorticoids, immunoglobulin infusion.

CHRONIC MYELOGENOUS LEUKEMIA (CML)

- CML is usually characterized by splenomegaly and production of increased numbers of granulocytes; course is initially indolent but eventuates in leukemic phase (blast crisis); rate of progression to blast crisis is variable; overall survival averages 3½ years from diagnosis.
- More than 95% of pts have characteristic chromosomal abnormality, Philadelphia chromosome.
- Blastic phase may involve cells of either lymphoid or myeloid origin.
- Treatment of chronic phase involves control of cell counts with alkylating agents or hydroxyurea; blast crisis is usually refractory to most regimens, but ALL or AML programs may be useful; bone marrow transplantation during chronic phase may improve prognosis in some pts.

HAIRY-CELL LEUKEMIA

Hairy-cell leukemia (HCL) is a lymphoid neoplasm marked by cytopenia, splenomegaly, and proliferation of typical cells (with characteristic cytoplasmic projections) in blood and bone marrow. Malignant cells are almost always B cells; T-cell variants are rare. Cells stain positively for tartrate-resistant acid phosphatase (TRAP). *Complications* include vasculitis and frequent infection.

Treatment   Splenectomy is the cornerstone of therapy; it ameliorates disease in majority of pts. Alpha-interferon is of therapeutic benefit for many pts. Conventional chemotherapy is contraindicated because of poor marrow reserve.

Disease can be quite indolent, and prognosis is variable; ≥50% of pts will survive more than 8 years from diagnosis.

For a more detailed discussion, see Champlin R, Golde DW: The Leukemias, Chap. 296, p. 1552; Adamson JW: The Myeloproliferative Diseases, Chap. 297, p. 1561, in HPIM-12

137 HODGKIN'S DISEASE AND OTHER LYMPHOMAS

DEFINITION Malignant lymphomas are tumors characterized by malignant transformation of lymphoid or monocytoid cells. Two major variants are *Hodgkin's disease* (HD) and *non-Hodgkin's lymphoma*. Diagnosis requires biopsy of affected tissue. Table 137-1 summarizes characteristics of two varieties of lymphomas.

CELLULAR ORIGINS Some 90% of non-Hodgkin's lymphomas are of B-cell origin; 10% are T cell–derived. The derivation of the malignant cells in Hodgkin's disease is unknown.

NON-HODGKIN'S LYMPHOMA

ETIOLOGY AND EPIDEMIOLOGY Etiology for most cases is unknown; EBV is associated with African Burkitt's lymphoma; HTLV-I is associated with adult T-cell lymphoma. There is increased incidence of non-Hodgkin's lymphomas in HIV infection. Pts previously treated with chemotherapy and radiation for malignancy are at higher risk.

CLINICAL MANIFESTATIONS

- Two-thirds present with painless peripheral lymphadenopathy. Biopsy of affected node necessary for diagnosis. ''B

TABLE 137-1 The malignant lymphomas

	Non-Hodgkin's	Hodgkin's
Cellular derivation	90% B Cell 10% T Cell Rare monocytic	Unresolved
Sites of disease		
Localized	Uncommon	Common
Nodal spread	Discontiguous	Contiguous
Extranodal	Common	Uncommon
Mediastinal	Uncommon	Common
Abdominal	Common	Uncommon
Bone marrow	Common	Uncommon
B systemic symptoms*	Uncommon	Common
Chromosomal translocation	Common	Yet to be described
Curability	<25%	>75%

* Fever, night sweats, weight loss of greater than 10% of body weight.
From Nadler L: HPIM-12, p. 1599.

symptoms'' (fever, sweats, weight loss) are less common than with Hodgkin's disease.
- Mediastinal adenopathy is present in approximately 20%. Superior vena cava syndrome may result.
- Involvement of retroperitoneal, mesenteric, pelvic nodes common. May arise in GI tract. Primary CNS site seen commonly in AIDS pts.

PATHOLOGIC CLASSIFICATION Classification schemes have evolved as histologic and immunologic methods of classifying tumors have improved. Table 137-2 compares the Working Formulation and Rappaport Classification systems.

APPROACH TO THE PATIENT
1. Biopsy diagnosis.
2. Establish stage of disease to assist in determining appropriate therapy and prognosis. Stages are summarized in Table 137-3.
   a. CBC, chemistry panels, serum protein electrophoresis.
   b. Laryngoscopy, GI studies.
   c. Chest and abdominopelvic CT.
   d. Bilateral bone marrow studies.
   e. Surgical staging (laparotomy) usually not needed.
3. Establish treatment regimen:
   a. Radiotherapy—role limited in non-Hodgkin's lymphoma; may be curative in stage I (any grade) or stage II low-grade lymphomas; useful palliative role for many pts.
   b. Chemotherapy—standard therapeutic approach for most stage II and all stage III and IV non-Hodgkin's lymphomas. Combination regimens including alkylating agents, vinca alkaloids, anthracyclines, and other agents are usually employed.
   c. Bone marrow transplantation—posttreatment infusion of autologous or HLA-matched marrow may permit use of more aggressive chemotherapy regimens for resistant or relapsing disease.
   d. Immunotherapy and use of growth factors are being investigated.

PROGNOSIS Varies with histologic type and stage; complete remission rates in excess of 80% possible with combination chemotherapy of low- and intermediate-grade lymphomas.

HODGKIN'S DISEASE

CLINICAL MANIFESTATIONS Histological classification is summarized in Table 137-4.

- Usually presents with asymptomatic lymph node enlargement or with adenopathy associated with fever, night

TABLE 137-2 Histologic classification of non-Hodgkin's lymphoma

Working formulation, malignant lymphoma	Rappaport terminology	Cellular origin, % B	T	Chromosomal abnormalities
LOW-GRADE				
A. Small lymphocytic cell	Diffuse well-differentiated lymphocytic (DWDL)	98	2	Trisomy 12 t(11;14) t(14;19)
B. Follicular, predominantly small cleaved cell	Nodular poorly differentiated lymphocytic (NPDL)	100		t(14;18)
C. Follicular mixed, small cleaved and large cell	Nodular mixed lymphocytic histiocytic (NM)	100		t(14;18) Trisomy 8
INTERMEDIATE-GRADE				
D. Follicular, predominantly large cell	Nodular histiocytic (NH)	100		Trisomy 7
E. Diffuse small cleaved cell	Diffuse poorly differentiated lymphocytic (DPDL)	80	20	
F. Diffuse mixed, small and large cell	Diffuse mixed lymphocytic-histiocytic (DM)	90	10	Trisomy 3
G. Diffuse large cell	Diffuse histiocytic (DH)	80	20	Trisomy 7, 18 t(14;18)
HIGH-GRADE				
H. Large cell immunoblastic	Diffuse histiocytic (DH)	80	20	
I. Lymphoblastic	Diffuse lymphoblastic (LL)	10	90	
J. Small noncleaved cell; Burkitt's	Diffuse undifferentiated (DUL)	95	5	t(8;14)

From Nadler L: HPIM-12, p. 1600.

sweats, weight loss, and sometimes pruritus. mediastinal adenopathy (common in nodular sclerosing HD) may produce cough.
- SVC obstruction or spinal cord compression may be presenting manifestation.
- Visceral involvement of bone marrow, liver, etc., may be seen, especially in advanced disease.

TABLE 137-3 Ann Arbor staging system

Stage I	Involvement of single lymph node region or single extralymphatic site.
Stage II	Involvement of two or more lymph node regions on the same side of the diaphragm. Can also include localized involvement of extralymphatic site (stage IIE).
Stage III	Involvement of lymph node regions or extralymphatic sites on both sides of the diaphragm.
Stage IV	Disseminated involvement of one or more extralymphatic organs with or without lymph node involvement.

NOTE: Substage A = asymptomatic pts; substage B = pts with history of fever, sweats, or weight loss of greater than 10% bodyweight.
From Nadler L: HPIM-12, p. 1604.

DIFFERENTIAL DIAGNOSIS

- Infection—mononucleosis, viral syndromes, toxoplasma, histoplasma, primary tuberculosis.
- Other malignancies—especially head and neck cancers.
- Sarcoidosis—mediastinal and hilar adenopathy.

IMMUNOLOGIC AND HEMATOLOGIC ABNORMALITIES

- Defects in cell-mediated immunity (remains even after successful treatment of lymphoma); cutaneous anergy; diminished antibody production to capsular antigens of *Haemophilus* and pneumococcus.
- Anemia; elevated ESR; leukemoid reaction; eosinophilia; lymphocytopenia; fibrosis and granulomas in marrow.

STAGING Important to determine extent of disease and guide choice of treatment protocol; should include thorough physical exam, CXR, lymphangiogram, abdominal CT and ultrasound examinations. Bone marrow biopsy, laparoscopy, or staging laparotomy should be used in certain selected cases.

TREATMENT More than 70% of pts with HD are curable with radiotherapy, combination chemotherapy, or both. Therapy should be performed by experienced clinicians in centers with appropriate facilities. Treatment and prognosis depend on stage and cell type. Generally, stages I and II are treated with radiotherapy, whereas stages III and IV receive chemotherapy. However, treatment protocols vary, and combinations of radio- and chemotherapy may be employed.

COMPLICATIONS OF LYMPHOMAS AND THEIR THERAPIES

- Infection—opportunistic organisms common.
- Obstruction of SVC, airways, esophagus, urinary or GI tracts. Infiltration of CNS, lung, skin, and other organ systems.

TABLE 137-4 Rye classification of Hodgkin's disease

Histologic subgroup	Incidence, %	Pathology RS*	Other	Prognosis
Lymphocyte-predominant	2–10	Rare	Predominance of normal-appearing lymphocytes	Excellent
Nodular sclerosis	40–80	Frequent "lacunae"	Lymphoid nodules, collagen bands	Very good
Mixed cellularity	20–40	Numerous	Pleomorphic infiltrate	Good
Lymphocyte-depleted	2–15	Numerous, often bizarre	Paucity of lymphocytes, pleomorphic, fibrosis	Poor

* RS = Reed-Sternberg cell.
From Nadler L: HPIM-12, p. 1609.

- Anemia, leukopenia, leukocytosis, thrombocytopenia, or thrombocytosis.
- Metabolic abnormalities—hypercalcemia, hyperuricemia.
- Radiation toxicity to susceptible organs.
- Secondary malignancies, especially AML, may follow therapy.

For a more detailed discussion, see Nadler LM: The Malignant Lymphomas, Chap. 302, in HPIM-12, p. 1599

Plasma cell disorders are monoclonal malignancies of the B-lymphocyte system characterized by excessive proliferation of plasma cells (antibody-secreting descendants of B lymphocytes) and secretion of cell products (immunoglobulin molecules or subunits or lymphokines).

Serum from pts with plasma cell tumors frequently contains a monoclonal protein that represents the immunoglobulin molecule (or heavy or light chain) produced by the malignant cells. This protein is called the M component (M for monoclonal), and in any given pt the amount of M component in the serum represents a measure of the pt's tumor burden. Some pts may excrete light chains in their urine (Bence Jones protein); this may be the only evidence of the abnormal protein in certain individuals. M components also may be seen in other neoplasms as well as in some infectious or immune-mediated diseases.

MULTIPLE MYELOMA

Multiple myeloma (also called simply myeloma) is a malignant proliferation of plasma cells chiefly in the bone marrow but also other organ systems. Cells may form solitary tumor masses known as plasmacytomas.

PATHOGENESIS AND CLINICAL MANIFESTATIONS

- Bone pain most common symptom; bone lesions are osteolytic without osteoblastic new bone formation, so are not well-visualized on radioisotopic bone scanning. Pathologic fractures may develop; vertebral body collapse may lead to spinal cord compression.
- Infection—recurrent infection may be presenting complaint in 25% of pts; may be significant *hypogammaglobulinemia* (when M component is excluded).
- Hypercalcemia.
- Renal failure—related to hypercalcemia and toxic effects of light chains on renal tubules.
- Neuropathies may be due to amyloid infiltration of nerves.
- Hyperviscosity syndrome—causes fatigue, headache, visual disturbances, and retinopathy.
- Hematologic disturbances—anemia in approximately 80%; granulocytopenia and thrombocytopenia are rare; clotting abnormalities may be present; cryoglobulins may be present.

DIAGNOSIS   Classic triad of myeloma is (1) marrow plasmacytosis (>10%), (2) lytic bone lesions, and (3) a serum and/or urine M component. Studies to determine diagnosis and staging should include:

• CBC, platelet count.   • Bone marrow aspiration and biopsy.   • Serum and urine electrophoresis and immunoelectrophoresis to detect and quantitate M component. • Skeletal radiographic survey—"punched out" lesions are characteristic of myeloma.   • Serum calcium.   • Serum viscosity.

Staging systems (see Table 265-2, in HPIM-12) correlate with survival.

Differential diagnosis   Includes benign monoclonal gammopathy (or monoclonal gammopathy of uncertain significance). 11% of pts with monoclonal gammopathy of uncertain significance will go on to develop myeloma.

TREATMENT   It is generally felt that cure is not possible in myeloma, so therapy must be tailored to individual case. Some pts will have a very indolent course and not require therapy, but majority will require therapy for an indefinite period of time. Standard therapy usually involves pulses of an alkylating agent (such as L-phenylalanine mustard, cyclophosphamide, or chlorambucil) and prednisone for 4–7 d every 4–6 weeks. Response to treatment may be judged by symptomatic improvement and decrease in serum M component (may lag behind symptomatic relief). Optimal duration of initial course of treatment is uncertain but usually is 1–2 years.

Supportive care of complications also must be given. Prognosis relates to stage of disease and response to treatment. Approximately 25% of pts may die of diseases unrelated to their myeloma.

WALDENSTRÖM'S MACROGLOBULINEMIA

Also a malignancy of lymphoplasmacytoid cells, but in contrast to myeloma is associated with lymphadenopathy and hepatosplenomegaly; cells secrete IgM; hyperviscosity is main clinical manifestation; bony lesions and hypercalcemia not seen; renal disease not common because size of IgM M component prevents glomerular filtration; cryoglobulinemia occurs in about 10% of pts.

TREATMENT   Identical to that of myeloma; plasmapheresis may be necessary for serious hyperviscosity symptoms; absence of serious organ system involvement in Waldenström's improves prognosis compared to that for myeloma.

HEAVY CHAIN DISEASES

Rare lymphoplasmacytic malignancies; clinical manifestations vary with heavy chain isotype secreted.

GAMMA HEAVY CHAIN DISEASE (FRANKLIN'S DISEASE) Characterized by lymphadenopathy, fever, anemia, malaise, hepatosplenomegaly, weakness; palatal edema may result from node involvement of Waldeyer's ring; usually demonstrates rapid downhill course with death from infection; chemotherapy may prolong survival.

ALPHA HEAVY DISEASE (SELIGMANN'S DISEASE) Most common of heavy chain diseases; lymphoplasmacytoid infiltration of intestinal lamina propria causes diarrhea, malabsorption, weight loss, mesenteric and paraaortic adenopathy; clinical course very variable.

MU HEAVY CHAIN DISEASE Appears to be a rare subset of chronic lymphocytic leukemia; tumor cells may have a defect in assembly of heavy and light chains.

For a more detailed discussion, see Longo DL: Plasma Cell Disorders, Chap. 265, in HPIM-12, p. 1410

---

139 CANCER CHEMOTHERAPY

BIOLOGY OF TUMOR GROWTH An understanding of the biologic principles of tumor growth is essential to rational therapy of malignancies. The malignant phenotype of a cell is the end result of a series of changes in various aspects of mechanisms controlling growth and cellular development. Among these changes is increased or abnormal expression of certain highly conserved genes known as proto-oncogenes. These genes are found in the normal human genome, their products show partial homology with some growth factors and growth factor receptors, and alterations in their structure or relocation in the genome may have profound effects on control of cellular growth.

In addition to uncontrolled growth, malignant cells have the ability to metastasize. This capacity appears to be related to deregulation of genetic mechanisms once responsible for normal cell adhesion and migration, the ability of malignant cells to express receptors for basement membrane components, and the power of enzymes to disrupt the basement membrane and allow cells to escape from the primary site.

Once cells are malignant, their growth kinetics are similar to those of normal cells. Tumor growth kinetics are expressed by a Gompertzian function: as the tumor mass increases, the growth is matched by an exponential retardation of growth. Cancer cells proceed through the same cell-cycle stages as normal cycling cells: G_1 (period of normal cell metabolism without DNA synthesis), S (DNA synthesis), G_2 (tetraploid phase preceding mitosis), and M (mitosis). Some noncycling cells may remain in a G_0 phase for long periods. Certain chemotherapeutic agents are specific for cells in certain phases of the cell cycle, a fact that is important in designing effective chemotherapeutic regimens.

DEVELOPMENT OF DRUG RESISTANCE Drug resistance of cancer cells may be viewed as either temporary or permanent. *Temporary resistance* refers to an inability of drugs to kill cells because cells are in the wrong phase of the cell cycle, are in pharmacologic sanctuaries such as the CNS or testis, or are in the center of a poorly vascularized tumor. *Permanent resistance* arises because of fundamental changes in the way in which the cell transports, activates, deactivates, or repairs damage caused by the drug in question.

The Goldie-Coldman hypothesis postulates that, as in bacteria, permanent drug resistance occurs in tumor cells as the result of random genetic mutations at a rate of perhaps

542

1 in 10^6 cells. Thus in a tumor of minimally detectable size of approximately 10^9 cells there is a good chance of occurrence of singly or even doubly resistant cell lines. As tumor size and cell number increase, the number of multiply drug-resistant cell lines will increase as well. This is consistent with the observations that reduction of tumor bulk often improves responsiveness to chemotherapy and that initially responsive tumors will regrow during continued exposure to drug therapy. Implications of the Goldie-Coldman hypothesis explain the usefulness of multidrug regimens in overcoming problems of resistance and the importance of early treatment in improving success of chemotherapy.

DISEASES WITH MAJOR ROLE FOR CHEMOTHERAPY

Acute lymphocytic leukemia (ALL)
Acute myelocytic leukemia (AML)
Anal cancer
Medulloblastoma
Adult gliomas
Breast cancer
Choriocarcinoma
Embryonal rhabdomyosarcoma
Ewing's sarcoma
Hairy-cell leukemia
Hodgkin's disease
Small cell lung cancer
Lymphocytic lymphomas
Mycosis fungoides
Ovarian carcinoma
Osteogenic sarcoma
Soft tissue sarcomas
Testicular carcinomas
Wilms' tumor

DISEASES WITH MODERATE ROLE FOR CHEMOTHERAPY

Adrenocortical carcinoma
Bladder carcinoma
Cervical carcinoma
Chronic lymphocytic leukemia
Chronic myelocytic leukemia
Endometrial carcinoma
Gastric carcinoma
Head and neck carcinoma, squamous cell
Islet cell carcinoma
Kaposi's sarcoma (epidemic)
Non-small-cell lung cancer
Multiple myeloma
Neuroblastoma
Prostate carcinoma
Retinoblastoma

DISEASES WITH MINOR ROLE FOR CHEMOTHERAPY

Colorectal carcinoma
Esophageal carcinoma
Hepatic carcinoma
Melanoma
Pancreatic carcinoma
Renal cell carcinoma

CATEGORIES OF CHEMOTHERAPEUTIC AGENTS AND MAJOR TOXICITIES
(*Note:* List of toxicities is partial; some toxicities may apply only to certain members of a group of drugs.)

Alkylating agents	**Toxicity**
Busulfan	Nausea and vomiting, bone
Chlorambucil	marrow depression,
Cyclophosphamide	pulmonary fibrosis,
Dacarbazine (DTIC)	sterility, hemorrhagic
L-Phenylalanine mustard	cystitis, secondary
Mechlorethamine (nitrogen	malignancies, alopecia
mustard)	
Nitrosoureas	
Thiotepa	

Antimetabolites	
Azathioprine	Nausea and vomiting, bone
Cytarabine	marrow depression, oral
Fluorouracil	and GI ulceration, hepatic
Methotrexate	toxicity, alopecia,
6-Mercaptopurine	neurologic defects
6-Thioguanine	

Vinca alkaloids	
Vinblastine	Nausea and vomiting, local
Vincristine	pain upon extravasation,
	bone marrow depression,
	peripheral neuropathy,
	alopecia, inappropriate
	ADH secretion, paralytic
	ileus

Antibiotics	
Bleomycin	Nausea and vomiting, bone
Dactinomycin (actinomycin	marrow depression,
D)	cardiotoxicity, pulmonary
Daunorubicin	fibrosis, hypocalcemia,
Doxorubicin	alopecia, hypersensitivity
Mithramycin	reactions
Mitomycin	

Enzymes	
L-Asparaginase	Nausea and vomiting,
	fever, anaphylaxis, CNS
	changes, pancreatitis,
	thrombosis, renal and
	hepatic damage

Miscellaneous agents	
Alpha interferon	Nausea and vomiting, bone
Cisplatin	marrow depression, fever,
Etoposide	chills, renal damage,
Hydroxyurea	antiestrogen effects
Tamoxifen	

COMPLICATIONS OF THERAPY While the effects of cancer chemotherapeutic agents may be exerted primarily on the malignant cell population, virtually all currently employed regimens have profound effects on normal tissues as well. Every side effect of treatment must be balanced against potential benefits expected, and pts must always be fully apprised of the risks they may undertake. While the duration of certain adverse effects may be short-lived, others, such as sterility and the risk of secondary malignancy, obviously have long-term implications; consideration of these effects s of importance in the use of regimens as adjuvant therapy. The combined toxicity of regimens involving radiotherapy and chemotherapy must be weighed in designing these programs. Teratogenesis is a special concern in treating women of childbearing years with radiation or chemotherapy.

For a more detailed discussion, see Cadman EC, Durivage HJ: Cancer Chemotherapy, Chap. 301, in HPIM-12, p. 1587

SECTION 10   ENDOCRINOLOGY AND METABOLISM

140   APPROACH TO THE PATIENT WITH ENDOCRINE AND METABOLIC DISEASES

Endocrinopathy can result from hormone deficiency, hormone excess, or resistance to hormone action, and abnormalities in more than one endocrine system may coexist in the same individual. The history and physical exam often lead directly to the current diagnosis. However, endocrinology differs from most subspecialties in that it is not oriented to a specific organ system. In common with infectious disease, it encompasses the entire body and hence its disorders can produce virtually all signs and symptoms of medicine. Consequently, few endocrine disorders have pathognomonic signs and symptoms, at least in the early phases of disease. For example, Graves' disease and acromegaly—among the easiest diagnoses in the advanced state—are difficult to recognize early in the course. Consequently, at the clinical level, endocrinology relies on the recognition of symptom patterns and combinations and, perhaps more than any other branch of medicine, on laboratory assessment.

Endocrine status is assessed by measuring plasma hormone levels, the urinary excretion of hormones (or metabolites), the rates of secretion of hormones into the circulation, hormone reserve and regulation of hormone secretion by dynamic testing, the levels of hormone receptors, selected effects of hormone action in target tissues, or appropriate combinations of these tests. Developments in diagnostic imaging have had a profound impact in endocrinology and provide better means of identifying abnormalities in almost every endocrine system. Indeed, nonfunctioning adenomas of the pituitary, the adrenals, and the testes are now frequently diagnosed with such techniques and must be differentiated from functioning and/or malignant masses.

141 DISORDERS OF THE ANTERIOR PITUITARY AND HYPOTHALAMUS

The anterior pituitary produces six major hormones: growth hormone (GH), prolactin (PRL), luteinizing hormone (LH), follicle-stimulating hormone (FSH), thyroid-stimulating hormone (TSH), and corticotropin (ACTH). Their production is under feedback control by target glands, and hence hormone levels in blood increase when target glands fail (e.g., elevated TSH in primary hypothyroidism). The pituitary is also under control of the hypothalamus via chemical mediators synthesized in the hypothalamus and transported to the pituitary via the portal vessels of the pituitary stalk. With hypothalamic ablation, the levels of GH, LH, FSH, TSH, and ACTH fall, whereas PRL levels increase, indicating that the major hypothalamic influence on the latter is inhibitory. Disorders of the anterior pituitary can cause three distinct syndromes.

ENLARGEMENT OF THE SELLA AND SUPRASELLAR MASSES

Enlargement of the sella may be an incidental finding on skull series, or may produce headache or visual disturbances (bitemporal hemianopsia). Differential diagnosis includes tumors (pituitary adenomas, craniopharyngiomas, meningiomas, metastatic lesions), granulomas, and empty sella syndrome (nontumorous enlargement resulting from protrusion of arachnoid cavity and CSF into the sella). Anterior pituitary hormone production is usually not impaired in the latter. CT scan with contrast and MRI with gadolinium contrast are the most reliable imaging tools available. Evaluation of pituitary function must be done on all pts with a pituitary mass.

The *hypothalamus* produces many regulatory hormones and controls many nonendocrine functions (food intake and feeding behavior, temperature regulation, sleep-wake cycling, short-term memory, thirst regulation, and autonomic nervous system function).

Craniopharyngiomas arise from remnants of Rathke's pouch and are usually manifested in childhood. Children present with signs of increased intracranial pressure due to hydrocephalus (80%) such as headache, vomiting, papilledema; visual abnormalities (60%) including field cuts and vision loss; short stature (7–40%); and delayed sexual development (20%). Adults present with visual complaints (80%), headache (40%), personality change (26%), or hypogonadism (35%). Diabetes insipidus and panhypopituitarism may develop. Skull x-ray abnormalities include calcification, sellar enlargement, and signs of increased intracranial pressure. CT scan and MRI are also useful. Therapy often results in major functional deficits. The currently favored approach is biopsy and partial resection followed by conventional radiation.

PITUITARY HORMONE HYPERSECRETION

May involve one or more pituitary hormones and can be caused by microadenomas (<1 cm) and/or macroadenomas that cause enlargement of the sella.

PROLACTIN (PRL)   Prolactin is essential for lactation. Prolactin secretion is under tonic inhibition by dopamine and is stimulated by thyroid hormone–releasing hormone (TRH) (although TSH and PRL are under independent control in most physiologic states). *Prolactin excess* has many causes (Table 141-1). Prolactin secreting adenomas are the most common functioning pituitary tumor (approximately 50%). Clinical features include galactorrhea, oligomenorrhea or amenorrhea (primary or secondary), and infertility in women. Men may be impotent and infertile but rarely have gynecomastia or galactorrhea. Serum prolactin levels should be measured in all patients with hypogonadism or galactorrhea. A prolactin level >300 μg/L is diagnostic of pituitary adenoma. Modest prolactin elevation may result from pituitary stalk compression and impairment of delivery of dopamine (prolactin inhibitory factor) to the gland. Hypogonadism results from inhibition by prolactin of hypothalamic release of LH-releasing hormone (LHRH) and subsequent decreased gonadotropin production. Dopamine agonists such as bromocriptine lower prolactin levels in virtually all hyperprolactinemic pts. Therapy should begin with 1.25 mg PO qhs, increasing gradually until serum prolactin is normal. The maximum dosage is usually 25 mg/d. Tumor mass usually shrinks, but residual tumor or unresponsive tumors may require surgical debulking or radiation therapy. Recurrence rate following surgery is about 17%.

Prolactin deficiency is manifested as an inability to lactate, which may be the first clue to panhypopituitarism. TRH normally causes an increase in serum prolactin by ≥200% of baseline. The presence of prolactin deficiency requires evaluation of other pituitary hormones.

TABLE 141-1   Causes of hyperprolactinemia

I. Physiologic states
   A. Pregnancy
   B. Nursing (early)
   C. "Stress"
   D. Sleep
   E. Nipple stimulation
II. Drugs
   A. Dopamine receptor antagonists
      1. Phenothiazines
      2. Butyrophenones
      3. Thioxanthenes
      4. Metoclopramide
   B. Dopamine-depleting agents
      1. Methyldopa
      2. Reserpine
   C. Estrogens
   D. Opiates
III. Disease states
   A. Pituitary tumors
      1. Prolactinomas
      2. Adenomas secreting GH and prolactin
      3. Adenomas secreting ACTH and prolactin (Nelson's syndrome and Cushing's disease)
      4. Nonfunctioning chromophobe adenomas with pituitary stalk compression
   B. Hypothalamic and pituitary stalk disease
      1. Granulomatous diseases especially sarcoidosis
      2. Craniopharyngiomas and other tumors
      3. Cranial irradiation
      4. Stalk section
      5. Empty sella
      6. Vascular abnormalities including aneurysm
      7. Lymphocytic hypophysitis
   C. Primary hypothyroidism
   D. Chronic renal failure
   E. Cirrhosis
   F. Chest wall trauma (including surgery, *herpes zoster*)
   G. Seizures

From Daniels GH, Martin JB: HPIM-12, p. 1658.

GROWTH HORMONE (GH, SOMATOTROPIN)   Growth hormone is necessary for linear growth, acting indirectly by stimulating the formation of other growth factors [insulin-like growth factors or somatomedins (IGF-1/SM-C)]. Hypothalamic inhibition of release is mediated by somatostatin, and hypothalamic stimulation of GH release is mediated by growth hormone–releasing hormone (GRH). GH deficiency in children leads to short stature and in adults causes minimal changes (fine wrinkling of facial skin and increased sensitivity to insulin in pts with diabetes mellitus). Evaluation of deficiency and excess is found in Table 141-2. GH excess in children leads to gigantism and in adults to acromegaly. Acromegaly results in soft tissue and bony overgrowth manifested by increased hand, foot, jaw, and cranial size; enlargement of the tongue; wide spacing of teeth; and coarsening of facial features. Thickening of the palms, increased skin tags, acanthosis nigricans, and oily skin are common. Obstructive sleep apnea may cause hypersomnolence. Neurologic symptoms include headaches, paresthesias (including carpal tunnel syndrome), muscle weakness, and arthralgias. Insulin resistance is common, with frank diabetes mellitus in one-sixth of pts. Basal or random GH determinations may be elevated in normal persons and should not be used as screening test. The standard diagnostic test is measurement of GH 60–120 min after 100 g oral glucose. Serum GH <5 μg/L is considered normal; GH <2 μg/L is a more rigorous criterion. Acromegalics usually have GH >10 μg/L. Serum IGF-1/SM-C concentrations correlate with disease activity. CT scan with contrast or MRI is recommended to define tumor size. Transsphenoidal surgery is the treatment of choice with apparent cure rates between 35 and 75%. Heavy-particle pituitary radiation is also used. Bromocriptine may be useful as an adjunct to other modalities in dosages of 20–60 mg/d. A long-acting somatostatin analogue (octreotide) 50–250 μg q 6–8 h SC lowers GH levels to normal in two-thirds of acromegalics and may cause partial tumor regression. It is of particular use as an adjunct to surgery and/or radiation.

GONADOTROPINS   FSH regulates spermatogenesis and growth of the ovarian follicular granulosa cell, while LH controls testosterone production in Leydig cells and ovarian steroidogenesis. LHRH is the hypothalamic hormone that regulates gonadotropin release. In postmenopausal women and in men with primary hypogonadism, FSH and LH are markedly elevated. Congenital isolated gonadotropin deficiency is a hereditary disorder (Kallman's syndrome). Ectopic gonadotropin (usually hCG) is sometimes produced by nonseminoma germ-cell tumors, lung carcinomas, hepatomas, and other tumors. *FSH-secreting pituitary adenomas* are large tumors most often diagnosed in men with decreased libido, decreased serum testosterone, and normal prolactin levels. No distinct syndrome is produced in women. TRH stimulates FSH release in such pts. *LH-secreting pituitary adenomas* are characterized by increased testosterone, elevated LH levels, normal or low FSH levels, and often partial hypopituitarism. Testicular response to hCG is preserved

TABLE 141-2 Pituitary hormone evaluation

Hormone	Excess	Deficiency

Growth hormone (GH)	1. Measurement of plasma GH 1 h after glucose PO	1. Measurement of plasma GH 30, 60, and 120 min after one of the following:
		   a. Regular insulin 0.1 to 0.15 unit/kg IV
		   b. Levodopa 10 mg/kg PO
		   c. L-Arginine 0.5 mg/kg intravenously over 30 min

	2. Measurement of IGF-1/SM-C	2. ?Measurement of IGF-1/SM-C

Prolactin	1. Measurement of basal serum prolactin	1. Measurement of serum prolactin 10 to 20 min after one of the following:
		   a. TRH 200 to 500 µg IV
		   b. Chlorpromazine 25 mg IM

TSH	1. Measurement of T₄, free T₄ index, T₃, TSH	1. Measurement of T₄, free T₄ index, TSH
Gonadotropins	1. Measurement of FSH, LH, testosterone, FSH beta, FSH response to TRH	1. Measurement of basal LH, FSH in postmenopausal women; no measurements in menstruating, ovulating women
		2. Testosterone, FSH, and LH in men
ACTH	1. Measurement of urine free cortisol*	1. Measurement of serum cortisol at 30 and 60 min following regular insulin 0.05 to 0.15 units per kilogram IV

	2. Dexamethasone suppression by one of the following:
	   a. Measurement of 8 A.M. plasma cortisol after administration of 1 mg dexamethasone at midnight
	   b. Measurement of 8 A.M. plasma cortisol or 24-h urine 17-hydroxysteroids or free cortisol after 0.5 mg dexamethasone PO q 6 h for 8 doses
		2. Metyrapone response by one of the following:
		   a. Measurement of plasma 11-deoxycortisol at 8 A.M. after 30 mg/kg metyrapone at midnight (maximal dose 2 g)
		   b. Measurement of 24-h urinary 17-hydroxycorticoids or plasma 11-deoxycortisol day of and day after 750 mg metyrapone q 4 h for 6 doses

$^{(T_4 = \text{thyroxine})}$

3. High-dose dexamethasone suppression by one of the following:

    a. Measurement of plasma cortisol after 8 mg dexamethasone PO at midnight

    b. Measurement of 8 A.M. plasma cortisol or 24 h urine 17-hydroxysteroids or free cortisol after 2 mg dexamethasone q 6 h for 8 doses

    c. Measurement of 24-h urinary 17-hydroxycorticoids day of and day after 500 mg metyrapone q 2 h for 12 doses

4. Metyrapone response (same protocol as for deficiency testing)

5. Response of plasma ACTH to ovine corticotropin-releasing hormone (1 μg/kg body wt)

3. ACTH stimulation test: Measurement of plasma cortisol and aldosterone at 0 and 60 min after IM or IV administration of 0.25 mg cosynitropin

Arginine vasopressin (AVP)

1. Measurement of serum sodium and osmolality, urine osmolality in presence of normal renal, adrenal, thyroid function

2. Simultaneous measurement of serum osmolality and AVP levels.

1. Comparison of urine osmolality and serum osmolality under conditions of increased AVP secretion†

2. Simultaneous measurement of serum osmolality and AVP levels.

* Tests 1 and 2 establish the diagnosis of Cushing's syndrome. Tests 3, 4, and 5 localize the Cushing's disease to the pituitary gland. Occasionally bilateral inferior petrosal sinus catheterization will be necessary.
† May be achieved by water deprivation or saline administration.
From Daniels GH, Martin JB: HPIM-12, p. 1671.

with gonadotropin-secreting adenomas and may help differentiate these tumors from primary hypogonadism.

THYROTROPIN (TSH)   Thyroid gland failure results in compensatory hypertrophy of thyrotrophs (increased TSH) and may also cause modest elevations in serum PRL. The diagnosis of hypothyroidism due to TSH deficiency is made with the supersensitive TSH assay. Pituitary (TSH-induced) hyperthyroidism can be caused by TSH-secreting adenomas (hallmark is overproduction of TSH alpha subunit with a ratio of >1:1 alpha:intact TSH). TSH and TSH alpha production decrease with octreotide. Pituitary resistance to thyroid hormone can result in hyperthyroidism secondary to TSH overproduction. See Chap. 143 for a discussion of thyroid diseases.

CORTICOTROPIN (ACTH)   Corticotropin-releasing hormone is the major (but not exclusive) regulator of ACTH release. ACTH controls the release of cortisol from the adrenal cortex and acutely causes release of aldosterone. ACTH is highest at 4 A.M. and lowest in late evening. Pituitary hypersection of ACTH (*Cushing's disease*) is caused by a microadenoma in 90% of cases. Clinical manifestations of cortisol excess are described in Chap. 144. Once the presence of cortisol excess is established (Chap. 144), a high-dose overnight dexamethasone (8 mg at midnight) or a 2-d dexamethasone suppression test (2 mg q 6 h for 8 doses) results in suppression of urine 17-hydroxycorticosteroids and free cortisol and of plasma cortisol, usually by >50% in cases of ACTH-secreting adenomas. Transsphenoidal surgery is successful therapy in about 75% of pts. Of pts who have undergone bilateral adrenalectomy, 10–30% develop Nelson's syndrome, an ACTH-producing pituitary adenoma with increased skin pigmentation. Ectopic ACTH production is discussed in Chap. 144. ACTH deficiency may be isolated or occur in association with other pituitary hormone deficiencies. Reversible isolated ACTH deficiency is common after prolonged glucocorticoid administration. Pts with ACTH deficiency are not hyperkalemic because cortisol is not needed for potassium excretion. For evaluation of ACTH deficiency see Table 141-2.

HYPOPITUITARISM

Hypopituitarism refers to deficiency of one or more pituitary hormones and has many etiologies (see Table 141-3). When diabetes insipidus is present the primary defect is almost invariably in hypothalamus or high in the pituitary stalk, often in conjunction with mild hyperprolactinemia and anterior pituitary hypofunction. Diagnosis is based upon mul-

TABLE 141-3   **Causes of hypopituitarism**

A. Isolated hormone deficiencies
    1. Congenital or acquired deficiencies
B. Tumors
    1. Large pituitary adenomas
    2. Pituitary apoplexy
    3. Hypothalamic tumors, e.g., craniopharyngiomas, germinomas, chordomas, meningiomas, gliomas, and others
C. Inflammatory diseases
    1. Granulomatous disease, e.g., sarcoidosis, tuberculosis, syphilis, granulomatous hypophysitis
    2. Eosinophilic granuloma
    3. Lymphocytic hypophysitis (autoimmune)
D. Vascular diseases
    1. Sheehan's postpartum necrosis
    2. ? Diabetic peripartum necrosis
    3. Carotid aneurysm
E. Destructive-traumatic events
    1. Surgery
    2. Stalk section
    3. Radiation (conventional—hypothalamus; heavy-particle—pituitary)
    4. Trauma
F. Developmental anomalies
    1. Pituitary aplasia
    2. Basal encephalocoele
G. Infiltration
    1. Hemochromatosis
    2. Amyloidosis
H. "Idiopathic" causes
    1. ? Autoimmune disease

From Daniels GH, Martin JB: HPIM-12, p. 1673.

tiple hormonal tests (see Table 141-2) and requires replacement of missing hormones. Cortisol is the most important and is commonly given as cortisone acetate (20–37.5 mg/d) or prednisone (5–7.5 mg/d). In emergent situations hydrocortisone hemisuccinate 75 mg IM/IV q 6 h or methylprednisolone sodium succinate 15 mg IM/IV q 6 h is given. Thyroid hormone replacement is with levothyroxine (0.1–0.2 mg/d); *glucocorticoid* replacement should *always precede levothyroxine* therapy to avoid precipitation of adrenal crisis. Hypogonadism in women is treated with estrogen-progestogen combinations and in men with testosterone esters by injection (see Chap. 147). GH deficiency is not treated in adults. See Chap. 142 for treatment of diabetes insipidus.

SHORT STATURE Screening laboratory investigations for evaluation of *short stature* can be found in Table 141-4.

TABLE 141-4   Screening laboratory investigations in short stature

Test or x-ray	Disorder
Serum thyroxine	Hypothyroidism
IGF-I	GH deficiency
Bone age	Constitutional delay, hypothyroidism, GH deficiency
Lateral skull film	Craniopharyngioma or other central nervous system lesion
Serum calcium	Pseudohypoparathyroidism
Serum phosphate	Vitamin D–resistant rickets
Serum bicarbonate	Renal tubular acidosis
Blood urea nitrogen	Renal failure
Complete blood count	Anemia, nutritional disorder
Sedimentation rate	Inflammatory disease of bowel
Chromosomal karyotype	Gonadal dysgenesis or other abnormality

From Daniels GH, Martin JB: HPIM-12, p. 1681.

For a more detailed discussion, see Daniels GH, Martin JB: Neuroendocrine Regulation and Diseases of the Anterior Pituitary and Hypothalamus, Chap. 313, p. 1655, and Hintz RL: Disorders of Growth, Chap. 314, p. 1679, in HPIM-12

DIABETES INSIPIDUS

Arginine vasopressin (AVP, antidiuretic hormone, ADH) functions to concentrate urine and hence to conserve water. In *central diabetes insipidus,* insufficient AVP is released in response to physiologic stimuli; it must be distinguished from other types of polyuria (Table 142-1). Causes include (1) neoplastic or infiltrative lesions of hypothalamus such as pituitary tumors that extend upward, metastatic tumors,

TABLE 142-1 **Major polyuric syndromes**

I. Primary disorders of water intake or output
  A. Excessive water intake
    1. Psychogenic polydipsia
    2. Hypothalamic disease: histiocytosis X, sarcoidosis
    3. Drug-induced polydipsia
      a. Thioridazine
      b. Chlorpromazine
      c. Anticholinergic drugs (dry mouth)
  B. Inadequate tubular reabsorption of filtered water
    1. Vasopressin deficiency
      a. Central diabetes insipidus
      b. Drug-induced inhibition of AVP release
        (1) Narcotic antagonists
    2. Renal tubular unresponsiveness to AVP
      a. Nephrogenic diabetes insipidus (congenital and familial)
      b. Nephrogenic diabetes insipidus (acquired)
        (1) Several chronic renal diseases, after obstructive uropathy, unilateral renal arterial stenosis, after renal transplantation, after acute tubular necrosis
        (2) Potassium deficiencies, including primary aldosteronism
        (3) Chronic hypercalcemias, including hyperparathyroidism
        (4) Drug-induced: lithium, methoxyflurane anesthesia, demeclocycline
        (5) Various systemic disorders: multiple myeloma, amyloidosis, sickle cell anemia, Sjögren's syndrome
II. Primary disorders of renal absorption of solutes (osmotic diuresis)
  A. Glucose: diabetes mellitus
  B. Salts, especially sodium chloride
    1. Various chronic renal diseases, especially chronic pyelonephritis
    2. After various diuretics, including mannitol

From Moses AM, Streeten DHP: HPIM-12, p. 1682.

leukemia, germinomas, pinealomas, histiocytosis X, and sarcoidosis; (2) pituitary or hypothalamic surgery; (3) severe head injury, usually associated with skull fracture; (4) ruptured cerebral aneurysms; and (5) idiopathic. The onset of polyuria, excessive thirst, and polydipsia may be sudden, and urine volume may be as high as 16–24 L/d. Urine osmolality (<290 mosmol/kg; specific gravity <1.010) is less than that of serum. Increase in serum osmolality stimulates thirst, and dehydration is unusual as long as pts have free access to water. When water intake is inadequate (postoperatively, head trauma, or other CNS dysfunction), rising serum sodium level and osmolality can cause weakness, fever, mental disturbances, prostration, and death.

Comparison of urinary osmolality after dehydration with that after AVP administration (Table 142-2) is a reliable way of defining the cause of polyuria. Urinary osmolality normally rises by ≤9% after injection of vasopressin. In central diabetes insipidus, the increase in urinary osmolality after vasopressin is >9%. In *nephrogenic diabetes insipidus* or potassium depletion little change occurs in urine osmolality with dehydration and there is no further rise with vasopressin.

In absence of brain tumor or systemic disease, treatment is usually successful. For acute therapy of unconscious pts after head trauma or neurosurgery, aqueous vasopressin should be given subcutaneously in doses of 5–10 U q 3–6 h. For long-term therapy see Table 142-3. Chlorpropamide may be useful in patients with partial AVP deficiency.

SYNDROME OF INAPPROPRIATE VASOPRESSIN SECRETION (SIADH)

Causes hyponatremia because of inability to dilute urine; ingested fluids are retained, and extracellular fluid volume is expanded *without edema*. It may occur by three mechanisms: (1) AVP is synthesized and autonomously released from tumors (usually oat cell carcinoma of lung); (2) nontumorous tissue acquires capacity to synthesize and release AVP autonomously or to stimulate AVP release by pituitary (as in pulmonary tuberculosis, pneumonias, and other pulmonary diseases); (3) pituitary AVP is released inappropriately due to inflammation, neoplasm, vascular lesions, or drugs such as morphine (see Table 142-4).

TABLE 142-2 Dehydration test

---

1. Withhold fluids until urinary osmolality becomes stable (an increase of <30 mosmol/kg/h for at least 3 h); body weight usually decreases by 1 kg.
2. Administration of 5 U aqueous vasopressin or 1 μg desmopressin by SC injection or 10 μg desmopressin intranasally.
3. Measure urine and plasma osmolality before and 1 h after the injection.

TABLE 142-3 Agents used in treatment of diabetes insipidus

	Dose form	Usual dose	Duration of action, h
CENTRAL DIABETES INSIPIDUS			
Hormone replacement:			
Aqueous vasopressin	10 or 20 units/ampul	5–10 units subcutaneously	3–6
Desmopressin	2.5-mL intranasal preparation, 100 µg/mL; 1- or 10-mL ampul, for injection, 4 µ/mL	10–20 µg intranasally or 1–4 µg subcutaneously	12–24
Lypressin	5-mL bottle, 50 units/mL	2–4 units intranasally	4–6
Vasopressin tannate in oil	5 units/ampul	5 units intramuscularly	24–72
Nonhormonal agents:			
Chlorpropamide	100- and 250-mg tablets	200–500 mg daily	
Clofibrate	500-mg capsules	500 mg four times daily	
Carbamazepine	200-mg tablets	400–600 mg daily	
NEPHROGENIC DIABETES INSIPIDUS			
Hydrochlorothiazide	50-mg tablets	50–100 mg daily	
Chlorthalidone	50-mg tablets	50 mg daily	

From Moses AM, Streeten DHP: HPIM 12, p. 1688.

TABLE 142-4   **Causes of inappropriate vasopressin secretion (SIADH)**

I. Malignant neoplasms with autonomous AVP release
   A. Oat cell carcinoma of lung
   B. Carcinoma of pancreas
   C. Lymphosarcoma, reticulum cell sarcoma, Hodgkin's disease
   D. Carcinoma of duodenum
   E. Thymoma
II. Nonmalignant pulmonary diseases
   A. Tuberculosis
   B. Lung abscess
   C. Pneumonia
   D. Viral pneumonitis
   E. Empyema
   F. Chronic obstructive airways disease
III. Central nervous system disorders
   A. Skull fracture
   B. Subdural hematoma
   C. Subarachnoid hemorrhage
   D. Cerebral vascular thrombosis
   E. Cerebral atrophy
   F. Acute encephalitis
   G. Tuberculous meningitis
   H. Purulent meningitis
   I. Guillain-Barré syndrome
   J. Lupus erythematosus
   K. Acute intermittent porphyria
IV. Drugs
   A. Chlorpropamide
   B. Vincristine
   C. Vinblastine
   D. Cyclophosphamide
   E. Carbamazepine
   F. Oxytocin
   G. General anesthesia
   H. Narcotics
   I. Tricyclic antidepressants
V. Miscellaneous causes
   A. Hypothyroidism
   B. Positive pressure respiration

From Moses AM, Streeten DHP: HPIM-12, p. 1689.

Symptoms   Weight gain, weakness, lethargy, and mental confusion, ultimately progressing to convulsion and coma.

Laboratory features   Low BUN, creatinine, uric acid, and albumin; serum Na <130 mmol/L and plasma osmolality <270 mosmol/kg; urine almost always hypertonic to plasma, and urinary Na usually >20 mmol/L.

SIADH should be suspected in hyponatremic pts with urine that is hypertonic to plasma.

Differential diagnosis   (1) Depletional hyponatremias, especially due to adrenal insufficiency, salt-losing nephritis, diarrhea, or diuretic therapy; (2) hyponatremic edematous states (CHF, cirrhosis, nephrosis); (3) pseudohyponatremia from hyperlipidemia or severe hyperglycemia; (4) hypothyroidism; and (5) primary polydipsia in which the urine is invariably dilute. Assessment of response to water loading may be useful in establishing diagnosis.

In pts with mild SIADH, fluid intake should be restricted to 0.8–1 L/day. If severe SIADH is life-threatening, 200–300 mL 5% sodium chloride solution should be given IV over *several hours* to raise the serum Na to a level at which symptoms will improve. Demeclocycline interferes with renal action of AVP and may be useful when fluid restriction is impractical, but it has delayed onset of action.

For a more detailed discussion, see Moses AM, Streeten DHP: Disorders of the Neurohypophysis, Chap. 315, in HPIM-12, p. 1682

The thyroid secretes thyroxine (T_4) and triiodothyronine (T_3), which influence basal metabolic rate and cardiac and neurologic function. Diseases of the thyroid may be manifest by quantitative or qualitative alterations in hormone secretion, enlargement of the gland, or both.

The hypothalamus releases thyrotropin-releasing hormone (TRH), which traverses the pituitary stalk and stimulates release of thyroid-stimulating hormone (TSH) from the anterior pituitary. TSH is released into the circulation and controls production and release of T_4 and T_3, which in turn inhibit further TSH release from the pituitary (see Chap. 141).

Some T_3 is secreted by the thyroid, but most is produced by deiodination of T_4 in peripheral tissues. Both T_4 and T_3 are bound to carrier proteins (principally thyroid-binding globulin, TBG) in the circulation.

Under- or overproduction of thyroid hormones is usually reflected in ↓ or ↑ of serum T_4 and T_3 levels. When TBG is elevated or low, the free thyroxine index (FTI) corrects serum T_4 for alterations in binding protein and thus provides an index of thyroid status (see Table 143-1).

HYPOTHYROIDISM

Insufficient thyroid hormone secretion can result from thyroid failure (primary hypothyroidism) or from pituitary or hypothalamic disease (secondary hypothyroidism). *Symptoms* of lethargy, constipation, cold intolerance, stiffness and cramping of muscles, carpal tunnel syndrome, and menorrhagia may be insidious in onset. Intellectual and motor activity

TABLE 143-1 **Altered TBG concentration**

Increased	Decreased
Pregnancy	Androgens
Newborn state	Large doses of glucocorticoids
Oral contraceptives and other estrogens	Chronic liver disease
Tamoxifen	Severe systemic illness
Infections and chronic active hepatitis	Active acromegaly
Biliary cirrhosis	Nephrosis
Acute intermittent porphyria	L-asparaginase
Perphenazine	Inherited trait
Inherited trait	

slows, appetite declines, weight increases, hair and skin become dry, and the voice deepens. Obstructive sleep apnea may occur. Cardiomegaly can be due to dilatation or pericardial effusion. Relaxation phase of deep tendon reflexes is prolonged. The ultimate picture is a dull, expressionless face, sparse hair, periorbital puffiness, large tongue, and pale, doughy, cool skin. Pts may progress into a hypothermic, stuporous state (myxedema coma). Factors predisposing to myxedema coma include cold exposure, trauma, infection, and administration of narcotics. Respiratory depression may cause rise in arterial P_{CO_2}.

Decreased serum T_4 is common to all varieties of hypothyroidism. Serum TSH is ↑ in primary and normal or ↓ in secondary hypothyroidism. Increases in serum cholesterol, creatinine phosphokinase, and lactic dehydrogenase are common, as are bradycardia, low-amplitude QRS complexes, and flattened or inverted T waves on ECG.

Levothyroxine is preferred *treatment*. In adults the initial daily dose of 25 μg/d is increased by 25–50 μg/d at 2–3 week intervals until serum TSH is within normal range (an average dose of 150 μg/d). When secondary hypothyroidism is suspected, thyroxine should not be administered until adrenal insufficiency has been treated. *Myxedema coma* is a life-threatening emergency requiring rapid administration of levothyroxine 200–300 μg IV over 5 min along with dexamethasone 2 mg PO/IV q 6 h. Levothyroxine 100 μg/d can then be given IV/PO until the pt stabilizes. Primary adrenal insufficiency must be evaluated with an ACTH stimulation test (Chap. 144).

THYROTOXICOSIS

Symptoms include nervousness, palpitations, emotional lability, inability to sleep, tremors, frequent bowel movements, excessive sweating, heat intolerance, oligomenorrhea, amenorrhea, and weight loss despite a well-maintained or increased appetite. Pt appears anxious, restless, and fidgety. Skin is warm, moist, and velvety; palms are erythematous; and fingernails may separate from the nail bed (Plummer's nails). Hair is fine and silky, and a fine tremor may involve fingers and tongue. Eye signs include a stare with widened palpebral fissures, infrequent blinking, and lid lag. Cardiovascular findings include a wide pulse pressure, especially atrial fibrillation, systolic murmurs, and cardiac enlargement.

Several disorders can produce thyrotoxicosis: *Graves' disease* is manifested by a diffuse goiter and infiltrative ophthalmopathy (with variable ophthalmoplegia, proptosis, and periorbital swelling) and dermopathy (pretibial myxedema). *Treatment* is directed at limiting the amount of hormone the gland can produce. Antithyroid drugs interpose a chemical blockage to hormone synthesis (propylthiouracil 150 mg every 6 or 8 h). Leukopenia is the principal side effect. Propranolol can alleviate adrenergic symptoms (40–120 mg/d in divided doses). Ablation of thyroid tissue can be effected by surgery or radioiodine. Radioiodine affords a simple, effective, and economic means of treating thyrotoxicosis and is the treatment of choice in many institutions for all age groups; as many as 40–70% of pts eventually become hypothyroid after radioiodine. Pts should be followed every 6 weeks after therapy until the residual thyroid function is known with certainty. Radioactive iodine is contraindicated in pregnancy.

Pts with severe thyrotoxicosis (*thyroid storm*) require rapid reduction in circulating thyroid hormone levels. Propylthiouracil (PTU) 1 g, followed by 300 mg q 6 h is given along with dexamethasone 2 mg PO/IV q 6 h. Potassium iodide (SSKI) 4–5 drops q 6 h for 2 d is initiated 2 h after the first dose of PTU. Propranolol 10–20 mg IV/PO q 6 h can be titrated to control tachycardia. Special care in the use of beta blockers is required in the setting of CHF.

Treatment of hyperthyroidism during pregnancy is difficult. PTU in dosages <300 mg/d may be effective. Pts not controlled may require subtotal thyroidectomy during the middle trimester.

Treatment of ophthalmopathy is frequently unsatisfactory. Corneal drying can be prevented during sleep by taping lids closed and using ocular wetting agents. In severe cases with progressive exophthalmos, chemosis, ophthalmoplegia, or vision loss, large doses of prednisone (120–140 mg/d) are given. Some pts benefit from orbital radiation or surgical decompression. Hypothyroidism should be avoided.

Toxic multinodular goiter can cause excess thyroid hormone production, usually in the elderly. The thyrotoxicosis is less severe than in Graves' disease, but impact on the cardiovascular system may be great. Radioactive iodine is the treatment of choice.

Thyrotoxicosis associated with *acute* and *subacute thyroiditis* is due to leakage of preformed thyroid hormone from the inflamed gland. Thyroid function eventually returns to normal. Mild cases may be treated with aspirin; prednisone (20–40 mg/d) is reserved for severe cases. Propranolol may control symptoms of thyrotoxicosis.

Rarely, source of excess thyroid hormone is from outside the thyroid, e.g., *thyroid hormone ingestion* or *metastatic thyroid carcinoma* (see Table 143-2).

TABLE 143-2 Varieties of thyrotoxicosis

  I. Disorders associated with thyroid hyperfunction*
    A. Excess production of TSH (rare)
    B. Abnormal thyroid stimulator
        1. Graves' disease
        2. Trophoblastic tumor
    C. Intrinsic thyroid autonomy
        1. Hyperfunctioning adenoma
        2. Toxic multinodular goiter
 II. Disorders not associated with thyroid hyperfunction†
    A. Disorders of hormone storage
        1. Subacute thyroiditis
        2. Chronic thyroiditis with transient thyrotoxicosis
    B. Extrathyroid source of hormone
        1. Thyrotoxicosis factitia
        2. Ectopic thyroid tissue
            a. Struma ovarii
            b. Functioning follicular carcinoma

---

* Associated with increased RAIU unless body iodine burden is excessive.
† Associated with decreased RAIU.
From Wartofsky L, Ingbar SH: HPIM-12, p. 1702.

SICK EUTHYROID SYNDROME

Severe illness, physical trauma, or physiologic stress can alter peripheral binding and metabolism of thyroid hormones and regulation of TSH secretion. The most consistent feature is low serum T_3, and serum T_4 may be ↓, normal, or rarely ↑. Condition is due to a combination of inhibition of conversion of T_4 to T_3 and inhibition of serum binding of hormones. The importance of this syndrome is that is has to be distinguished from mild hyperthyroidism. Measurements of serum T_4 or T_3 in conjunction with assessment of hormone binding are generally the most reliable means of making this distinction. Primary alterations in TBG produce changes in T_3 uptake that are inverse to those in serum T_4 and T_3, and as a result, free levels of the hormone and the FTI remain normal. By contrast, hyper- and hypothyroidism cause changes in free hormone levels in the same directions as those in total serum thyroxine. When the FTI is low (e.g., in severely ill patients), euthyroid state can be confirmed by measuring TSH.

THYROIDITIS

   SUBACUTE THYROIDITIS Can be due to any of several viruses, including mumps. *Symptoms* usually follow URI, are due to stretching of the thyroid capsule, and are principally pain over the thyroid or pain referred to lower jaw, ear, or occiput. Onset may be acute, with severe pain over thyroid, accompanied by fever and nodularity over thyroid. ESR may be $\uparrow$, and radioactive iodine uptake may be $\downarrow$. Early, many pts are mildly thyrotoxic owing to leakage of T_4 from gland. After glandular hormone is depleted, a hypothyroid phase may ensue. Normal thyroid function eventually returns. In mild cases, aspirin controls symptoms. In more severe cases, prednisone is generally effective. Propranolol can be used to control associated thyrotoxicosis. When RAIU returns to normal, therapy can be withdrawn without recurrence of symptoms.

HASHIMOTO'S THYROIDITIS (LYMPHADENOID GOITER)   A chronic inflammation of thyroid, probably autoimmune in nature. It may coexist with other autoimmune diseases, including pernicious anemia, Sjögren's syndrome, chronic hepatitis, SLE, rheumatoid arthritis, adrenal insufficiency, and diabetes mellitus. Goiter may be asymmetric. Pt may be metabolically normal, but thyroid failure usually supervenes. The latter is evident first in a rise in serum TSH concentration, serum T_4 then declines, and when serum T_3 concentration falls, frank hypothyroidism ensues. High titers of thyroid antimicrosomal antibody are almost always present. Such antibodies may cause simultaneous thyroiditis and hyperthyroidism (so-called Hashitoxicosis). Treatment with replacement doses of levothyroxine is indicated. In some pts, such therapy is associated with regression of goiter.

THYROID NEOPLASMS

THYROID ADENOMAS   These are classified into three types: papillary, follicular, and Hurthle cell. Follicular adenomas are the most common and most likely to function autonomously. Thyrotoxicosis may occur including T_3 toxicosis. Surgery or ^{131}I is curative. Hyperfunctioning nodules are rarely malignant.

THYROID CARCINOMAS   These arise from follicular epithelium or from parafollicular (C) cells. Carcinomas of follicular epithelium can be anaplastic, follicular, or papillary. Anaplastic carcinoma is rare, highly malignant, and rapidly fatal. Follicular carcinoma may undergo hematogenous spread and is more common in older age groups. Papillary carcinoma has a bimodal frequency with a peak during the second and third decades and again later in life.

The diagnostic approach to the solitary thyroid nodule is shown in Fig. 143-1. Features suggesting carcinoma include recent or rapid growth of a nodule or mass, history of neck irradiation, and fixation to surrounding tissues.

FIGURE 143-1

DIAGNOSTIC APPROACH TO THE SOLITARY NODULE
Fine Needle Aspiration (FNA)[1]

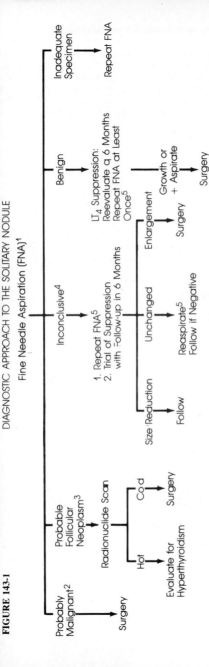

1 22–25 gauge needle with repeat using 18 gauge needle if fluid is obtained.
2 Evidence of carcinoma (papillary, medullary, poorly differentiated, follicular) or lymphoma.
3 eg., sheets of follicular cells.
4 eg., small groups of uniform follicular cells with little colloid.
5 Changes in cytologic findings redirect clinician to the appropriate arm of the algorithm.

From Wartofsky L, Ingbar SH: HPIM-12, p. 1710.

567

Near-total thyroidectomy is recommended, with regional lymph node exploration. Levothyroxine therapy is instituted, and approximately 3 weeks after surgery, liothyronine (50–75 μg/d) is substituted since it permits a more rapid return of TSH secretion when *withdrawn* 3 weeks later. When the TSH is ≥50 mU/L, a large scanning dose is given of ^{131}I [1850 MBq (50 mCi)]. Suppression therapy with levothyroxine is reinstituted 24–48 h later, and a follow-up scan is done 1 week later. Ablation may be repeated if more functioning tissue is found. Pts are maintained on levothyroxine therapy and have biannual whole-body scans for the first 3 years and then at 5 years posttherapy. 6 weeks before the scan, levothyroxine is changed to liothyronine, then discontinued after 3 weeks of therapy. Once the scan and any additional therapy is complete, levothyroxine is reinstituted 24–48 h later. Measurement of serum thyroglobulin assists in this evaluation since elevated levels in pts on suppressive therapy signal metastatic disease. Also, a rising level should prompt reevaluation.

NONTOXIC GOITER

Enlargement of thyroid gland (normally 15–25 g) may be generalized or focal and may be associated with ↑, normal, or ↓ hormone secretion. Most commonly, a cause cannot be found. In the case of a nontoxic (euthyroid) goiter, clinical manifestations arise solely from the large gland itself when the metabolic state is normal. Mechanical sequelae include compression and displacement of trachea or esophagus and obstructive symptoms. *Treatment* is generally aimed at reduction in goiter size or prevention of further growth by suppression of TSH and is achieved by graduated dosages of levothyroxine to a maximum of 150–200 μg/d. Surgical resection is rarely indicated.

For a more detailed discussion, see Wartofsky L, Ingbar SH: Diseases of the Thyroid, Chap. 316, in HPIM-12, p. 1692

HYPERFUNCTION OF ADRENAL GLAND

CUSHING'S SYNDROME Distinct clinical syndromes are produced when excess adrenocortical hormones are produced. However, the most common cause of glucocorticoid excess is iatrogenic administration. Excess production of cortisol by the adrenal (Cushing's disease) is usually due to bilateral adrenal hyperplasia secondary to hypersecretion of pituitary ACTH (micro- or macroadenomas) or production of ACTH by nonendocrine tumors (small cell carcinoma of lung, medullary carcinoma of thyroid, or tumors of thymus, pancreas, or ovary). Approximately 25% is due to adrenal neoplasm, half of which is malignant.

Glucocorticoid excess causes muscle weakness, cutaneous striae, and easy bruisability and promotes fat deposition in face (moon facies), interscapular areas (buffalo hump), and mesenteric bed (truncal obesity), along with muscle wasting. Hypertension and emotional changes are common, and diabetes mellitus occurs in $\geq 10\%$.

Plasma and urine cortisol and urinary 17-hydroxycorticoid levels are elevated. Hypokalemia, hypochloremia, and metabolic alkalosis are prominent, particularly with ectopic production of ACTH.

The diagnosis requires demonstration of increased cortisol production and of failure to suppress cortisol secretion normally by dexamethasone (see Table 141-2). Overnight dexamethasone test or measurement of urinary free cortisol is an appropriate screening test. Definitive diagnosis requires demonstration of failure of suppression of urinary cortisol to <30 μg/d or plasma cortisol to <5 mg/dL after 0.5 mg dexamethasone q 6 h for 48 h. Once diagnosis is established, further testing is required to determine cause (Table 141-2). Demonstration of low levels of plasma ACTH suggests an adrenal adenoma or carcinoma, but a high plasma ACTH and/or failure of adrenal suppression by high-dose dexamethasone suggests an ACTH-producing tumor (pituitary or ectopic). A head CT scan can be used to differentiate pituitary from ectopic sources of ACTH.

Surgery of adrenal neoplasms requires pre- and postoperative glucocorticoid therapy and adrenal exploration with excision of the tumor. Transsphenoidal surgery can be

TABLE 144-1   Causes of secondary hyperaldosteronism

I. Normotensive states
   A. Pregnancy
   B. Diuretic therapy
II. Hypertensive states
   A. Primary reninism (renin secreting tumors)
   B. Secondary reninism
      1. Renal artery stenosis (atherosclerotic, fibromuscular type)
      2. Arteriolar nephrosclerosis (malignant hypertension)
      3. Accelerated hypertension
   C. Diuretic therapy
III. Bartter's syndrome
IV. Edematous states
   A. Cirrhosis
   B. Nephrotic syndrome

---

curative for pituitary hypersecretion (see Chap. 141). Metastatic adrenocortical carcinoma is treated with mitotane (*o,p'*-DDD) in doses gradually increased to 8–10 g/d given in three to four divided doses. On occasion, debulking of lung carcinoma can cause remission of ectopic Cushing's disease.

Adrenal masses are common findings on abdominal CT or MRI scans. The first step in evaluating such masses is to determine the functional status. 90% are nonfunctional. The frequency of adrenal carcinomas is less than 1% the frequency of benign adrenal adenomas. Surgery should be performed on nonfunctional masses >3 cm in diameter and on all functional masses. If surgery is not performed, CT scans should be repeated every 3–6 months.

ALDOSTERONISM   Aldosteronism is a syndrome associated with hypersecretion of the major adrenal mineralocorticoid aldosterone. *Primary* refers to adrenal hypersecretion, *secondary* refers to an extraadrenal stimulus. Most pts with primary hyperaldosteronism have headaches and mild diastolic hypertension. Hypokalemia may be severe, and hypernatremia can be due both to Na retention and water loss due to polyuria (impairment of concentration of urine). Metabolic alkalosis and elevated serum HCO_3 are due to H^+ movement intracellularly and H^+ loss in urine. The ECG shows signs of potassium depletion (U waves, arrhythmias, premature contractions). The criteria for diagnosis are (1) diastolic hypertension with edema, (2) hyposecretion of renin (as judged by low plasma renin activity levels) that fails to increase appropriately during volume depletion (upright posture, sodium depletion), and (3) hypersecretion of aldosterone that fails to suppress appropriately during volume expansion (salt loading). Abdominal CT/MRI or percutaneous transfemoral bilateral adrenal vein catheterization with simultaneous

TABLE 144-2   Causes of hirsutism in women

I. Familial
II. Idiopathic
III. Ovarian
    A. Polycystic ovaries; hilus-cell hyperplasia
    B. Tumor arrhenoblastoma, hilus cell, adrenal rest
IV. Adrenal
    A. Congenital adrenal hyperplasia
    B. Noncongenital adrenal hyperplasia (Cushing's)
    C. Tumor: virilizing carcinoma or adenoma

From Williams GH, Dluhy RG: HPIM-12, p. 1713.

adrenal venography can localize the adenoma. Surgery can be curative in pts with adrenal adenoma. Sodium restriction and spironolactone (25–100 mg/d) may be effective in pts with bilateral adrenal hyperplasia. Secondary hyperaldosteronism is associated with elevated plasma renin activity (see Table 144-1). Rarely, hypertensive pts with hypokalemic alkalosis have deoxycorticosterone (DOC)-secreting adenomas. Such pts have low renin levels and normal or reduced aldosterone levels.

ADRENAL ANDROGEN EXCESS   The syndromes of adrenal androgen excess result from overproduction of dehydroepiandrosterone and androstenedione. Signs and symptoms in women include hirsutism, oligomenorrhea, acne, and virilization. These syndromes can result from hyperplasia, adenoma, or carcinoma. *Congenital adrenal hyperplasia* is caused by various enzymatic defects in the steroid hormone pathway inherited as an autosomal recessive trait. C-21 hydroxylase deficiency is the most common, resulting in virilization of female infants and cortisol deficiency, with or without an associated salt-losing tendency. Other enzyme defects result in a range of phenotypes. The diagnosis should be considered in any infant with "failure to thrive," esp. if there is saltwasting or abnormal genitalia. Therapy consists of daily prednisone 5–7.5 mg. *Late onset adrenal hyperplasia* (partial C-21 hydroxylase deficiency) is characterized by elevated urinary 17-ketosteroids and plasma DHEA sulfate. Diagnosis can be confirmed by high basal levels of 17-hydroxyprogesterone, or elevation of 17-hydroxyprogesterone after ACTH stimulation (1–4 h infusion). Therapy consists of daily glucocorticoids (prednisone 2.5–5 mg/night). For adenoma and carcinoma see above.

Hirsutism in women is most often idiopathic. The differential diagnosis is found in Table 144-2, and evaluation in Table 144-3.

TABLE 144-3 Laboratory evaluation of hirsutism-virilizing syndromes

	Ovarian		Adrenal			Idiopathic
	PCO	Ovarian tumor	CAH	Adrenal neoplasm	Cushing's syndrome	
Urinary 17-ketosteroids, plasma DHEA sulfate	N↑	N	N↑	↑↑	N↑	N
Plasma testosterone	N↑	↑↑	N↑	N↑	N	N
LH/FSH ratio	N↑	N	N	N	N	N
Precursors of cortisol biosynthesis:						
Basal	N	N	N↑	N↑	N	N
Following ACTH infusion	N	N	↑↑	N↑	N	N
Cortisol following overnight dexamethasone suppression test	N	N	N	↑	↑	N

NOTE: CAH, congenital adrenal hyperplasia; PCO, polycystic ovary syndrome; N, normal; ↑, elevated.
From Williams GH, Dluhy RG: HPIM-12, p. 1729.

HYPOFUNCTION OF THE ADRENAL GLAND

ADDISON'S DISEASE   Occurs when $\geq 90\%$ of adrenal tissue is destroyed, either by tuberculosis, histoplasmosis, coccidioidomycosis and cryptococcosis, or autoimmune mechanisms. Bilateral tumor metastases, amyloidosis, and sarcoidosis are rare causes.

Clinical manifestations   Include fatigability, weakness, anorexia, nausea and vomiting, cutaneous and mucosal pigmentation, hypotension, and occasionally, hypoglycemia. Routine laboratory parameters may be normal, or serum Na, Cl, and HCO_3 can be reduced while serum K is increased. Extracellular fluid depletion accentuates hypotension.

Diagnosis   Requires assessment of adrenal capacity for steroid production. A rapid screening test is to administer 25 U ACTH (cosyntropin) intravenously and measure plasma cortisol levels at baseline, then 30 and 60 minutes later. An increment of <7 µg/dL above baseline suggests adrenal insufficiency. To differentiate primary from secondary adrenal insufficiency, cosyntropin is infused at a rate of 2 U/h for 24 h. In normal subjects, 17-hydroxysteroid excretion is increased by 25 mg/d, and plasma cortisol levels >40 µg/dL. In secondary disease, the maximal urinary 17-hydroxysteroid is 3–20 mg/d, and the plasma cortisol ranges from 10–40 mg/dL. Pts with primary disease have smaller responses.

Treatment   Hydrocortisone: in periods of stress, the dosage should be 100–200 mg/d, tapered for long-term replacement to 25–37.5 mg/d. Fludrocortisone (0.1 mg/d) also may be necessary. In emergencies, a bolus of 100 mg IV cortisol is followed by a continuous infusion of 10 mg/h.

HYPOALDOSTERONISM   Isolated aldosterone deficiency accompanied by normal cortisol production occurs with hyporeninism, as an inherited biosynthetic defect, postoperatively following removal of aldosterone-secreting adenomas, during protracted heparin or heparinoid administration, in pretectal disease of the nervous system, and in severe postural hypotension. Most pts present with unexplained hyperkalemia, often exacerbated by salt restriction.

Hyporeninemic hypoaldosteronism is most commonly seen in adults with mild renal failure and diabetes mellitus in association with disproportionate hyperkalemia and metabolic acidosis. Oral fludrocortisone (0.1–0.2 mg daily) restores electrolyte balance if salt intake is adequate. Some pts may require higher doses to correct hyperkalemia.

CLINICAL USE OF GLUCOCORTICOIDS

Glucocorticoids are pharmacologic agents for a variety of disorders. Replacement therapy is indicated for pts with

Addison's disease (hydrocortisone 20–30 mg/d regardless of size). Steroids are also used in rheumatologic diseases (rheumatoid arthritis, SLE, vasculitis, temporal arteritis), hematologic diseases (hemolytic anemia, leukemia), neurologic (cerebral edema) and pulmonary disorders (sarcoidosis, COPD), and endocrine states (hypercalcemia). As little as 10 mg/d of prednisone for 3 weeks can suppress the adrenal axis for up to 1 year. Stress can precipitate adrenal crisis in such patients even months after discontinuation, and these individuals should carry this information in case of emergency. "Stress doses" of glucocorticoids are the equivalent of 80–160 mg/d of hydrocortisone. Long-term glucocorticoid therapy in pharmacologic doses can result in weight gain, hypertension, Cushingoid facies, diabetes mellitus, osteoporosis, myopathy, increased intraocular pressure, ischemic bone necrosis, infection, hypercholesterolemia, type IV hyperlipoproteinuria, and other effects. See Table 144-4 for dosage equivalents of glucocorticoids in common use.

PHEOCHROMOCYTOMA (see Chap. 69).

TABLE 144-4 Glucocorticoid preparations

Generic name	Relative potency		Dose equivalent
	Glucocorticoid	Mineralocorticoid	
Short-acting			
Hydrocortisone (cortisol)	1.0	1.0	20.0
Cortisone	0.8	0.8	25.0
Intermediate-acting			
Prednisone	4.0	0.8	5.0
Methylprednisolone	5.0	0.5	4.0
Triamcinolone	5.0	0	4.0
Long-acting			
Dexamethasone	25.0	0	0.75
Betamethasone	25.0	0	0.6

For a more detailed discussion, see Williams GH, Dluhy RG: Diseases of the Adrenal Cortex, Chap. 317, in HPIM-12, p. 1713

145 DIABETES MELLITUS

Diabetes mellitus is the most common endocrine disorder. The diagnosis requires a fasting plasma glucose of ≥7.8 mmol/L (>140 mg/dL) on two occasions. Following ingestion of 75 g of glucose, the finding of a venous plasma glucose ≥11.1 mmol/L (≥200 mg/dL) after 2 h and on at least one other occasion during the 2-h test is suggestive of the diagnosis. Pts with insulin-dependent diabetes (IDDM) develop ketoacidosis in absence of insulin. Those with non-insulin-dependent diabetes (NIDDM) do not develop ketoacidosis and may be treated with diet, oral hypoglycemics, or insulin. Secondary forms of diabetes occur in chronic pancreatitis, pheochromocytoma, acromegaly, Cushing's syndrome and exogenous glucocorticoid administration. Hyperglycemia usually causes <u>polyuria</u>, <u>polydipsia</u>, <u>polyphagia</u>, and <u>weight loss</u>, but the first symptom may be ketoacidosis or hyperosmolar nonketotic coma.

Once diagnosis is established, a diet should be instituted that includes an appropriate number of calories based on ideal body weight, adequate protein, and a carbohydrate intake of about 40–60% of total energy. In IDDM appropriate distribution of intake is also important to avoid hypoglycemia. When hyperglycemia in NIDDM cannot be controlled by diet, sulfonylureas may be administered (see Table 145-1). Insulin is required for pts with IDDM and many with NIDDM (see Table 145-2). Conventional therapy involves the administration of an intermediate-acting insulin (NPH) once or twice a day with or without small amounts of regular insulin. Adults with NIDDM can be started on NPH 20 U/d given in the A.M. Markedly obese patients can be started on 25–30 U/d of NPH. Changes in therapy are usually made in 5 to 10-U increments. Two injections per day are generally used when the total dose reaches 50–60 U/d. Goals for blood glucose control are found in Table 145-3.

Recommendations regarding the use of regular insulin in combination with NPH insulin once the blood sugar is in a reasonable range on NPH alone can be found in Table 145-4.

LONG-TERM COMPLICATIONS These cause serious morbidity and mortality. <u>*Peripheral atherosclerosis*</u> may cause intermittent claudication, gangrene, coronary artery disease, and stroke. <u>*Cardiomyopathy*</u> can cause heart failure, despite angiographically normal coronary arteries. <u>*Diabetic retinopathy*</u> can be divided into simple (background) and proliferative

(more often Type II)* (more often Type I)* 575

TABLE 145-1   The sulfonylureas

Agent	Daily dose, mg	Doses/d	Duration of hyperglycemic action, h
Acetohexamide	250–1500	1–2	12–18
Chlorpropamide	100–500	1	60
Tolazamide	100–1000	1–2	12–14
Tolbutamide	500–3000	2–3	6–12
Glyburide	1.25–20	1–2	Up to 24
Glipizide	2.5–40	1–2	Up to 24
Glibornuride	12.5–100	1–2	Up to 24

SOURCE: Modified from RH Unger, DW Foster, Diabetes mellitus, in *Williams' Textbook of Endocrinology*, 8th ed, JD Wilson, DW Foster (eds). Philadelphia, Saunders, 1990.

forms. New vessel formation and scarring can cause vitreal hemorrhage and retinal detachment, so that it is leading cause of blindness. _Renal disease_ is a major cause of death and disability. The kidneys are initially enlarged with "superfunction." Microalbuminuria then appears with excretion of albumin in the range of 20–200 mg/d. Once macroalbuminuria begins (>200 mg/d), GFR declines at a rate of about 1 mL/min per month. Ordinarily azotemia begins about 10–12 years after onset of diabetes and may be preceded by nephrotic syndrome. No specific treatment is available, but the rate of progression may be slowed with the use of ACE inhibitors. Hypertension must be aggressively controlled. Low-protein diets may be useful. Chronic dialysis and renal transplantation are routine in these pts. Hyporeninemic hypoaldosteronism, associated with renal tubular acidosis, may require alkalinizing solutions (Shohl's) and avoidance of external potassium loads.

TABLE 145-2   Insulin preparations available * note differences b
human + beef/po

	Onset of action, h	Peak effect, h	Duration of action, h
Rapid-acting:			
Regular	0.25–1	2–6	4–12
Semilente	0.25–1	3–6	8–16
Intermediate-acting:			
NPH	1.5–4	6–16	12–24
Lente	1–4	6–16	12–28
Long-acting:			
Ultralente	3–8	14–24	24–48
Protamine zinc	3–8	14–24	24–48

TABLE 145-3   Goals for blood glucose in the control of diabetes*

	Acceptable		Ideal	
Goal	mmol/L	mg/dL	mmol/L	mg/dL
Fasting	3.3–7.2	60–130	3.9–5.6	70–100
Preprandial	3.3–7.2	60–130	3.9–5.6	70–100
Postprandial (1 h)	<11.1	<200	<8.9	<160
3 A.M.	>3.6	>65	>3.6	>65

* Values for healthy patients below the age of 65. Goals may be shifted upward in older patients.
From Foster DW: HPIM-12, p. 1747.

Peripheral sensory neuropathy causes numbness, paresthesias, severe hypesthesias, and pain that may be deep-seated and severe and is often worse at night. Absent stretch reflexes and diminished vibratory sensation are early signs. A special problem is foot ulcers. Diabetics should be instructed about proper foot care to prevent ulcers. _Autonomic neuropathy_ may cause GI complaints (esophageal dysfunction, delayed gastric emptying, constipation, or diarrhea), orthostatic hypotension, bladder dysfunction, incontinence, and (in men) erectile impotence.

TABLE 145-4   Adjusting insulin dosage in conventional insulin therapy*

		Regular insulin, units	
Blood glucose		Breakfast (to be mixed with intermediate dosage)	Supper
mmol/L	mg/dL		
2.8–5.5	51–100	8	4
5.6–8.3	101–150	10	5
8.4–11.1	151–200	12	6
11.2–13.9	201–250	14	7
14.0–16.6	251–300	16	8
>16.6	>300	20	10

* Once the patient has most blood sugars in the reasonable range, a prescription can be written for varying the regular insulin dosage as illustrated. The prescription in this case was for a patient in reasonable control on 25 units of NPH plus 10 units of regular before breakfast and 10 units of NPH plus 5 units of regular before supper. Change in metabolic status may require adjustments in both intermediate insulin and the sliding scale of regular insulin.
From Foster DW: HPIM-12, p. 1745.

For a more detailed discussion, see Foster DW: Diabetes
Mellitus, Chap. 319, in HPIM-12, p. 1739

Diabetic retinopathy:
1) Background - microaneurysms (dots), microhemorrhages (blots), hard exudate
2) Pre-proliferation - cotton-wool exudates (small retinal infarcts), extensive microh
3) Proliferative - new vessels (worst in optic disc)
4) Maculopathy - more common in Type II DM, impaired visual acuity

Samogyi phenomenon:
  - rebound hyperglycemia following an episode of hypoglycemia
  due to counter-regulatory hormone (glucagon, epinephrine) release
  - suspect whenever wide swings in plasma glucose occur over
  short time intervals even if no S_x
  - check 3 am b.g. - should be low
  ∴ ↓ insulin (intermediate)

Dawn phenomenon:
  - early morning rise in plasma glucose requiring ↑ insulin
  - due to nocturnal surge of growth hormone - major factor
  - also ↑ insulin clearance in early morning hours

The diagnosis requires a plasma glucose <2.5–2.8 mmol/L (<45–50 mg/dL) in men and <1.9–2.2 mmol/L (<35–40 mg/dL) in women, symptoms consistent with the diagnosis, and improvement of symptoms with an increase of plasma glucose (Whipple's triad). When diagnosis is strongly suspected, glucose should be administered after drawing blood for diagnostic studies.

Catecholamine secretion causes sweating, tremor, tachycardia, anxiety, and hunger. CNS symptoms include dizziness, visual abnormalities, diminished mental acuity, convulsions, and syncope. In diabetics hypoglycemic symptoms may be masked if severe autonomic neuropathy is present or if treated with beta blockers.

POSTPRANDIAL (REACTIVE) HYPOGLYCEMIA Results when gastrectomy, gastrojejunostomy, pyloroplasty, or vagotomy causes rapid gastric emptying and when brisk absorption of glucose in turn causes excessive insulin release. Plasma glucose falls more rapidly than insulin levels, and hypoglycemia results. Additional causes include fructose intolerance, galactosemia, and leucine sensitivity.

FASTING HYPOGLYCEMIA Results from an imbalance between hepatic production and peripheral glucose utilization. Increased utilization (glucose demand of >200 g/d) usually results from hyperinsulinism (insulinoma, exogenous insulin, sulfonylurea ingestion, or insulin autoimmunity). Glucose overutilization with low plasma insulin can be due to extrapancreatic tumors (fibromas, sarcomas, hepatomas, carcinomas of GI tract, and adrenal tumors). Such tumors either produce insulin-like factors or utilize glucose directly. Hypoglycemia with low plasma insulin also may occur when free fatty acids are not available for oxidation, as in carnitine deficiency and carnitine palmitoyltransferase deficiency. Diminished hepatic glucose production can be due to alcoholism, adrenal insufficiency, or liver disease (i.e., CHF) (see Table 146-1).

Diagnosis of fasting hypoglycemia is established by the simultaneous measurement of serum glucose, insulin, and C-peptide and urine sulfonylurea metabolites during an episode of symptoms consistent with hypoglycemia. If history is suggestive but fasting plasma glucose is normal, hospitalization for a 72-h fast is required; serial measurements of glucose and insulin are made until symptoms develop or fast is completed. Diagnosis of insulinoma requires a low plasma

TABLE 146-1   Major causes of fasting hypoglycemia

I. Conditions primarily due to underproduction of glucose
  A. Hormone deficiencies
      1. Hypopituitarism
      2. Adrenal insufficiency
      3. Catecholamine deficiency
      4. Glucagon deficiency
  B. Enzyme defects
      1. Glucose-6-phosphatase
      2. Liver phosphorylase
      3. Pyruvate carboxylase
      4. Phosphoenolpyruvate carboxykinase
      5. Fructose-1, 6-diphosphatase
      6. Glycogen synthetase
  C. Substrate deficiency
      1. Ketotic hypoglycemia of infancy
      2. Severe malnutrition, muscle wasting
      3. Late pregnancy
  D. Acquired liver disease
      1. Hepatic congestion
      2. Severe hepatitis
      3. Cirrhosis
      4. Uremia (probably multiple mechanisms)
      5. Hypothermia
  E. Drugs
      1. Alcohol
      2. Propranolol
      3. Salicylates
II. Conditions primarily due to overutilization of glucose
  A. Hyperinsulinism
      1. Insulinoma
      2. Exogenous insulin
      3. Sulfonylureas
      4. Immune disease with insulin or insulin receptor antibodies
      5. Drugs: quinine in falciparum malaria, disopyramide, pentamidine
      6. Endotoxic shock
  B. Appropriate insulin levels
      1. Extrapancreatic tumors
      2. Systemic carnitine deficiency
      3. Deficiency in enzymes of fat oxidation
      4. 3-Hydroxy-3-methylglutaryl-CoA lyase deficiency
      5. Cachexia with fat depletion

From Foster DW, Rubenstein AH: HPIM-12, p. 1761.

glucose and inappropriately high insulin. Exogenous insulin is excluded by the simultaneous measurement of C peptide, and a screen for sulfonylureas eliminates the possibility of oral hypoglycemic agents. The presence of an extrapancreatic tumor is suggested by low glucose and insulin levels (see Table 146-2).

TABLE 146-2 Differential diagnosis of insulinoma and factitious hyperinsulinism

Test	Insulinoma	Exogenous insulin	Sulfonylurea
Plasma insulin	High	Very high*	High
Insulin/glucose ratio	High	Very high	High
Proinsulin	Increased	Normal or low	Normal
C peptide	Increased	Normal or low†	Increased
Insulin antibodies	Absent	± Present‡	Absent
Plasma or urine sulfonylurea	Absent	Absent	Present

* Total plasma insulin in patients with insulinoma is rarely above 1435 pmol/L (200 μU/mL) in the basal state and often much lower. Values greater than 7175 pmol/L (100 μU/mL) are highly suggestive of exogenous insulin injection.
† C peptide may be normal in absolute terms, but low in relation to the increased insulin value. See text for C peptide suppression test.
‡ Insulin bodies may not be present if only a few injections have been given, especially with purified insulins.
From Foster DW, Rubenstein AH: HPIM-12, p. 1764.

THERAPY Initial rapid IV administration of 50 mL 50% glucose in water followed by infusion of 10% glucose to keep plasma glucose >5.6 mmol/L (>100 mg/dL) in serious hypoglycemia. Pts with glucose overutilization may require >10 g/h (or a diet containing more than 300 g carbohydrate/ d if the pt can eat). Glucagon (1 mg) is less desirable because its transient effects are blunted when hepatic glycogen is depleted. Hypoglycemia caused by sulfonylureas may be prolonged, and pts must be carefully monitored. Surgical excision is the treatment of choice for insulinoma. Localization should be attempted by CT scan, sonography, or arteriography. Medical therapy is indicated only in preparation for surgery or after failure to localize the tumor at surgery. Diazoxide IV or orally in doses of 300–1200 mg/d plus a diuretic may be used, or octreotide is given SC in divided doses of 150–450 μg/d.

Therapy of other forms of hypoglycemia is dietary. Pts should avoid fasting and should ingest frequent small meals.

For a more detailed discussion, see Foster DW, Rubenstein AH: Hypoglycemia, Chap. 320, in HPIM-12, p. 1759

Inadequate production of sperm can occur as an isolated defect, whereas inadequate formation of testosterone by the interstitial (Leydig) cells usually impairs spermatogenesis secondarily. Classification of abnormalities of testicular function in adults is found in Table 147-1.

DISORDERS OF ANDROGENS Assessment of androgen status should include documenting timing and extent of sexual maturation at puberty, rate of beard growth, testicular size, current libido, sexual function, and general strength and energy. If Leydig cell dysfunction occurs prior to onset of puberty, sexual maturation will not occur (eunuchoidism), evidenced by an infantile amount and distribution of body hair, poor development of skeletal muscles, and failure of closure of the epiphyses so that the arm span is >5 cm greater than height and the lower body segment is >5 cm longer than the upper body segment (pubis to crown).

At the completion of puberty, plasma testosterone levels reach the adult level of 10–35 nmol/L (3–10 ng/mL) throughout the day, and plasma LH and FSH levels are 5–20 IU/L each. Testicular failure after puberty can be due either to hypothalamic-pituitary defects (secondary hypogonadism) or testicular failure (primary hypogonadism). Detection of Leydig cell failure that occurs after puberty requires a high index of suspicion, commonly presenting as gynecomastia or diminished virilization and libido.

Kallman's syndrome (hypogonadotropic hypogonadism) The most frequent cause of secondary hypogonadism. It is characterized by familial occurrence, low FSH and LH levels, and (in some) anosmia, midline skeletal defects, mental retardation, and cryptorchidism. The defect appears to be in the synthesis or release of LH-releasing hormone (LHRH) with the resulting gonadotropin pattern ranging from absence of pulsatile LH secretion to defects in amplitude and frequency of LH secretion. If untreated, these pts usually remain in the prepubertal state indefinitely. Destruction of pituitary gland by tumors, infections, trauma, or metastatic disease ordinarily causes hypogonadism as a component of panhypopituitarism. Pts with Cushing's syndrome, congenital adrenal hyperplasia, hemochromatosis, and hyperprolactinemia (due to either pituitary adenomas or drugs such as phenothiazines) may have suppressed levels of LH with resultant low testosterone levels.

TABLE 147-1 Classification of abnormalities of testicular function in the adult

Site of defect	Presentation	
	Infertility with underandrogenization	Infertility with normal virilization
Hypothalamic-pituitary	Panhypopituitarism	
	Hypogonadotropic hypogonadism	Isolated FSH deficiency
	Cushing's syndrome	Congenital adrenal hyperplasia
	Hyperprolactinemia	Hyperprolactinemia
	Hemochromatosis	Androgen use
Testicular	Developmental and structural defects:	
	Klinefelter's syndrome*	Germinal cell aplasia
		Cryptorchidism
	XX male	Varicocele
		Immotile cilia syndrome
	Acquired defects:	
	Viral orchitis*	*Mycoplasma* infection
	Trauma	
	Radiation	Radiation
	Drugs (spironolactone, alcohol, ketoconazole, cyclophosphamide)	Drugs (cyclophosphamide) Environmental toxins
	Autoimmunity	Autoimmunity
	Granulomatous disease	
	Associated with systemic diseases:	
	Liver disease	Febrile illness
	Renal failure	Celiac disease
	Sickle cell disease	
	Neurologic diseases (myotonic dystrophy and paraplegia)	Neurologic disease (paraplegia)
	Androgen resistance	Androgen resistance
Sperm transport		Obstruction of the epididymis or vas deferens (cystic fibrosis, diethylstilbestrol exposure, congenital absence)

* The common testicular causes of underandrogenization and infertility in adults—Klinefelter's syndrome and viral orchitis—are associated with small testes.

From Griffin JE, Wilson JD: HPIM-12, p. 1771.

In men with primary hypogonadism, testosterone levels are lowered and gonadotropin levels are raised.

Klinefelter's syndrome   Most frequent cause of primary testicular failure; due to the presence of one or more extra X chromosomes, usually 47,XXY karyotype. The testes are small and contain sclerosed tubules; azoospermia is usual. Gynecomastia is common, and variable features include a eunuchoid habitus, mental retardation, and diabetes mellitus.

Acquired primary testicular failure   Usually results from *viral orchitis*, most frequently mumps, but also may be due to trauma, radiation damage, or systemic diseases such as amyloidosis, Hodgkin's disease, and sickle cell anemia. Testicular failure also may result from malnutrition, renal failure, liver disease, and toxins such as lead, alcohol, marijuana, heroin, methadone, and antineoplastic and chemotherapeutic agents. Spironolactone and ketoconazole block the synthesis of testosterone, and spironolactone and cimetidine act as antiandrogens by competing for binding to the androgen receptor. Testicular failure also occurs as part of a generalized disorder of autoimmunity in which multiple primary endocrine deficiencies coexist (polyglandular autoimmune failure). Granulomatous diseases can also destroy the testes (leprosy is the most common).

The aim of androgen therapy in hypogonadal men is to restore normal male secondary sexual characteristics (beard, body hair, external genitalia), male sexual behavior, and somatic development (hemoglobin, muscle mass). Parenteral administration of a long-acting testosterone ester (100–200 mg testosterone enanthate at 1- to 3-week intervals) causes a return of testosterone levels to normal.

MALE INFERTILITY   Normal sperm production is dependent on both FSH and testosterone. When damage occurs to seminiferous tubule prior to puberty, testes are small and firm, whereas testes are usually soft following postpubertal damage (the capsule once enlarged does not contract to its previous size). Normal ejaculate volume should be >2 mL, with 20–100 million sperm/mL, >60% of which should be mobile. Plasma FSH usually correlates inversely with spermatogenesis.

In addition to secondary impairment of spermatogenesis by androgen deficiency, isolated spermatogenic tubule dysfunction and impaired spermatogenesis can arise from alterations of temperature of testes (varicocele), cryptorchism, cystic fibrosis, or immotile cilia syndrome. Kartagener's syndrome is a subgroup of the latter with situs inversus. Varicocoele may be of etiologic importance in one-third of all male infertility.

Defects in the androgen receptor cause resistance to the action of androgen usually associated with defective male phenotypic development as well as infertility and underandrogenization. Disorders of sperm transport may also cause infertility in as many as 6% of infertile men with normal virilization. Ejaculatory obstruction may be congenital (idiopathic, cystic fibrosis, in utero DES exposure) or acquired (tuberculosis, leprosy, gonorrhea).

IMPOTENCE Simply defined, impotence is the failure to achieve erection, ejaculation, or both. Men with sexual dysfunction may complain of loss of libido, inability to initiate or maintain an erection, ejaculatory failure, premature ejaculation, or inability to achieve orgasm. Sexual dysfunction can be secondary to systemic disease, specific urogenital or endocrine disorders, or psychologic disturbances. Some organic causes of erectile impotence in men can be found in Table 147-2. Evaluation includes a detailed general as well as genital physical exam. Penile abnormalities (Peyronie's disease), testicular size, and gynecomastia are of particular importance. Palpation of all pulses and auscultation for bruits are essential. Neurologic exam includes assessment of anal sphincter tone, perineal sensation, and bulbocavernosus reflex. Penile arteriography, electromyography, or pulsed-Doppler analyses with high-resolution ultrasound are occasionally performed. Pooled serum testosterone, LH, and prolactin should be measured.

Treatment includes correction (if possible) of the underlying cause, injection of vasoactive substances into the corpora cavernosa (papaverine with or without phentolamine), vacuum devices, or penile prostheses.

TESTICULAR CARCINOMA Once universally fatal, now usually curable by excision and/or chemotherapy with cisplatin-based regimens. Manifestations range from an asymptomatic nodule or swelling detected while performing testicular self-examination to symptoms caused by metastases. Any testicular mass in a man requires prompt evaluation to exclude testicular carcinoma. Testicular biopsy is performed via an inguinal approach. Alpha fetoprotein and beta human chorionic gonadotropin are common tumor markers produced by nonsemenomatous testicular tumors.

PROSTATIC HYPERPLASIA Common in men aged >50, and 40% or more of men eventually develop urinary tract obstruction. Symptoms can be minimal if compensatory hypertrophy of detrusor musculature of bladder compensates for resistance to urine flow. With increasing obstruction, diminution in caliber and force of urinary stream, hesitancy in initiating voiding, postvoiding dribbling, sensation of incomplete emptying, and on occasion, urinary retention su-

TABLE 147-2   Some organic causes of erectile impotence in men

I. Endocrine causes
    A. Testicular failure (primary or secondary)
    B. Hyperprolactinemia
II. Drugs
    A. Antiandrogens
        1. H-2 blockers (e.g., cimetidine)
        2. Spironolactone
        3. Ketocanazole
    B. Antihypertensives
        1. Central-acting sympatholytics (e.g., clonidine and methyl-
           dopa)
        2. Peripheral acting sympatholytics (e.g., guanadrel)
        3. Beta blockers
        4. Thiazides
    C. Anticholinergics
    D. Antidepressants
        1. Monoamine oxidase inhibitors
        2. Tricyclic antidepressants
    E. Antipsychotics
    F. Central nervous system depressants
        1. Sedatives (e.g., barbiturates)
        2. Antianxiety drugs (e.g., diazepam)
    G. Drugs of habituation or addiction
        1. Alcohol
        2. Methadone
        3. Heroin
III. Penile diseases
    A. Peyronie's disease
    B. Previous priapism
    C. Penile trauma
IV. Neurologic diseases
    A. Anterior temporal lobe lesions
    B. Diseases of the spinal cord
    C. Loss of sensory input
        1. Tabes dorsalis
        2. Disease of dorsal root ganglia
    D. Disease of nervi erigentes
        1. Radical prostatectomy and cystectomy
        2. Rectosigmoid operations
    E. Diabetic autonomic neuropathy and various polyneuropathies
V. Vascular disease
    A. Aortic occlusion (Leriche syndrome)
    B. Atherosclerotic occlusion or stenosis of the pudendal and/or
       cavernosal arteries
    C. Venous leak
    D. Disease of the sinusoidal spaces

From McConnell JD, Wilson JD: HPIM-12, p. 29.

pervene. These obstructive symptoms must be distinguished from irritative symptoms such as dysuria, frequency, and urgency that can result from inflammatory, infectious, or neoplastic causes. As residual urine increases, nocturia and overflow incontinence may develop.

The prostate is palpated during digital rectal examination. Hyperplasia produces a smooth, firm, elastic enlargement. Bladder neck obstruction is evaluated by cystourethroscopy. Obstruction to outflow is assessed by measurement of urine flow rate and/or residual urine. Treatment may be surgical (usually transurethral prostatectomy). When surgery is contraindicated, medical castration with LHRH agonists may improve urine outflow.

PROSTATIC CARCINOMA Cancer of the prostate is second most common malignancy in men. It can be asymptomatic at diagnosis, but most pts have extensive disease at diagnosis. Common presenting complaints include dysuria, difficulty in voiding, increased urinary frequency, complete urinary retention, back or hip pain, and hematuria.

Importance of the rectal exam in the physical exam of men cannot be stressed too strongly. The posterior surfaces of the lateral lobes, where carcinoma usually begins, are palpable on rectal examination. Carcinoma is characteristically hard, nodular, and irregular.

Biopsy is indicated when a palpable abnormality is detected or when lower urinary tract symptoms occur in men who have no known cause of obstruction. Core-needle biopsy may be performed transperineally or transrectally. Elevated serum acid phosphatase level is present in some localized disease but more commonly with extensive disease. Prostate-specific antigen is also commonly elevated and is a more specific test.

Surgical staging is the usual modality for identifying lymph node involvement and determining therapy. Radiation therapy and androgen deprivation (orchiectomy or diethylstilbestrol) are indicated for palliation of metastatic disease.

For a more detailed discussion, see McConnell JD, Wilson JD: Impotence, Chap. 52, p. 296; Griffin JE III, Wilson JD: Disorders of the Testis, Chap. 321, p. 1765; and Sagalowsky AI, Wilson JD: Hyperplasia and Carcinoma of the Prostate, Chap. 306, p. 1629, in HPIM-12

MENSTRUAL DISORDERS **Abnormal uterine bleeding** When uterine bleeding is suspected, other sources such as rectum, bladder, cervix, and vagina must be excluded. In premenarche period, abnormal uterine bleeding may result from trauma, infection, or precocious puberty. When vaginal bleeding develops following menopause, malignancy must be excluded.

In absence of pregnancy, abnormal uterine bleeding during reproductive years is associated with either ovulatory or anovulatory cycles. Menstrual bleeding with ovulatory cycles is spontaneous, regular in onset, predictable in duration and amount of flow, and usually painful. Abnormal but nevertheless regular cycles are usually due to organic obstruction of uterus, usually leiomyomas, adenomyosis, endometrial polyps, or on occasion, uterine synechiae or scarring. Bleeding between cyclic ovulatory menses can be due to cervical or endometrial lesions.

Menstrual bleeding unassociated with ovulation (dysfunctional uterine bleeding) is painless, irregular in occurrence, and unpredictable as to amount and duration. Transient disruption of hypothalamic-pituitary-ovarian cycle is a common cause of failure of ovulation in menarchial years. Persistent dysfunctional uterine bleeding in reproductive years is usually due to continuous estrogenization of uterus uninterrupted by cyclic progesterone withdrawal, most commonly due to polycystic ovarian disease.

Amenorrhea All women of childbearing age with amenorrhea should be assumed to be pregnant until proven otherwise. Even when history and physical exam are not suggestive, it is prudent to exclude pregnancy by a suitable screening test.

Primary amenorrhea is defined as failure of menarche by age 16 regardless of the presence or absence of secondary sexual characteristics, and *secondary amenorrhea* is failure of menstruation for 6 months in a woman with previous periodic menses. However, the causes of primary and secondary amenorrhea overlap, and it is generally more useful classifying the disorder according to etiology (Fig. 148-1). Initial workup involves careful physical exam, serum prolactin assay, and evaluation of estrogen status.

Anatomic defects of reproductive tract Defects that prevent vaginal bleeding include absence of vagina, imper-

FIGURE 143-1 Flow diagram for the evaluation of women with amenorrhea. The most common diagnosis for each category is shown in parenthesis. The dotted lines indicate that in some instances a correct diagnosis can be reached on the basis of history and physical exam alone. (Reproduced from Carr BR, Wilson JD; HPIM-12, p. 1830.)

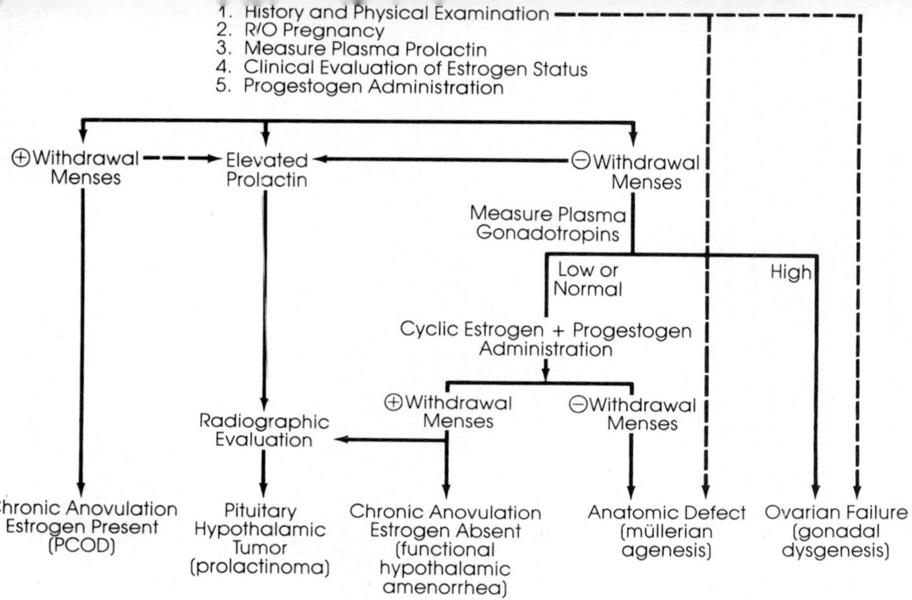

forate hymen, transverse vaginal septae, and cervical stenosis; presence is usually suggested by physical exam. When findings are indeterminate, diagnosis can be established by administration of medroxyprogesterone acetate 10–20 mg/d PO for 5 d or 100 mg progesterone in oil IM. If estrogen levels are adequate (and outflow tract is intact), menstrual bleeding should occur within 1 week of ending progestogen treatment, and hence diagnosis is *chronic anovulation with estrogen present*, usually *polycystic ovarian disease*. If no withdrawal bleeding occurs and the serum prolactin level is normal in the anovulatory woman with absent estrogen, plasma gonadotropins should be measured. If plasma gonadotropins are increased, the diagnosis is *ovarian failure (gonadal dysgenesis, resistant ovary syndrome*, or *premature ovarian failure)*. Chromosomal karyotyping is useful when gonadal dysgenesis is suspected.

If gonadotropins are normal or decreased, the diagnosis is either *hypothalamic-pituitary disorder* or an anatomic defect of outflow tract (see above). When physical findings are not clear-cut, it is useful to administer cyclic estrogen plus progestogen (1.25 mg oral conjugated estrogens qd for 3 weeks with 10 mg medroxyprogesterone acetate added for the last 5–7 d of treatment) followed by 10 d of observation. If no bleeding occurs, the diagnosis of *Asherman's syndrome* or *other anatomic defects* of outflow tract is confirmed by hysteroscopy or hysterosalpingogram. If withdrawal bleeding occurs following estrogen-progesterone combination, the diagnosis is *chronic anovulation with estrogen absent (functional hypothalamic amenorrhea)*; causes include Kallman's syndrome (hypogonadotropic hypogonadism), extreme emotional stress, anorexia nervosa, chronic debilitating disease, pituitary adenomas, craniopharyngiomas, and panhypopituitarism. Radiologic evaluation of pituitary-hypothalamic region may be indicated.

Pelvic pain may be associated with normal menstrual periods as well as abnormal menstrual cycles. Many women experience abdominal discomfort with ovulation ("mittelschmerz"), a dull, aching pain at midcycle lasting minutes to hours. In addition, ovulatory women may experience somatic symptoms during the few days prior to menses, including edema, breast engorgement, abdominal discomfort, and a symptom of cyclic irritability, depression, and lethargy known as *premenstrual syndrome*. Severe or incapacitating cramping in women with ovulatory menses in the absence of demonstrable disorders of the pelvis is termed *primary dysmenorrhea* and is best treated with NSAIDs or oral contraceptive agents. Pelvic pain due to organic causes may be classified as uterine (leiomyomas, adenomyosis, cervical stenosis, infections, cancer), adnexal (salpingo-oophoritis, cysts, neoplasms, torsion, endometriosis), vulvar or vaginal (*Monilia, Trichomonas, Gardnerella, Herpes,* condyloma acuminatum, cysts or abscesses of Bartholin's glands) and pregnancy-associated (threatened or incomplete abortion, ectopic pregnancy). Evaluation includes history, pelvic exam, human chorionic gonadotropin measurement, pelvic ultrasound, and laparoscopy or laparotomy in some cases.

MENOPAUSE The interval between the reproductive years up to and beyond the last menstrual period. During this time there is a progressive loss of ovarian function accompanied by endocrine, somatic, and psychological changes. The same symptoms may result from surgical ablation of the ovaries and include those of vasomotor instability (hot flash), atrophy of urogenital epithelium and skin, decreased size of breasts, and osteoporosis. Additional symptoms include nervousness, anxiety, irritability, and depression. Plasma gonadotropins are elevated.

Estrogen therapy in menopause relieves vasomotor instability (hot flashes), prevents atrophy of urogenital epithelium and skin, and prevents osteoporosis. The risks of endometrial adenocarcinoma, venous thromboembolism, and hypertension may be minimized by low-dose cyclic estrogen administration (0.625 mg/d conjugated estrogen for 25 d/month with daily progestogen for the last 10 d) and close clinical monitoring. Pts who have had a hysterectomy can be treated with conjugated estrogen (0.625 mg/d).

ORAL CONTRACEPTIVE AGENTS Widely used to prevent pregnancy and control dysmenorrhea and anovulatory bleeding. The ideal contraceptive contains the lowest amount of steroid to minimize side effects but sufficient to prevent pregnancy or breakthrough bleeding. Combination oral contraceptive agents contain synthetic estrogen (mestranol or ethinyl estradiol) and synthetic progestogen (norethindrone, norethindrone acetate, norethynodrel, norgestrel, or ethynodiol diacetate). Biphasic or triphasic formulations utilize different agents at different times of the cycle.

Despite overall safety, users are at risk for deep venous thrombosis, pulmonary embolism, thromboembolic stroke, hypertension, glucose intolerance, and cholelithiasis. Risks are increased with smoking and increasing age, and the drugs should be discontinued in women who experience visual complaints or headaches. Other side effects include minor dyspepsia, breast discomfort, weight gain, pigmentation of the face (chloasma), and psychological effects such as depression and changes in libido. Oral contraceptives are not associated with an increased incidence of cancer of the uterus, cervix, or breast.

Absolute contraindications to the use of oral contraceptives include previous thromboembolic disorders, cerebral vascular or coronary artery disease, known or suspected carcinoma of breasts or other estrogen-dependent neoplasia, undiagnosed genital bleeding, or known or suspected pregnancy. Relative contraindications include hypertension, migraine headaches, diabetes mellitus, uterine leiomyomas, sickle cell anemia, hyperlipidemia, and elective surgery.

For a more detailed discussion, see Carr BR, Wilson JD: Disorders of the Ovary and Female Reproductive Tract, Chap. 322, in HPIM-12, p. 1776

The breasts are the site of fatal and preventable disease in women and frequently provide clues to underlying systemic disease in both men and women. As a consequence, examination of the breasts is a vital part of the physical exam.

GALACTORRHEA Whereas small amounts of fluid can be commonly expressed from the breasts of parous women, secretions from the breasts of nulliparous women are always abnormal and require evaluation. Spontaneous leakage of milk is of particular concern. When secretion is milky or white, assume that it contains milk constituents; brown or green secretions rarely contain normal milk constituents. Bloody breast secretions suggest malignancy. Although enhanced prolactin secretion is necessary for initiation of milk production, the elevation need not be sustained in long-standing galactorrhea.

Galactorrhea is generally the result of failure of normal hypothalamic inhibition of prolactin release (sarcoidosis, craniopharyngioma, pinealoma, encephalitis, meningitis, hypothalamic tumors) or of autonomous secretion of prolactin (pituitary adenomas, hypothyroidism). Likewise, drugs (psychotropic agents, metoclopramide, methyldopa, reserpine, antiemetics) may enhance prolactin release (see Chap. 141).

Once drug causes and hypothyroidism are excluded, workup of hyperprolactinemia is that of a pituitary tumor. *Treatment* is aimed at removing the source of elevated prolactin level, by resection or suppression of the pituitary tumor, withdrawal of causative drugs, or correction of hypothyroidism. Bromocriptine may cause disappearance of galactorrhea even when plasma prolactin levels are normal.

Normal lactation can be suppressed by the administration of estrogens or diethylstilbestrol, which inhibits milk production at the level of the breast, or bromocriptine, which inhibits prolactin secretion by the pituitary.

GYNECOMASTIA Growth of the breast in men and women is mediated by estrogen, and breast enlargement in men is believed to result from disturbances of the normal ratio of active androgen to estrogen or from increases in estrogen formation. In ≥50% of men with gynecomastia, no cause is found after extensive workup. Presumably, in these pts the elevation of estrogen is transient or remains unidentified, but in such cases the gynecomastia has no serious import for health. In other cases, gynecomastia results from major endocrine disturbances, including deficiency in testosterone production or action, increase in estrogen production, or drugs (Table 149-1).

Evaluation (1) A careful drug history; (2) measurement and examination of testes (if both are small, a chromosomal karyotype should be obtained; if they are asymmetric, a testicular tumor should be considered); (3) evaluation of liver

TABLE 149-1   Differential diagnosis of gynecomastia

PHYSIOLOGIC GYNECOMASTIA

Newborn
Adolescence
Aging

PATHOLOGIC GYNECOMASTIA

Deficient production or action of testosterone:
  Congenital defects:
    Congenital anorchia
    Klinefelter syndrome
    Androgen resistance (testicular feminization and Reifenstein syndrome)
    Defects of testosterone synthesis
  Secondary testicular failure:
    Viral orchitis
    Trauma
    Castration
    Neurologic and granulomatous diseases
    Renal failure
Increased estrogen production:
  Estrogen secretion:
    True hermaphroditism
    Testicular tumors
    Carcinoma of the lung and other tumors producing hCG
  Increased substrate for extraglandular aromatase:
    Adrenal disease
    Liver disease
    Starvation
    Thyrotoxicosis
  Increase in extraglandular aromatase
Drugs:
  Estrogens (diethylstilbestrol, birth control pills, digitalis, estrogen-containing cosmetics, estrogen-contaminated foods)
  Drugs that enhance endogenous estrogen secretion (gonadotropins, clomiphene)
  Inhibitors of testosterone synthesis and/or action (ketoconazole, metronidazole, alkylating agents, cisplatin, spironolactone, cimetidine)
  Unknown mechanisms (busulfan, isoniazid, methyldopa, tricyclic antidepressants, penicillamine, diazepam, marijuana, heroin)
Idiopathic

From Wilson JD: HPIM-12, p. 1797.

function; (4) measurement of plasma androstenedione or 24-h urinary 17-ketosteroids, plasma estradiol, plasma luteinizing hormone (LH), and plasma testosterone. If LH is increased and testosterone decreased, diagnosis is usually testicular failure; if both LH and testosterone are decreased, diagnosis is likely enhanced estrogen production; and if both LH and testosterone are increased, diagnosis is either androgen resistance or a gonadotropin-secreting tumor.

When primary cause of overestrogenization can be identified and corrected, breast enlargement usually subsides promptly and eventually disappears. *Indications for surgery* include severe psychological and/or cosmetic problems, continued growth, or suspected malignancy.

BREAST CANCER   Breast cancer is a major disease. At particular risk are women whose mothers had breast cancer prior to menopause, women with first-degree relatives with postmenopausal breast cancer, nulliparous women above age 50, women whose first parity occurred after age 30, women with a history of chronic breast disease, women exposed to ionizing radiation, and obese women. Increased risk for breast carcinoma in men includes feminizing states (such as Klinefelter syndrome) and testicular atrophy from viral orchitis or injury.

Breast cancer is frequently multicentric (13% of pts show microscopic foci in contralateral breast). Size of primary tumor can be estimated by palpitation combined with mammography. Tumor <2 cm in size are associated with most favorable outcome. Another prognostic factor is presence or absence of estrogen receptor (ER) and progesterone receptor (PR), the degree of positivity being proportional to cellular differentiation and responsiveness of tumor to hormonal deprivation.

Most breast masses are found by the pt either accidentally or during self-examination. Annual mammograms are recommended for all women over 50 and for high-risk women ages 40–49. Disease usually presents with a hard, circumscribed mass in breast. Most lumps are benign, but if mass is fixed to skin or muscle or there is edema of skin or retraction of nipple, breast cancer is more likely. Once a mass is detected, metastatic disease should be searched for, and the mass should then be biopsied.

The current trend in management aims at minimal disfigurement by surgical or radiation therapy and control of metastatic disease with adjuvant systemic chemotherapy.

Skeletal metastases can cause both pain and fractures, including vertebral collapse. Limited-field irradiation of metastases and narcotics may be effective in control of pain.

Hypercalcemia is also common in metastatic disease (see Chap. 150).

For a more detailed discussion, see Henderson C: Breast Cancer, Chap. 303, p. 1612; Wilson JD: Endocrine Disorders of the Breast, Chap. 323, in HPIM-12, p. 1795

---

150 HYPER- AND HYPOCALCEMIC DISORDERS

HYPERCALCEMIA

The causes of hypercalcemia are listed in Table 150-1. Hyperparathyroidism and malignancy account for 90% of cases.

PARATHYROID-RELATED HYPERCALCEMIA **Primary hyperparathyroidism** This is a generalized disorder of bone metabolism that results from increased secretion of parathyroid hormone (PTH), because of either an adenoma (81%), carcinoma (4%) in a single gland, or hyperplasia of all four glands (15%). Familial hyperparathyroidism may be part of multiple endocrine neoplasia type I (MEN I), which also includes tumors of pituitary and pancreatic islets and hypergastrinemia with peptic ulcer disease (Zollinger-Ellison syndrome), or MEN II, in which hyperparathyroidism occurs with pheochromocytoma and medullary carcinoma of the thyroid.

Half or more of pts with hyperparathyroidism are asymptomatic. Specific manifestations involve primarily the kidneys (nephrolithiasis and nephrocalcinosis) and the skeletal system

TABLE 150-1 Classification of causes of hypercalcemia

Parathyroid-related:
1. Primary hyperparathyroidism
   a. Solitary adenomas
   b. Multiple endocrine neoplasia
2. Lithium therapy
3. Familial hypocalciuric hypercalcemia

Malignancy-related:
1. Solid tumor with metastases (breast)
2. Solid tumor with humoral mediation of hypercalcemia (lung, kidney)
3. Hematologic malignancies (multiple myeloma, lymphoma, leukemia)

Vitamin D–related:
1. Vitamin D intoxication
2. ↑ 1,25(OH)₂D; sarcoidosis and other granulomatous diseases
3. Idiopathic hypercalcemia of infancy

Associated with high bone turnover:
1. Hyperthyroidism
2. Immobilization
3. Thiazides
4. Vitamin A intoxication

Associated with renal failure:
1. Severe secondary hyperparathyroidism
2. Aluminum intoxication
3. Milk-alkali syndrome

From Potts JT Jr.: HPIM-12, p. 1902.

(rarely osteitis fibrosa cystica, in which normal cellular and marrow elements are replaced by fibrous tissue). Resorption of phalangeal tufts, subperiosteal resorption of bone in the digits, and tiny "punched out" lesions in the skull also may be present. Other features include CNS dysfunction (neuropsychiatric), peripheral neuromuscular disease (proximal muscle weakness, fatigability, atrophy), GI manifestations (abdominal discomfort, peptic ulcer disease, pancreatitis), chondrocalcinosis, and pseudogout. Symptoms can be seen at levels >2.9 mmol/L (>11.5 mg/dL); nephrocalcinosis and renal failure occur at calcium levels >3.2 mmol/L(>13 mg/dL).

Diagnosis is made on clinical grounds and confirmed by demonstration of an inappropriately high PTH level for degree of hypercalcemia. The immunoradiometric assay (IRMA) for PTH is the most reliable. Hypercalcemia may be intermittent or sustained. Serum phosphate is usually low, may be normal. Serum K may be normal or low. Serum Cl is often raised with a reduced serum bicarbonate. Cl $\uparrow$ and K $\downarrow$ (reflecting acidosis and renal phosphate wasting) can be a diagnostic clue. Hypercalciuria is a common feature and helps to distinguish this disorder from familial hypocalciuric hypercalcemia. ECG may reveal a short QT interval and arrhythmias. Treatment of parathyroid adenomas requires the initial management of hypercalcemia if severe and symptomatic. General recommendations that apply to the acute management of hypercalcemia from any cause can be found in Table 150-2. Curative therapy involves surgical parathyroidectomy, though no uniform recommendations can be made. In pts <50 years old, surgery is usually performed (with one normal gland transplanted to the forearm in some centers). In older pts who are asymptomatic, conservative observation is appropriate as long as bone loss is not progressive. If neck exploration does not reveal an abnormal gland, ultrasound, CT, radio thallium and technetium studies, or intraarterial digital angiography may help localize the abnormal tissue.

Postoperative management requires close monitoring of calcium and phosphorous. Calcium supplementation is given for symptomatic hypocalcemia [calcium gluconate or chloride 1 mg/mL in 5% dextrose in water at 0.5–2 (mg/kg)/h or 30–100 mL/h]. Hypomagnesemia should be corrected (deficiency impairs PTH release).

Lithium   Lithium causes hypercalcemia in 10% of pts by causing hyperfunctioning of the parathyroid glands (not adenoma). Elevation of calcium is dependent upon continued administration of lithium, and the drug may be continued if hypercalcemia is asymptomatic. If hypercalcemia and elevated PTH persist off lithium, parathyroidectomy may be indicated.

Familial hypocalciuric hypercalcemia (FHH) This is an autosomal dominant trait in which most pts exceed 99% renal calcium resorption, whereas most pts with hyperparathyroidism have less than 99% resorption. Hypercalcemia may be detectable in affected family members before age 10 (rare in hyperparathyroid/MEN syndromes). The immunoreactive PTH levels are usually normal in FHH. Most pts are detected on routine screening and are asymptomatic. Surgery does not reverse the hypercalcemia unless all parathyroid tissue is removed. No medical or surgical intervention is advocated.

HYPERCALCEMIA OF MALIGNANCY This is common (involving 10–15% of tumors such as lung carcinoma), often severe, and difficult to manage. Malignancies may cause hypercalcemia by local bone destruction (myeloma, breast carcinoma), by increased synthesis of $1,25(OH)_2$ vitamin D $[1,25(OH)_2D]$ (lymphoma), or by elaborating other humoral mediators of bone resorption (lung, kidney, squamous cell carcinomas).

VITAMIN D–RELATED HYPERCALCEMIA Sarcoidosis and other granulomatous disease (such as tuberculosis and histoplasmosis) cause hypercalcemia by increasing synthesis of $1,25(OH)_2D$, thus enhancing calcium and phosphorus absorption from the GI tract. Vitamin D intoxication results from chronic ingestion of large doses of vitamin D (50–100 × normal physiologic requirements, i.e., 50,000–100,000 U/d). Diagnosis can be documented by finding elevated 25(OH)D levels. Treatment is hydration, restriction of vitamin D intake, and in some cases glucocorticoids (100 mg/d hydrocortisone).

HIGH BONE TURNOVER STATES Hyperthyroidism commonly produces a mild elevation of serum calcium with hypercalciuria. Immobilization in adults is rarely associated with hypercalcemia in absence of associated disease. Thiazides can aggravate hypercalcemia in primary hyperparathyroidism and in high bone turnover states as well. It augments PTH responsiveness in target cells of bone and renal tubule. Vitamin A intoxication is a rare cause of hypercalcemia, caused by ingestion of 10–20 × the minimum daily requirement (50,000–100,000 U/d). Therapy is the same as for vitamin D intoxication.

RENAL FAILURE Severe secondary hyperparathyroidism may complicate end-stage renal disease. Pts may have hypercalcemia, hyperphosphatemia, bone pain, ectopic calcification pruritus, concomitant osteomalacia (vitamin D and calcium deficiency), and osteitis fibrosa cystica (excessive PTH action on bone) may be seen. Aluminum intoxication occurs in some pts on chronic dialysis. Hypercalcemia

TABLE 150-2 Summary of treatments for hypercalcemia

Therapy	Therapeutic details
MOST GENERALLY USEFUL THERAPIES	
Hydration	2 L or more
High salt intake	Until urine Na $\geq$ 300 mmol/d
Furosemide	40–160 mg/d
or ethacrynic acid	50–200 mg/d
Forced diuresis	4–6 L fluid IV/day containing 600–900 mmol Na plus furosemide q 1–2 h, plus at least 60 mmol K/d, plus at least 60 mmol Mg/d
Oral phosphate	250 mg P q 6 h PO
Plicamycin	10–25 g/kg body weight IV, repeat prn
Diphosphonate (etidronate)	15–30 mg IV q 2–6 h for 3–6 d or 1200 mg/d PO for 6 days
Prednisone or equivalent	5–15 mg q 6 h
SPECIAL THERAPIES FOR PARTICULAR USES	
IV phosphate	1500 mg P q 12 h until P is 2 mmol/L (6 mg/dL) or less
Calcitonin	2 U/kg body weight q 4 h subcutaneously
Indomethacin	25 mg q 6 h PO
Hemodialysis	Lo-Ca bath

develops when they are treated with vitamin D or calcitriol. Failure to recognize this syndrome can be fatal. Milk-alkali syndrome is characterized by hypercalcemia, alkalosis, and renal failure. Treatment involves dialysis, and discontinuing ingestions.

HYPOCALCEMIA

Symptoms include muscle spasms, carpopedal spasm, facial grimacing, laryngeal spasm, seizure, and respiratory arrest. Increased intracranial pressure and papilledema may occur

Indications	Complications	Precautions
Universal	—	—
Universal	Edema	—
Universal	↓ K and ↓ Mg	Measure serum K and Mg
Universal	Pulmonary edema; ↓ K and ↓ Mg	Intensive monitoring, including venous pressure and serum Mg and K
Universal if serum P < 3 mg/dL	Ectopic calcification	Keep serum P below 5–6 mg/dL
Increased bone resorption	Liver, kidney; marrow toxicity	Monitor platelets, CBC, BUN, SGOT
Increased bone resorption		
Breast cancer, lymphomas, leukemias, multiple myeloma, vitamin D poisoning, sarcoidosis	Cushing's syndrome if chronic Rx	Alternate-day Rx for chronic use
Severe hypercalcemia: diuresis or mithramycin contraindicated	Ectopic calcification: severe hypocalcemia	Monitor serum Ca and P closely
Adjunct in presence of bone reabsorption; paralysis; immobilization	—	—
Certain types of pseudohyperparathyroidism	Na retention: GI bleeding; headache	Careful clinical monitoring
Acute renal failure	Multiple	Monitor serum P after dialysis

Modified from Potts JT Jr.: HPIM-12, p. 1914.

with long-standing hypocalcemia. Other manifestations include irritability, depression, psychosis, intestinal cramps, and chronic malabsorption. Chvostek's and Trousseau's signs are frequently positive, and the QT interval on ECG is prolonged.

The differential diagnoses are listed in Table 150-3, and other considerations include critically ill pts who experience transient hypocalcemia (sepsis, burns, acute renal failure,

TABLE 150-3   Differential diagnosis of hypercalcemia: Laboratory criteria

	Blood*			
	Ca	P_i	$1,25(OH)_2D$	iPTH
Primary hyperparathyroidism	↑	↓	↑,↔	↑(↔)
Malignancy-associated hypercalcemia:				
Humorally mediated (HHM)	↑ ↑	↓	↓,↔	↓↔
Local destruction (osteolytic metastases)	↑	↔	↓,↔	↓↔

* Symbols in parentheses refer to values rarely seen in the particular disease.

NOTE: P_i = inorganic phosphate; iPTH = immunoreactive parathyroid hormone.

From Potts JT Jr.: HPIM-12, p. 1911.

states (reduced total calcium), certain medications (protamine, heparin, glucagon), and pancreatitis (etiology unclear).

PTH ABSENT   *PTH deficiency* may be *hereditary* (isolated deficiency, DiGeorge syndrome), *acquired* (surgery, radiation therapy, hemochromatosis), or part of an autoimmune syndrome (adrenal, ovarian and parathyroid failure, mucocutaneous candidiasis, alopecia, vitiligo, and pernicious anemia). Treatment involves replacement of calcium (calcium citrate 950 mg, 2 tablets tid) and vitamin D or calcitriol (0.5 μg/d), adjusted according to serum calcium levels and urinary excretion. Avoid excessive hypercalciuria to prevent nephrolithiasis. (Thiazide diuretics may reduce urinary calcium excretion if a low-sodium diet is followed.) *Severe hypomagnesemia* [<0.4 mmol/L (<1.0 mg/dL)] can cause hypocalcemia due to impaired PTH secretions and reduced peripheral responsiveness. Restoration of total-body magnesium stores leads to rapid reversal of hypocalcemia.

PTH INEFFECTIVE   *Chronic renal failure* results in phosphate retention and impaired $1,25(OH)_2D$ production and action leading to hypocalcemia and secondary hyperparathyroidism. Phosphate binders (aluminum hydroxide), calcium supplements (1–2 g/d), and calcitriol (0.25–1.0 μg/d) are integral to proper management. *Vitamin D deficiency* is occasionally diagnosed in the elderly. Concentrations of 25(OH)D are low or low normal. Bone biopsy reveals osteomalacia. Treatment is with vitamin D 1000–2000 U/d and calcium 1–1.5 g/d. *Defective vitamin D metabolism* may result from *anticonvulsant therapy* (phenytoin), and responds to vitamin D 50,000 U/week and calcium 1 g/d. *Vitamin D–dependent rickets type I* is autosomal recessive disorder due to a defect in conversion of 25(OH)D to 1,25(OH)$_2$D. Calcitriol in physiologic doses is curative. *Intestinal malabsorption* may result in hypocalcemia, secondary hyperparathyroidism, and severe hypophosphatemia. *Vitamin D–dependent rickets type II* is due to defective response to 1,25(OH)$_2$D. Plasma levels of 1,25(OH)$_2$D are elevated at least 3 × normal. High doses of vitamin D are required. *Pseudohypoparathyroidism* is due to end-organ unresponsiveness to PTH. A working classification is found in Table 150-4. Treatment is similar to that of hypoparathyroidism, but vitamin D and calcium doses are lower.

PTH OVERWHELMED   Occasionally loss of calcium from extracellular fluid is so severe that PTH cannot compensate (rhabdomyolysis, hypothermia, massive hepatic failure, hematologic malignancies with acute tumor lysis, and acute renal failure). Osteitis fibrosa cystica is now an infrequent manifestation of hyperparathyroidism. After parathyroidectomy in pts with osteitis fibrosis, hypocalcemia may result, requiring parenteral calcium and calcitriol.

MANAGEMENT OF HYPOCALCEMIA   Symptomatic hypocalcemia of all types may be treated with intravenous calcium chloride or calcium gluconate. Management of chronic hypocalcemia usually requires a vitamin D preparation, commonly calcitriol, and an oral calcium preparation (see Table 150-5).

TABLE 150-4   Classification of pseudohypoparathyroidism (PHP) and pseudo-pseudohypoparathyroidism (PPHP)

	PHP-1a	PHP-1b	PHP-II	PPHP
Hypocalcemia, hyperphosphatemia	Yes	Yes	Yes	No
Response of urinary cyclic AMP to PTH	↓	↓	Normal	Normal
Serum PTH	↑	↑	↑	Normal
G$_s$ subunit deficiency	Yes	No	No	Yes
Albright's hereditary osteodystrophy	Yes	No	No	Yes
Resistance to hormones in addition to PTH	Yes	No	No	±

Modified from Pott JT Jr.: HPIM-12, p. 1919.

TABLE 150-5 Elemental calcium content of various oral calcium preparations

Calcium preparation	Elemental calcium content
Calcium citrate	40 mg/300 mg
Calcium carbonate	400 mg/g
Calcium lactate	80 mg/600 mg
Calcium gluconate	40 mg/500 mg
Calcium carbonate + 5 μg vitamin D_2 (Os-Cal 250)	250 mg/tablet

From Potts JT Jr.: HPIM-12, p. 1926.

For a more detailed discussion, see Potts JT Jr.: Diseases of the Parathyroid Gland and Other Hyper- and Hypocalcemic Disorders, Chap. 340, in HPIM-12, p. 1902

OSTEOPOROSIS A reduction of bone density below level required for mechanical support. Remodeling of bone (formation and resorption) is continuous, and density decreases whenever rate of resorption exceeds formation. Vertebrae, wrist, hip, humerus, and tibia are particularly prone to fracture.

In *type I osteoporosis* disproportionate loss of trabeculae is associated with fractures of vertebrae and distal forearm in middle-aged, postmenopausal women. *Type II osteoporosis* occurs in men and women above age 75 and is associated with fractures of femoral neck, proximal humerus, proximal tibia, and pelvis.

Vertebral collapse is common in lower dorsal and upper lumbar regions after sudden bending, lifting, or jumping movements. Pain usually subsides after days, and patients may be ambulatory in 4–6 weeks. Collapse unassociated with pain can cause dorsal kyphosis and exaggerated cervical lordosis (widow's hump).

Blood levels of calcium, phosphorus, and alkaline phosphatase are normal. Mild hypercalciuria may be present. In absence of fractures, a 30% decrease in bone mass may not be evident on standard x-rays. More sensitive studies such as single and dual photon bone densitometry, quantitative CT, and neutron activation analysis may suggest whether pt is at risk for fracture.

The differential diagnosis is listed in Table 144-1. Other disorders known to reduce bone mass include acromegaly, hyperparathyroidism, and malignancies (multiple myeloma, lymphoma, leukemia, carcinomas). Cigarette smoking and glucocorticoids contribute to bone loss.

Treatment Directed toward prevention of further loss of bone mass or to an increase in bone density. White postmenopausal women who are small, sedentary, and smokers are at high risk of developing osteoporosis. Estrogen administration to postmenopausal women decreases rate of bone resorption, but bone mass does not increase and eventually usually decreases. The minimum effective dosage of conjugated estrogen is 0.625 mg/d given with or without progestogens on a variety of schedules. Oral calcium (1–1.5 g/d elemental calcium) is recommended to decrease bone resorption. Thiazide diuretics are useful in high-turnover osteoporosis with hypercalciuria and secondary hyperparathyroidism. Fluoride increases new bone formation, but is recommended only for treatment of established vertebral osteoporosis with symptomatic crush fractures because of the increased incidence of hip fracture in some series. These therapies not only retard loss of bone density, but also result in decreased fracture rate in subjects at risk.

OSTEOMALACIA Defective mineralization of organic matrix of bone; may result from inadequate intake or malabsorption of vitamin D (chronic pancreatic insufficiency, gastrectomy, and steatorrhea of other causes), acquired or inherited disorders of vitamin D metabolism (anticonvulsant therapy or chronic renal failure), chronic acidosis (renal tubular acidosis, acetazolamide ingestion), renal tubular defects that produce hypophosphatemia (Fanconi's syndrome), and chronic administration of aluminum-containing antacids.

Clinical manifestations May be subtle in adults. Skeletal deformities may be overlooked until fractures occur after minimal trauma. Symptoms include diffuse skeletal pain and bony tenderness. Pain in hips may result in an altered gait. Proximal muscle weakness may mimic primary muscle disorders. Decrease in bone density is usually associated with loss of trabeculae and thinning of cortices. Characteristic x-ray finding is radiolucent bands (Looser's zones or pseudofractures) ranging from a few millimeters to several centimeters in length, usually perpendicular to surface of femur, pelvis, scapula, upper fibula, or metatarsals. Changes in serum calcium, phosphorus, 25(OH)D, and 1,25(OH)$_2$D vary with underlying causes.

Treatment In osteomalacia due to vitamin D deficiency 2000–4000 IU/d vitamin D$_2$ (cholecalciferol) or D$_3$ (ergocalciferol) is given PO for 6 12 weeks, followed by daily supplements of 200–400 IU. Healing of pseudofractures may be evident within 3–4 weeks. Osteomalacia due to malabsorption requires large doses of vitamin D (up to 100,000 IU/d) and calcium (calcium carbonate 4 g/d). In pts on anticonvulsants, it is usually necessary to continue drugs while administering sufficient vitamin D to bring serum calcium and serum 25(OH)D to the normal range. Dihydrotachysterol (0.2–1.0 mg/d) or calcitrol (0.25 µg/d) are effective in treating hypocalcemia and osteodystrophy of chronic renal failure.

For a more detailed discussion, see Krane SM, Holick MF: Metabolic Bone Disease, Chap. 341, in HPIM-12, p. 1921

REGULATION OF PLASMA LIPIDS

LIPID TRANSPORT   **Exogenous pathway**   In the intestinal wall, dietary triglycerides and cholesterol are incorporated into large lipoproteins (chylomicrons), which are transported via lymph to the circulation. Chylomicrons contain apoprotein CII, which activates lipoprotein lipase in capillaries, thus liberating fatty acids and monoglycerides from the chylomicron. Fatty acids pass through the endothelial cells into adipocytes or muscle. The chylomicron remnants in the circulation are taken up by liver. The net result is to deliver triglycerides to adipose tissue and cholesterol to the liver.

Endogenous pathway   The liver synthesizes triglycerides and secretes them into the circulation together with cholesterol in the form of very low density lipoproteins (VLDL). VLDL particles are large, carry 5–10 times more triglycerides than cholesterol esters, and like other lipoproteins, are coated with apoproteins that direct them to tissues where lipoprotein lipase hydrolyzes triglycerides. VLDL remnants either return to the liver for reutilization or are processed to low-density lipoprotein (LDL). LDL supplies cholesterol to extrahepatic cells, such as adrenal cortex, lymphocytes, muscles, and kidney. LDL binds to specific receptors on cell surfaces and then undergoes endocytosis and digestion by lysosomes. The liberated cholesterol is used for membrane synthesis and metabolic requirements. In addition, some LDL is degraded by a scavenger system in phagocytic cells in the reticuloendothelial system. As cell membranes undergo turnover, unesterified cholesterol is released into plasma, where it initially binds to high-density lipoprotein (HDL) and is esterified with fatty acid by lecithin:cholesterol acyltransferase (LCAT). HDL cholesterol esters are transferred to VLDL and eventually to LDL. By this cycle LDL delivers cholesterol to cells and cholesterol returns from extrahepatic sites via HDL.

HYPERLIPOPROTEINEMIA (See Table 152-1.)

In adults, hyperlipoproteinemia is defined as plasma cholesterol >5.2 mmol/L (>200 mg/dL) or triglyceride levels >2.2 mmol/L (>200 mg/dL). An isolated increase in plasma tri-

TABLE 152-1 **Characteristics of the primary hyperlipoproteinemias resulting from single-gene mutations**

Genetic disorder	Primary biochemical defect	Plasma lipoprotein elevation (pattern)
Familial lipoprotein lipase deficiency	Deficiency of lipoprotein lipase	Chylomicrons (1)
Familial apoprotein CII deficiency	Deficiency of apoprotein CII	Chylomicrons and VLDL (1 or 5)
Familial type 3 hyperlipoproteinemia	Abnormal apoprotein E of VLDL	Chylomicron remnant and IDL (3)
Familial hypercholesterolemia	Deficiency of LDL receptor	LDL (2a, rarely 2b)
Familial hypertriglyceridemia	Unknown	VLDL (rarely chylomicrons) (4, rarely 5)
Multiple lipoprotein-type hyperlipidemia (familial combined hyperlipidemia)	Unknown	LDL and VLDL (2a, 2b, or 4, rarely 5)

From Brown MS, Goldstein JL: HPIM-12, p. 1817.

glycerides indicates that chylomicrons, VLDL, and/or remnants are increased. An isolated increase of plasma cholesterol indicates elevated LDL. Elevations of both triglycerides and cholesterol are caused by elevations in chylomicrons or VLDL, in which case the triglyceride/cholesterol ratio $\geq 5:1$. Alternatively, elevations of both VLDL and LDL are associated with a triglyceride/cholesterol ratio $< 5:1$ (see Table 152-2).

FAMILIAL LIPOPROTEIN LIPASE DEFICIENCY Rare autosomal recessive disorder that results from absence or deficiency in liproprotein lipase, which in turn retards metabolism of chylomicrons. Accumulation of chylomicrons in plasma causes recurrent bouts of pancreatitis, beginning usually in childhood. Eruptive xanthomas occur on buttocks, trunk, and extremities. Plasma is milky or creamy (lipemic). Symptoms and signs recede when pt is placed on a fat-free diet (<20 g/d). Accelerated atherosclerosis is not a feature.

FAMILIAL APOPROTEIN CII DEFICIENCY Rare autosomal recessive disorder due to absence of apoprotein CII, an essential cofactor for lipoprotein lipase. As a result, chylomicrons and triglycerides accumulate and cause manifestations similar to those in lipoprotein lipase deficiency. *Diagnosis* requires demonstration of absence of apoprotein CII by protein electrophoresis. *Treatment* involves the use of fat-free diet.

Typical clinical findings	Lipoprotein pattern in affected relatives	Drug therapy First choice	Other
...uptive xanthomas, ...ncreatitis	1	None	None
...ncreatitis	1 or 5	None	None
	3, 2a, 2b, or 4	Gemfibrozil; clofibrate	Nicotinic acid
...mar and tuberous ...nthomas; premature ...erosclerosis	2a (rarely 2b)	Bile acid-binding resin plus lovastatin	Nicotinic acid; probucol
...ndon xanthomas; ...emature atherosclerosis	4 (rarely 5)	Gemfibrozil; nicotinic acid	Clofibrate
...ruptive xanthomas; ...emature atherosclerosis)	2a, 2b, or 4 (rarely 5)	Gemfibrozil; nicotinic acid	Lovastatin

FAMILIAL DYSBETALIPOPROTEINEMIA Transmitted as a single-gene mutation, but expression requires additional environmental and/or genetic factors. Plasma cholesterol and triglycerides are increased due to accumulation of remnant-like particles derived from VLDL. Severe atherosclerosis involves coronary arteries, internal carotids, and abdominal aorta and causes premature MI, intermittent claudication, and gangrene. Cutaneous xanthomas are distinctive: xan-

TABLE 152-2 Patterns of lipoprotein elevation in plasma (lipoprotein types)

Lipoprotein pattern	Major elevation in plasma Lipoprotein	Lipid
Type 1	Chylomicrons	Triglycerides
Type 2a	LDL	Cholesterol
Type 2b	LDL and VLDL	Cholesterol and triglycerides
Type 3	Chylomicron remnants and IDL	Triglycerides and cholesterol
Type 4	VLDL	Triglycerides
Type 5	VLDL and chylomicrons	Triglycerides and cholesterol

From Brown MS, Goldstein JL: HPIM-12, p. 1817.

TABLE 152-3 Lipid lowering agents

Agent	Mechanism of action	Dosage	Clinical use	Side effects
Bile acid sequestrants (colestipol cholestyramine)	Bind bile acids in intestinal lumen, interrupt enterohepatic circulation of bile acids	20 g/d 16 g/d	Primary hypercholesterolemia; elevated LDL cholesterol only (most effective for heterozygous familial hypercholesterolemia)	Constipation, bloating, epigastric fullness, nausea, flatulence, hyperchloremic acidosis; binds thyroxine, coumadin, and thiazides; increases triglycerides
Nicotinic acid (niacin)	Reduces LDL and VLDL; reduces hepatic synthesis of VLDL; can cause 15–40% reduction of LDL with concurrent 10–20% rise in HDL	Start 100–250 tid after meals; increase every 7 d up to 3 g/d total	Primary hypercholesterolemia (first-line therapy); familial combined hyperlipidemia	Cutaneous flushing (prevented with ASA 325 mg prior to dose), nausea, diarrhea, abdominal discomfort; contraindicated in pts with liver disease, PUD, or hyperuricemia; LFTs and uric acid must be monitored periodically
Probucol	Reduces LDL (15–25%) and HDL (8–10%) by incompletely understood mechanisms	500 mg bid with meals	Second-line therapy for primary hypercholesterolemia; no role in treatment of hypertriglyceridemia	Diarrhea, flatulence, abdominal pain, nausea, fetid sweat, hyperhydrosis, angioedema; contraindicated in pts with prolonged QT interval
Lovastatin	Lowers LDL cholesterol by inhibiting HMG Co-A reductase and enhancing receptor-mediated catabolism of LDL	20–40 mg bid	Primary hypercholesterolemia (familial hypercholesterolemia); familial combined hyperlipidemia, nephrotic syndrome; effects are potentiated when used with bile acid–binding resins	Change in bowel function, headache, nausea, fatigue, insomnia, skin rash, elevated LFTs, myositis with increased CPK

Drug	Mechanism	Dose	Indications	Side Effects
Gemfibrozil	Reduces synthesis of VLDL triglyceride, and apoprotein B with concurrent increased rate of triglyceride-rich lipoprotein clearance from plasma; consistently reduces VLDL 50–75%; less consistently reduces LDL 25–5%; raises HDL 10–15%	600 mg bid	Severe hypertriglyceridemia (type 4 phenotype); also useful for type 2b and 3	Abdominal pain, diarrhea, nausea, muscle tenderness, skin rash, elevated LFTs; potentiates coumadin; increased risk of gallstones
Clofibrate	Actual mechanism unclear; increases rate of metabolism of triglyceride-rich lipoproteins due to increased lipoprotein lipase deficiency; reduces VLDL cholesterol and plasma tryglycerides by 75%	1 g bid	Drug of choice for type 3 phenotype; second-line therapy for severe hypertriglyceridemia in pts who cannot take gemfibrozil or nicotinic acid; no role in treatment of primary hypercholesterolemia	Nausea, abdominal discomfort, decreased libido, breast tenderness, myositis; rare arrhythmia or lupus-like syndrome, transient LFT increases, increased risk of gallstones, potentiates coumadin; contraindicated in pts with chronic renal failure or nephrotic syndrome

thoma striata palmaris and tuberous or tuberoeruptive xanthomas. Levels of triglyceride and cholesterol are similarly
elevated. *Diagnosis* is established by finding of a broad beta
band on lipoprotein electrophoresis. *Treatment* is either
clofibrate or gemfibrozil. If present, hypothyroidism and
diabetes mellitus must be treated.

FAMILIAL HYPERCHOLESTEROLEMIA   Autosomal dominant
disorder that affects 1 in 500 individuals. Heterozygotes
manifest a 2- to 3-fold increase in plasma cholesterol and
LDL. Accelerated atherosclerosis causes premature MI,
particularly in men. Xanthomas of tendons and arcus cornea
are common. Diagnosis is suggested by finding an isolated
increase of plasma cholesterol with normal triglycerides.
Every effort should be made to lower plasma cholesterol
concentration to normal. *Treatment* is restriction of dietary
cholesterol and bile acid–binding resins (cholestyramine or
colestipol) plus lovastatin.

FAMILIAL HYPERTRIGLYCERIDEMIA   Autosomal dominant disorder in which increased plasma VLDL causes plasma
triglyceride concentration to range from 2.2–5.6 mmol/L
(200–500 mg/dL). Obesity, hyperglycemia, and hyperinsulinemia are characteristic, and diabetes mellitus, ethanol consumption, oral contraceptives, and hypothyroidism may exacerbate the condition. Because atherosclerosis is accelerated,
vigorous attempts should be made to control all exacerbating
factors, and intake of saturated fat should be minimal. If
dietary measures fail, clofibrate or gemfibrozil should be
administered.

MULTIPLE LIPOPROTEIN-TYPE HYPERLIPIDEMIA   Inherited disorder that can cause different lipoprotein abnormalities in
affected subjects, including hypercholesterolemia (type 2a
lipoprotein pattern), hypertriglyceridemia (type 4), or simultaneous hypercholesteremia and hypertriglyceridemia (type
2b). Atherosclerosis is accelerated. *Therapy* should be directed at predominant lipid abnormality. Restriction of dietary fat and cholesterol and avoidance of alcohol and oral
contraceptives are appropriate for all pts. Triglyceride elevation may respond to clofibrate or gemfibrozil, and a bile
acid–binding resin plus lovastatin may be used when cholesterol is elevated.

SECONDARY HYPERLIPOPROTEINEMIAS   Diabetes mellitus,
ethanol consumption, oral contraceptives, and hypothyroidism can either cause secondary hyperlipoproteinemias or
worsen prior hyperlipoproteinemic states. In either case,
control of aggravating or inciting cause is essential for
management.

TREATMENT   Options available for pharmacologic intervention can be found in Table 152-3.

For a more detailed discussion, see Brown MS, Goldstein JL: The Hyperlipoproteinemias and Other Disorders of Lipid Metabolism, Chap. 326, in HPIM-12, p. 1814

153 INHERITED METABOLIC DISEASES

HEMOCHROMATOSIS

Hemochromatosis is an iron-storage disorder that occurs when increased intestinal iron absorption causes Fe deposition, fibrosis, and organ failure of liver, heart, pancreas, and pituitary. Causes include single-gene mutations, impaired hematopoiesis (as in sideroblastic anemia and thalassemia), or excessive Fe ingestion. Alcoholic liver disease also may be associated with a moderate increase in hepatic Fe and elevated body Fe stores (Table 153-1).

Symptoms Include weakness, lassitude, weight loss, darkening of skin, abdominal pain, and loss of libido. Hepatomegaly occurs in 95% of pts, sometimes in the presence of normal LFTs. Other signs include bronze pigmentation, spider angiomas, splenomegaly, arthropathy, ascites, cardiac arrythmias, CHF, loss of body hair, palmar erythema, gynecomastia, and testicular atrophy. The latter is due to pituitary involvement and gonadotropin deficiency. Diabetes mellitus occurs in about 65%, usually in pts with family history of diabetes. Adrenal insufficiency, hypothyroidism, and hypoparathyroidism rarely occur.

Serum Fe, percent transferrin saturation, and serum ferritin levels are increased. Liver biopsy is the definitive test and should be performed in suspected cases. Once diagnosis is established, family members at risk should be screened with the combined measurements of (1) percent transferrin saturation and (2) serum ferritin level. If either test is abnormal a liver biopsy should be done.

Treatment Involves removal of excess body Fe, usually by intermittent phlebotomy. Since 1 unit of blood contains about 250 mg Fe, and since 25 g or more of Fe must be removed, phlebotomy is performed weekly for 2–3 years. Less frequent phlebotomy is then used to maintain serum Fe at <27 μmol/L (<150 μg/dL).

Causes of death in untreated pts include cardiac failure (30%), cirrhosis (25%), and hepatocellular carcinoma (30%); the latter may develop despite adequate Fe removal.

WILSON'S DISEASE

Wilson's disease is an autosomal recessive disorder that causes accumulation of copper in liver, brain, and other

TABLE 153-1 Representative iron values in normal subjects, patients with hemochromatosis, and patients with alcoholic liver disease

Determination	Normal	Symptomatic hemochromatosis	Homozygotes with early, asymptomatic hemochromatosis	Alcoholic liver disease
Plasma iron, μmol/L (μg/dL)	9–27 (50–150)	32–54 (180–300)	Usually elevated	Often elevated
Total iron-binding capacity, μmol/L (μg/dL)	45–66 (250–370)	36–54 (200–300)	36–54 (200–300)	45–66 (250–370)
Transferrin saturation, percent	22–46	50–100	50–100	27–60
Serum ferritin, μg/L	10–200	900–6000	200–500	10–500
Urinary iron,* mg/24 h	0–2	9–23	2.5	Usually <5
Liver iron, μg/100 ng dry wt	30–140	600–1800	200–400	30–200

* After intramuscular administrationom of 0.5 g deferoxamine.
From Powell LW, Isselbacher K: HPIM-12, p. 1827.

615

organs. The underlying defect is an inability to excrete Cu cleaved from ceruloplasmin into bile. Excessive Cu inhibits formation of ceruloplasmin from apoceruloplasmin and Cu, and when capacity to store Cu in liver is exceeded, it is released into blood and deposited in extrahepatic sites. Pathologic consequences in liver include necrosis, inflammation, fibrosis, and cirrhosis. On occasion, death can occur from the CNS effects when liver dysfunction is minimal.

Disease may present as acute hepatitis, cirrhosis, or asymptomatic hepatomegaly. Green or golden deposits in the cornea (Kayser-Fleischer rings) can be demonstrated by slit-lamp examination. Neurologic manifestations include resting and intention tremors, spasticity, rigidity, chorea, drooling, dysphagia, and dysarthria. Schizophrenia, manic depressive psychosis, and neuroses may occur.

Diagnosis   Should be suspected in any pt of age <40 with unexplained CNS disease, chronic active hepatitis, or cirrhosis of unknown etiology. Diagnosis is confirmed by demonstration of (1) a serum ceruloplasmin <200 mg/L and Kayser-Fleischer rings or (2) a serum ceruloplasmin <200 mg/L and a Cu level in a liver biopsy specimen >250 μg/g dry weight.

Treatment   Lifelong; penicillamine is given in an initial dose of 1 g PO before meals and at bedtime. WBC and platelet counts, UA, and body temperatures should be monitored several times weekly for the first month of therapy. Hypersensitivity reactions to penicillamine are common and should be treated with prednisone. Serum-free Cu should be kept <2 μmol/L (<10 μg/dL).

PORPHYRIAS

The porphyrias are inherited or acquired disturbances in heme biosynthesis, each of which causes a unique pattern of overproduction, accumulation, and excretion of intermediates of heme synthesis. Manifestations include intermittent nervous system dysfunction and/or sensitivity of skin to sunlight.

INTERMITTENT ACUTE PORPHYRIA   This is an autosomal dominant disorder with variable expressivity. Manifestations include colicky abdominal pain, fever, leukocytosis, vomiting, constipation, port-wine colored urine, and neurologic and psychiatric disturbances. Acute attacks rarely occur before puberty and may last from days to months. Photosensitivity does not occur. Clinical and biochemical manifestations may be precipitated by barbiturates, anticonvulsants, estrogens, oral contraceptives, or alcohol. Diagnosis is established by the Watson-Swartz test. Fresh urine may darken on standing because porpholinogens polymerize spontaneously to uroporphyrin and porphobilin. Treatment involves administration of IV glucose at rates up to 20 g/h. If symptoms do not improve in 48 h, hematin (4 mg/kg) should be infused every 12 h for 3–6 d.

PORPHYRIA CUTANEA TARDA The most common porphyria; characterized by chronic skin lesions and (usually) hepatic disease. It is due to deficiency (inherited or acquired) of uroporphyrinogen decarboxylase. Photosensitivity causes enhanced facial pigmentation, increased fragility of skin, erythema, and vesicular and ulcerative lesions, typically involving face, forehead, and forearms. Liver disease and hepatic siderosis may be related to alcoholism. Diabetes mellitus, SLE, and other autoimmune diseases may coexist. Urine uroporphyrin and coproporphyrin are increased. Abstinence from alcohol leads to improvement, and decrease in hepatic iron may ameliorate skin lesions. Chloroquine may be used in pts unable to undergo phlebotomy.

CONGENITAL ERYTHROPOIETIC PORPHYRIA A rare autosomal recessive defect that causes chronic photosensitivity, mutilating skin lesions, and hemolytic anemia. Death may occur in childhood. Exposure to sunlight should be avoided.

For a more detailed discussion, see Powell LW, Isselbacher KI: Hemochromatosis, Chap. 327, p. 1825; Scheinberg IH: Wilson's Disease, Chap. 330 p. 1843; and Meyer UA: Porphyrias, Chap. 328, p. 1829, in HPIM-12

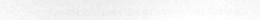

SECTION 11 NEUROLOGY

154 THE NEUROLOGIC EXAMINATION

MENTAL STATUS EXAM

Tests are designed to evaluate pt's attention, orientation, memory, insight, judgment, and grasp of general information. A series of numbers can be recited and the pt asked to respond every time a specific item recurs (attention). The pt should be asked about his or her name, the place, the day, and date. Retentive memory and immediate recall can be tested by determining the number of digits the pt can repeat in sequence. Recent memory is evaluated by testing recall of a series of objects after defined times (e.g., 5 and 15 min). More remote memory is evaluated by assessing pt's ability to provide a cogent chronologic history of his or her illness or personal life events. Recall of major historical events or dates or of major current events may provide insight into fund of general knowledge. Evaluation of language function should include assessment of spontaneous speech, naming, repetition, reading, writing, and comprehension. Additional tests such as ability to draw and copy, perform calculations, interpret proverbs or logic problems, identify right vs. left, name and identify body parts, etc. are also important.

CRANIAL NERVE (CN) EXAM

CN I Occlude each nostril sequentially and use a mild test stimulus, such as soap, toothpaste, coffee, or lemon oil, to see if pt can detect the odor and correctly identify it.

CN II Check visual acuity with and without correction using a Snellen chart (distance) and Jaeger's test type (near). Map visual fields (VFs) by confrontation testing in each quadrant of visual field for each eye individually. The best method is to sit facing pt (2–3 ft apart), have him or her cover one eye gently, and fix uncovered eye on examiner's nose. A small white object (e.g., a cotton-tipped applicator) is then moved slowly from periphery of field toward center until pt appreciates its presence. The pt's VF should be mapped against examiner's for comparison. Formal perimetry and tangent screen exam are essential to identify and delineate small defects. Optic fundi should be examined with an ophthalmoscope and the color, size, and degree of swelling or elevation of the optic disc recorded. The retinal vessels should be checked for size, regularity, AV nicking at crossing points, hemorrhage, exudates, aneurysms, etc. The retina, including the macula, should be examined for abnormal pigmentation and other lesions.

CNs III, IV, VI   Describe size, regularity, and shape of pupils as well as their reaction (direct and consensual) to light and convergence of eyes. Check for lid drooping, lag, or retraction. Ask pt to follow your finger as you move it horizontally to left and right and vertically with each eye first fully adducted then fully abducted. Check for failure to move fully in particular directions and for presence of regular, rhythmic, involuntary oscillations of eyes (nystagmus). Test quick voluntary eye movements (saccades) as well as pursuit (e.g., follow the finger).

CN V   Feel the masseter and temporalis muscles as pt bites down and test jaw opening, protrusion, and lateral motion against resistance. Examine sensation over entire face as well as response to touching each cornea lightly with a small wisp of cotton.

CN VII   Look for asymmetry of face at rest and with spontaneous as well as emotion-induced (e.g., laughing) movements. Test eyebrow elevation, forehead wrinkling, eye closure, smiling, frowning, cheek puff, whistle, lip pursing, and chin muscle contraction. Look particularly for differences in strength of lower and upper facial muscles. Taste on the anterior two-thirds of tongue can be affected by lesions of the seventh CN proximal to the chorda tympani. Test taste for sweet (sugar), salt, sour (lemon), and bitter (quinine) using a cotton-tipped applicator moistened in appropriate solution and placed on lateral margin of protruded tongue about halfway back from tip.

CN VIII   Check ability to hear tuning fork, finger rub, watch tick, and whispered voice at specified distances with each ear. Check for air vs. mastoid bone conduction (Rinne) and lateralization of a tuning fork placed on center of forehead (Weber). Accurate, quantitative testing of hearing requires formal audiometry. Remember to examine tympanic membranes.

CNs IX, X   Check for symmetric evaluation of palate-uvula with phonation ("*ahh*"), as well as position of uvula and palatal arch at rest. Sensation in region of tonsils, posterior pharynx, and tongue also may require testing in specific pts. Pharyngeal ("gag") reflex is evaluated by stimulating posterior pharyngeal wall on each side with a blunt object (e.g., tongue blade). Direct examination of vocal cords by laryngoscopy is necessary in some situations.

CN XI Check shoulder shrug (trapezius muscle) and head rotation to each side (sternocleidomastoid muscle) against resistance.

CN XII Examine bulk and power of tongue. Look for atrophy, deviation from midline with protrusion, tremor, and small flickering or twitching movements (fibrillations, fasciculations).

MOTOR EXAM

Power should be systematically tested for major movements at each joint (see Table 154-1). Strength should be recorded using a reproducible scale (e.g., 0 = no movement, 1 = flicker or trace of contraction with no associated movement at a joint, 2 = movement present but cannot be sustained against gravity, 3 = movement against gravity but not applied resistance, 4 = movement against some degree of resistance, and 5 = full power; values can be supplemented with the addition of + and − signs to provide additional gradations). The speed of movement, the ability to promptly relax contractions, and fatigue with repetition all should be noted. Loss in bulk and size of muscle (atrophy) should be checked for, as well as the presence of irregular involuntary contraction (twitching) of groups of muscle fibres ("fasciculations"). Involuntary movements should be looked for while pt is at rest, during maintained posture, and with voluntary action. Rhythmic involuntary movements are referred to as "tremors," whereas more irregular movements generally fall into categories of choreoathetosis, ballismus, myoclonus, or tics.

REFLEXES

Important muscle-stretch reflexes to test routinely and the spinal cord segments involved in their reflex arcs include biceps C5,6, triceps C6,7,8, brachioradialis C5,6, patellar L2,3,4, Achilles L5,S1. A common grading scale is 0 = absent, 1 = present but diminished, 2 = normal, 3 = hyperactive, and 4 = hyperactive with clonus (repetitive rhythmic contractions with maintained stretch). The plantar reflex should be tested by using a blunt-ended object such as the point of a key to stroke the outer border of the sole of the foot from the heel toward the base of the great toe. An abnormal response (Babinski sign) is extension (dorsi-

TABLE 154-1 Muscles that move joints

	Muscle	Nerve	Segmental innervation
Shoulder	Supra- and infra-spinati	Suprascapular n.	
	Deltoid	Axillary n.	C4,5
Forearm	Biceps	Musculocutanoeus n.	C5,6
	Brachioradialis	Radial n.	C5,6
	Triceps	Radial n.	C6,7,8
	Ext. carpi radialis	Radial n.	C5,6,7
	Ext. carpi ulnaris	P. interosseous n.	C6,7,8
	Ext. digitorum	P. interosseous n.	C6,7,8
	Flex. carpi radialis	Median n.	C6,7
	Flex. carpi ulnaris	Ulnar n.	C7,8,T1
	Supinator	Radial n.	C6,7
	Pronator teres	Median n.	C6,7
Hand	Lumbricals	Median + ulnar n.	C8,T1
	Interossei	Ulnar n.	C8,T1
Thumb	Opponens pollicis	Median n.	C8,T1
	Ext. pollicis	P. interosseous n.	C7,8
	Add. pollicis	Ulnar n.	C8,T1
	Flex. pollicis br.	Ulnar n.	C8,T1
Pelvis	Iliopsoas	Femoral n.	
	Glutei	Sup. + inf. gluteal n.	L1,2,3
			L4,5,S12
Thigh	Quadriceps	Femoral n.	L2,3,4
	Adductors	Obturator n.	L2,3,4
	Hamstrings	Sciatic n.	L5S12
Leg	Gastrocnemius	Tibial n.	S12
	Tibialis ant.	Deep peroneal n.	L4,5
	Peronei	Deep peroneal n.	L5S1
	Tibialis post.	Tibial n.	L4,5
Foot	Ext. hallucis l.	Deep peroneal n.	L5S1

flexion) of the great toe at the metatarsophalangeal joint. In some cases this may be associated with abduction (fanning) of other toes and variable degrees of flexion at ankle, knee, and hip. (Normal response is slow plantar flexion of great toe.) Abdominal, anal, and sphincteric reflexes are important in certain situations, as are additional muscle stretch reflexes.

SENSORY EXAM

For most purposes it is sufficient to test sensation to pinprick, touch, position, and vibration in each of the four extremities (see Figs. 154-1 and -2). Specific problems often require more painstaking evaluation. Pts with cerebral lesions may have abnormalities in "discriminative sensation" such as the ability to perceive double simultaneous stimuli, to localize

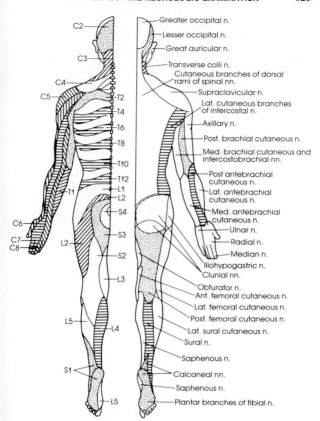

FIGURE 154-1 *(Reproduced from Asbury AK: HPIM-12, p 179.)*

stimuli accurately, to identify closely approximated stimuli as separate (two-point discrimination), to identify objects by touch alone (stereognosis), or to judge weights, evaluate texture, or identify letters or numbers written on the skin surface (graphesthesia).

COORDINATION AND GAIT

The ability to move the index finger accurately from the nose to the examiner's outstretched finger and the ability to slide the heel of each foot from the knee down the shin are tests

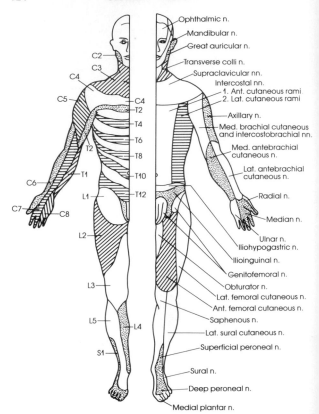

FIGURE 154-2   *(Reproduced from Asbury AK: HPIM-12, p 179.)*

of coordination. Additional tests (drawing objects in the air, following a moving finger, tapping with index finger against thumb or alternately against each individual finger) also may be useful in some pts. The pt's ability to stand with feet together and eyes closed (Romberg test), to walk a straight line (tandem walk), and to turn should all be observed.

For a more detailed discussion, see Asbury AK: Numbness, Tingling, and Sensory Loss, Chap. 28, in HPIM-12, p. 176

155 DIAGNOSTIC METHODS IN NEUROLOGY

Clinical neurophysiologic techniques provide objective, quantitative measures of central and peripheral and/or autonomic nervous system function. Because of time constraints and cost, they should be used only to provide data otherwise unavailable or to monitor progression and/or recovery in certain neurologic disorders.

ELECTROMYOGRAPHY   EMG is useful as an extension of the clinical neurologic exam to differentiate diseases of neuromuscular junction from primary myopathy or from those secondary to demyelination and/or denervation (see Chapter 167). CNS disorders can also be evaluated by EMG, e.g., to distinguish types of tremor, cerebellar vs. sensory ataxias, asterixis, as well as different types of myoclonus.

EMG techniques include measurement of latencies of F responses, H reflexes and blink reflexes to determine conduction times in nerves from periphery (limbs or face) to CNS and back again.

F response: Time required for a stimulus to propagate antidromically up an alpha motor neuron to the spinal cord and return orthodromically down the same axon.

H reflex: Time required for orthodromic conduction up group 1A sensory fibers through the monosynaptic connection with the spinal cord and then orthodromically down the alpha motor axon. With these techniques, recognition of abnormal conduction velocity in peripheral neuropathy is 80–90%. They can also demonstrate conduction block in proximal nerve segments in inflammatory and/or demyelinating neuropathies (e.g., Guillain-Barré syndrome).

Blink reflexes: Times required for conduction in branches of trigeminal and facial nerves tested by using stimuli of supraorbital branches of fifth cranial nerve and measuring latency to blink response.

Single fiber and macro EMG   Single-fiber techniques record jitter (variation in single potentials) in individual fibers and measure function of individual neuromuscular junctions. Characteristic abnormalities are found in myasthenia gravis, Lambert-Eaton syndrome, and other disorders of neuromuscular transmission. Macro EMG techniques measure summated electrical activity of all fibers of a motor unit. Amplitude and area are increased in reinnervation (more fibers subserved by a given nerve) and decreased in primary muscle disease (reduced number of fibers per motor unit).

AUTONOMIC TESTING   *Sympathetic skin response (SSR):*
Voltage changes recorded from skin evoked by electrical
stimuli, loud noise, or deep inspiration. SSR abnormalities
are more common in axonal neuropathies than demyelination.
Absence of the SSR is due to loss of unmyelinated fibers.

ELECTROENCEPHALOGRAPHY (EEG)   Used principally for diagnosis of seizure disorders, but also may be used to assess
cerebral cortical disease or CNS effects of many medical
illnesses.

Normal EEG rhythms in adults   Include alpha—8–12
Hz, 50 μV sinusoidal waves seen in occipital and parietal
regions; beta—>13 Hz, 10–20 μV waves seen in frontal
regions; in sleep, symmetric slowing with characteristic
waveforms, e.g., vertex sharp waves and sleep spindles.

Abnormal EEG rhythms in adults   Awake recordings
include: theta—<4 Hz, 50–350 μV waves (the higher the
voltage, the more abnormal are theta and delta slowing);
spike or sharp waves—faster, higher-voltage waveforms
which, when paroxysmal, are suggestive of epilepsy; characteristic epileptiform patterns such as the 3-Hz spike-and-
wave complexes of absence (petit mal) seizures. The most
pathologic finding of all is the disappearance of EEG pattern
("electrocerebral silence"), which in the absence of extreme
hypothermia [<21°C (<70°F)] or acute intoxication with
anesthetic levels of drugs, is suggestive of irreversible coma
or brain death.

EVOKED RESPONSES   The amplitude of these potentials
ranges from 0.5–20 μV so that detection of the time-locked
evoked response requires summation in order to separate
the wave form from background by signal averaging.

Visual evoked responses (VER)   A checkered pattern
shift (PSVER) produces a characteristic waveform recorded
from the posterior scalp with a positive peak at 95–115 ms.
Latency, duration, and amplitude of response are measured.
Can be used in evaluation of glaucoma; compression of optic
nerve, chiasm, or tract; optic degenerative disease; or, most
commonly, optic neuritis. One-half of pts with multiple
sclerosis (MS) and *no* history of visual symptoms show
PSVER abnormalities, so that PSVERs often support an
apparent diagnosis of first episode of MS.

Brainstem auditory evoked responses (BAERs)   Using
earphones, clicks presented to one ear produce seven wave
forms (I–VII) recorded from the scalp. These represent
successive activation of the auditory nerve (I) and brainstem
auditory pathways (cochlear nucleus, II; superior oblivary
complex, III; lateral lemniscus, IV; inferior colliculus, V;
and higher auditory centers, VI, VII). Lesion at or between
any of these levels delays or obliterates the waves that follow.

It is the most sensitive screening test for acoustic neuroma. Other applications: localization of level of the lesion in coma or other suspected brainstem pathology, hearing evaluation of infants.

Somatosensory evoked responses (SERs) Small, painless electrical stimuli to large sensory fibers of hand or leg produce afferent volleys recorded at many levels of the somatosensory pathway to reflect successive activity in peripheral nerve trunks, spinal cord tracts, gracile and cuneate nuclei, pontine and/or cerebellar structures, thalamus, thalamocortical radiations, and primary sensory cortex. SERs are of localizing value analogous to BAERs.

LUMBAR PUNCTURE **Indications** (1) To obtain pressure measurements and secure a sample of CSF for cellular, chemical, and bacteriologic examination (see table of normal values in Appendix; (2) for administration of spinal anesthesia, antibiotics, or antitumor agents; and (3) to inject contrast agents for myelography.

Complications (1) Cerebellar or transtentorial herniation when puncture performed in setting of markedly elevated intracranial pressure (ICP) or strategically placed space-occupying lesion. When the possibility of raised ICP exists, it is prudent to exclude a mass lesion by CT before obtaining CSF. In such cases a fine-bore needle (no. 22 or 24) should be used and if opening pressure is >400 mmHg, the minimum amount of fluid required is taken, the needle withdrawn, and a unit of mannitol may be given. (2) Introduction of bacteria into CNS.

For a more detailed discussion, see Chiappa KH, Shahani B, and Martin JB: Clinical Electrophysiology and Other Diagnostic Methods, Chap. 349, in HPIM-12, p. 1963

OLFACTORY NERVE (I)

The sense of smell may be impaired by (1) interference with access of odorant to olfactory neuroepithelium (*transport loss*), e.g., by swollen nasal mucous membrane in URI, allergic rhinitis, or structural changes in naval cavity such as with a deviated septum, nasal polyps, or neoplasm; (2) injury to receptor region (*sensory loss*), e.g., destruction of olfactory neuroepithelium by viral infections, neoplasms, inhalation of toxic chemicals, or radiation to head; and (3) damage to central olfactory pathways (*neural loss*), e.g., by head trauma with or without fractures of cribriform plate, neoplasms of anterior cranial fossa, neurosurgical procedures, neurotoxic drugs, or congenital disorders such as Kallmann's syndrome.

OPTIC NERVE (II)

Visual disturbances may be localized upon examination of globe, retina, or optic disc or may require careful visual field testing to pinpoint. Retinal lesions cause arcuate, central, or centrocecal scotomas. Chiasmal lesions produce bitemporal hemianopsias. Homonymous hemianopsias arise behind the chiasm and, if complete, are of no further localizing value. When incomplete, an incongruous homonymous hemianopsia suggests a lesion in the tract or radiations (tract lesions may have associated optic atrophy and an afferent pupillary defect, whereas pupils in postgeniculate lesions are normal). A congruous (identical) homonymous hemianopsia implies a lesion in calcarine cortex.

AQUEOUS HUMOR AND GLAUCOMA Glaucoma is a condition in which elevated intraocular pressure (>22 mmHg) transmitted through aqueous humor damages the optic nerve. It is the leading cause of blindness in the U.S.

Open-angle glaucoma Rarely causes ocular pain or corneal edema. Visual loss occurs first in the periphery, and visual acuity remains normal until late in the course. *Treatment*: topical cholinergic (pilocarpine or carbachol) and beta-blocking (timolol) agents with or without carbonic anhydrase inhibitors (acetazolamide or methazolamide).

Angle-closure glaucoma May be precipitated by drugs to dilate the pupil. *Symptoms*: visual loss, pupillary dilation, pain, and when acute, erythema. This is a medical emergency, to be treated with IV mannitol, parenteral acetazolamide, and topical pilocarpine or timolol.

Congenital glaucoma Rare.

Secondary glaucoma May be associated with leukemia, sickle cell disease, Waldenström's macroglobulinemia, ankylosing spondylitis, rheumatoid arthritis, sarcoidosis, congenital rubella, onchocerciasis, amyloidosis, osteogenesis imperfecta, neoplastic metastases, neurofibromatosis, Sturge-Weber syndrome, chronic glucocorticoid use, amphetamines, hexamethonium, reserpine, anticholinergics, ocular trauma, and dislocation of the lens (homocystinuria and Marfan's syndrome).

RETINA Causes of retinal disease include *vasculopathies* associated with major medical illnesses (e.g., hypertension, diabetes mellitus); *central retinal artery occlusion* (CRA) (with boxcar segmentation of blood flow in retinal veins, milky white retina, and cherry red spot from preserved vascularity of choroid) due to emboli, temporal arteritis, arteriosclerosis, collagen-vascular disease, hyperviscosity states; *transient monocular blindness* (amaurosis fugax) due to episodic retinal ischemia, usually associated with ipsilateral carotid artery stenosis or embolism of the retinal arteries. May be distinguished from transient blindness of classic migraine as the latter often begins with unformed light flashes (photopsia) or zigzag lines (fortification spectra or teichopsia) moving across visual field for several minutes leaving scotomatous/hemianopic defect (although pts may report monocular symptoms); exam usually reveals homonymous defects. Retinal disease may also ensue from degeneration due to retinitis pigmentosa and associated multisystem diseases and toxic effects of drugs, e.g., phenothiazines or chloroquine.

OPTIC NERVE Retrobulbar optic neuropathy Characterized by rapid development (hours to days) of impaired vision in one or both eyes, usually due to acute optic nerve demyelination. Most cases occur in childhood, adolescence, or young adulthood. Total blindness is rare. PE: acutely, optic disc and retina are normal or there is papillitis; eye movement or pressure on globe produces pain; affects central more than peripheral vision, and the pupillary light reflex is impaired (swinging flashlight test). CSF is normal or has WBCs (10–$20/\mu L$) with or without oligoclonal bands. 50% will develop signs of multiple sclerosis within 15 years. Other causes: postinfectious or disseminated encephalomyelitis, posterior uveitis, vascular lesions of the optic nerve, tumors (optic nerve glioma, neurofibromatosis, meningioma, metastases), and fungal infections.

Anterior ischemic optic neuropathy (AION) Caused by atherosclerotic or inflammatory disease of ophthalmic artery or its branches. Presents as acute painless monocular visual loss with an altitudinal defect. Optic disc is pale and swollen with splinter peripapillary hemorrhages and normal macula and retina. Evaluation should aggressively rule out temporal arteritis. Occasionally microemboli (e.g., following cardiac surgery) may cause AION.

Toxic or nutritional optic neuropathy Presents as simultaneous impairment of vision in both eyes with central or centrocecal scotomas, developing over days to weeks. Agents: methyl alcohol intoxication, chloramphenicol, ethambutol, isoniazid, streptomycin, sulfonamides, digitalis, ergot, disulfiram, and heavy metal.

Bitemporal hemianopsia Caused by suprasellar extension of a pituitary tumor or saccular aneurysm of circle of Willis, tuberculum sellae meningioma, or rarely, sarcoid, metastases, and Hand-Schüller-Christian disease.

OCULOMOTOR, TROCHLEAR, AND ABDUCENS NERVES (III, IV, VI)

Isolated third or sixth nerve palsies May be due to diabetes mellitus, neoplasm, increased ICP (sixth nerve), pontine glioma in children or metastatic nasopharyngeal tumor in adults (sixth nerve), tumor at base of brain (third nerve), ischemic infarction of nerve, aneurysms in the circle of Willis. In compressive third nerve lesions the pupil is usually dilated, whereas pupils are spared in infarction of the nerve.

Third, fourth, and sixth nerve lesions May occur at level of their nuclei, along their course from brainstem through subarachnoid space, cavernous sinus, or superior orbital fissure (see Table 156-1).

Tolosa-Hunt syndrome Painful, combined unilateral palsies due to parasellar granuloma.

Pituitary apoplexy Acute onset of uni- or bilateral ophthalmoplegia and visual field defect with headache and/or drowsiness.

Migrainous ophthalmoplegia Attacks of ocular palsy in conjunction with typical migraine.

TRIGEMINAL NERVE (V)

Trigeminal neuralgia (tic douloureux) Frequent, excruciating paroxysms of pain in lips, gums, cheek, or chin (rarely in ophthalmic division of fifth nerve) lasting seconds to

TABLE 156-1 Cranial nerve syndromes

Site	Cranial nerves involved	Usual cause
Sphenoid fissure (superior orbital)	III, IV, first division V, VI	Invasive tumors of sphenoid bone, aneurysms
Lateral wall of cavernous sinus	III, IV, first division V, VI, often with proptosis	Aneurysms or thrombosis of cavernous sinus, invasive tumors from sinuses and sella turcica, sometimes benign granuloma responsive to steroids
Retrosphenoid space	II, III, IV, V, VI	Large tumors of middle cranial fossa
Apex of petrous bone	V, VI	Petrositis, tumors of petrous bone
Internal auditory meatus	VII, VIII	Tumors of petrous bone (dermoids, etc.), infectious processes, acoustic neuroma
Pontocerebellar angle	V, VII, VIII, and sometimes IX	Acoustic neuroma, meningioma
Jugular foramen	IX, X, XI	Tumors and aneurysms
Posterior latero-condylar space	IX, X, XI, XII	Tumors of parotid gland, carotid body, and metastatic tumor
Posterior retro-parotid space	IX, X, XI, XII and Horner syndrome	Tumors of parotid gland, carotid body, metastatic tumor, lymph node tumors, tuberculous adenitis

Modified from Victor M, Martin JB: HPIM-12, p 2080.

minutes. Appears in middle or old age. Pain is often stimulated at trigger points. Sensory deficit cannot be demonstrated. Must be distinguished from other forms of facial pain arising from diseases of jaw, teeth, or sinuses. Tic is rarely caused by herpes zoster or a tumor. *Treatment*: carbamazepine (1–1.5 g qd in divided doses) is effective in 75% of cases; follow CBC for rare complications of aplastic anemia. When medications fail, surgical gangliolysis or suboccipital craniectomy for decompression of trigeminal nerve are options.

Trigeminal neuropathy May be caused by a variety of rare conditions, usually presenting with facial sensory loss or weakness of jaw muscles. These include tumors of middle cranial fossa, trigeminal nerve, or metastases to base of skull, lesions in cavernous sinus (affecting first and second divisions of fifth nerve) or superior orbital fissure (affecting first division of fifth nerve).

FACIAL NERVE (VII)

Lesions of the seventh nerve or nucleus produce hemifacial weakness that includes muscles of forehead and orbicularis oculi; if lesion is in middle ear portion, taste is lost over the anterior two-thirds of tongue and there may be hyperacusis; if lesion is at internal auditory meatus, there may be involvement of auditory and vestibular nerves, whereas pontine lesions usually affect abducens nerve and often corticospinal tract as well. Peripheral nerve lesions with incomplete recovery may result in diffuse continuous contraction of affected facial muscles ± associated movements (synkinesis) of other facial muscle groups and facial spasms.

Bell's palsy   Most common form of idiopathic facial paralysis, found in 23/100,000 annually. Weakness evolves over 12–48 h, sometimes preceded by retroaural pain. Fully 80% recover within several weeks or months. *Treatment:* involves protection of eye during sleep. Prednisone (60–80 mg qd over 5 d, tapered off over the next 5 d) may be beneficial, but this has not been firmly established.

Ramsay Hunt syndrome   Caused by herpes zoster infection of geniculate ganglion; distinguished from Bell's palsy by a vesicular eruption in pharynx, external auditory canal, and other parts of the cranial integument.

Acoustic neuromas   Often compress the seventh nerve.

Pontine tumors or infarcts   May cause a lower motor neuron facial weakness.

Bilateral facial diplegia   May appear in Guillain-Barré, sarcoidosis, Lyme disease, and leprosy.

Hemifacial spasm   May appear either as a result of Bell's palsy, with irritative lesions (e.g., acoustic neuroma, basilar artery aneurysm, or aberrant vessel compressing the nerve) or as an idiopathic disorder.

Blepharospasm   Involuntary recurrent spasm of both eyelids occurring in the elderly ± facial spasm. May spontaneously subside. *Treatment:* in severe cases, differential facial nerve section or nerve decompression. Recently, local injection of botulinum toxin into orbicularis occuli has been effective, even with repeated treatment, without morbidity.

VESTIBULAR NERVE (VIII)

Vertigo due to a lesion in the vestibular component of N. VIII is discussed in Chap. 8. Lesions of the auditory nerve cause hearing impairment which can be either *conductive*, caused by structural abnormalities in external auditory canal or middle ear due to tumor, infection, trauma, etc., or *sensorineural*, due to damage to hair cells of the organ of

Corti secondary to excessive noise, viral infections, ototoxic drugs, temporal bone fractures, meningitis, cochlear otosclerosis, Ménière's disease, or neural damage due largely to cerebellar angle tumors or vascular, demyelinating, or degenerative diseases affecting the central auditory pathways. Brainstem auditory evoked responses (BAERs) are a sensitive and accurate test for distinguishing sensory from neural hearing losses. Audiometry can distinguish conductive from sensorineural hearing losses. Most pts with conductive and asymmetric sensorineural hearing losses should have CT scans of the temporal bone. Sensorineural hearing losses should be evaluated with electronystagmography and caloric testing.

GLOSSOPHARYNGEAL NERVE (IX)

Glossopharyngeal neuralgia   Paroxysmal, intense pain in tonsillar fossa of throat that may be precipitated by swallowing. There is no demonstrable sensory or motor deficit. *Treatment* with carbamazepine or phenytoin is often effective, but surgical division of the ninth nerve near the medulla is sometimes necessary. Other diseases affecting this nerve include herpes zoster or compressive neuropathy when found in conjunction with vagus and accessory nerve palsies due to tumor or aneurysm in region of jugular foramen.

VAGUS NERVE (X)

Lesions of vagus nerve cause symptoms of dysphagia and dysphonia. Unilateral lesions produce drooping of soft palate, loss of gag reflex, and "curtain movement" of lateral wall of pharynx with hoarse, nasal voice. Diseases that may involve the vagus include diphtheria (toxin), neoplastic and infectious processes at the meningeal level, tumors and vascular lesions in the medulla, or compression of the recurrent laryngeal nerve by intrathoracic processes.

HYPOGLOSSAL NERVE (XII)

The twelfth cranial nerve supplies the ipsilateral muscles of the tongue. Lesions affecting the motor nucleus may occur in the brainstem (tumor, poliomyelitis, or motor neuron disease), during the course of the nerve in the posterior fossa (platybasia, Paget's disease), or in the hypoglossal canal.

For a more detailed discussion, see Victor M, Martin JB: Disorders of the Cranial Nerves, Chap. 360, in HPIM-12, p. 2076

157 EPILEPSY

ETIOLOGY Both seizure type and age of pt provide important clues to etiology. Important causes of seizures by age group are shown in Table 157-1.

MEDICAL HISTORY Seizures may begin in a localized area of cortex ("partial" or "focal") or diffusely ("generalized"). Partial seizures may be associated with loss or alteration in consciousness ("complex") or not affect mentation ("simple"). Simple partial seizures may be motor, sensory, autonomic, or psychic. In complex partial seizures there is alteration in consciousness coupled with automatisms (e.g., lip smacking, chewing, aimless walking, or other complex motor activities). Generalized seizures may result from secondary generalization of a partial seizure or as a primary disorder. Tonic-clonic seizures ("grand mal") result in sudden loss of consciousness, loss of postural control, tonic muscular contraction producing teeth-clenching and rigidity

TABLE 157-1 The causes of seizures

Infant (0–2)	Paranatal hypoxia and ischemia
	Intracranial birth injury
	Acute infection
	Metabolic disturbances (hypoglycemia, hypocalcemia, hypomagnesemia, pyridoxine deficiency)
	Congenital malformation
	Genetic disorders
Child (2–12)	Idiopathic
	Acute infection
	Trauma
	Febrile convulsion
Adolescent (12–18)	Idopathic
	Trauma
	Drug, alcohol withdrawal
	Arteriovenous malformations
Young adult (18–25)	Trauma
	Alcoholism
	Brain tumor
Older adult (>35)	Brain tumor
	Cerebrovascular disease
	Metabolic disorders (uremia, hepatic failure, electrolyte abnormality, hypoglycemia)
	Alcoholism

From Dichter MA: HPIM-12, p. 1471.

in extension (*tonic phase*), followed by rhythmic muscular jerking (*clonic phase*).

Recovery of consciousness is typically gradual with an intervening period of confusion and disorientation. Headache and somnolence are common postictal phenomena (see Chap. 4). Tongue biting and incontinence may occur during the seizure. In absence seizures ("petit mal") there is sudden cessation, without warning, of ongoing mental activity which rarely lasts longer than 30 s. Minor motor symptoms are common, but complex automatisms and clonic activity do not occur. Return of consciousness is abrupt, and there is no postictal somnolence or confusion. Other types of generalized seizures include atypical absence, infantile spasms, tonic, atonic, and myoclonic seizures.

PHYSICAL EXAMINATION   Vital signs may provide a clue to malignant hypertension or infection. Gum hyperplasia suggests chronic phenytoin therapy. Skin lesions can occur in Sturge-Weber (port-wine facial nevus), tuberous sclerosis (adenoma sebaceum, shagreen patches), and neurofibromatosis (café-au-lait spots, neurofibroma). The general exam also may provide evidence of drug or alcohol abuse, trauma, hepatic or renal failure, or acute CNS infection. Asymmetries in the neurologic exam can suggest a brain tumor, stroke, or other focal lesion. During a generalized seizure, the pupils may be nonreactive, the corneal reflexes absent, and hyperreflexia and Babinski signs may be transiently present.

LABORATORY FINDINGS   Serum glucose, electrolytes, and calcium should be obtained immediately. LFTs, BUN, CBC, toxic screen, and alcohol level can add valuable information in specific pts. If pt takes anticonvulsant medication, drug levels should be measured. An MRI or CT scan should be obtained in all pts with an unexplained first seizure, and a follow-up study (at 3–6 months) is often advisable. An LP is indicated in all pts where infection is suspected. An EEG with activation procedures (hyperventilation, photic stimulation, sleep) often helps in diagnosis and classification of seizures.

THERAPY   Acutely, pt should be placed in semiprone position, head down, to avoid aspiration. Oxygen should be given via face mask. Pt should not be forcibly restrained, and no attempt should be made to insert a tongue blade or other object between teeth. Reversible metabolic disorders (hypoglycemia, hyponatremia, hypertension, drug or alcohol withdrawal) should be promptly corrected. A principle of drug therapy (Table 157-2) is that pts are placed on a single drug (dose optimized by serum levels), and only if high therapeutic levels fail to give control is a second drug begun. If control is then obtained, the first drug is slowly tapered.

TABLE 157-2   Commonly used antiepileptic drugs

Generic name	Phenytoin (diphenylhydantoin)	Carbamazepine	Phenobarbital	Primidone
Trade name	Dilantin	Tegretol	Luminol	Mysoline
Principal uses	Tonic-clonic (grand mal) Focal Complex partial	Tonic-clonic Focal Complex partial	Tonic-clonic Focal	Tonic-clonic Focal
Dosage	300–400 mg/d (3–5 mg/kg, adult; 4–7 mg/kg, child)	600–1200 mg/d (20–30 mg/kg, child)	60–120 mg/d (1–5 mg/kg, adult; 3–6 mg/kg, child)	750–1000 mg/d (10–25 mg/kg
Half-life	24 h (wide variation)	13–17 h	90 h (shorter in children)	8 h
Therapeutic range	10–20 µg/mL	4–12 µg/mL	10–50 µg/mL	2–10 µg/mL
% Protein bound	90	80	40–60	Small
Toxic effects				
Neurologic	Ataxia Incoordination Confusion Skin rash	Ataxia Dizziness Diplopia Vertigo	Sedation Ataxia Confusion Dizziness ↓ Libido Depression	Same as phenobarbital
Systemic	Gum hyperplasia Lymphadenopathy Hirsutism Osteomalacia Facial coarsening	Bone marrow suppression GI irritation Hepatotoxicity	Skin rash	
Drug interactions	Level increased by isoniazid, dicumarol, sulfonamides Level decreased by carbamazepine, phenobarbital	Level decreased by phenobarbital, phenytoin	Level increased by valproic acid, phenytoin Enhances metabolism of other drugs via liver enzyme induction	

ium val-roate (val-roic acid)	Ethosuximide	Methsuximide	Clonazepam	Trimethadione
akane akote	Zarontin	Celontin	Clonopin	Tridione
ence pical ab-ence oclonic ic-tonic	Absence (petit mal)	Absence (complex partial)	Absence Atypical absence Myoclonic	Absence Atypical absence (intractable seizures only)
-1250 mg/d 0–60 mg/kg)	750–1250 mg/d (20–40 mg/kg)	600–1200 mg/d	1–12 mg/d (0.1–0.2 mg/kg)	900–2100 mg/d (20–60 mg/kg)
	60 h, adult 30 h, child	38–50 h	24–48 h	6–13 days (for dimethadione)
00 μg/mL	40–100 μg/mL	10–30 μg/mL (N-desmethyl methsuximide)	5–70 ng/mL	700 μg/mL (for dimethadione)
4	Small	Small	50	Small
sia ation nor	Ataxia Lethargy	Ataxia Lethargy	Ataxia Sedation Lethargy	Sedation Blurred vision
atotoxicity e marrow ppression ritation erammo-mia	GI irritation Skin rash Bone marrow suppression	Same as ethosuximide	Anorexia	Skin rash Bone marrow suppression Nephrosis Hepatitis
ot give th clonaze-m ases carba-azepine me-olites		Increases phenytoin level Increases phenobarbital from primidone	May precipitate absence status if given with valproic acid	

For a more detailed discussion, see Dichter MA: The Epilepsies and Convulsive Disorders, Chap. 350, in HPIM-12, p. 1968

PATHOGENESIS The process may: (1) be intrinsic to a vessel (atherosclerosis, lipohyalinosis, inflammation, amyloid deposition, arterial dissection, developmental malformation, aneurysmal dilation, or venous thrombosis); (2) originate remotely (embolus from heart or extracranial circulation lodges in an intracranial vessel); (3) result from decreased perfusion pressure or increased blood viscosity with inadequate blood flow; (4) result from rupture of a vessel in the subarachnoid space or intracranial tissue.

Stroke The acute neurologic injury resulting from these pathologic processes. Evidence suggests that an ischemic zone surrounds an infarct and secondary phenomena (e.g., excitotoxins from damaged neurons, cerebral edema, altered local blood flow) can serve to increase the severity of permanent deficit. Therapy has three goals: (1) reduce risk factors (attenuate pathologic process); (2) prevent recurrent stroke by removing underlying cause; (3) minimize secondary brain damage by maintaining adequate perfusion to marginally ischemic areas and limiting edema.

CLINICAL PRESENTATION Abrupt, dramatic onset of focal neurologic symptoms. Temporal pattern is an indicator of underlying pathophysiology (see Table 158-1).

Stroke in evolution A neurologic deficit that progresses or fluctuates while under observation. Possible mechanisms include (1) propagating thrombus obliterating collateral branches with enlarging territory of ischemic brain, (2) progressive narrowing of a vessel by thrombus, (3) cerebral edema, (4) enlarging intracerebral hematoma from continued hemorrhage, (5) emboli propagating, migrating, lysing, and dispersing, and (6) recurrent artery-to-artery embolization.

Completed stroke A neurologic deficit that does not progress over several days after pt is under observation.

Transient ischemic attack (TIA) A focal neurologic deficit that resolves fully within 24 h. However, when a deficit persists beyond 1 h, some infarction of tissue has probably occurred. Repetitive, short-lived (<15 min), stereotyped focal neurologic deficits attributable to a vascular territory suggest a proximal vascular stenosis or occlusion with inadequate collateral circulation to maintain appropriate perfusion. A single episode of focal neurologic deficit persisting longer than 30 min but less than 24 h suggests an embolic TIA. Other causes of transient neurologic deficit (e.g., seizure manifestation or migraine accompaniment) should be ruled out by history or appropriate testing.

Ischemic stroke   A neurologic deficit produced by interruption of blood supply to a brain region due to an intravascular occlusion or low-flow state. Deficit is consistent with vascular territory supplied.

Embolic stroke   Suggested by abrupt appearance of a neurologic deficit that is maximal at onset.

Intracranial hemorrhage   Most common forms are *hypertensive* and *lobar* intracerebral hemorrhages (50%), ruptured saccular aneurysm, and ruptured AV malformation. Vomiting occurs in most cases and headache in about one-half. Signs and symptoms are not usually confined to a single vascular territory. Hypertensive hemorrhage typically occurs in the (1) putamen, adjacent internal capsule, and central white matter; (2) thalamus; (3) pons; and (4) cerebellum. A neurologic deficit that evolves relentlessly over 5–30 min is strongly suggestive of intracerebral bleeding. Ocular signs are important in the localization of these hemorrhages: (1) putaminal—eyes deviated to side opposite paralysis (toward lesion); (2) thalamic—eyes deviated downward, sometimes with unreactive pupils; (3) pontine—reflex lateral eye movements impaired and small (1–2 mm), reactive pupils; (4) cerebellar—eyes deviated to side opposite lesion (early on, in absence of paralysis).

Lacunar stroke   An infarct that can be pinpointed to an anatomic locus of up to 0.5–1.0 cm in diameter, resulting from local small vessel disease.

RISK FACTORS   (1) Systemic atherothrombotic disease—ischemic stroke/TIA; (2) source of emboli (e.g., atrial fibrillation, valvular heart disease, MI, infective endocarditis, etc.)—embolic stroke/TIA; (3) severe hypertension—lacunar stroke with small vessel lipohyalinotic disease, atherothrombotic lesions of large and medium-sized vessels, and deep intracerebral hemorrhages; (4) smoking and familial hyperlipidemia—atherothrombotic ischemic stroke/TIA.

COMPLICATIONS   (1) Occlusive atherothrombotic disease: increased risk of embolization from distal stump until endothelialization occurs; continued propagation of thrombus to occlude collateral circulation. (2) Embolic stroke: recurrent embolism. (3) Ischemic stroke: intracerebral hemorrhage, particularly in large strokes, as infarcted tissue undergoes necrosis; seizures in 5–10%. (4) Large cortical or cerebellar strokes: cerebral edema—this is particularly critical in cerebellar infarcts because expansion in the posterior fossa can rapidly cause brainstem compression and may require emergency cerebellectomy for lifesaving intervention; period of maximal risk is 12–72 h after infarct. (5) Intracerebral hem-

TABLE 158-1 Anatomic localization of cerebral lesions in stroke

Signs and symptoms	Structures involved
CEREBRAL HEMISPHERE, LATERAL ASPECT (MIDDLE CEREBRAL A.)	
Hemiparesis	Contralateral parietal and frontal motor cortex
Hemisensory deficit	Contralateral somatosensory cortex
Motor aphasia (Broca's)—hesitant speech with word-finding difficulty and preserved comprehension	Motor speech area, dominant frontal lobe
Central aphasia (Wernicke's)—anomia, poor comprehension, jargon speech	Central, perisylvian speech area, dominant hemisphere
Unilateral neglect, apraxias	Nondominant parietal lobe
Homonymous hemianopsia or quadrantanopsia	Optic radiation in inferior parietal or temporal lobe
Gaze preference with eyes deviated to side of lesion	Center for lateral gaze (frontal lobe)
CEREBRAL HEMISPHERE, MEDIAL ASPECT (ANTERIOR CEREBRAL A.)	
Paralysis of foot and leg with or without paresis of arm	Leg area with or without arm area of contralateral motor cortex
Cortical sensory loss over leg	Foot and leg area of contralateral sensory cortex
Grasp and sucking reflexes	Medial posterior frontal lobe
Urinary incontinence	Sensorimotor area, paracentral lobule
Gait apraxia	Frontal cortices
CEREBRAL HEMISPHERE, INFERIOR ASPECT (POSTERIOR CEREBRAL A.)	
Homonymous hemianopsia	Calcarine occipital cortex
Cortical blindness	Occipital lobes, bilaterally
Memory deficit side	Hippocampus, bilaterally or dominant
Dense sensory loss, spontaneous pain dysesthesias, choreoathetosis	Thalamus plus subthalamus
BRAINSTEM, MIDBRAIN (POSTERIOR CEREBRAL A.)	
Third nerve palsy and contralateral hemiplegia	Third nerve and cerebral peduncle (Weber's syndrome)
Paralysis/paresis of vertical eye movement	Supranuclear fibers to third nerve
Convergence nystagmus, disorientation	Top of midbrain, periaqueductal
BRAINSTEM, PONTOMEDULLARY JUNCTION (BASILAR A.)	
Facial paralysis	Seventh nerve, ipsilateral
Paresis of abduction of eye	Sixth nerve, ipsilateral

TABLE 158-1   Anatomic localization of cerebral lesions in stroke *(continued)*

Signs and symptoms	Structures involved
BRAINSTEM, PONTOMEDULLARY JUNCTION (BASILAR A.) *(Cont.)*	
Paresis of conjugate gaze	"Center" for lateral gaze, ipsilateral
Hemifacial sensory deficit	Tract and nucleus of V, ipsilateral
Horner's syndrome	Descending sympathetic pathways
Diminished pain and thermal sense over half body (with or without face)	Spinothalamic tract, contralateral
Ataxia	Middle cerebellar peduncle and cerebellum
BRAINSTEM, LATERAL MEDULLA (VERTEBRAL A.)	
Vertigo, nystagmus	Vestibular nucleus
Horner's syndrome (miosis, ptosis, decreased sweating)	Descending sympathetic fibers, ipsilateral
Ataxia, falling toward side of lesion	Cerebellar hemisphere or fibers
Impaired pain and thermal sense over half body with or without face	Contralateral spinothalamic tract

orrhage: in addition to cerebral edema, continued expansion of the hematoma with resultant compression; seizures (in <10%, most likely when hemorrhage extends to the cortical–white matter junction).

LABORATORY EVALUATION   CT   Without contrast, immediately excludes hemorrhage as the cause of focal stroke, can detect surrounding edema, and, less reliably, hemorrhagic infarction. Provides an estimate of extent and location of supratentorial infarctions as small as 0.5–1 cm. It cannot detect most infarcts for at least 48 h and often doesn't detect lesions in the cortical surface or brainstem.

MRI   Reveals more than CT in nonhemorrhagic stroke. Infarcts are seen within hours, including those in the cortical surface, posterior fossa, and lacunes <0.5 cm. Hemorrhagic components of infarcts can be detected, and blood flow in many intracranial arteries can be imaged.

Noninvasive carotid tests   Ophthalmodynamometry, oculoplethysmography, directional supraorbital Doppler, transcranial Doppler, and carotid ultrasound techniques.

Cerebral angiography   Usually performed by retrograde femoral artery catheterization.

ECG, cardiac ultrasound, and 24-h Holter monitor For evaluation of suspected embolic stroke/TIA.

Coagulation studies To include PT and PTT, particularly in pts receiving anticoagulation therapy, as well as in cerebral hemorrhage.

TREATMENT Ischemic stroke or TIA (1) *Anticoagulation*—in the absence of objective clinical data, use of this therapy is empirical. IV heparin is used when atherothrombotic vascular occlusion is suspected, particularly in ischemic stroke in evolution or in posterior circulation involvement. Warfarin may be used for atherothrombotic disease when surgery is not an option or for cardiac sources of embolism (anterior MI, AF, or valvular disease). (2) *Antiplatelet agents* may reduce risk of further TIAs and strokes in symptomatic pts and provide an alternative to anticoagulation. (3) *Surgical endarterectomy*—for carotid stenosis (particularly ≤1.0-mm lumen) below the siphon.

Lacunar stroke Aggressive management of hypertension.

Intracerebral hemorrhage (1) Aggressive correction of any coagulopathy; (2) neurosurgical evaluation for possible emergent evacuation of hematoma, especially in cases of cerebellar hemorrhage; (3) prophylactic anticonvulsant therapy in supratentorial hemorrhage, particularly when extending to cortical surface.

Fluid management in acute stroke Governed by consideration of relative risk of developing cerebral edema or extending thrombotic occlusion (or propagation) by intravascular volume depletion. In general, restrict fluids and use isotonic IV maintenance fluids (with or without hyperosmotic agents) in cases of large supratentorial or cerebellar strokes (maintain serum osmolality of 290–310 mosmol/L); when basilar thrombosis is suspected, use only isotonic IV fluids; mild fluid restriction may be advisable if cerebellar infarction is present, but *avoid* intravascular volume depletion.

Blood pressure management in acute stroke Adequate cerebral perfusion pressure must be maintained in face of a critical stenosis, vasospasm, or developing cerebral edema with increasing intracranial pressure; therefore, hypotension (and probably systolic BP <140 mmHg) should be avoided; because of a risk of new or continued intracerebral hemorrhage, sustained systolic BP >210 mmHg should be lowered with caution (usually gentle diuresis will suffice).

SUBARACHNOID HEMORRHAGE (SAH)

ETIOLOGY Most common causes (1) rupture of an intracranial aneurysm, (2) AV malformation. *Mycotic aneurysms* may occur in pts with infective endocarditis, systemic infection, or immunocompromise.

CLINICAL PRESENTATION Begins with rapid loss of consciousness in 45% of cases. In another 45%, the initial symptom is excruciating headache, often described as "the worst headache of my life." Vomiting is a prominent symptom and, in combination with severe headache, suggests SAH. A progressive third or sixth nerve palsy may herald SAH. Occasionally, an aneurysm may rupture into subdural space or into basal cisterns of subarachnoid space to form a clot large enough to produce focal neurologic symptoms by mass effect.

COMPLICATIONS (1) Communicating hydrocephalus; (2) recurrent rupture, especially in first 3 weeks after SAH; (3) cerebral ischemia and infarction due to vasospasm, usually 4–14 d after SAH, the major cause of delayed morbidity and death; (4) cerebral edema; (5) seizures; and (6) others: thrombophlebitis with pulmonary embolism, perforated stress-induced duodenal ulcer, ECG changes suggestive of MI or ischemia, cardiac arrhythmias, and hyponatremia due to inappropriate ADH secretion.

LABORATORY EVALUATION   CT Noncontrast first, to evaluate presence of blood in subarachnoid space; then with contrast in an effort to visualize an aneurysm or AVM. More than 75% of SAH cases are detectable by CT if obtained within the first 72 h.

Lumbar puncture To demonstrate presence of blood in subarachnoid space; should be obtained only if CT fails to make diagnosis *and* shows no evidence of mass or obstructive hydrocephalus; CSF should be examined for xanthochromia.

Cerebral angiography To establish diagnosis firmly, localize and characterize anatomy of aneurysm or AV malformation, and assess presence of vasospasm prior to surgery.

ECG ST changes, prolonged QRS complex, increased QT interval, and prominent or inverted T waves are often secondary to the SAH rather than myocardial ischemia.

Serum electrolytes and osmolality Should be followed because of hyponatremia secondary to inappropriate ADH secretion.

TREATMENT (1) *Strict bed rest* in a quiet room; stool softeners to prevent constipation, and analgesics to prevent rebleeding while awaiting surgery. (2) *Emergency surgical intervention* to evacuate intracerebral or subdural hematoma or to place intraventricular drains if obstructive or communicating hydrocephalus develops. (3) *Anticonvulsants* to prevent seizures. (4) *Assisted ventilation* for stuporous or comatose pt to control elevated intracranial pressure and ensure adequate oxygenation. (5) *Blood pressure* is monitored and controlled to maintain adequate cerebral perfusion pressure while avoiding excessive elevation. (6) *Aminocaproic acid (Amicar)* (antifibrinolytic therapy) to prevent rerupture; efficacy has not been established; reports suggest that it increases risk of ischemic complications of SAH. (7) *Symptomatic cerebral vasospasm*: increase cerebral perfusion pressure by increasing mean arterial pressure through plasma volume expansion and pressor agents; calcium channel blockers (e.g., nimodipine) may prevent or minimize development of vasospasm. (8) *Surgical clipping of aneurysm* or *resection of AV malformation*. Surgery is typically delayed at least 10–14 d after SAH in an effort to stabilize pt and minimize risk of symptomatic vasospasm in postoperative period; however, surgery may be attempted within the first 48 h if pt is neurologically intact and aneurysm is easily accessible.

For a more detailed discussion, see Kistler JP, Ropper AH, Martin JB: Cerebrovascular Disease, Chap. 351, in HPIM-12, p. 1977

159 NEOPLASTIC DISEASES OF THE CENTRAL NERVOUS SYSTEM

Care of pts with primary or metastatic tumors in the CNS requires (1) accurate diagnosis of tumor and exclusion of other causes of symptoms (abscess, demyelinating and vascular disease); (2) proper use of CT scan, MRI, myelography, arteriography, and surgical biopsy; (3) control of edema and seizures; (4) exclusion of systemic malignancy prior to referring pt for intracranial biopsy; and (5) management of the medical complications of the tumor and its therapy.

SYMPTOMS AND SIGNS OF CNS TUMORS

INTRACRANIAL TUMORS Pts with intracranial tumors present because of nonfocal symptoms due to increased intracranial pressure (ICP) (see Chap. 26) or focal symptoms that are dependent on location of the lesion (see Chaps. 174 and 176). Constant headache is common in pts with CNS tumors, especially headache that is worsened by lying down, coughing, sneezing, or Valsalva. Papilledema and sixth nerve palsies also occur frequently if ICP is elevated. A sudden onset of symptoms can result from hemorrhage into a tumor. Slow-growing tumors in relatively "silent" brain areas (unilateral prefrontal) can attain a large size with few symptoms. Occasionally, diencephalic and frontal or temporal lobe tumors present with prominent psychiatric disorders. New-onset epilepsy in adults often heralds the diagnosis of CNS malignancy. In such pts over 35 years of age, a series of MRI or contrast-enhanced CT scans every 2–4 months should be performed to document presence or absence of a tumor.

Tumors that occur in the third ventricle region include pituitary adenomas, craniopharyngiomas, germ cell neoplasms, pineal tumors, and astrocytomas. They give rise to neuroendocrine abnormalities, optic nerve or chiasmal compression, obstructive hydrocephalus, and Parinaud's syndrome (paralysis of upward gaze and accommodation with fixed pupils). Specific syndromes also are associated with acoustic nerve schwannomas (hearing loss, tinnitus, intermittent vertigo followed by facial weakness and facial sensory loss) and cerebellar hemangioblastomas (headache, head tilt, recurrent emesis, and ataxia, sometimes associated with polycythemia and renal tumors).

SPINAL TUMORS Tumors of the cord or spinal canal can cause neurologic dysfunction due to infiltration, compression, or interference with cord blood supply. Extramedullary tumors (outside the substance of the cord), such as schwannoma, spinal metastases, and meningioma, compress nerve roots, cause back and radicular pain, and produce spastic paresis with sensory loss below a spinal level. Bowel and bladder dysfunction also occur with loss of perineal sensation and rectal tone. Spinal epidural cancer should be suspected in pts with back pain and known systemic malignancy. Intramedullary tumors are less common and usually extend over many levels; their presentation is more varied, usually gradual, and they can be associated with syringomyelia.

Idiopathic syringomyelia, B_{12} deficiency, paraneoplastic syndromes, transverse myelitis, arachnoiditis, spinal AV malformation, and meningeal carcinomatosis may be difficult to distinguish from an intrinsic cord tumor on clinical grounds. Pts with slow-growing cord tumors who accumulate patchy cord deficits over time are often misdiagnosed as suffering from multiple sclerosis. MRI, myelography, and CSF exam are essential for accurate diagnosis in many cases.

Melanoma, lymphoma, leukemia, and adenocarcinoma of breast, GI tract, and lung commonly invade the meninges. Leptomeningeal spread of tumor causes headache and cranial and spinal nerve root deficits, sometimes with spinal cord signs. The CSF shows an elevated protein, low glucose, and pleocytosis. Repeated CSF exam may be necessary to obtain positive cytology.

GENERAL AND RADIOLOGIC EVALUATION

Initial evaluation of pts suspected of having a brain tumor should include a search for a primary tumor; this should include careful examination for melanotic lesions, a search for enlarged lymph nodes, breast masses, bony tenderness, abdominal or rectal masses, and organomegaly. Urine and stool should be examined for occult blood. Chest films often reveal the site of primary or secondary tumor. MRI is the most sensitive study to detect brain tumor. CT scan with contrast will detect brain masses greater than 0.5 cm in diameter and is the technique of choice in radiation planning. Most tumors enhance after radiographic or paramagnetic contrast administration. Low density surrounding the mass on CT scan or extensive T_2 signal abnormality on MRI scan usually represents edema; central low density indicates cavitation. Pts with tumors that shift midline structures to the opposite side or compress midbrain structures are prone to acute neurologic deterioration. MRI can define brainstem and intrinsic spinal cord tumors that are only poorly defined by CT scan. Angiography can show an abnormal vascular blush with early draining veins, characteristic of some tumors. It also provides important information to the neurosurgeon contemplating biopsy or resection. MRI, myelography, and CT scan after injection of metrizamide into the subarachnoid space are essential radiologic procedures in the diagnosis of spinal cord tumors; these studies may detect deposits of tumor on nerve roots or on the cord itself in pts with leptomeningeal metastases.

MANAGEMENT OF CNS TUMORS

INITIAL MANAGEMENT   Dexamethasone, 32–48 mg/d, in 4–6 divided doses reduces cerebral edema due to tumor. Restriction of free water intake may be necessary to prevent edema formation. A mannitol infusion (1 g/kg) may be necessary if pt is deteriorating due to raised ICP (see Chap. 26). Anticonvulsants are sometimes used prophylactically. Surgical biopsy affords a definitive diagnosis of the tumor along with prognostically important pathologic features. Partial resection of large, surgically incurable tumors still enables decompression of intracranial contents and better seizure control.

Tumors that compress the pathway of CSF outflow can cause severe hydrocephalus. Urgent placement of a ventricular-atrial or ventricular-peritoneal shunt in such pts may be lifesaving. Shunts placed into expanding tumor cavities also can help decrease mass effect.

CEREBRAL METASTASES   Melanoma has the highest likelihood of any single tumor type to spread to the CNS. Lung and breast cancers are more prevalent and account for the largest percentage of CNS metastases. Pts with lung cancer should have a brain CT scan prior to undergoing curative pulmonary lobectomy. The surgical removal of a single brain metastasis may improve the quality of life for the cancer pt depending on the nature and stage of the systemic disease. Radiation therapy is often palliative and can cause neurologic improvement. Unfortunately, melanoma, GI tract, and lung cancer tend to be relatively resistant to the doses of radiation permissible in the CNS. Treatment of meningeal metastases requires combination of radiation and intrathecal chemotherapy.

PRIMARY BRAIN TUMORS   Malignant astrocytoma or glioblastoma accounts for 75% of adult glial tumors. Biopsy with resection of accessible tumors combined with radiation improves survival, but the gains are short-lived. Meningiomas are common benign tumors arising from cells of the pia-arachnoid. Schwannomas usually arise from cranial nerves close to their foramina. Resection can be curative for these benign tumors in addition to ependymomas, oligodendrogliomas, hemangioblastomas, and low-grade astrocytomas. Radiation can be reserved for a time of deterioration. Primary CNS lymphoma may be multifocal, simulating metastases or plaques of demyelination. Primary lymphoma is more frequent in pts with AIDS, IgM or IgA deficiencies, or otherwise immunosuppressed. Marked shrinkage of the CNS lymphoma can occur after short courses of glucocorticoids. Radiation is also effective in reducing tumor size. Unfortunately, recurrence and eventual therapeutic resistance are the common pattern.

SPINAL CORD TUMORS   Rapid radiologic diagnosis and treatment of cord compression are mandatory to avert permanent neurologic disability. Glucocorticoids, radiation, and surgical decompression may prevent progression of deficits. Radiation therapy is palliative in some cases. Intrinsic cord tumors in children may be successfully resected even if they extend over multiple cord levels.

For a more detailed discussion, see Hochberg F, Pruitt A: Neoplastic Diseases of the Central Nervous System, Chap. 353, in HPIM-12, p. 2010

ACUTE BACTERIAL MENINGITIS

Etiology

- *Streptococcus pneumoniae* (see Chap. 42): 30–50% of cases in adults, 10–20% in children, up to 5% in infants; ↑ risk: acute otitis media, pneumonia, head injury with CSF leak, sickle cell, Hodgkin's, multiple myeloma, alcoholism.
- *Neisseria meningitidis* (see Chap. 47): most often children and adolescents (25–40% cases), also 10–35% of cases in adults, rare in infants; epidemics.
- *Haemophilus influenzae,* type B (see Chap. 48): most frequent meningeal infection between 2 months and 3 years (40–60% of cases in children); rare in adults except with anatomic defect (dermal sinus tract, skull fracture), immunodeficient, diabetes, alcoholism.
- *Staphylococcus aureus*: follows neurosurgery or penetrating head wound.
- *Staphylococcus epidermidis*: 75% of CSF shunt infections.
- Gram-negative bacilli: associated with brain abscess, epidural abscess, neurosurgical procedures, cranial thrombophlebitis.
- *Listeria monocytogenes*: predisposed in elderly, debilitated, immunosuppressed, alcoholics, diabetics.

Clinical Manifestations

- Fever, headache, seizures, vomiting, impaired consciousness, stiff neck and back; 25% fulminant onset over 24 h; 50% over 1–7 d following respiratory symptoms.
- Children: onset often nonspecific with fever and vomiting, ↑ seizures.
- Infants: fever, irritability, lethargy, anorexia.
- Stiff neck or positive Kernig's and Brudzinski's signs may be absent in the very young, very old, or severely obtunded pt.
- 50% with meningococcal meningitis have skin rash; may also occur with *H. influenzae, S. pneumoniae,* echovirus type 9, *S. aureus.*

Laboratory Findings

- CSF leukocytes: 1000–100,000 (avg. 5000–20,000); >50,000 suspicious for ruptured brain abscess; early ↑ PMNs with

↑ mononuclear cells as infection continues. • Pressure: consistently >180 mmH$_2$O. • Protein: average 1.5–5.0 g/L (150–500 mg/dL). • Glucose: usually <40% of blood glucose. • Gram's stain: + in three-quarters if untreated. • Cultures: + in 70–80%; in partially treated meningitis, latex agglutination for *H. influenzae* type B, *S. pneumoniae*, *N. meningitidis* groups A, B, C, Y. • Blood cultures: + in 40–60% with *H. influenzae*, meningococcus, and pneumococcus.

Treatment

- Pneumococcal or meningococcal: penicillin G, 18–24 million U IV qd in 4–6 divided doses × 10 d; cefotaxime 2 g IV q 4 h, ceftriaxone 2 g IV qd, or chloramphenicol 4–6 g IV qd in penicillin-allergic pts.
- *H. influenzae*: children—cefotaxime 200 (mg/kg)/d IV divided in 4–6 doses or ceftriaxone 100 mg/kg IV qd (max 2 g/d); if ampicillin-sensitive organism, ampicillin 300–400 (mg/kg)/d IV divided in 4–6 doses; dexamethasone 0.15 mg/kg IV q 6 h for the first 4 d may reduce nerve deafness in children. Adults—cefotaxime or ceftriaxone as for pneumococcal meningitis, or ampicillin 12–18 g/d divided in 4–6 doses. Alternatively, can initiate treatment with ampicillin and chloramphenicol 100–200 (mg/kg)/d in children or 4–6 g/d in adults until sensitivities known.
- Community-acquired gram-negative: cefotaxime 2 g IV q 4 h; in hospital following head trauma or neurosurgery, ↑ risk *Pseudomonas aeruginosa* or *Acinetobacter*, add tobramycin 5 mg/kg qd IV and 8–10 mg intrathecally.
- *S. aureus*: Nafcillin or oxacillin 2.0 g IV q 4 h.
- Unknown etiology: adults—ampicillin 12–18 g IV qd or penicillin G 18–24 million U IV qd, plus either cefotaxime or ceftriaxone; children—cefotaxime or ceftriaxone as for *H. influenzae*; substitute chloramphenicol for penicillin or ampicillin in penicillin-allergic pts; neonates—ampicillin 100–200 mg/kg IV qd + gentamicin 5 mg/kg IV qd.

SUBDURAL EMPYEMA

Etiology

• Primary from extension from sinuses, osteomyelitis, brain abscess. • Secondary from neurosurgical drainage of a subdural hematoma. • Usually polymicrobial: aerobic streptococci > staphylococci > microaerophilic and anaerobic streptococci > aerobic GNR > other anaerobes.

Symptoms   Chronic sinusitis or otitis with recent flare → headache, fever, vomiting, depressed sensorium → focal motor seizures, hemiplegia, aphasia over several days; 50% papilledema.

Diagnosis
• Laboratory: ↑ WBC and ESR.   • LP contraindicated (risk of herniation) but if done, shows ↑ pressure, WBC of 50–1000, ↑ protein [0.75–3.0 g/L (75–300 mg/dL)], normal sugar.   • CT scan is the procedure of choice.

Treatment
• Early surgical drainage.   • Empiric antibiotics: penicillin 20 million U IV qd + metronidazole 500 mg IV q 6 h (or chloramphenicol 4 g qd) × 3–6 weeks. Adjust antibiotics as indicated by results of culture and sensitivities.

BRAIN ABSCESS

Etiology
• Most from chronic ear, sinus, or pulmonary infection.
• Streptococci > *Bacteroides* > Enterobacteriaceae (ear infections) > *S. aureus* (penetrating head trauma or bacteremia). Anaerobic organisms present in about 50% of cases, singly or as mixed infection.

Clinical manifestations
• Reactivation of chronic ear, sinus, or pulmonary infection → headache, vomiting, ↑ CSF pressure over <2 weeks; fever > 50%.
• Frontal lobe: headache, drowsiness, inattention, hemiparesis, unilateral seizures.
• Temporal lobe: unilateral headache, aphasia, and anomia if in dominant hemisphere; homonymous upper quadrant field defect.
• Cerebellar: postauricular or suboccipital headache, nystagmus, gaze weakness, ipsilateral arm and leg weakness.

Diagnosis
• Demonstration of infection in ears, sinuses, lungs or right-to-left cardiac shunt; ↑ ICP, focal cerebral or cerebellar signs.   • LP dangerous; if suspect, get CT scan → ring-enhancing mass lesion (radionuclide brain scan if CT unavailable). MRI may reveal multiple lesions better than CT.
• CT-guided stereotactic needle aspiration for Gram stain and culture.

Treatment
• If focal cerebritis, may cure with antibiotics alone—penicillin 20–30 million U IV qd + metronidazole 500 mg IV q 6 h × 6–8 weeks. Can add cefotaxime or ceftriaxone in doses as for meningitis empirically; chloramphenicol 4–6 g/d for penicillin-allergic adult pts.
• Surgical drainage if large and encapsulated, if multiple, deep, concomitant meningitis, or underlying debilitating disease → antibiotics alone.

• Control of ICP with mannitol or dexamethasone.

For a more detailed discussion, see Harter DH, Petersdorf RG: Bacterial Meningitis and Brain Abscess, Chap. 354, in HPIM-12, p. 2023

ASEPTIC MENINGITIS

- *Epidemiology:* 90% <30 years old; peak in late summer; majority by coxsackie- and echoviruses (see Chap. 54).
- *Clinical picture:* prodromal "flulike" illness; then intense headache, malaise, nausea, vomiting, photophobia, stupor rare; temperature 38–40°C; neck stiffness; parotitis → mumps; skin rash → consider coxsackie- or echovirus; herpangina (painful vesicles in posterior third of oropharynx) → coxsackie viruses.
- *Diagnosis:* CSF—10–100 WBCs, >¾ lymphs (PMNs early), normal protein and glucose (glucose rarely ↓ with mumps, HSV); positive CSF cultures rare except mumps; diagnosis by serology.
- *Treatment:* symptomatic; fever usually resolves in 3–5 d; CSF WBC may be ↑ for several weeks.

VIRAL ENCEPHALITIS See Chap. 57.
MYELITIS

- Infection localizing to parenchyma of spinal cord. • Spinal paralytic disease: polio, coxsackie- and echoviruses (see Chap. 54). • Herpes viruses: genital HSV → paralysis of sphincter tone; varicella-zoster virus → bilateral leg weakness with sphincter disturbances (see Chap. 55).

SUBACUTE SCLEROSING PANENCEPHALITIS

- *Epidemiology:* 80% <11 years old; 3–10 times more likely in males; years after clinical measles.
- *Clinical picture:* well, then insidious mental deterioration → incoordination, ataxia → death.
- *Diagnosis:* abnormal EEG, ↑ measles antibody in CSF and serum; pts lack antibody to measles virus protein M.
- *Treatment:* none uniformly effective; isoprinosine controversial.

PROGRESSIVE MULTIFOCAL LEUKOENCEPHALOPATHY (PML)

- *Epidemiology:* ↑ risk—leukemia, lymphoma, carcinomatosis, AIDS.
- *Clinical picture:* insidious onset, organic mental changes, hemiplegia, hemianopsia, aphasia, visual field abnormalities; death in 1–6 months.

- *Diagnosis:* CSF normal; CT or MRI shows white matter destruction; brain biopsy → viral particles of JC virus (polyomavirus).

NEUROLOGIC CONDITIONS IN AIDS

- ↑ risk: herpes, CMV, PML (JC virus).
- Human immunodeficiency virus may cause acute encephalopathy or aseptic meningitis with recent seroconversion. AIDS dementia—insidious onset of difficulty concentrating, decreased recall, decreased ability to perform complex tasks (differentiate from depression) → gait unsteadiness, weakness; MRI shows cerebral atrophy and patchy ↑ signal in central white matter; rule out cryptococcal meningitis, toxoplasma brain abscess, PML. Zidovudine may benefit some pts.

CREUTZFELDT-JAKOB DISEASE

- *Etiology:* peak 50–75 years old; incubation as long as 20 years; transmission by corneal transplants, EEG electrodes, growth hormone from cadaveric pituitary glands; causative agent not identified.
- *Clinical picture:* progressive mental deterioration, disturbances of gait, vision, balance → myoclonic jerks, cortical blindness, confusion; majority die within 6 months.
- *Diagnosis:* distinct EEG; rapid progressive atrophic changes on CT suggestive; no serologic tests.

For a more detailed discussion, see Harter DH, Petersdorf RG: Viral Diseases of the Central Nervous System: Aseptic Meningitis and Encephalitis, Chap. 355, in HPIM-12, p. 2031

PATHOLOGY Characterized pathologically by focal regions of demyelination ("plaques") of varying size and age scattered throughout the white matter of the CNS, with a propensity to involve the periventricular and subpial white matter of the cerebrum, the optic nerves, brainstem, cerebellum, and spinal cord.

CLINICAL MANIFESTATIONS Onset in third to fourth decades of recurrent attacks of focal neurologic dysfunction occurring at erratic and nonpredictable intervals, typically lasting weeks, and with subsequent variable recovery. Less commonly, slowly progressive neurologic deterioration occurs. Symptoms may be exacerbated by fatigue, stress, exercise, and heat. The manifestations of MS are protean but commonly include <u>weakness and/or sensory symptoms involving a limb</u>, <u>visual difficulties, abnormalities of gait and coordination</u>, and <u>urinary urgency or frequency</u>. Motor involvement can make a limb seem heavy, stiff, weak, or clumsy. Localized tingling, "pins and needles," or "deadness" are common sensory complaints. <u>Optic neuritis</u> can result in blurring or misting of vision, especially in the central visual field, often with associated retro-orbital pain accentuated by eye movement. Involvement of the brainstem may result in diplopia, nystagmus, vertigo, facial pain (including tic douloureux), facial numbness, facial weakness, or hemispasm. Problems with coordination, ataxia, tremor, and dysarthria may reflect cerebellar disease.

PHYSICAL EXAMINATION Check for abnormalities in visual fields, loss of visual acuity, disturbed color perception, optic pallor or papillitis, abnormalities in pupillary reflexes, nystagmus, internuclear ophthalmoplegia (slowness or loss of adduction in one eye with nystagmus in the abducting eye on lateral gaze), facial numbness or weakness, dysarthria, incoordination, ataxia, weakness and spasticity, hyperreflexia, loss of abdominal reflexes, ankle clonus, upgoing toes, sensory abnormalities.

LABORATORY FINDINGS MRI scans are the most sensitive means of detecting demyelinating lesions. (See Fig. 348-3, p. 1958, of HPIM-12.) IV administration of gadolinium DPTA can enhance detection of lesions. CT scan, especially with high contrast doses and delayed imaging, also may show plaques. Visual, auditory, and somatosensory evoked response tests are of value in identifying lesions that are clinically silent. Abnormalities in the CSF may include

oligoclonal bands, elevated IgG or myelin basic protein, mild
lymphocytic pleocytosis, and slight elevation of total protein.
Analysis of T-lymphocyte subpopulations in serum or CSF
may demonstrate reduced numbers of cells with the "sup-
pressor" phenotype during or immediately preceding attacks.
Urodynamic studies often aid in investigation and management of bladder symptoms. CT scan, MRI, and myelography
may help exclude other processes that can mimic MS.

TREATMENT   No definitive therapy is currently available.
Glucocorticoids (ACTH, prednisone) are of value in ameliorating the severity of acute attacks, although they do not
appear to increase the ultimate degree of recovery or alter
the extent of subsequent disability. Immunosuppressive therapy (cyclophosphamide) is thought by some to decrease the
frequency of attacks and stabilize progressive disease but no
consensus about the optimum use of this therapy currently
exists. A number of other therapies including use of antibodies
against specific lymphocyte subpopulations, plasma exchange, cyclosporine A, α- and β-interferon, 4-aminopyri-
dine, and hyperbaric oxygen treatment are under research.
Useful supportive therapy may include anticholinergics, smooth
muscle relaxants, and self-catheterization for bladder symptoms; diazepam, baclofen, and dantrolene for spasticity and
flexor spasms; and phenytoin and carbamazepine for dysesthesia. Clonazepam benefits some pts with intention tremor.

For a more detailed discussion, see Antel JP, Arnason BGW:
Demyelinating Diseases, Chap. 356, in HPIM-12, p. 2038

163 PARKINSON'S DISEASE

ETIOLOGY Degeneration of dopaminergic neurons of the substantia nigra. Parkinsonian syndromes may follow the use of major tranquilizers and other medications that interrupt dopaminergic functions (e.g., phenothiazines, reserpine, alpha-methyldopa), CO poisoning, intoxications with manganese and other heavy metals, and the use of illicit synthetic drugs (e.g., MPTP; see HPIM-12, p. 1954). Rare cases follow viral encephalitis or occur in association with focal lesions of substantia nigra and striatum. Parkinsonism also occurs in other degenerative neurologic disease (e.g., striatonigral degeneration, olivopontocerebellar atrophy, and progressive supranuclear palsy).

CLINICAL MANIFESTATIONS Onset between ages 40 and 70 with subsequent chronic progression. Presenting symptoms include tremor, stiffness and slowness of movement, loss of dexterity, deterioration in handwriting, difficulty arising from a chair or turning in bed, and abnormalities in gait and posture. Additional complaints may include excessive sweating and salivation, postural hypotension, subtle dementia (in up to one-third of pts), and depression.

PHYSICAL EXAMINATION Tremor at rest (4–7 Hz) is first noticed in the hands and fingers ("pill rolling") but later may involve legs, face, and tongue. A faster "action tremor" may be present. Slowness and poverty of movement (bradykinesia) can be detected by testing quick movements (e.g., "slap my hand!") and rapid alternating movements; the superimposition of tremor on passive movements creates a sense of "cogwheeling" most easily demonstrated at the wrist. Rigidity produces resistance to passive limb displacement. Postural abnormalities result in flexion of head and trunk, flexion of knees and elbows, and positional deformities of hands. Pts have infrequent eye blinking, a fixed, expressionless face ("masked"), and decreased spontaneous and associated movements (e.g., arm-swing while walking). Abnormalities of gait include short, shuffling steps, difficulty in getting started and in turning, festination, and frequent falls. Additional signs may include micrographia, hypophonia, hypometric saccades, drooling, excess salivation, and seborrhea. Some degree of intellectual deterioration is common in advanced cases. Paralysis, alterations in tendon reflexes, and objective sensory findings do not occur.

COMPLICATIONS Aspiration pneumonia, bedsores, and other problems secondary to inanition and general enfeeblement occur in advanced cases.

LABORATORY FINDINGS Diagnosis is based on history and clinical findings. CT scan, MRI, EEG, and CSF profile are typically normal. Neuropsychologic testing may help to define intellectual impairment. Recording of tremor rate, rhythm, and amplitude may be useful in some pts.

TREATMENT Drug-induced parkinsonism is treated by reducing dose of drug or by administrating an anticholinergic. Anticholinergics [e.g., trihexyphenidyl (Artane) 1–5 mg tid or benztropine (Cogentin) 0.5–2 mg tid] are used for treatment of mild cases of idiopathic Parkinson's disease to suppress resting tremor (see Table 163-1). Beta blockers (e.g., propranolol 40–80 mg tid, metoprolol) are helpful for action tremor. Primidone may also be of value. Sinemet (carbidopa/levodopa) is the mainstay of therapy in most cases. Dopamine receptor agonists (e.g., bromocriptine) and amantadine are useful adjuncts. Recent studies suggest that Eldepryl (selegiline HCl, L-deprenyl) (5 mg bid) may delay the development of symptoms in some Parkinsonian patients. Stereotactic

TABLE 163-1 Doses of drugs used in Parkinson's disease

Drug	Trade name	Dose	Side effects
Trihexyphenidyl	Artane	1–5 mg tid	Dry mouth, blurred vision, confusion
Benztropine	Cogentin	0.5–2 mg tid	Dry mouth, confusion
Procyclidine	Kemadrin	2.5–5 mg tid	Dry mouth, blurred vision, GI complaints
Carbidopa/levodopa	Sinemet	10/100 to 25/250 mg; increase slowly to tid or qid	Orthostatic hypotension, GI complaints, hallucinations, confusion, chorea
Amantadine	Symmetrel	100 mg bid	Depression, orthostatic hypotension, psychosis, urinary retention
Bromocriptine	Parlodel	10–100 mg daily in divided doses	Orthostatic hypotension, nausea and vomiting, hallucinations, psychosis
L-Deprenyl	Eldepryl	5 mg bid	Nausea, dizziness, confusion, hallucinations

surgery to place lesions in the ventrolateral thalamus may be beneficial in cases of severe tremor. Recent studies of the effect of adrenal medullary transplants to the striatum failed to confirm earlier enthusiastic reports of favorable responses. The procedure must currently be considered an experimental approach of unproven efficacy.

For more detailed discussion, see Beal MF, Richardson EP Jr, Martin JB: Alzheimer's Disease, Parkinsonism, and Other Degenerative Diseases of the Nervous System, Chap. 359, p. 2060, in HPIM-12

164 ALZHEIMER'S DISEASE (AD) AND OTHER DEMENTIAS

ETIOLOGY About 70% of progressive dementias occurring in adults are due to AD. Other causes in descending order of frequency are multiinfarct dementia (MID), metabolic/nutritional/endocrine disorders (including Wernicke-Korsakoff syndrome), brain tumors, chronic CNS infection, and normal-pressure hydrocephalus (NPH). Less common causes are Huntington's disease (HD), Creutzfeldt-Jakob disease (see Chap. 161), and Pick's disease. AIDS encephalopathy is emerging as an important cause of dementia in groups at risk.

CLINICAL MANIFESTATIONS Dementia is defined as a decline from a former level of cognitive function. Although effects on memory (particularly recent memory) are usually prominent, all aspects of cortical functions may be affected, leading to disorientation, poor judgment, poor concentration, aphasia, apraxia, and alexia. Level of consciousness is usually normal, and hallucinations or agitated confusion should lead to consideration of toxic/metabolic/drug-related or infectious etiologies.

AD Presents initially with memory loss, but soon also alters other cognitive functions with evidence of aphasia, apraxia, or impaired judgment. Pt's personality is preserved, and superficial assessment may miss extent of dementia. Symptoms are usually noted first by family members; pt is often unaware of serious degree of memory loss. Disease is characterized by neuropathologic changes of neurofibrillary tangles and senile plaques, found most prominently in hippocampus and association cortex. Familial AD (FAD) (10%) has been linked in some early onset pedigrees to chromosome 21q. Down's syndrome is also associated with neuropathologic changes identical to AD. The senile (neuritic) plaque contains an extracellular amyloid core formed from an amyloid precursor protein (APP) that is encoded by a gene distal to the FAD locus on 21q. APP is a membrane-spanning glycoprotein that may be abnormally processed in AD, leading to abnormal deposition.

MID Pts with hypertension, diabetes mellitus, and hypercholesterolemia are susceptible to multiple CNS infarcts of varying sizes. History of strokes, asymmetrical neurologic signs, and pseudobulbar palsy are clues to diagnosis. CT and MRI reveal multiple lesions.

Toxic/metabolic/nutritional Pts should be assessed for systemic signs of vitamin deficiency (thiamine, B_{12}), for endocrine disturbance (hypothyroidism, hypercalcemia), and for history of drug use (iatrogenic or illicit). Pts with Wernicke's encephalopathy (B_1 deficiency) present with memory loss and confusion, abnormal eye movements (sixth nerve palsy, nystagmus), and ataxia. The persistent deficit in memory is called Korsakoff's syndrome. Pts with this condition have permanent inability to learn or memorize new material, show confabulation, but have near normal preservation of other higher cortical functions (language, calculations), etc.

Brain tumors (see Chap. 159) **and subdural hematoma** CT or MRI will clarify diagnosis.

CNS infections Cryptococcus (torula), neurosyphilis, and other chronic infections can be sought by CSF examination. AIDS can present first as an aseptic meningitis followed by a progressive dementia. CSF is abnormal (WBC pleocytosis), and HIV can be cultured from CSF or brain.

NPH Should be suspected in elderly pts with combination of gait disorder, dementia, and urinary incontinence. Diagnosis may be difficult in elderly pts with cortical atrophy and *hydrocephalus ex vacuo*. Diagnostic studies in hospital are required to make the diagnosis.

HD An autosomal dominant disorder (gene on chromosome 4p16) that presents in pts aged 20–50, with depression, choreiform movements, and *subcortical* dementia—abulia, inattention, poor concentration, but less striking memory loss. Abnormal CT or MRI with caudate atrophy is found. Genetic presymptomatic testing is now available with restriction fragment length polymorphisms (RFLPs).

Limbic encephalitis See Chap. 176.

Creutzfeldt-Jakob disease See Chap. 161.

LABORATORY INVESTIGATION Pts with diagnosis of dementia should have (1) CBC, ESR; (2) serum calcium, electrolytes, B_{12}, and folate levels, and liver, renal, and thyroid function tests; (3) CT or MRI; (4) CSF examination for cell count, protein, and cytology; and (5) serology to exclude syphilis should always be measured; HIV antibody testing should be obtained when indicated.

DIFFERENTIAL DIAGNOSIS *Pseudodementia of depression* may be difficult to distinguish from true dementia. Pts over age 60 commonly complain of subtle memory loss—usually due to *benign senescent forgetfulness*. In both these cases, a clinical assessment of memory functions usually reveals no serious deficit. A useful test is the Mini-mental scale (see Table 164-1). Pts with Parkinson's disease (see Chap. 163) may become demented.

TABLE 164-1 Mini-mental status examination

EXAMINATION

		Patient ————————————
		Examiner ————————————
		Date ————————————

Maximum score	Score	Orientation
5	( )	What is the (year) (season) (date) (day) (month)?
5	( )	Where are we? (state) (county) (town) (hospital)(floor)

		Registration
3	( )	Name 3 objects: 1 s to say each. Then ask the patient all 3 after you have said them. Give 1 point for each correct answer. Then repeat them until he learns all 3. Count trials, and record: Trials ————————————

		Attention and calculation
5	( )	Serial 7s. 1 point for each correct. Stop after 5 answers. Alternative: Spell "world" backwards.

		Recall
3	( )	Ask for the 3 objects repeated above. Give 1 point for each correct.

		Language
9	( )	Name a pencil and wristwatch (2 points) Repeat the following: "No ifs, and, or buts." (1 point) Follow a 3-stage command: "Take a paper in your right hand, fold it in half, and put it on the floor." (3 points) Read and obey the following: Close your eyes (1 point)

Write a sentence (1 point)

Copy design (1 point)

Total score ————————————

Assess level of consciousness along a continuum

Alert   Drowsy   Stupor   Coma

INSTRUCTIONS FOR ADMINISTRATION

Orientation
Ask for the date. Then ask specifically for parts omitted, e.g., "Can you also tell me what season it is?" One point for each correct.
Ask in turn "Can you tell me the name of this hospital?" (town, country, etc.). One point for each correct.

Registration
Ask the patient if you may test his memory. Then say the names of 3 unrelated objects, clearly and slowly, about 1 s for each. After you have said all 3, ask him to repeat them. This first repetition determines his score (0–3), but keep saying them until he can repeat all 3, up to 6 trials. If he does not eventually learn all 3, recall cannot be meaningfully tested.

Attention and calculation
Ask the patient to begin with 100 and count backwards by 7. Stop after 5 subtractions (93, 86, 79, 72, 65). Score the total number of correct answers.
If the patient cannot or will not perform this task, ask him to spell the word "world" backwards. The score is the number of letters in correct order: e.g., dlorw = 5, dlorw = 3.

Recall
Ask the patient if he can recall the 3 words you previously asked him to remember. Score 0–3.

Language
Naming: Show the patient a wristwatch and ask him what it is. Repeat for pencil. Score 0–2.
Repetition: Ask the patient to repeat the sentence after you. Allow only one trial. Score 0–1.
3-Stage command: Give the patient a piece of plain blank paper and repeat the command. Score 1 point for each part correctly executed.
Reading: On a blank piece of paper print the sentence "Close your eyes," in letters large enough for the patient to see clearly. Ask him to read it and do what it says. Score 1 point only if he actually closes his eyes.
Writing: Give the patient a blank piece of paper and ask him to write a sentence for you. Do not dictate a sentence; it is to be written spontaneously. It must contain a subject and verb and be sensible. Correct grammar and punctuation are not necessary.
Copying: On a clean piece of paper, draw intersecting pentagons, each side about 1 in, and ask him to copy it exactly as it is. All 10 angles must be present and 2 must intersect to score 1 point. Tremor and rotation are ignored.

Estimate the patient's level of sensorium along a continuum, from alert on the left to coma on the right.

SOURCE: Reproduced with permission from Folstein et al., J. Psychiatr Res 12: 189, 1975.

TREATMENT The treatable cases will emerge from the laboratory evaluation. NPH can be improved in two-thirds of cases by CSF shunting. Nontreatable causes of dementia include AD, HD, Creutzfeldt-Jakob.

For a more detailed discussion, see Cassem EH: Behavioral and Emotional Disturbances, Chap. 29, p. 180; Brown MM, Hachinski VC: Acute Confusional States, Amnesia, and Dementia, Chap. 30, p. 183; and Beal MF, Richardson EP Jr, Martin JB: Alzheimer's Disease, Parkinsonism, and Other Degenerative Diseases of the Nervous System, Chap. 359, p. 2060, in HPIM-12

---

165 AMYOTROPHIC LATERAL SCLEROSIS (ALS)

ETIOLOGY A disorder caused by degeneration of motor neurons at all levels of the CNS including anterior horns of the spinal cord, brainstem motor nuclei, and motor cortex. Syndromes clinically indistinguishable from classic ALS may result rarely from intoxication with mercury or lead and in hyperparathyroidism, thyrotoxicosis, paraproteinemias, and hexosaminidase A deficiency. Tumors near the foramen magnum, high spinal cord tumors, cervical spondylosis, chronic polyradiculopathies, polymyositis, spinal muscle atrophies, and diabetic, syphilitic, and postpolio amyotrophies can all produce signs and symptoms similar to those seen in ALS and should be carefully considered in differential diagnosis (see Table 165-1).

CLINICAL HISTORY Onset is usually midlife, with most cases progressing to death in 3–5 years. Common initial symptoms are <u>weakness, muscle wasting, stiffness and cramping, and twitching in muscles of hands and arms.</u> Legs are less severely involved than arms, with complaints of leg stiffness, cramping, and weakness common. Symptoms of brainstem involvement include <u>dysarthria and dysphagia.</u>

PHYSICAL EXAMINATION Lower motor neuron disease results in weakness and wasting that often first involves intrinsic hand muscles but later becomes generalized. <u>Fasciculations</u> occur in involved muscles, and <u>fibrillations</u> may be seen in the tongue. Hyperreflexia, spasticity, and upgoing toes in weak, atrophic limbs provide evidence of upper motor neuron disease. Brainstem disease produces wasting of the tongue, difficulty in articulation, phonation, and deglutition, and pseudobulbar palsy (e.g., involuntary laughter, crying). Important additional features that characterize ALS are <u>preservation of intellect, lack of sensory abnormalities,</u> and absence of bowel or bladder dysfunction.

LABORATORY FINDINGS EMG provides objective evidence of muscle denervation, as well as of involvement of muscles innervated by different peripheral nerves and nerve roots. Myelography, CT, or MRI may be useful to exclude compressive lesions. <u>CSF is normal.</u> Muscle enzymes (e.g., CK) may be elevated. Serum antibodies to the gangliosides GM_1 and GD_{1b} have been reported in a variable percentage of pts. Pulmonary function studies may aid in management of ventilation. Useful tests to exclude other diseases can include urine and serum screens for heavy metals, thyroid functions,

TABLE 165-1 Etiology and investigation of secondary motor neuron disorders

Diagnostic categories	Investigations
I. Structural lesions	
A. Parasagittal or foramen magnum tumors	MRI/CT scan—head, spine including foramen magnum
B. Cervical spondylosis	MRI/CT scan or myelogram
C. Chiari malformation or syrinx	
D. Spinal cord arteriovenous malformation	
II. Infections	
A. Bacterial—tetanus, syphilis	CSF exam, VDRL
B. Viral—poliomyelitis, herpes zoster	Antibody titers
III. Intoxications, physical agents	
A. Toxins—lead, aluminum, other metals	24-h urine for lead, mercury, arsenic, thallium, aluminum; serum lead and aluminum
B. Drugs—strychnine, phenytoin, dapsone	
C. Electric shock	
D. X-irradiation	
IV. Immunologic mechanisms	
A. Plasma cell dyscrasias	Complete blood count, sedimentation rate
B. Autoimmune polyradiculoneuropathy	Immuno-electrophoresis, ANA, cryoglobulins ($\pm$), bone marrow biopsy
V. Paraneoplastic	
A. Paracarcinomatous	
B. Paralymphomatous; Hodgkin's disease	
VI. Metabolic	
A. Hypoglycemia	Fasting blood sugar (FBS)
B. Hyperparathyroidism	Routine chemistries including calcium, magnesium, phosphate
C. Hyperthroidism	Thyroid functions
D. Vitamin B_{12}, Vitamin E deficiency	Vitamin B_{12}, folate, vitamin E levels
E. Malabsorption	Stool fat (72-h; spot), carotene, prothrombin time (PT)
VII. Hereditary biochemical disorders	
A. Hexosaminidase A deficiency	Lysosomal enzyme screen
B. α-Glucosidase deficiency (Pompe's)	
C. Hyperlipidemia	Lipid electrophoresis
D. Hyperglycinuria	Urine and serum amino acids
E. Methylcrotonylglycinuria	CSF amino acids

From Beal MF, Richardson EP Jr, Martin JB: HPIM-12, p. 2073.

serum immunoelectrophoresis, lysosomal enzyme screens, B_{12} levels, VDRL, CBC, ESR, and serum chemistries.

COMPLICATIONS Weakness of ventilatory muscles leads to respiratory insufficiency; dysphagia may result in aspiration pneumonia and compromised energy intake.

TREATMENT There is no effective treatment. IV or intrathecal infusions of thyrotropin-releasing hormone (TRH) can produce transitory improvement of motor function in some pts, but do not appear to be of long-term benefit. Supportive care can include home care ventilation and pulmonary support, speech therapy, nonverbal, electronic or mechanical communication systems for anarthric patients, and dietary management to ensure adequate energy intake. Attention to use of rehabilitative devices (braces, splints, canes, walkers, mechanized wheelchairs) is essential to improve care.

For a more detailed discussion, see Beal MF, Richardson EP Jr., Martin JB: Alzheimer's Disease, Parkinsonism, and Other Degenerative Diseases of the Nervous System, Chap. 359, in HPIM-12, p. 2060

SYMPTOMS AND SIGNS Principal clinical signs of spinal cord disease are loss of sensation below a horizontal meridian on trunk (''sensory level''), accompanied by weakness and spasticity of limbs.

Sensory symptoms Often paresthesias; may begin in one or both feet and ascend. Sensory level to pin sensation or vibration often correlates well with location of transverse lesion.

Motor impairment Disruption of corticospinal tracts causes quadriplegia or paraplegia with increased muscle tone, hyperactive deep tendon reflexes, and Babinski signs.

Segmental signs These are approximate indicators of level of lesion—e.g., band of hyperalgesia/hyperpathia, isolated flaccidity, atrophy, or single lost tendon reflex.

Autonomic dysfunction Primarily urinary retention; should raise suspicion of spinal cord disease when associated with spasticity and/or a sensory level.

Pain Midline back pain is of localizing value; interscapular pain may be first sign of midthoracic cord compression; radicular pain may mark site of more laterally placed spinal lesion; pain from lower cord (conus medullaris) lesion may be referred to low back.

Lesions at or below L1 vertebra Affect cauda equina to produce flaccid, areflexic, asymmetric paraparesis with bladder and bowel dysfunction and sensory loss in saddle distribution up to L1; pain is common and projected to perineum or thighs.

Lesions at foramen magnum Classically, weakness of shoulder and arm is followed by ipsilateral and then contralateral leg and finally contralateral arm; a Horner's syndrome suggests presence of a cervical lesion.

Extramedullary lesions Associated with radicular pain, Brown-Séquard syndrome, asymmetric segmental lower motor neuron signs, early corticospinal signs, sacral sensory loss, early prominent CSF abnormalities.

Intramedullary lesions Associated with poorly localized burning pain, loss of pain sensation with preserved joint position sense, spared perineal/sacral sensation, less prominent corticospinal signs, normal or mildly abnormal CSF.

ETIOLOGY Spinal cord compression

1. *Tumors of spinal cord:* Primary or metastatic, extra or intradural; most are epidural metastases from adjacent vertebra; malignancies commonly responsible: prostate

breast, lung, lymphoma, and plasma cell dyscrasias; initial symptom commonly back pain, worse when recumbent, with local tenderness, preceding other symptoms by many weeks.

2. *Epidural abscess:* Initially, unexplained fever with dull spinal ache and local tenderness followed by radicular pain are common; once neurologic signs appear, cord compression rapidly ensues.

3. *Spinal epidural hemorrhage and hematomyelia:* Present as acute transverse myelopathy evolving over minutes or hours with severe pain. Causes: minor trauma, LP, anticoagulation, hematologic disorder, AV malformation, hemorrhage into tumor—most are idiopathic.

4. *Acute disk protrusion:* Thoracic and cervical disk herniation are less common than lumbar. See Chap. 5.

5. *Acute trauma with spinal fracture/dislocation:* May not produce myelopathy until mechanical stress further displaces destabilized spinal column.

Noncompressive neoplastic myelopathies Intramedullary metastasis, paracarcinomatous myelopathy, complication of radiation therapy.

Inflammatory myelopathies

1. *Acute myelitis, transverse myelitis, necrotic myelopathy:* Onset over days of sensory and motor symptoms, often with bladder involvement. May be first sign of multiple sclerosis.

2. *Infectious myelopathy:* Herpes zoster, preceded by radicular symptoms, most common viral agent; also seen in HTLV-I and HIV infections, poliomyelitis.

Vascular myelopathies Spinal cord infarction, vascular malformation.

Chronic myelopathies Spondylosis, degenerative and inherited myelopathies, subacute combined degeneration (B_{12} deficiency), syringomyelia, tabes dorsalis.

LABORATORY EVALUATION Plain x-rays or CT of spine to assess presence of fractures and alignment of vertebral column or detect possible metastases to vertebrae. MRI affords rapid evaluation with higher resolution, particularly for intramedullary lesions, and is preferred over conventional myelography. CSF analysis for infectious processes, multiple sclerosis, carcinoma. Somatosensory evoked responses may be abnormal.

TREATMENT Tumor-related compression For epidural metastases, high-dose glucocorticoids (to reduce edema) and local irradiation of metastasis, with or without chemotherapy; surgery is used when tumor is known to be insensitive to radiation or a maximal dose has already been delivered. Surgery is indicated for removal of neurofibromas, meningiomas, or other extramedullary tumors.

Epidural abcess Usually requires emergency surgery for abscess drainage and culture of organism, followed by IV antibiotic course.

Epidural hemorrhage or hematomyelia Where appropriate, emergency evacuation of clot. Bleeding dyscrasias should be identified and corrected. An AV malformation may be diagnosed by MRI, myelography, or arteriography of segmental spinal arteries.

Acute disk protrusion or spinal fracture/dislocation Requires surgical intervention.

COMPLICATIONS Damage to urinary tract due to urinary retention with bladder distention and injury to detrusor muscle; paroxysmal hypertension or hypotension with volume aberrations; ileus and gastritis; in high cervical cord lesions, mechanical respiratory failure; severe hypertension and bradycardia in response to stimuli or bladder or bowel distention; UTI; pressure sores; pulmonary emboli.

For a more detailed discussion, see Ropper AH, Martin JB: Diseases of the Spinal Cord, Chap. 361, in HPIM-12 p. 2081

167 PERIPHERAL NEUROPATHIES INCLUDING GUILLAIN-BARRÉ SYNDROME

Peripheral nerve disorders may be primarily *axonal* (affecting metabolic function of the neuron distally) or *demyelinating* (with loss of myelin sheath). A wide array of processes can produce these lesions.

CLINICAL FEATURES (pts presenting with peripheral neuropathy alone) **Symmetric, distal sensorimotor neuropathy** Acquired toxic or metabolic neuropathies are typical. Initial symptoms tend to be sensory: tingling, prickling, burning, or bandlike, such as dysesthesias in distal extremities, first feet, later hands in a "stocking-glove" distribution. Onset is usually symmetric. If mild, sensorimotor signs may be absent. Worsening proceeds centripetally to muscle atrophy, pansensory loss, areflexia, motor weakness greater in extensor than corresponding flexor groups. In extreme cases, respiratory compromise or sphincteric dysfunction may develop. Time course, distribution, and severity vary widely with etiology.

Mononeuropathy Confined to a single peripheral nerve. Raises possibility of mechanical entrapment that may require surgical release.

Mononeuropathy multiplex Simultaneous or sequential involvement of isolated, noncontiguous nerve trunks. Raises possibility of a multifocal axonopathy (as in a vasculitis) or an acquired multifocal form of demyelinating neuropathy.

Polyneuropathy A widespread process that is usually symmetric, distal, and graded, often a "stocking-glove" distribution. Presents with considerable variability of tempo, severity, mix of sensory/motor features, presence of positive symptoms. When *demyelinating:* acute, suggests Guillain-Barré syndrome (see below); chronic, suggests chronic inflammatory demyelinating polyradiculopathy (CIDP), disproteinemia, or carcinoma. When *axonal:* acute, suggests porphyric neuropathy or massive intoxications; subacute, suggests toxic exposure, associated systemic disease (myeloma, carcinoma, diabetes, etc.), or alcoholism; chronic (years), suggests possible genetic/familial disorder. A *mixed* axonal/demyelinating picture is often seen in diabetes mellitus.

LABORATORY STUDIES Begin with CBC, ESR, UA, CXR, blood glucose, B_{12}, and folate levels, and serum protein

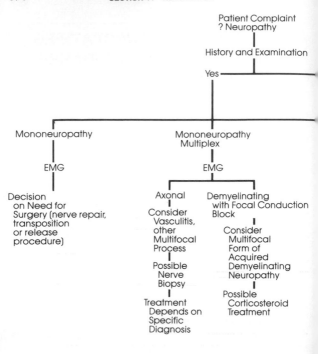

FIGURE 167-1 Flowchart approach to the evaluation of peripheral neuropathies. (*After Asbury AK, Harrison's Principles of Internal Medicine, Update IV, McGraw-Hill, New York, 1983, pp. 211–239.*)

electrophoresis. EMG and nerve conduction studies aid in further evaluation (see Fig. 167-1 and Tables 167-1 and -2). Nerve biopsy may be of value, e.g., mononeuropathy multiplex of unclear etiology. Considerations for biopsy include vasculitis, amyloidosis, leprosy, sarcoidosis, when cutaneous nerves are palpably enlarged, or in diagnosis of certain genetic disorders.

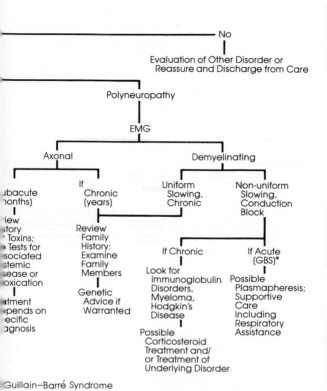

No

Evaluation of Other Disorder or
Reassure and Discharge from Care

Polyneuropathy

EMG

Axonal — Demyelinating

ubacute
nonths)

iew
story
Toxins;
e Tests for
sociated
stemic
ease or
oxication

tment
pends on
ecific
agnosis

If
Chronic
(years)

Review
Family
History:
Examine
Family
Members

Genetic
Advice if
Warranted

Uniform
Slowing,
Chronic

If Chronic

Look for
Immunoglobulin
Disorders,
Myeloma,
Hodgkin's
Disease

Possible
Corticosteroid
Treatment and/
or Treatment of
Underlying Disorder

Non-uniform
Slowing,
Conduction
Block

If Acute
(GBS)*

Possible
Plasmapheresis;
Supportive
Care
Including
Respiratory
Assistance

Guillain–Barré Syndrome

GUILLAIN-BARRE SYNDROME (GBS)   GBS is an acute, often
ascending, predominantly motor neuropathy that may follow
infection, trauma, or surgery. It has been described after
EBV, infectious hepatitis, CMV, *Mycoplasma* and HIV
infection. There is proximal nerve fiber (radicular) demyelination and monocyte infiltration: the disease is likely an
autoimmune sensitization to peripheral nerve myelin.
   Clinical manifestations   There is often myalgia and
sensory complaints (paresthesia). The weakness progresses

TABLE 167-1 Patterns of electrical activity in muscle

	At rest	Slight contraction	Maximal contraction
Normal muscle	Short-lived activity after needle insertion	Bi–triphasic potentials, amplitude: 2–5 mV, duration: 2–10 ms	Continuous activity of multiple motor units ("full" interference pattern)
Denervated muscle	Prolonged insertional activity; fibrillation potentials	High-amplitude (5–15 mV) polyphasic potentials ("giant motor units")	Reduced interference pattern with gaps in activity
Myopathic muscle	Prolonged insertional activity; fibrillation potentials	Small-amplitude (0.2–0.5 mV) polyphasic potentials	"Full" interference pattern of small amplitude

rapidly over days, reaching a maximum deficit in 7–10 d in most pts. Symmetrical weakness, loss of tendon reflexes, and relatively well preserved sensation are typical. Bilateral facial paralysis is common. One variant (Miller-Fisher syndrome) has ophthalmoplegia, bilateral facial weakness, and severe ataxia.

Diagnosis The CSF protein is usually elevated, but the fluid contains no or only a few (<10) cells. Nerve conduction velocities are prolonged and F-responses are slowed (see Chap. 155).

Treatment and prognosis 90% of pts recover completely, and no treatment has been shown to improve the prognosis (except plasmapheresis, which in some studies diminishes clinical severity if given early, i.e., within the first week). Persistent severe weakness occurs in about 10% of pts. Glucocorticoids are not beneficial.

SYSTEMIC DISEASES ASSOCIATED WITH POLYNEUROPATHY Diabetes mellitus, uremia, porphyria (three types), hypoglycemia, vitamin deficiencies (B_{12}, folate, thiamine, pyridoxine, pantothenic acid), chronic liver disease, primary biliary cirrhosis, primary systemic amyloidosis, hypothyroidism, chronic obstructive lung disease, acromegaly, malabsorption (sprue, celiac disease), carcinoma (sensory, sensorimotor, axonal, or demyelinating neuropathies), lymphoma, polycythemia vera, multiple myeloma, benign monoclonal gammopathy, macroglobulinemia, cryoglobulinemia.

DRUGS OR TOXINS ASSOCIATED WITH POLYNEUROPATHY Amiodarone, aurothioglucose, cisplatin, dapsone, disulfiram, hy-

TABLE 167-2 Nerve conduction studies

	Conduction velocity	Distal latency
Normal motor nerve	42–74 m/s, depending on nerve	2–6 m/s, depending on nerve
Axonopathies with "dying back" or wallerian degeneration of selected fibers (diabetic, alcoholic, uremic, carcinomatous, nutritional neuropathies, etc.)	Mild slowing (35–40 m/s)	Prolonged
Axonopathies with segmental demyelination of all fibers (Guillain-Barré syndrome, diphtheria, metachromatic leukodystrophy, Krabbe's, Charcot-Marie-Tooth, etc.)	Marked slowing (10–15 m/s)	Prolonged
Focal compressive (entrapment) neuropathies (e.g., median n. in carpal tunnel syndrome)	Focal conduction slowing at site of compression	Prolonged (>4.5 m/s for median n.)

dralazine, isoniazid, metronidazole, misonidazole, perhexilene, phenytoin, thalidomide, vincristine, acrylamide (flocculant, grouting agent), arsenic (herbicide; insecticide), buckthorn (toxic berry), carbon disulfide (industrial), diphtheria, dimethylaminopropionitrile (industrial), γ-diketone hexacarbons (solvents), inorganic lead, organophosphates, thallium (rat poison), pyridoxine (vitamin).

GENETICALLY DETERMINED NEUROPATHIES Peroneal muscular atrophy (HMSN-I, HMSN-II), Déjerine-Sottas (HSMN-III), hereditary amyloid neuropathies, hereditary sensory neuropathy (HSN-I, HSN-II), porphyric neuropathy, hereditary liability to pressure palsy, Fabry's disease, adrenomyeloneuropathy, Refsum's disease, ataxia-telangiectasia, abetalipoproteinemia, giant axonal neuropathy, metachromatic leukodystrophy, globoid cell leukodystrophy, Friedreich's ataxia.

CAUSES OF MONONEUROPATHY Differential is implied by location of lesion as determined by physical exam and EMG (i.e., how distal to nerve root electrophysiologic abnormalities are first found). Considerations include nerve entrapment (carpal tunnel, meralgia paresthetica, etc.), direct trauma or dislocation, compression from tumor (Pancoast, in the case of brachial plexus; pelvic or retroperitoneal, in the case of lumbosacral plexus lesions), direct tumor infiltration of nerve sheath, compression from a retroperitoneal hematoma, plexitis, diabetes mellitus, peripheral nerve tumors, herpes zoster, Bell's palsy, sarcoidosis, leprous neuritis.

For a more detailed discussion, see Asbury AK: Diseases of the Peripheral Nervous System, Chap. 363, in HPIM-12, p. 2096

168 DISORDERS OF THE AUTONOMIC NERVOUS SYSTEM

The autonomic nervous system (ANS) innervates vascular and visceral smooth muscle, exocrine and endocrine glands, and selected parenchymal cells. The ANS regulates blood pressure, blood flow and tissue perfusion, volume and composition of extracellular fluid, metabolic processes, sweat glands, and visceral smooth muscle. Central functions in the hypothalamus regulate food intake (hunger and satiety), temperature, thirst, and circadian rhythms.

ANATOMY The ANS is divided anatomically and functionally into two components, the sympathetic and parasympathetic nervous systems. Preganglionic neurons of the sympathetic nervous system are located in the intermediolateral column of the eighth cervical to the first lumbar segments of the spinal cord. Neurons of the parasympathetic nervous system are located in the brainstem and sacral spinal cord and exit the CNS via the third, seventh, ninth, and tenth cranial nerves and the second, third, and fourth sacral nerves. Responses to sympathetic and parasympathetic activation are frequently opposite, e.g., their opposing effects on heart rate and gut motility. These antagonistic functions reflect highly coordinated interactions within the CNS.

NEUROTRANSMITTERS Acetylcholine (ACh) is the neurotransmitter in preganglionic neurons of both divisions of the ANS and the transmitter of parasympathetic postganglionic neurons and of sympathetic neurons that innervate the sweat glands. Norepinephrine (NE) is the neurotransmitter of sympathetic postganglionic neurons. The adrenal medulla releases epinephrine (E) into blood under cholinergic regulation by the sympathetic nervous system.

SYNTHESIS AND METABOLISM OF THE CATECHOLAMINES Catecholamines are synthesized from tyrosine [(1) hydroxylated to levodopa, (2) decarboxylated to dopamine, (3) hydroxylated to NE] (see Fig. 67-1, HPIM-12, p. 381). Tyrosine hydroxylation is the rate-limiting step in biosynthesis. E is formed by *N*-methylation of NE in the adrenal medulla. The major metabolites of the catecholamines are 4-hydroxy-3-methoxymandelic acid (from NE and E) and homovanillic acid (HVA) from dopamine. Catecholamines are stored in secretory vesicles in the adrenal medulla and in sympathetic nerve endings and are released on cellular depolarization. Released neurotransmitter from nerve endings is inactivated in part by reuptake into the nerve terminal. Uptake inhibitors (tricyclic antidepressants) facilitate catecholamine function by enhancing neurotransmitter levels in the synapse.

SYNTHESIS AND METABOLISM OF ACh   Parasympathetic neurons and preganglionic sympathetic neurons make ACh from choline and acetate. It is stored in small synaptic vesicles and is released on depolarization. Most ACh is metabolized in the synaptic cleft and reuptake mechanisms are of little importance.

RECEPTORS   Catecholamines exert their effects on two types of receptors, alpha and beta. Distinct alpha$_1$ and alpha$_2$ subtypes exist. The alpha$_1$ receptor mediates vasoconstriction (phenylephrine and methoxamine are selective agonists; prazosin is a selective antagonist). The alpha$_2$ receptor mediates presynaptic inhibition of NE release from adrenergic nerves, inhibits ACh release from cholinergic nerves, inhibits lipolysis in adipocytes, inhibits insulin secretion, and stimulates platelet aggregation. Specific agonists of alpha$_2$ receptors are clonidine and alpha-methylnorepinephrine; yohimbine is a specific antagonist.

Beta receptors are subdivided into two types. The beta$_1$ receptor responds to both NE and E and mediates cardiac stimulation and lipolysis. The beta$_2$ receptor is more responsive to E than NE and mediates vasodilation and bronchodilation. Isoproterenol stimulates both receptors and propranolol blocks both types. Selective antagonists for the beta$_1$ receptor include metoprolol and atenolol. Several subtypes of both alpha$_1$ and alpha$_2$ receptors have been sequenced and each shows a typical seven-element transmembrane-spanning structure (see Fig. 67-3, HPIM-12, p. 383). ACh acts on nicotinic (neuromuscular and ganglionic) and muscarinic receptors, each of which has several molecular subtypes.

Pharmacologic uses of catecholamine agonists and antagonists are summarized in Table 168-1. For a more complete listing see HPIM-12, pp. 388–9.

DISORDERS OF THE ANS   Hypothalamic disorders   Disturbances of temperature regulation, food intake (anorexia nervosa, obesity), circadian rhythm, and sexual function can result from diseases that affect the hypothalamus (congenital or inherited, tumors, trauma, subarachnoid hemorrhage). Childhood conditions include the Prader-Willi syndrome (obesity, hypogonadism, muscular hypotonia, and mild mental retardation), Kleine-Levin syndrome (adolescent hypersomnia, hypersexuality, and bulimia), and craniopharyngioma. In adults trauma, aneurysm with subarachnoid hemorrhage (anterior communicating artery aneurysm), and hypothalamic gliomas can cause central ANS disorders.

TABLE 168-1 Some commonly used autonomic drugs[a,b,c]

Agent	Indication	Dose and route
ADRENERGIC AGONISTS[d]		
Epinephrine	Anaphylaxis	100–500 μg SC or IM (0.1–0.5 mL of 1/1000 solution of hydrochloride salt); 25–50 μg IV (slowly) every 5–15 min; titrate as needed
Norepinephrine	Shock Hypotension	2–4 μg of NE base/min IV; titrate as needed
Isoproterenol	Cardiogenic shock Bradyarrhythmias AV block	0.5–5.0 μ/min IV; titrate as needed
	Asthma	Inhalation
Terbutaline	Asthma	2.5–5.0 mg PO tid; 0.25–0.5 mg SC; inhalation every 4–5 h
Albuterol	Asthma	2.0–4.0 mg PO tid or qid; inhalation every 4–6 h
DOPAMINERGIC AGONISTS		
Dopamine	Shock	2–5 (μ/kg)/min IV (dopaminergic range) 5–10 (μg/kg)/min IV (dopaminergic and beta range) 10–20 (μg/kg)/min IV (beta range) 20–50 (μg/kg)/min IV (alpha range)
Bromocriptine	Amenorrhea-galactorrhea	2.5 mg PO bid or tid
	Acromegaly	5–15 mg PO tid or qid
	Parkinson's disease	15–75 mg qd
INHIBITORS OF CENTRAL SYMPATHETIC OUTFLOW		
Clonidine	Hypertension	0.1–0.6 mg PO bid
ADRENERGIC NEURON BLOCKING AGENTS		
Guanethidine	Hypertension	10–100 mg PO qd
BETA BLOCKING AGENTS[e]		
Propranolol	Hypertension	40–160 mg PO bid (or higher)
	Angina	10–40 mg PO tid or qid
	Myocardial infarction	60–80 mg PO tid
	Arrhythmias	10–30 mg PO tid or qid; 1–3 mg IV

TABLE 168-1   Some commonly used autonomic drugs[a,b,c] **(continued)**

Agent	Indication	Dose and route
	Hypertrophic cardiomyopathy	20–40 mg PO tid or qid
	Pheochromocytoma	10–20 mg PO tid or qid; 0.5–2.0 mg IV
	Essential tremor	20–80 mg PO tid
	Migraine	20–80 mg PO bid or tid
	Hyperthyroidism	10–60 mg PO tid or qid
Metoprolol	Hypertension	50–200 mg PO bid
	Myocardial infarction	100 mg PO bid
Nadolol	Hypertension	80–320 mg PO qd
	Angina	80–240 mg PO qd
Timolol	Hypertension	10–30 mg PO bid
	Myocardial infarction	10 mg PO bid
Atenolol	Hypertension	50–100 mg PO qd

ALPHA BLOCKING AGENTS

Agent	Indication	Dose and route
Phenoxybenzamine	Pheochromocytoma	10–60 mg PO bid; titrate as needed
Phentolamine	Pheochromocytoma	5 mg IV (after test dose of 0.5 mg)
Prazosin	Hypertension	1–5 mg PO bid or tid
	CHF	2–7 mg PO qid

GANGLIONIC BLOCKING AGENT

Agent	Indication	Dose and route
Trimethaphan	Hypertensive crisis (aortic dissection)	1–3 mg/min IV

CHOLINERGIC AGONIST

Agent	Indication	Dose and route
Bethanechol	Urinary retention (nonobstructive)	10–100 mg PO tid or qid; 5 mg SC

ANTICHOLINESTERASE AGENTS

Agent	Indication	Dose and route
Physostigmine	Central cholinergic blockade	1–2 mg IV (slow)
Pyridostigmine bromide	Myasthenia gravis	60–120 mg bid or tid

CHOLINERGIC BLOCKING AGENTS[f]

Agent	Indication	Dose and route
Atropine	Bradycardia and hypotension	0.4–1.0 mg IV every 1–2 h

[a] Consult complete prescribing information.   [b] Doses for children not given.   [c] Only the common indications and routes are given.   [d] Dopamine, at high doses, is an adrenergic agonist as well.   [e] Clinical efficacy of most beta blockers appears similar for major indications. When discontinuing them, reduce dose gradually.   [f] Many synthetic atropine derivatives are available for (1) diminishing GI tract motility and secretion and (2) increasing urinary bladder capacity. Usefulness is limited by anticholinergic side effects. Some may be used adjunctively in peptic ulcer disease.

POSTURAL HYPOTENSION   Primary disorders that cause postural hypotension act either at the central or peripheral nervous system level. The Shy-Drager syndrome results from CNS system degeneration (multisystem disease) that includes loss of neurons in the basal ganglia, brainstem, and intermediolateral cell column of the spinal cord. Postural hypotension sometimes occurs with a fixed heart rate and signs of CNS dysfunction (tremor, parkinsonism, and cerebellar ataxia). Incontinence is common in the later stages. Treatment includes modest volume expansion and administration of fludrocortisone, 0.05–0.1 mg qd. Peripheral degeneration of ANS neurons can also lead to postural hypotension. This can occur as an acute manifestation in Guillain-Barré syndrome, in degeneration of postganglionic autonomic neurons (of unknown cause), or as a chronic manifestation of small-fiber neuropathy (diabetes mellitus, amyloid neuropathy). Tumors of the adrenal medulla (pheochromocytomas) lead to episodic hypertension and tachycardia.

OTHER DISEASES OF THE ANS   Disorders of bladder function are common. They can result from lesions of the spinal cord above the sacral innervation level; in this condition the bladder can empty reflexly but voluntary control of micturition is lost. Lesions that destroy the spinal cord below T12 (meningomyelocele, necrotic myelopathy) result in an atonic, reflex-insensitive bladder that cannot empty. Lesions of the motor innervation (sacral neurons, nerve roots, or peripheral nerves) cause a lower motor neuron disorder in which there is difficulty in urination but normal sensation. Sensory denervation of the bladder results in loss of sense of fullness with atonic bladder (diabetes mellitus, tabes dorsalis).

For a more detailed discussion, see Beal MF, Richardson EP Jr, Martin JB: Degenerative Diseases of the Nervous System, Chap. 359, p. 2060

A neuromuscular disorder resulting in weakness and fatigability of skeletal muscles, due to an autoimmune-mediated decrease in number of acetylcholine receptors (AChRs) at neuromuscular junctions (NMJs).

PATHOPHYSIOLOGY Specific anti-AChR antibodies reduce the number of AChRs at the NMJ. Repetitive activation of NMJs produces a normal decrease in release of ACh and because AChR numbers are low, fewer muscle fibers are activated, producing myasthenic fatigue. Anti-AChR antibodies are detected in 80% of myasthenics (50% with only ocular symptoms). Thymus is abnormal in 75% (65% hyperplasia, 10% thymoma). Other associated autoimmune diseases appear in 10%.

CLINICAL FEATURES May present at any age. Symptoms fluctuate throughout the day and are provoked by exertion. Characteristic distribution: cranial muscles (lids, extraocular muscles, facial weakness, "nasal" or slurred speech, dysphagia) and in 85% limb muscles (often proximal and asymmetric) become involved. Tendon reflexes are preserved in weak muscles.

LABORATORY Anticholinesterase (edrophonium) test—look for improvement in muscle strength; electrodiagnostics (decremental response on repetitive nerve stimulation, increased jitter on single-fiber recording); anti-AChR antibodies—levels do not correspond to severity of disease; CT or MRI for thymoma; thyroid function tests (elevated in 3–8% of MG and may exacerbate symptoms); rheumatoid factor and antinuclear antibodies (associated autoimmune disease).

DIFFERENTIAL DIAGNOSIS (1) Lambert-Eaton syndrome (LES)—autoantibody to calcium channel in motor nerve terminal results in reduced ACh release; increased muscle strength with exertion; association with carcinoma (small cell of lung); (2) Botulism—toxin from *Clostridium botulinum* interferes with calcium facilitation of ACh; like LES, repetitive stimulation gives incremental response; (3) drug-induced myasthenia—most unmask a preexisting myasthenia: penicillamine (true MG), polymyxin, tetracycline, aminoglycoside antibiotics, procainamide, propranolol, phenothiazines, lithium, anticholinesterase insecticides; (4) neurasthenia; (5) hyperthyroidism; (6) intracranial mass lesion affecting extraocular muscles.

TREATMENT Anticholinesterase medication (pyridostigmine); thymectomy for all MG pts from puberty to 55 years;

immunosuppression (alternate-day prednisone, azathioprine, cyclosporin); plasmapheresis.

COMPLICATIONS Most severe is respiratory compromise as thoracic and diaphragmatic musculature weaken (myasthenic crisis); aspiration pneumonia when bulbar muscles are affected; cholinergic crisis from anticholinesterases; acute exacerbation with intercurrent illness requiring therapy with drugs affecting the NMJ (see above).

For a more detailed discussion, see Drachman DB: Myasthenia Gravis, Chap. 366, in HPIM-12, p. 2118

ETIOLOGY   A disparate group of disorders that are all inherited progressive degenerations of muscle but vary widely in their clinical and pathologic features and mode of inheritance. Recent advances in molecular genetics have enabled identification of the gene and its product (dystrophin) involved in Duchenne and Becker dystrophy on the short arm of the X chromosome (Xp21). The mutant gene responsible for myotonic dystrophy has been localized to the long arm of chromosome 19.

CLINICAL FEATURES OF INDIVIDUAL DISORDERS   Duchenne dystrophy   An X-linked recessive disorder that affects males almost exclusively. Onset is by age 5; symmetric and relentlessly progressive weakness in hip and shoulder girdle muscles leading to difficulty in climbing, running, jumping, hopping, etc. By age 8–10, most children require leg braces; by age 12, the majority are nonambulatory. Survival beyond age 25 is rare.

Associated problems include tendon and muscle contractures (e.g., heel cords), progressive kyphoscoliosis, impaired pulmonary function, cardiomyopathy, and intellectual impairment. Muscle weakness is conjoined with palpable enlargement and firmness of some muscles (e.g., calves) resulting initially from hypertrophy and later from replacement of muscle by fat and connective tissue.

Laboratory findings include massive elevations of muscle enzymes (CK, aldolase), a myopathic pattern on EMG testing, and evidence of groups of necrotic muscle fibers with regeneration, phagocytosis, and fatty replacement of muscle on biopsy. ECG abnormalities (increased net RS in V_1, deep Q in precordial leads) reflect the presence of cardiomyopathy.

Carrier detection   Serum CK is elevated in 50% of female carriers. Since the gene and its product (dystrophin) have now been identified, complementary DNA probes are now available for use in detecting carriers and in prenatal diagnosis. Genetic probes for restriction fragment length polymorphisms (RFLPs) involving the dystrophin gene are also available and can be used in diagnostic studies.

Complications include respiratory failure and infections, aspiration, and acute gastric dilatation. CHF and cardiac arrhythmias may complicate the cardiomyopathy. Passive stretching of muscles, tenotomy, bracing, physiotherapy, mechanical assistance devices, and avoidance of prolonged immobility may all be of symptomatic benefit.

Treatment   No specific therapy is available, although glucocorticoids are used by some clinicians.

Becker dystrophy (benign pseudohypertrophic)   A less severe and rarer dystrophy than Duchenne with a slower course and later age of onset (5–15) but similar clinical and laboratory features. This disorder also results from defects in the dystrophin gene.

Myotonic dystrophy   An autosomal dominant disorder in which weakness typically becomes obvious in the second to third decade and initially involves the muscles of the face, neck, and distal extremities. This results in a distinctive facial appearance ("hatchet face") characterized by ptosis, temporal wasting, drooping of the lower lip, and sagging of the jaw. Myotonia manifests as a peculiar inability to rapidly relax muscles following a strong exertion (e.g., after tight hand grip), as well as by sustained contraction of muscles following percussion (e.g., of tongue or thenar eminence).

Associated problems can include frontal baldness, posterior subcapsular cataracts, gonadal atrophy, respiratory and cardiac problems, endocrine abnormalities, intellectual impairment, and hypersomnia.

Laboratory studies show normal or mildly elevated CK, characteristic myotonia and myopathic features on EMG, and a typical pattern of muscle fiber injury on biopsy. Cardiac complications, including complete heart block, may be life-threatening. Respiratory function should be carefully followed, as chronic hypoxia may lead to cor pulmonale.

Early diagnosis   Early disease detection and prenatal diagnosis may be possible in selected families using genetic linkage techniques employing RFLPs as genetic markers.

Treatment   Phenytoin, procainamide, and quinine may help myotonia, but they must be used carefully in pts with heart disease as they may worsen cardiac conduction.

Facioscapulohumeral dystrophy   Typically a slowly progressive, mild disorder with onset in the third to fourth decade. Weakness involves facial, shoulder girdle, and proximal arm muscles and can result in atrophy of biceps, triceps, scapular winging, and slope shoulders. Facial weakness results in inability to whistle and loss of facial expressivity. Foot drop and leg weakness may cause falls and progressive difficulty with ambulation.

Laboratory studies include normal or slightly elevated CK and mixed myopathic-neuropathic features on EMG and muscle biopsy. Orthoses and other stabilization procedures may be of benefit for selected patients.

LESS COMMON DYSTROPHIES **Scapuloperoneal dystrophy**
Clinical features are generally similar to facioscapuloperoneal
dystrophy, although facial weakness does not occur and
cardiomyopathy may be present. Most cases are of midlife
onset and autosomal dominant inheritance, but an early-
onset X-linked recessive form with prominent joint contractures and cardiomyopathy (Emery-Dreifuss type) can occur.

**Oculopharyngeal dystrophy (progressive external
ophthalmoplegia)** Onset in the fifth to sixth decade of
ptosis, limitation of extraocular movements, and facial and
cricopharyngeal weakness. Cricopharyngeal muscle weakness results in achalasia, dysphagia, and aspiration. Chronic
nature of the eye movement disorder rarely results in diplopia.
Most pts are Hispanic or of French-Canadian descent.

Limb-girdle dystrophy Probably a constellation of diseases with proximal muscle weakness involving the arms and
legs as the core symptom. Age of onset, rate of progression,
severity of manifestations, and associated complications
(e.g., cardiac, respiratory) vary with the specific subtype of
disease. Laboratory findings include elevated CK and myopathic features on EMG and muscle biopsy.

Distal dystrophy A rare group of disorders with several
variants that have differing ages of onset and patterns of
inheritance. Typically there is weakness in the hands and
feet with slow progression to more proximal muscle groups.
CK is elevated, and EMG and muscle biopsy show myopathic
features.

METABOLIC MYOPATHIES These disorders result from abnormalities in utilization by muscle of glucose or fatty acids
as sources of energy. Pts present with either an acute
syndrome of myalgia, myolysis, and myoglobinuria or chronic
progressive muscle weakness. Definitive diagnosis requires
biochemical-enzymatic studies of biopsied muscle. However
muscle enzymes, EMG, and muscle biopsy are all typically
abnormal and may suggest specific disorders.

Infantile and childhood forms of glycogen storage disorders
often have associated disorders of cardiac, hepatic, and
endocrine function that overshadow the muscle disease.
Childhood and adult forms can mimic muscular dystrophy
or polymyositis. In some types the presentation is one of
episodic muscle cramps and fatigue provoked by exercise.
The ischemic forearm lactate test is helpful as normal post
exercise rise in serum lactic acid does not occur. Disorders
of fatty acid metabolism present with clinical pictures similar
to those described above. In some pts, exercise-induced
cramps, myolysis, and myoglobinuria are common; in others
the picture resembles polymyositis or muscular dystrophy.
Some pts have benefited from special diets (medium-chain

triglyceride-enriched), oral carnitine supplements, or glucocorticoids.

MISCELLANEOUS DISORDERS Myopathies may be associated with endocrine disorders, especially those involving hypo- or hyperfunction of the thyroid, parathyroid, and adrenal glands. Drugs (esp. glucocorticoids) and certain toxins (e.g., alcohol) are commonly associated with myopathies (see Table 170-1); In most cases weakness is symmetric and involves proximal limb girdle muscles. Weakness, myalgia, and cramps are common symptoms. Diagnosis often depends on resolution of signs and symptoms with correction of underlying disorder or removal of offending agent, as muscle enzymes, EMG, and even muscle biopsy may be unremarkable in individual pts.

TABLE 170-1 Toxic myopathies

FOCAL MYOPATHIES

Pentazocine, meperidine

GENERALIZED MYOPATHIES

Inflammatory:
  Cimetidine, D-penicillamine, procainamide
Muscle weakness and myalgias:
  Chloroquine, clofibrate, colchicine, glucocorticoids, emetine, ϵ-aminocaproic acid, labetalol, perhexiline, propranolol, vincristine
Rhabdomyolysis and myoglobinuria:
  Alcohol, azathioprine, heroin, amphetamine, clofibrate, ϵ-aminocaproic acid, phencyclidine, barbiturates, cocaine
Malignant hyperthermia:
  Halothane, ethylene, diethyl ether, methoxyflurane, ethyl chloride, trichloroethylene, gallamine, succinylcholine, lidocaine, mepivacaine

---

Modified from Mendell JR, Griggs RC: HPIM-12, p. 2117.

For a more detailed discussion, see Mendell JR, Griggs RC: Muscular Dystrophy, Chap. 365, in HPIM-12, p. 2112

171 POLYMYOSITIS

DEFINITION Polymyositis is an inflammatory condition of skeletal muscle in which muscle tissue is involved predominantly by lymphocytic infiltration. When polymyositis is accompanied by a characteristic skin rash, the term *dermatomyositis* may be used. Approximately a third of cases are associated with connective tissue diseases such as rheumatoid arthritis, SLE, or scleroderma; 10% are associated with malignancy.

ETIOLOGY In most instances, the etiology is not known. There are likely a variety of causes. Myositis may follow certain viral and parasitic infections, and the disease may represent an immune-mediated response to viral antigens; alternatively, autoimmune processes may be operative.

CLASSIFICATION One commonly used classification is as follows:

Group I: Primary idiopathic polymyositis
Group II: Primary idiopathic dermatomyositis
Group III: Dermatomyositis (or polymyositis) associated with neoplasia
Group IV: Childhood dermatomyositis (or polymyositis) associated with vasculitis
Group V: Polymyositis (or dermatomyositis) associated with collagen-vascular disease

CLINICAL MANIFESTATIONS
Group I: Primary idiopathic polymyositis

- Approximately a third of all cases of polymyositis; onset and course usually insidiously progressive; 2:1 female:male predominance.
- Proximal muscle weakness first noted; difficulty climbing steps, combing hair, arising from squatting position; ocular muscles rarely affected.
- Some pts have aching muscle pain or tenderness.
- Dysphagia in 25%, cardiac abnormalities in 30%, respiratory involvement in 5%.

Group II: Primary idiopathic dermatomyositis

- About 25% of all cases.
- Skin changes may precede or follow muscle findings; type of eruptions include (1) localized or diffuse erythema, (2) maculopapular eruption, (3) scaling eczematoid dermatitis, (4) exfoliative dermatitis, or (5) classic lilac-colored heliotrope rash on eyelids, nose, cheeks, forehead, trunk, extremities, nailbeds, knuckles.

• About 40% of all pts with myositis have dermatomyositis.

Group III: Polymyositis or dermatomyositis with neoplasia

• About 8% of all myositis; skin and muscle changes indistinguishable from other groups.
• <u>Malignancy</u> may precede or follow onset of myositis by up to 2 years.
• Chiefly in older pts.
• <u>Commonly associated malignancies include lung, ovary, breast, GI tract, and myeloproliferative disorders.</u>

Group IV: Childhood polymyositis and dermatomyositis associated with vasculitis

• About 7% of all myositis.
• Subcutaneous calcification common.
• Vasculitis may involve skin and visceral organs.

Group V: Polymyositis or dermatomyositis associated with a connective tissue disorder

• About 20% of myositis cases.
• Rheumatoid arthritis, scleroderma, SLE, mixed connective tissue disease most frequently associated; polyarteritis nodosa and rheumatic fever also seen.

OTHER DISORDERS ASSOCIATED WITH MYOSITIS Sarcoidosis, focal nodular myositis, infections (toxoplasma, coxsackievirus, trichinella, influenza), inclusion-body myositis.

DIAGNOSIS

• Typical clinical picture—weakness (proximal greater than distal), possible associated rash.
• Laboratory findings—elevated serum CK, aldolase, glutamic oxaloacetic transaminase (SGOT), lactic acid dehydrogenase (LDH), glutamic pyruvate transaminase (SGPT) levels; rheumatoid factor and ANA may be present; myoglobulinuria if muscle damage acute and extensive; elevated ESR.
• EMG—may show irritability and myopathic changes.
• ECG—abnormal in 5–10% at presentation.
• Muscle biopsy—usually diagnostic but may be normal in 10%.
• Workup for malignancy in older pts.

DIFFERENTIAL DIAGNOSIS Spinal muscular atrophies, amyotrophic lateral sclerosis, muscular dystrophies, metabolic myopathies, toxic myopathies, myasthenia gravis, Lambert-Eaton syndrome, Guillain-Barré syndrome, neurotoxin, enzyme-deficiency states, acute viral infections, polymyalgia rheumatica, fibrositis/fibromyalgia.

TREATMENT

- Prednisone 1–2 (mg/kg)/d is accepted treatment, but efficacy not proven. Improvement may be seen in first few weeks or may take up to 3 months to begin. Doses of prednisone should be decreased as disease activity permits.
- Indications for cytotoxic drugs: (1) severe disease, (2) response to steroids inadequate, (3) relapses frequent. Options include: azathioprine 2.5–3.5 (mg/kg)/d; cyclophosphamide 1–2 (mg/kg)/d; methotrexate 7.5–15 mg/week.
- Serum CK activity is important guide to efficacy of treatment, though early fall may overestimate initial response to prednisone.
- Elderly pts should have initial and yearly evaluation for malignancy.
- Physiotherapy and rehabilitation therapy are important adjunctive measures.

For a more detailed discussion, see Bradley WG, Tandan R: Dermatomyositis and Polymyositis, Chap. 364, in HPIM-12, p. 2108

Disturbed sleep is one of the most frequent complaints that physicians encounter. One-third of adults experience occasional or persistent sleep disturbances. A classification of the major sleep disorders is shown in Table 172-1. Sleep deprivation or disruption of the circadian timing system can lead to serious impairment of daytime functioning. Two systems govern the sleep-wake cycle: one that generates sleep and sleep-associated events and the other that times sleep within the 24-h day (circadian pacemaker).

Continuous monitoring of EEG, EMG, and eye movements during sleep (polysomnography) defines two stages of sleep: (1) rapid eye movement (REM) sleep, and (2) non-rapid eye movement (NREM). NREM is divided into four stages, progressing from stage 1 to deep or slow-wave sleep (stage 4).

DISORDERS OF SLEEP

INSOMNIA A disorder in initiating or maintaining sleep; also describes pt's feeling of inadequate sleep, which may be due to an impairment in onset, depth, duration, or restorative properties of sleep. It may be a primary disorder or secondary to psychiatric illness, anxiety, drug use, or medical conditions. It may be a temporary problem or lifelong. Treatment is difficult when the condition is chronic. Avoid overuse of sedatives that may temporarily alleviate symptoms but over time may worsen the problem.

HYPERSOMNIAS Typified by inappropriate sleepiness leading to sleep when pt wishes to be awake. Pt complains of an irresistable urge to sleep during the day or of decreased concentration. In clinical practice, two forms are likely to occur:

Sleep apnea syndrome A sleep-induced respiratory impairment characterized by snoring, respiratory pauses lasting 10–120 s, and often respiratory obstruction. In severe cases, more than 500 episodes of sleep apnea may occur in a single night. During working hours, pt notes attacks of drowsiness, poor concentration, and headaches. Men are affected 20 times as frequently as women, usually in the 40–65 age range. About two-thirds of pts are obese. In obstructive apnea there is narrowing of the oral pharynx

TABLE 172-1 International classification of sleep disorders

I. Dyssomnias
    A. Intrinsic sleep disorders
        1. Psychophysiologic insomnia
        2. Idiopathic insomnia
        3. Narcolepsy
        4. Sleep apnea syndromes
        5. Periodic limb movement disorder
        6. Restless legs syndrome
    B. Extrinsic sleep disorders
        1. Inadequate sleep hygiene
        2. Altitude insomnia
        3. Drug- or alcohol-dependent sleep disorders.
    C. Circadian rhythm sleep disorders
        1. Time-zone change (jet-lag) syndrome
        2. Shift-work sleep disorder
        3. Delayed sleep phase syndrome
        4. Advanced sleep phase syndrome

II. Parasomnias
    A. Arousal disorders
        1. Confusional arousals
        2. Sleepwalking
        3. Sleep terrors
    B. Sleep-wake transition disorders
        1. Sleep talking
        2. Nocturnal leg cramps
    C. Parasomnias usually associated with REM sleep
        1. Nightmares
        2. Sleep paralysis
        3. Impaired sleep-related penile erections
        4. Sleep-related painful erections
    D. Other parasomnias
        1. Sleep bruxism
        2. Sleep enuresis

III. Sleep disorders associated with medical/psychiatric disorders
    A. Associated with mental disorders
    B. Associated with neurologic disorders
        1. Cerebral degenerative disorders
        2. Parkinsonism
        3. Sleep-related epilepsy
        4. Sleep-related headaches
    C. Associated with other medical disorders
        1. Nocturnal cardiac ischemia
        2. Chronic obstructive pulmonary disease
        3. Sleep-related asthma
        4. Sleep-related gastroesophageal reflux

SOURCE: Modified from *International Classification of Sleep Disorders* prepared by the Diagnostic Classication Committee, Thorpy MJ, Chairman. American Sleep Disorders Association, 1990.

during respiration. A rare form of nonobstructive apnea is due to a central defect in respiratory control.

Treatment consists of weight loss and, in severe cases, positive pressure-assisted breathing or tracheostomy. Tricyclic antidepressants and progesterone are beneficial in some cases.

Narcolepsy-cataplexy Characterized by recurrent episodes of irresistible daytime sleepiness associated with abnormal manifestations of REM sleep. Associated symptoms are cataplexy (brief episodes of muscular paralysis), often precipitated by emotional events, hypnagogic hallucinations, and sleep paralysis.

The disorder is not rare (prevalence 40/100,000 population); men and women are equally affected; onset is usually in adolescence or early adulthood. Narcolepsy appears to have a genetic basis; nearly all pts are DR 2-positive. Sleep studies show the hallmark of disease to be rapid transition to REM sleep (shortened REM latency).

Treatment is a combination of stimulants (for narcolepsy) and tricyclic antidepressants (for cataplexy). Excessive hypersomnolence also can occur with metabolic or endocrine disorders—uremia, hypothyroidism, hypercalcemia, and chronic pulmonary disease (with hypercapnia).

DISORDERS OF CIRCADIAN RHYTHMICITY

Some pts with insomnia or hypersomnia have a disorder of sleep timing rather than sleep generation. Such disorders may be organic—due to an intrinsic defect in the circadian pacemaker (suprachiasmatic nucleus of the hypothalamus)—or environmental—due to a disruption of entraining stimuli. Assessment of pts with these disorders may require their study under controlled light-dark cycle conditions. Common transient disorders that affect many pts include jet-lag syndrome (60 million/year) and shiftwork sleep disorder (7 million workers in the U.S.). Delayed sleep phase syndrome is characterized by late sleep onset and awakening with otherwise normal sleep pattern. Pts respond to a rescheduling regimen in which bedtimes are successively delayed by about 3 h/d until the desired (earlier) bedtime is achieved. In the advanced sleep phase syndrome, which commonly affects the elderly, pts describe excessive daytime sleepiness during the evening hours. After sleep onset, awaking occurs at 3 to 5 A.M. Bright light phototherapy may benefit these pts as well as those with severe jet-lag sleep disturbance.

TREATMENT OF SLEEP AND CIRCADIAN DISORDERS

The most common medical problem is the tendency by physicians to overprescribe nighttime sedative or anxiolytic medications (benzodiazepines). The establishment of sleep-disorders clinics has made rational treatment more readily available. It is important to establish the diagnosis and to treat the underlying disorder with specific therapies.

For a more detailed discussion, see Czeisler CA, Richardson GS, Martin JB: Disorders of Sleep and Circadian Rhythms, Chap. 34, in HPIM-12, p. 209

Patients with disorders of language can present with several different syndromes.

GLOBAL APHASIA Etiology Occlusion of internal carotid artery (ICA) or middle cerebral artery (MCA) supplying dominant hemisphere (less commonly hemorrhage, trauma, or tumor), resulting in a large lesion of frontal, parietal, and superior temporal lobes.

Clinical manifestations All aspects of speech and language are impaired. Pt cannot read, write, or repeat and has poor auditory comprehension. Speech output is minimal and nonfluent. Usually hemiplegia, hemisensory loss, and homonymous hemianopsia are present.

BROCA'S APHASIA (MOTOR OR NONFLUENT APHASIA) Etiology
Core lesion involves dominant inferior frontal convolution (Broca's area), although cortical and subcortical areas along superior sylvian fissure and insula are often involved. Commonly caused by vascular lesions involving the superior division of the MCA, less commonly due to tumor, abscess, metastasis, subdural hematoma, encephalitis.

Clinical manifestations Speech output is sparse, slow, effortful, dysmelodic, poorly articulated, and telegraphic. Most pts have severe writing impairment. Comprehension of written and spoken language is relatively preserved. Pt is aware of and visibly frustrated by deficit.

With large lesions, a dense hemiparesis may occur and the eyes may deviate toward side of lesion. More commonly, lesser degrees of contralateral face and arm weakness are present. Sensory loss is rarely found, and visual fields are intact. Buccolingual apraxia is common, the pt having difficulty imitating movements with tongue and lips or performing these movements on command. An apraxia involving the ipsilateral hand may occur due to involvement of fibers in the corpus callosum.

WERNICKE'S APHASIA (SENSORY OR FLUENT APHASIA) Etiology Embolic occlusion of inferior division of dominant MCA (less commonly hemorrhage, tumor, encephalitis, or abscess) involving posterior perisylvian region.

Clinical manifestations Although speech sounds grammatical, melodic, and effortless ("fluent"), it is often virtually incomprehensible due to errors in word usage, structure, and tense and the presence of neologisms and paraphasia. Comprehension of written and spoken material is severely impaired, as are reading, writing, and repetition. Pt seems unaware of deficit. Associated clinical symptoms can include parietal lobe sensory deficits and homonymous hemianopsia. Motor disturbances are rare.

CONDUCTION APHASIA Comprehension of speech and writing is largely intact, and speech output is fluent, although paraphasia is common. *Repetition is severely affected.* Most cases are due to lesions involving supramarginal gyrus of dominant parietal lobe, dominant superior temporal lobe, or arcuate fasciculus. Lesions are typically due to an embolus to either the ascending parietal or posterior temporal branch of the dominant MCA. Associated symptoms include contralateral hemisensory loss and hemianopsia.

PURE WORD DEAFNESS Almost total lack of auditory comprehension with inability to repeat or write to dictation and relatively preserved spoken language and spontaneous writing. Comprehension of visual or written material is superior to that of auditory information. The lesion(s) are typically in or near the primary auditory cortex (Heschl's gyrus) in the superoposterior temporal lobe. Causes are infarction, hemorrhage, or tumor.

PURE WORD BLINDNESS Inability to read and often to name colors with preserved speech fluency, language comprehension, repetition, and writing to dictation (alexia without agraphia). Lesion usually involves left striate cortex and visual association areas as well as fibers in splenium of corpus callosum connecting right and left visual association areas. Most pts have an associated right homonymous hemianopsia, hemisensory deficit, and memory disturbance due to vascular lesions [involving the left posterior cerebral artery (PCA) territory]. Rarely tumor or hemorrhage may be the cause.

ISOLATION OF SPEECH AREA Hypotension, ischemia, or hypoxia may result in borderzone infarctions between the anterior cerebral–MCA–PCA territories that spare the sylvian region of the MCA. Pts are severely brain damaged and have parrot-like repetition of spoken words (echolalia) with little or no spontaneous speech or comprehension.

LABORATORY STUDIES IN APHASIA CT scan or MRI usually identify the location and nature of the causative lesion. Angiography helps in accurate definition of specific vascular syndromes.

THERAPY OF APHASIA Speech therapy may be helpful in treatment of certain types of aphasia.

For a more detailed discussion, see Mohr JP: Disorders of Speech and Language, Chap. 33, in HPIM-12, p. 203

174 FOCAL CEREBRAL LESIONS

Patients with focal cerebral lesions often present with a characteristic set of signs and symptoms that enable the astute physician to (1) recognize that a brain disorder exists; (2) localize the disorder to a specific brain region; and (3) together with the clinical history, develop a differential diagnosis. A lesion causes focal symptoms and signs by disrupting functional centers or pathways that connect them.

FRONT LOBE (See Table 174-1) Extensive anterior frontal lobe pathology may produce only subtle personality changes recognizable by family members or misdiagnosed as depression or thought disorder.

TEMPORAL LOBE (See Table 174-2) Temporal lobe centers are important for speech, memory, emotions. Left hemisphere coordinates speech in almost all right-handed and 60% of left-handed people.

PARIETAL LOBE (See Table 174-3) Parietal lobe lesions affect cortical sensation, i.e., two-point discrimination, ability to recognize objects by tactile cues (astereognosia), along with the more complicated sense of body's position in space.

OCCIPITAL LOBE Occipital lobes deal primarily with visual processing. Lesions of inferior calcarine cortex (or temporal lobe lesions that affect optic radiations to this area) cause contralateral superior quadrantanopia. Damage to superior

TABLE 174-1 Frontal lobe lesions

Site of lesion	Signs
Motor cortex, primary/secondary	Contralateral spastic paresis
Pre-motor cortex	Grasp reflex; left-sided lesions sometimes cause bilateral dyspraxia
Frontal eye fields	Gaze preference; eyes and sometimes head are turned toward the side of the lesion
Anterior (prefrontal)	May be relatively asymptomatic, but if large or bilateral damage, then cause lack of initiative, inappropriate jocularity, impulsivity, incontinence, perseveration, gait apraxia
Prerolandic	Lesions on dominant side cause mutism, expressive aphasia, often with bilateral apraxia

TABLE 174-2   Temporal lobe lesions

Site of lesion	Signs
Dominant superior convolution and adjacent inferior parietal convolution	Wernicke's receptive aphasia with jargon speech, inability to comprehend spoken or written language, often with agitation
Bilateral auditory cortex	Cortical deafness
Medial basal cortex	Emotional disorders, psychotic behavior; if bilateral, then Klüver-Bucy syndrome
Hippocampus	Short-term memory loss if dominant or bilateral

calcarine cortex or optic radiations through parietal lobe cause a contralateral inferior quadrantanopia. Bilateral lesions cause occipital blindness. Occasionally pt is unaware of his or her blindness.

THALAMUS   All somatosensory input is processed in thalamus on way to cortical centers. Unilateral thalamic lesions often cause contralateral total hemianesthesia. A disabling delayed pain syndrome may follow. Many neural circuits involve loops through thalamus, so that aphasia, asterixis, choreoathetosis, and mental aberrations also can occur in pts with thalamic lesions. Pupils may be miotic.

BRAINSTEM   (See Table 174-4)   All neural input and output must pass through compact brainstem. Relatively small lesions can be accurately diagnosed by neuroanatomic criteria.

TABLE 174-3   Parietal lobe lesions

Site of lesion	Signs
Post-central sensory cortex	Defect in sensory discrimination: extinction of double simultaneous stimulation, astereognosia, etc.
Dominant angular gyrus	Agraphia, acalculia, left-right disorientation, finger agnosia
Nondominant parietal	Contralateral visual inattention, neglect of contralateral side, constructional apraxia, lack of awareness of deficits

TABLE 174-4   Brainstem lesions

Site of lesion	Signs
Top of midbrain	Paralysis of upward gaze, convergence nystagmus, miosis, abulia, disorientation, third nerve palsy
Pontomedullary junction	Contralateral hemiplegia, sixth and seventh nerve palsy, ipsilateral loss of pain sense on face, contralateral sensory loss on body
Lateral medulla	Vertigo, nystagmus, ipsilateral ataxia, loss of facial pain, miosis, ptosis, anhidrosis, contralateral loss of pain sense on body

For a more detailed discussion, see Adams RD, Victor M: Syndromes due to Focal Cerebral Lesions, Chap. 32, in HPIM-12, p. 200

Global disruption of brain function occurs commonly in pts with serious medical illness. Such metabolic encephalopathies usually begin with an alteration in alertness (drowsiness), followed by agitation, confusion, delirium, or psychosis, and progressing to stupor and coma. These states are discussed in Chap. 9.

Evaluation of pt requires careful physical exam for underlying structural brain lesions, CNS infection, and general medical illness. Next, blood should be drawn, glucose and naloxone administered, and electrolytes, toxic screen, CBC, and renal, liver, and thyroid functions measured. A brain CT scan is sometimes necessary to exclude mass lesions, and CSF exam should be done to exclude meningitis or encephalitis. Common causes of metabolic encephalopathy are listed below with their salient features.

ELECTROLYTE DISORDERS Hyponatremia is often associated with seizures if the serum Na^+ <120 mmol/L. Too rapid or overcorrection of the serum Na^+ can cause central pontine myelinolysis. Extreme hyperosmolarity due to hypernatremia or hyperglycemia causes tremulousness, convulsions, and coma. Hypokalemia is associated with severe muscle weakness and confusion; hypercalcemia with inattentiveness, somnolence, and depression. Acidosis also produces stupor or coma; D-lactic acidosis produces encephalopathy in pts with jejunoileal shunts.

ENDOCRINE DISORDERS Confusional states, affective disorders, and psychosis occur commonly in *Cushing's disease* or in pts treated with glucocorticoids. *Hyperthyroidism* causes restlessness, insomnia, tremor, and agitated delirium. A syndrome of lethargy and depression termed *apathetic hyperthyroidism* occurs in elderly pts. Slowed mentation, depression, dementia, and coma occur in *hypothyroidism* and *Addison's disease*. An inappropriate jocularity and ataxia are sometimes seen in *hypothyroidism,* occasionally with paranoia and psychosis. *Hypoglycemia* causes convulsions and even focal neurologic findings if glucose falls below 1.4–1.7 mmol/L (25–30 mg/dL). Because of its variable clinical presentation and risk of permanent brain injury, hypoglycemia should be considered in all encephalopathies without known cause. Glucose level should be determined and IV dextrose administered. Recurrent hypoglycemia as occurs with islet cell tumor may present as episodic encephalopathy

MISCELLANEOUS ENCEPHALOPATHIES   Hypercapneic encephalopathy is frequently accompanied by headache, asterixis, coarse muscular twitching, and sometimes papilledema.

Hepatic encephalopathy also causes asterixis sometimes with fluctuating rigidity, Babinski signs, and seizures. Paroxysms of triphasic slow waves may be found on the EEG. Restriction of dietary protein, oral antibiotics, acidification of colonic contents with lactulose, and treatment of infection constitute the standard of therapy. Chronic or recurrent hepatic encephalopathy can lead to hepatocerebral degeneration. *Reye's syndrome* is a special form of hepatic encephalopathy seen in children and characterized by brain swelling.

Anoxic-ischemic encephalopathy occurring after insults severe enough to cause loss of consciousness is commonly seen after cardiorespiratory failure or arrest, CO poisoning, drowning, and asphyxia. If extreme and sustained, permanent brain injury will result. If brainstem reflexes and spontaneous respirations return, full recovery can occur. Incomplete recovery results in the postanoxic syndromes, i.e., persistent vegetative state, dementia, parkinsonism, cerebellar ataxia, intention myoclonus, Korsakoff's amnesia. Occasionally delayed cerebral degeneration occurs weeks after an initial recovery from an anoxic insult, especially in CO poisoning.

Renal disease with uremia leads to apathy, inattentiveness, and irritability progressing to delirium and stupor. There is usually myoclonus or seizures. Episodic encephalopathy with seizures, muscle cramps, and headache sometimes complicates hemodialysis. Dialysis dementia with prominent dysarthria, myoclonus, psychosis, and motor aphasia may be related to aluminum in the dialysate passing into the bloodstream.

Hypertensive encephalopathy with headache, retinopathy, and uremia can complicate pregnancy, renal failure, pheochromocytoma, or primary hypertension.

Nutritional encephalopathies occur in patients with B_{12}, thiamine, niacin, nicotinic acid, or pyridoxine deficiency. Peripheral neuropathy, spinal cord dysfunction, and mucocutaneous abnormalities are frequent accompaniments. Wernicke's encephalopathy is characterized by diplopia, nystagmus, and ataxia. Early treatment with thiamine can prevent a permanent Korsakoff's amnestic state. The encephalopathy of B_{12} deficiency is occasionally misdiagnosed as Alzheimer's dementia.

Toxic encephalopathies are common. A recent onset of an encephalopathic condition should lead to blood and urine screening for narcotics, salicylates, hypnotics, antidepressants, phenothiazines, lithium, anticonvulsants, amphetamines, alcohol, arsenic, lead, bismuth, and carbon monoxide.

Others Illnesses that can present as encephalopathy include bacterial endocarditis, thrombotic thrombocytopenic purpura, multiple fat emboli, typhoid fever, AIDS, multiple intracerebral metastases, hepatic porphyria, collagen-vascular disorders, and hyperproliferative hematologic disorders.

For a more detailed discussion, see Victor M, Martin JB: Nutritional and Metabolic Diseases of the Nervous System, Chap. 357, in HPIM-12, p. 2045

Patients with systemic neoplasia commonly develop neurologic disorders. These may result from local tumor (i.e., metastases, see Table 176-1) or leptomeningeal infiltration or follow compression or infiltration of cranial and peripheral nerves. Pts with systemic tumor are also at risk for *paraneoplastic syndromes* (see Table 176-2), disorders of central or peripheral nervous system structures that are distant from the tumor site. The paraneoplastic syndrome may present as the first sign of systemic malignancy.

Circulating antibodies that react with a Purkinje cell antigen are found in most cases of cerebellar degeneration associated with breast and ovarian cancer. Circulating antibodies that react with neuronal nuclei have been found in some cases of paraneoplastic neuropathy and limbic encephalitis. Occa-

TABLE 176-1 Metastases

Site	Clinical manifestations	Cancer	Evaluation
Cerebrum	Headache, focal signs, drowsiness papilledema, sixth nerve palsy, seizure	Breast, lung, GI tract, melanoma, treated ovarian	CT scan with contrast, or MRI scan
Posterior fossa	Ataxia, headache, cranial nerve palsy, head tilt, emesis, obstructive hydrocephalus	Same as above	CT scan with contrast, MRI scan
Spinal cord	Sensory level, bowel and bladder dysfunction, back pain, corticospinal tract signs	As above; also lymphoma, prostate cancer	MRI, CT scan with metrizamide, myelography, spine films
Leptomeninges	Cranial or peripheral nerve lesions (often painful), spinal cord signs	Melanoma, lymphoma, glioblastoma, adenocarcinoma	CSF cytology, myelography, MRI scan

TABLE 176-2 Paraneoplastic syndromes

Type	Clinical manifestations	Cancer	Evolution
Limbic encephalitis	Confusional state, memory loss, dementia, anxiety	Oat cell, lung	Weeks to months
Photoreceptor degeneration	Visual loss	Oat cell, cervical	Weeks to months
Subacute cerebellar degeneration	Ataxia, dysarthria, vertigo	Oat cell, ovarian, breast, Hodgkin's lymphoma	Weeks to months
Opsoclonus, myoclonus	Dancing eyes, ataxia (children)	Neuroblastoma, lung, breast	Weeks
Brainstem encephalitis	Nystagmus, vertigo, diplopia, dysarthria, ataxia, dysphagia	Lung tumors	Days to weeks
Necrotizing myelopathy	Paraplegia, quadriplegia, sensory level	Oat cell, lymphoma	Hours to weeks
Subacute motor neuronopathy	Flaccid weakness, muscular atrophy	Non-Hodgkin's lymphoma	Weeks to months
Subacute sensory neuronopathy	Severe sensory loss	Oat cell	Weeks to months
Guillain-Barré	Weakness, areflexia, minimal sensory abnormalities	Hodgkin's lymphoma	Days to weeks
Sensory motor neuropathy	Distal motor and sensory loss, distal areflexia	Oat cell, myeloma	Weeks to months
Myasthenia gravis	Weakness, fatigability	Thymoma	Weeks to months
Lambert-Eaton	Weakness, fatigability	Oat cell, breast, prostate, stomach	Week to months
Polymyositis	Proximal muscle weakness, CHF, tender muscles	Breast, ovarian, lung, lymphoma	Months to years

sional pts improve neurologically when treated with gluco-corticoids or plasmapheresis.

In addition to local tumor and paraneoplastic syndromes, delayed effects of radiation and chemotherapy can cause nervous system pathology.

For a more detailed discussion, see Brown RH Jr.: Paraneo-plastic Neurologic Syndromes, Chap. 310, in HPIM-12, p. 1641

SECTION 12 PSYCHIATRIC AND DEPENDENCY DISORDERS

177 APPROACH TO THE PATIENT WITH PSYCHIATRIC DISEASE

MAJOR AFFECTIVE DISORDERS AND PSYCHOSES

Primary disorders of affect and thought are considered psychobiologic manifestations of abnormal brain mechanisms. Pts also may present with depressive, manic, or psychotic disorders *secondary* to metabolic derangements, drug toxicity, focal cerebral lesions, epilepsy, or degenerative brain disease. Therefore, pts with newly diagnosed emotional or thought disorders should be carefully evaluated for underlying medical and neurologic illnesses. Pts with *primary* major affective disorders are divided into those with a history of depression alternating with mania (bipolar) and those with depression alone (unipolar). Schizophrenia is the major primary psychotic illness.

MAJOR DEPRESSION *Diagnosis* Dysphoric mood or anhedonia are always features in major depression but need not be the most prominent symptom. At least four of the following symptoms are also present: (1) change in appetite with corresponding change in weight; (2) insomnia (especially early morning awakening) or hypersomnia; (3) psychomotor retardation or its opposite, agitation; (4) loss of interest, pleasure, and decreased sexual drive; (5) loss of energy (fatigue); (6) feelings of worthlessness, self-reproach, or guilt; (7) diminished ability to concentrate and make decisions; (8) recurrent thoughts of death or suicide. Depression usually occurs in episodes lasting 5–12 months, and there is a tendency for periodicity and recurrence. Some pts are chronically depressed. Depressed pts commonly seek medical attention because of various subjective, unremitting somatic complaints, i.e., constant headache, diffuse achiness, fatigue. Some women note depressive symptoms prior to menses.

Pts with major depression often have disordered sleep patterns, abnormal monoamine neurotransmission, and abnormal neuroendocrine control.

Prevalence and suicide risk Depression is common; it occurs in children as well as in adults. In the adult population, prevalence is 3% in men and twice that in women. Risk increases with age >55. 70% of the 30,000 annual suicides in the U.S. occur in pts with major affective disorders. Many seek general medical attention just prior to their suicide attempt, so it is important that physicians directly question potentially depressed pts regarding suicide risk. Pts who have given detailed thought to possible methods of suicide, have concomitant alcoholism, are socially isolated, elderly males, or have serious medical illnesses have greater risk of suicide.

Treatment Pts with significant risk of suicide should be hospitalized. Antidepressants can produce remarkable amelioration of symptoms, usually over a period of weeks. The combination of psychotherapy with pharmacotherapy is significantly better than either alone. Electroshock therapy is used in those pts with life-threatening depression who require immediate benefit or in those refractory to antidepressants. Atypical depression with excessive anxiety, hypersomnia, overeating, and interpersonal rejection sensitivity responds well to monoamine oxidase inhibitors.

MANIC DISORDERS *Diagnosis* Pts with mania have elevated, expansive mood, although they are frequently hyperirritable. They experience (1) increase in activity or physical restlessness, (2) unusual talkativeness, (3) flight of ideas and the subjective impression that their thoughts are racing, (4) inflated self-esteem that may be delusional, (5) decreased need for sleep, (6) distractability, and (7) excessive involvement in risky activities, i.e., buying sprees, sexual indiscretion, foolish business investments.

Treatment Acutely manic pts may need hospitalization to reduce degree of environmental stimulation and to protect themselves and others from consequences of reckless behavior. Lithium therapy is the mainstay of treatment.

SCHIZOPHRENIA *Diagnosis* Schizophrenia usually presents in late teenage years or the third decade. Psychotic features last 6 months or more and include (1) bizarre delusions; (2) paranoid, jealous, somatic, grandiose, religious, nihilistic, or other delusions; (3) auditory hallucinations, often including a voice or voices maintaining a running commentary; and (4) incoherence, marked loosening of associations, markedly illogical thinking, inappropriate affect, delusions, hallucinations, and catatonic or grossly disorganized behavior. Pts with primary psychoses have normal memory, calculating abilities, and language function, but the insertion of bizarre thought may contaminate or even preclude accurate cognitive testing.

Treatment Acutely psychotic pts, especially those with violent "command hallucinations," may be dangerous to themselves or others. Such pts need psychiatric hospitalization. Antipsychotic medications are usually quite effective in ameliorating hallucinations and agitation, but are less effective in treating social isolation and anhedonia.

ANXIETY AND PERSONALITY DISORDERS

Anxiety refers to paroxysmal or persistent psychological feelings (dread, irritability, ruminations) and somatic symptoms (dyspnea, sweating, insomnia, trembling) that impair normal functioning. A variety of relatively distinct anxiety disorders have been described.

ANXIETY STATES Panic disorder Characterized by sudden, unexpected, and overwhelming feeling of terror or apprehension with associated somatic symptoms. Estimated to occur in 1–2% of population with a female-male ratio of 2:1. Tends to be familial, onset in second or third decade, and affective illness often coexists. The *Diagnostic and Statistical Manual,* third edition revised (DSM-IIIR), developed by the American Psychiatric Association, lists specific criteria for diagnosis: (1) at least 4 panic attacks within 4 weeks in nonthreatening or nonexertional settings that can be precipitated by other than circumscribed phobic stimuli; and (2) attacks manifested by discrete episodes of apprehension or fear and at least four of the following: dyspnea, palpitations, chest pain or discomfort, choking/smothering feelings, dizziness/vertigo/unsteady feelings, feelings of unreality, paresthesias, hot and cold flashes, sweating, faintness, trembling, and fear of dying, going crazy, or doing something uncontrolled during an attack.

Laboratory findings IV lactate precipitates panic attacks in about half of afflicted individuals.

Differential diagnosis The diagnostic challenge is to differentiate panic disorder from cardiovascular diseases it mimics. There may be an increased prevalence of mitral valve prolapse in pts with panic disorder. Symptoms associated with hyper- and hypothyroidism, pheochromocytoma, complex partial seizures, hypoglycemia, drug ingestions (amphetamines, cocaine, caffeine, sympathomimetic nasal decongestants), and drug withdrawal (alcohol, barbiturates, opiates, minor tranquilizers) may simulate panic attacks.

Treatment Tricyclic antidepressants or monoamine oxidase inhibitors have an 80–90% effectiveness in treatment and prevention of spontaneous attacks. Alprazolam (Xanax) given in high dose (2–4 mg qd) is as effective as antidepressants with fewer side effects and works in 1–2 d. Other benzodiazepines have not proven effective. Beta blockers may reduce somatic symptoms but are ineffective in preventing psychic fear or panic.

Generalized anxiety disorder These pts experience persistent anxiety, without the specific symptoms of phobic, panic, or obsessive-compulsive disorders. Common signs are motor tension (shakiness, trembling, restlessness, easy startle, etc.), autonomic hyperactivity, apprehensive expectation (anxiety, fear, rumination, anticipation of misfortune, etc.), and vigilance (distractibility, poor concentration, insomnia, impatience, irritability). Prevalence is estimated at 2–3%. A familial or genetic basis has not been established. High-affinity, stereospecific benzodiazepine receptors, coupled to GABA receptors, have been defined through which the anxiolytic actions of benzodiazepines are mediated. This suggests that endogenous anxiogenic compounds may be found in the brain.

Differential diagnosis Symptoms and signs resembling anxiety occur in coronary artery disease, thyroid disease, and drug intoxication or withdrawal. Anxiety may be present in depression, schizophrenia, and organic mental states.

Treatment Supportive or intensive psychotherapy or behavioral modification therapy. When generalized anxiety is severe enough to warrant treatment with drugs, anxiolytics are agents of choice. Buspirone, a non-benzodiazepine anxiolytic, may become the drug of choice because it lacks many of the problems associated with benzodiazepam.

Obsessive-compulsive disorder Characterized by recurrent obsessions (persistent intrusive thoughts) and compulsions (intrusive behaviors) that the pt experiences as involuntary, senseless, or repugnant. Common obsessions include thoughts of violence (e.g., killing a loved one), obsessive slowness, fears of germs or contamination, and doubt. Examples of compulsions include repeated checking to be assured that something was done properly, hand washing, extreme neatness, and counting rituals, as in numbering steps while walking.

Clinical features Obsessive-compulsive disorder usually begins in adolescence, with 65% of cases manifest before age 25. Clear precipitants are identified in 60% of cases. There are reports of an increased incidence of the disorder in monozygotic twins and first-degree relatives of probands. Most pts follow an episodic course with periods of incomplete remission. Depression, substance abuse, social impairment are common.

Treatment   Clomipramine and fluoxetine are recently released antidepressants that are now the drugs of choice in treating obsessive-compulsive disorders. Behaviorally oriented psychotherapy and psychopharmacology can be helpful.

Posttraumatic stress disorder   Refers to acute and chronic psychic distress following traumatic events. DSM-IIIR criteria include (1) existence of a recognizable stress that would evoke significant symptoms of distress in almost everyone; (2) reexperiencing the trauma by recurrent intrusive recollections, recurrent dreams, or sudden acting or feeling as if the traumatic event were recurring; (3) numbing of responsiveness to or reduced involvement with the external world, beginning sometime after the trauma; and (4) presence of at least two of the following symptoms: hyperalertness or exaggerated startle, sleep disturbance, guilt about having survived when others have not or about behavior required for survival, memory impairment or trouble concentrating, avoidance of activities that arouse recollection of traumatic event, and intensification of symptoms by exposure to events that symbolize or resemble traumatic event.

Treatment   Involves a combination of psychosocial support systems, psychotherapy, behavioral and conditioning techniques, and medications.

PHOBIC DISORDERS   This group has in common persistently recurring, irrational fear of specific objects, activities, or situations with secondary avoidance behavior of the phobic stimulus. The diagnosis is made only when avoidance behavior is a significant source of distress to the individual or interferes with social or occupational functioning.

Agoraphobia   Fear of being alone or in public places. May occur in absence of panic disorder but is almost invariably preceded by that condition.

Social phobias   Persistent irrational fear of and need to avoid any situation where there is risk of scrutiny by others, embarrassment, or humiliation. Common examples include excessive fear of public speaking or any public performance.

Simple phobias   Persistent irrational fears and avoidance of specific objects. Common examples include fear of heights (acrophobia), closed spaces (claustrophobia), and animals.

Treatment   *Social and simple phobias:* behavioral modification and relaxation techniques, systematic desensitization. Propranolol and/or alprazolam may be helpful in treating social phobias. *Agoraphobia:* as in treatment of panic disorder.

PERSONALITY DISORDERS Defined as the inappropriate, stereotyped, maladaptive use of a certain set of psychological characteristics; said to affect 5–23% of the population. In medical and surgical pts such disorders may underlie an ineffectual doctor-pt relationship. Medical disorders and neurologic disease may cause personality changes that mimic the following personality disorders. Pts may be characterized as:

- *Paranoid:* suspicious, hypersensitive, often hostile
- *Schizoid:* isolated, cold, indifferent
- *Schizotypal:* eccentric with ideas reference, magical thinking, suspiciousness
- *Borderline*: impulsive, with unpredictable and fluctuating intense moods, occasional psychosis
- *Histrionic:* dramatic, engaging, self-centered, attention seeking
- *Narcissistic:* inflated sense of self-importance
- *Antisocial*: engaging in deviant behavior with lack of remorse
- *Dependent:* fearing separation and engaging others to assume responsibility
- *Obsessive-compulsive:* perfectionistic and inflexible but often indecisive

---

For a more detailed discussion, see Judd LL, Braff DL, Britton KT, Risch SC, Gillin JC, Grant I: Psychiatry and Medicine, Chap. 368, in HPIM-12, p. 2123

178 PSYCHOTROPIC DRUGS

The four major classes of psychotropic drugs are (1) antidepressants, (2) anxiolytics, (3) antipsychotics, and (4) other mood-normalizing medications.

GENERAL PRINCIPLES OF DRUG ADMINISTRATION

1. Nonpsychiatric physicians should familiarize themselves with *one* drug in each of the four classes, so its indications, efficacy, and side effects become well known.
2. Avoid polypharmacy or drug combinations.
3. Previous history of positive response to a drug is usually an indication that positive response to the same drug will occur again.
4. Two common errors in prescribing psychotropic drugs are *undermedication* and *impatience;* effects from proper dosage levels may take weeks or months.
5. Pharmacokinetics of psychotropic drugs in elderly pts are different, with longer biologic half-lives.
6. Failure to respond to one drug in a class does not mean that pt will not respond to another drug in same class.
7. The physician should never withdraw a psychotropic drug abruptly; taper over 2–4 weeks.
8. Physicians who only infrequently prescribe psychotropic drugs should review the side effects each time a drug is prescribed; pts and family members should be informed of potential side effects.

ANTIDEPRESSANTS See Tables 178-1, 178-2, and 178-3.
ANXIOLYTICS See Table 178-4.
ANTIPSYCHOTICS See Table 178-5.

TABLE 178-1 Commonly used antidepressants

Drug	Daily oral therapeutic dose range, mg
Tricyclic derivatives:	
Amitriptyline (Elavil, etc.)	150–300
Nortriptyline (Aventyl, etc.)	50–150
Imipramine (Tofranil, etc.)	150–300
Desipramine (Norpramin)	150–250
Doxepin (Sinequan, etc.)	150–300
Monoamine oxidase inhibitors:	
Phenelzine (Nardil)	45–90
Tranylcypromine (Parnate)	10–30
Isocarboxazid (Marplan)	10–30

From Judd LL: HPIM-12, p. 2140.

TABLE 178-2 Common side effects of tricyclic antidepressants

Anticholinergic (atropine-like) responses:
 Dry mouth*; nausea and vomiting*; constipation*; urinary retention;
 blurred vision (mydriasis and cycloplegia)
Cardiovascular effects:
 Postural hypotension*; tachycardia; cardiotoxic side effects—can in-
 duce an arrythmia
Obstructive jaundice—more rare; is reversible when drug is removed
Drowsiness and sleepiness—may want to avoid driving a car meanwhile
Fine rapid tremor*
Dizziness, ataxia
Hematologic effects:
 Leukopenia

* Side effects seen most commonly.
From Judd LL: HPIM-12, p. 2140.

TABLE 178-3 Selected second-generation antidepressants

Drug	Daily oral therapeutic dose range, mg
Tricylic derivatives:	
Trimipramine (Surmontil)	100–250
Amoxapine (Asendin)	150–300
Tetracyclic derivatives:	
Mianserin (Bolvidon)	50–150
Maprotiline (Ludiomil)	150–300
Derivatives of other chemical classes:	
Nomifensine (Merital)	100–200
Trazodone (Desyrel)	100–600
Alprazolam (Xanax)	0.75–4
Bupropion (Wellbutrin)	350–750

From Judd LL: HPIM-12, p. 2141.

TABLE 178-4 Commonly used benzodiazepines

Drug	Daily oral dose range, mg	Half-life, h*
Anxiolytics:		
Chlordiazepoxide (Librium)	20–100†	7–28*
Diazepam (Valium)	5–40	20–90*
Lorazepam (Ativan)	1–10‡	10–20
Oxazepam (Serax)	30–120‡	3–20
Prazepam (Centrax)	20–60	40–70*
Alprazolam (Xanax)	0.75–4‡	12–15
Sedative-hypnotic:		
Flurazepam (Dalmane)	15–30§	24–100*
Temazepam (Restoril)	30§	8–10
Triazolam (Halcion)	0.5–1.0§	2–5

* Indicates long-acting active metabolites.
† Prescribed in a qd or bid regimen.
‡ Prescribed in a tid or qid regimen.
§ Prescribed in a qd or qhs regimen.
From Judd LL: HPIM-12, p. 2143.

OTHERS   Lithium   The administration of lithium is monitored by serum levels, best obtained in the morning approximately 10 h after the last dose of lithium. In treatment of acute mania, therapeutic efficacy is achieved at serum levels between 0.8 and 1.5 mmol/L. There is rarely necessity for pts to be treated at serum levels above 1.5 mmol/L. Oral dose range to sustain therapeutic serum levels ranges from 600 mg to approximately 3000 mg daily.

TABLE 178-5   Some of the more commonly used antipsychotic medications

Drug	Average daily oral dose range, mg	Potency ratio compared to 100 mg chlorpromazine
Phenothiazines:		
Aliphatics:		
Chlorpromazine (Thorazine)	400–800	1:1
Piperazines:		
Fluphenazine (Prolixin)	4–20	1:50
Fluphenazine enanthate or decanoate	25–100*	
Perphenazine (Trilafon)	8–32	1:10
Trifluoperazine (Stelazine)	6–20	1:20
Piperidines:		
Thioridazine (Mellaril)	200–600	1:1 (approx)
Butyrophenones:		
Haloperidol (Haldol)	8–32	1:50
Thioxanthenes:		
Chlorprothixene (Taractan)	400–800	1:1
Thiothixene (Navane)	15–30	1:25
Oxoindoles:		
Molindone (Moban, Lidone)	40–200	1:10
Dibenzoxazepines:		
Laxapine (Loxitane, Daxolin)	60–100	1:10

* IM injection, long-acting, q 1 to 3 weeks.
From Judd LL: HPIM-12, p. 2145.

For a more detailed discussion, see Judd LL: Therapeutic Use of Psychotropic Medications, Chap. 369, in HPIM-12, p. 2139

179 ALCOHOLISM

DEFINITION Regular and excessive use of alcohol with associated psychologic dependence on its use during daily life that results in social and occupational problems and physical impairment.

HISTORY Pts typically present with marital difficulties, job problems (including absenteeism), legal problems resulting from driving while intoxicated, disorderly behavior, etc. Medical Hx should be reviewed for presence of alcohol-related physical problems, which can be neurologic (blackouts, seizures, delirium tremens, Wernicke-Korsakoff's, cerebellar degeneration, neuropathy, myopathy), gastrointestinal (esophagitis, gastritis, pancreatitis, hepatitis, cirrhosis, GI hemorrhage), cardiovascular (hypertension, cardiomyopathy), hematologic (macrocytosis, folate deficiency, thrombocytopenia, leukopenia), endocrine (testicular atrophy, amenorrhea, infertility), skeletal (fractures, osteonecrosis), or infectious.

CLINICAL MANIFESTATIONS Behavioral, cognitive, and psychomotor changes may occur at blood alcohol levels as low as 4–7 mmol/L (20–30 mg/dL). Mild to moderate intoxication occurs at 17–43 mmol/L (80–200 mg/dL). Incoordination, tremor, ataxia, confusion, stupor, coma, and even death can occur at progressively higher blood alcohol levels. Signs of alcohol withdrawal may include tremulousness ("shakes" or "jitters"), autonomic hyperactivity (sweating, hypertension, tachycardia, tachypnea, fever), insomnia, nightmares, anxiety, and GI upset. Psychotic symptoms can include visual, auditory, tactile, and olfactory hallucinations. Seizures can occur ("rum fits"). Delirium tremens ("DTs") is a severe withdrawal syndrome characterized by extreme confusion, agitation, vivid delusions and hallucinations, and profound autonomic hyperactivity.

LABORATORY FINDINGS Clues to occult alcoholism include mild anemia with macrocytosis, folate deficiency, thrombocytopenia, granulocytopenia, abnormal LFTs (e.g., elevated γ-glutamyl transferase), hyperuricemia, elevated triglycerides. Decreases in serum K, Mg, Zn, and P levels are common. Diagnostic studies such as GI radiology or endoscopy, abdominal ultrasound or CT, liver-spleen scan, liver biopsy, ECG, echocardiogram, cranial CT, EEG, and nerve conduction studies may show evidence of alcohol-related organ dysfunction.

THERAPY Alcohol withdrawal is treated with thiamine (50–100 mg IV daily for 5 d), multivitamins, CNS depressant drugs, and in some cases, anticonvulsants. Many clinicians prefer to use benzodiazepines with longer half-lives (e.g., diazepam, chlordiazepoxide) as CNS depressants because they produce less fluctuation in drug blood levels and can be administered less frequently. These benefits must be weighed against the increased risk of oversedation, which occurs less commonly with shorter-acting agents (e.g., oxazepam, lorazepam). Fluid and electrolyte status and blood sugar levels should be closely followed. Cardiovascular and hemodynamic monitoring is crucial, because deaths have resulted from hemodynamic collapse and cardiac arrhythmias. Care should be taken to search for evidence of trauma or infection that may be masked by prominent withdrawal symptoms. Treatment of chronic alcoholism depends on recognition of the problem by pt. Rehabilitation programs and support groups (e.g., Alcoholics Anonymous) may be of value. Disulfiram (Antabuse), a drug that inhibits aldehyde dehydrogenase and results in toxic symptoms (nausea, vomiting, diarrhea, tremor) if pt consumes alcohol, is used in some centers.

For a more detailed discussion, see Schuckit MA: Alcohol and Alcoholism, Chap. 370, in HPIM-12, p. 2146

Opioid addiction creates major social and medical problems. Three groups of abusers can be identified: (1) pts with chronic pain syndromes, (2) medical staff with easy access to narcotics, and (3) street abusers.

ADDICTION AND THE OPIATE ABSTINENCE SYNDROME

Opiate tolerance, dependence, and withdrawal symptoms are considered to be related phenomena with common underlying mechanisms. The euphoric, analgesic, or anxiolytic effects of opiates initially attract the user. Family history of substance abuse and a variety of psychologic factors influence the development of drug dependence. Acute, uncomfortable abstinence syndromes begin to occur as the opiate effects wane. The former include diarrhea, coughing, lacrimation, rhinorrhea, diaphoresis, twitching muscles, piloerection, fever, tachypnea, hypertension, diffuse body pain, insomnia, and yawning. Relief of these exceedingly unpleasant symptoms by narcotic administration leads to more frequent narcotic use. Eventually, chronic addiction is established, and all the person's efforts are consumed by drug-seeking behavior.

TREATMENT OF THE ABSTINENCE SYNDROME Pts who present with any manifestation of drug abuse should be examined for signs of the life-threatening complications. Effective treatment of withdrawal requires admitting pt to hospital or drug withdrawal center for initial administration of opiates followed by gradual reduction over 5–10 d. Long-acting oral methadone is most convenient: 1 mg methadone is equivalent to 3 mg morphine, 1 mg heroin, or 20 mg meperidine. Most pts receive 10–25 mg methadone bid, and higher doses are given if withdrawal symptoms break through. Clonidine is effective in decreasing sympathetic nervous system hyperactivity. Withdrawal syndromes in newborns of street abusers are fatal in 3–30%.

EFFECTS ON BODY SYSTEMS Opioid effects on the CNS can result in sedation, euphoria, decreased pain perception, decreased respiratory drive, and vomiting. The adulterants added to "cut" street drugs (quinine, phenacetin, strychnine, antipyrine, caffeine, powdered milk) may contribute to more permanent neurologic damage, including peripheral neuropathy, amblyopia, and myelopathy. The shared use of contaminated needles is a major cause of brain abscess, in addition to acute endocarditis, hepatitis B, AIDS, septic arthritis, and soft tissue infections. At least 25% of street abusers die with 10–20 years of active abuse.

TREATMENT **Overdose** High doses, taken in suicide attempt or accidentally if the potency is misjudged, are frequently lethal. Toxic syndrome occurs immediately after IV administration, with a variable delay after oral ingestion. Symptoms include miosis, shallow respirations, bradycardia, hypothermia, and stupor or coma; less commonly pulmonary edema. Treatment requires cardiorespiratory support and administration of the opiate antagonist naloxone (0.4 mg IV and repeated in 3 min if no or partial response). Because effects of naloxone diminish in 2–3 h compared to longer-lasting effects of heroin (up to 24 h) or methadone (up to 72 h), it is important to observe these pts for reappearance of toxic state.

Patient with chronic pain Physicians should avoid establishing narcotic addiction in pts with chronic pain syndromes. If physical dependence is established, then abstinence syndromes will intensify the pain and confuse an already difficult problem. Drugs should be used to minimize effects of pain on function and not to abolish pain. Oral administration of the least potent drug able to take the edge off the pain should be used. Nonmedicinal approaches to pain control should be part of the pt's program.

Medical staff Doctors are advised never to prescribe opiates for themselves or members of their families. Medical organizations need to identify and rehabilitate substance-impaired physicians before problems escalate to the point of licensure revocation.

The street abuser Identification of any chronic narcotic user is possible by blood and urine screens or the opiate antagonist challenge test (0.4 mg naloxone given slowly IV over 5 min, after which the pt is observed for 1–2 h for signs of withdrawal). For any realistic expectation of rehabilitation, the pt must be motivated to make a long-term commitment to a drug-free lifestyle. Special vocational, counseling, and peer programs are often helpful. Chronic use of opiate antagonists (naltrexone, 50–100 mg/d) blocks the "high" of moderate doses of narcotics and is sometimes helpful. Addicts who fail drug-free programs and who still wish to improve function within the family, social structure, etc. can do so on chronic methadone treatment. A relatively low dose (30–40 mg/d) may control abstinence symptoms and help curb drug-seeking behavior. The drug is administered orally at a program center.

For a more detailed discussion, see Schuckit MA, Segal DS: Opioid Drug Use, Chap. 371, p. 2151; and Mendelson JH, Mello NK: Commonly Abused Drugs, Chap. 372, p. 2155, in HPIM-12

SECTION 13 DERMATOLOGY

181 GENERAL EXAMINATION OF THE SKIN

Physical examination usually provides more useful information than history. Examination of skin with precise description of lesion(s) should generate a differential diagnosis regardless of Hx; narrowing the differential is then aided by pertinent facts from the Hx. Examination of skin should take place in a well-illuminated room with pt completely disrobed. Ancillary helpful equipment includes a hand lens and a pocket flashlight to provide peripheral illumination of lesions.

GENERAL EXAMINATION History Onset, duration, progression of lesions, prior treatment, allergies, personal or family Hx of atopic disease, occupation, predisposing or aggravating factors (including underlying diseases, exposure to cosmetics or irritating chemicals, etc.).

PHYSICAL EXAMINATION Distribution Sun-exposed (SLE, photoallergic, phototoxic, polymorphous light eruption, porphyria cutanea tarda); dermatomal (herpes zoster); generalized (systemic diseases); extensor surfaces (elbows and knees in psoriasis); flexural surfaces (antecubital and popliteal fossae in atopic dermatitis). As illustrated in Fig. 181-1, the distribution of skin lesions can provide valuable clues to the identification of the disorder.

Configuration *Linear*—contact dermatitis such as poison ivy or lesions that appear at sites of local skin trauma (Koebner phenomenon), such as psoriasis, lichen planus, and lichen nitidis; *annular*—"ring-shaped" lesion with an active border and central clearing (erythema chronicum migrans, erythema annulare centrificum, and tinea corporis); *circinate*—circular lesion (urticaria, herald patch of pityriasis rosea); *nummular*—"coin-shaped" (nummular eczema); *guttate*—"droplike" (guttate psoriasis); *morbilliform*—"measles-like" with small confluent papules coalescing into unusual shapes (measles, drug eruption); *reticulated*—"netlike" (livedo reticularis); *herpetiform*—grouped vesicles, papules, or erosions (herpes simplex); *iris* or *target lesion*—two or

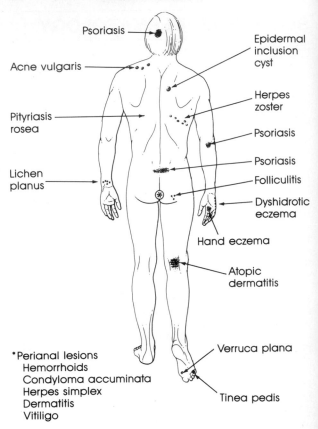

A

FIGURE 181-1   The distribution of some common dermatologic diseases and lesions.

three concentric circles of differing hue (erythema multiforme).

PRIMARY LESIONS   Cutaneous changes caused directly by disease process.

Macule—a flat circumscribed lesion of a different color, allowing for differentiation from surrounding skin; *patch*—

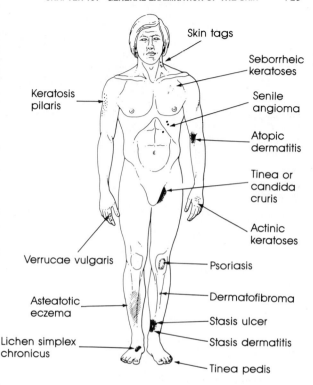

B

FIGURE 181-1B

macule >1 cm in diameter; *papule*—elevated, circumscribed lesion of any color <1 cm in diameter, with the major portion of lesion projecting above surrounding skin; *nodule*—palpable lesion similar to a papule but >1 cm in diameter; *plaque*—an elevated lesion >2 cm in diameter; *vesicle*—sharply marginated elevated lesion <1 cm in diameter filled with clear fluid; *bullae*—vesicular lesion >1 cm in diameter; *pustule*—a well-marginated focal accumulation of inflammatory cells within skin; *wheal*—a transient elevated lesion due to accumulation of fluid in upper dermis; *cyst*—lesion consisting of liquid or semisolid material contained within limits of cyst wall (true cyst).

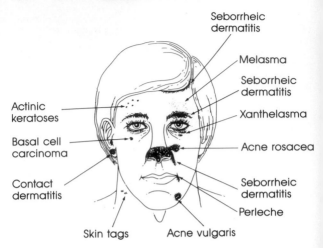

C

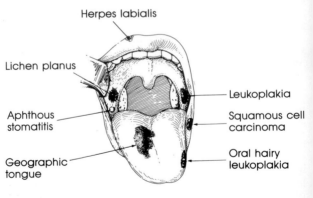

D

FIGURE 181-1C and 1D

SECONDARY LESIONS   Changes in area of primary pathology often due to secondary events, e.g., scratching, secondary infection, bleeding.

Scale—a flaky accumulation of excess keratin that is partially adherent to skin; *crust*—a circumscribed collection of inflammatory cells and dried serum on skin surface; *erosion*—a circumscribed, usually depressed, moist lesion resulting from loss of overlying epidermis; *ulcer*—a deeper erosion involving not only epidermis but also underlying papillary dermis; may leave a scar on healing; *atrophy:* (1) epidermal—thinning of skin with loss of normal skin surface markings, (2) dermal—depression of skin surface due to loss of underlying collagen or dermal ground substance; *lichenification*—thickening of skin with accentuation of normal skin surface markings most commonly due to chronic rubbing; *scar*—collection of fibrous tissue replacing normal dermal constituents.

OTHER DESCRIPTIVE TERMS   *Verrucous*—"wartlike"; *poikiloderma*—a combination of atrophy, hypo- and hyperpigmentation, and telangiectasia; *umbilicated*—containing a central depression; *color terms*—(i.e., violaceous, erythematous); *pedunculated*—on a stalk; *eczematous*—a crusted, weeping, erythematous, scaly patch with vesicles or erosions.

ROUTINE DIAGNOSTIC PROCEDURES   Potassium hydroxide preparation   Useful for detection of dermatophyte or yeast. Scale is collected from advancing edge of a scaling lesion by gently scraping with side of a microscope slide. Nail lesions are best sampled by trimming back nail and scraping subungual debris. A drop of 10–15% potassium hydroxide is added to slide and cover slip is applied. The slide may be gently heated and examined under microscope. Positive preparations show translucent, septate branching hyphae among keratinocytes.

Tzanck preparation   Useful for determining presence of herpes viruses. Optimal lesion to sample is an early vesicle. Lesion is gently unroofed with no. 15 scalpel blade and base of vesicle is gently scraped with belly of blade (keep blade perpendicular to skin surface to prevent laceration). Scrapings are transferred to slide and stained with Wright's or Giemsa stain. A positive preparation has multinucleate giant cells.

For a more detailed discussion, see Lawley TJ, Yancey KB: Examination of the Skin, Chap. 55, in HPIM-12, p. 304

PAPULOSQUAMOUS DISORDERS

Disorders exhibiting papules and scale.

PSORIASIS A chronic, recurrent disorder. Classic lesion is a well-marginated, erythematous plaque with silvery-white surface scale. Distribution includes extensor surfaces (i.e., knees, elbows, and buttocks); may also involve palms and scalp (particularly anterior scalp margin). Associated findings include psoriatic arthritis and nail changes (onycholysis, pitting or thickening of nail plate with accumulation of subungual debris).

Treatment Maintain cutaneous hydration; topical glucocorticoids; coal tar ointment; UV light (psoralens); methotrexate for severe advanced disease.

PITYRIASIS ROSEA A self-limited condition lasting 4–8 weeks. Initially, there is a single round or oval erythematous to salmon-colored patch (herald patch) with a peripheral rim of scale. Within 5–7 d, a generalized eruption involves the trunk and proximal extremities. Individual lesions are similar to but smaller than the herald patch and are arranged in symmetric fashion with long axis of each individual lesion along skin lines of cleavage. Appearance may be similar to that of secondary syphilis.

Treatment Disorder is self-limited, so treatment is directed at symptoms; oral antihistamines for pruritus; topical glucocorticoids; UV-B phototherapy in some cases.

LICHEN PLANUS Chronic disorder of unknown cause; can follow administration of certain drugs and in chronic graft-versus-host disease; lesions are pruritic, polygonal, flat-topped, and violaceous.

Treatment Topical glucocorticoids.

ECZEMATOUS DISORDERS

ATOPIC DERMATITIS One aspect of atopic triad of hayfever, asthma, and eczema. Usually an intermittent, chronic, severely pruritic, eczematous dermatitis with scaly erythematous patches, vesiculation, crusting, and fissuring. Lesions are most commonly on flexures with prominent involvement of antecubital and popliteal fossae; generalized erythroderma in severe cases. Most pts with atopic dermatitis are chronic carriers of *Staphylococcus aureus* in anterior nares and on skin.

Treatment   Avoidance of irritants; hydration; topical glucocorticoids; treatment of infected lesions. Systemic glucocorticoids only for severe exacerbations.

RHUS **DERMATITIS (POISON IVY, OAK, SUMAC)**   A common, vesicular, weeping, crusting dermatitis secondary to a delayed hypersensitivity reaction to resin of plants in the genus *Rhus*. Lesions occur at sites of contact with resin; linear arrangement of vesicles is common.

Treatment   Avoidance of sensitizing agent; topical (or, if severe, systemic) glucocorticoids.

SEBORRHEIC DERMATITIS   A chronic noninfectious process characterized by erythematous patches with greasy yellowish scale. Lesions are generally on scalp, eyebrows, nasolabial folds, axillae, central chest, and posterior auricular area.

Treatment   Nonfluorinated topical glucocorticoids; shampoos containing coal tar, salicylic acid, or selenium sulfide.

INFECTIONS AND INFESTATIONS

IMPETIGO   A superficial infection of skin secondary to either *S. aureus* or more commonly beta-hemolytic streptococci (group A). The hallmark is an eruption that begins as small vesicles progressing to erosions covered by a "honey-colored" crust. A bullous variety is most often associated with *S. aureus* infection. Lesions may occur anywhere but commonly on face.

Treatment   Improved hygiene; appropriate oral antibiotics depending on organism (see Chap. 38).

ERYSIPELAS   Superficial cellulitis, most commonly on face, characterized by a bright red, warm plaque sharply demarcated from surrounding normal skin. Because of superficial location of infection and associated edema, surface of plaque may exhibit a *peau d'orange* (orange peel) appearance. Most commonly due to infection with gram-positive cocci (frequently beta-hemolytic streptococci) occurring at sites of trauma or other breaks in skin.

Treatment   Appropriate antibiotics depending on organism (see Chap. 38).

SCABIES   A common infestation of children and adults due to the mite *Sarcoptes scabiei*. Often presents as pruritus, commonly worse at night. Typical lesions include burrows (short linear lesions often in web spaces of fingers) and small vesiculopapular lesions in intertriginous areas. Excoriations often with bleeding may be prominent.

Treatment   Topical lindane (e.g., Kwell).

HERPES SIMPLEX   Recurrent eruption characterized by grouped vesicles on an erythematous base that progress to erosions; often secondarily infected with staphylococci or streptococci. Tzanck preparation of an unroofed early vesicle reveals multinucleate giant cells.

Treatment   Oral or topical acyclovir; appropriate antibiotics for secondary infections depending on organism (see Chap. 38).

HERPES ZOSTER   Eruption of grouped vesicles on an erythematous base usually limited to a single dermatome; disseminated lesions also can occur, especially in immunocompromised pts. Tzanck preparation reveals multinucleate giant cells; indistinguishable from herpes simplex except by culture. Postherpetic neuralgia, lasting months to years, may occur, especially in elderly.

Treatment   No antiviral therapy indicated for localized lesions; glucocorticoids may help prevent postherpetic neuralgia.

DERMATOPHYTE INFECTION   May involve any area of body; due to infection of stratum corneum, nail plate, or hair by a skin fungus. Appearance may vary from mild scaliness to florid inflammatory dermatitis. Classic lesion of tinea corporis ("ring worm") is an erythematous papulosquamous patch often with central clearing and scale along peripheral advancing border. Hyphae are seen on potassium hydroxide preparation.

Treatment   Topical (e.g., tolnaftate or undecylenic acid) or systemic (griseofulvin 500 mg/d) antifungals.

VASCULAR DISORDERS

ERYTHEMA NODOSUM   Characterized by erythematous, warm, tender subcutaneous nodular lesions typically over anterior tibia. Lesions are usually flush with skin surface but are indurated and have appearance of an erythematous/violaceous bruise. Commonly seen in sarcoidosis, leprosy, tuberculosis, streptococcal infections, during treatment with some drugs (e.g. oral contraceptives, sulfonamides, and estrogens); may be idiopathic.

ERYTHEMA MULTIFORME   A reaction pattern of skin consisting of a variety of lesions but most commonly erythematous papules and bullae. "Target" or "iris" lesion is characteristic and consists of concentric circles of erythema and normal flesh-colored skin often with a central vesicle or bulla. Distribution of lesions classically acral, esp. palms and soles. Three most common causes include drug reaction (particularly penicillins and sulfonamides) or concurrent herpetic or *Mycoplasma* infection. Systemic glucocorticoids may be useful, but efficacy is unproven.

URTICARIA   A common disorder, either acute or chronic, characterized by evanescent (individual lesions lasting <24 h), pruritic, edematous, pink to erythematous plaques with a whitish halo around margin of individual lesions. Lesions range in size from papules (several mm in diameter) to giant coalescent lesions (10–20 cm in diameter). Often due to drugs, systemic infection, or foods (esp. shellfish). Food additives such as tartrazine dye (F.D. & C yellow no. 5), benzoate, or salicylates also have been implicated. If individual lesions last >24 h, consider diagnosis of urticarial vasculitis. See Chap. 115 for treatment.

VASCULITIS   Palpable purpura (nonblanching, elevated lesions) is the cutaneous hallmark of vasculitis. Other lesions include petechiae (esp. early lesions), necrosis with ulceration, bullae, and urticarial lesions (urticarial vasculitis). Lesions usually most prominent on lower extremities. Pathogenic factors include bacterial infections, underlying collagen-vascular disease or malignancy, hepatitis B, drugs (esp. thiazides), and inflammatory bowel disease. See Chap. 119 for therapy.

ACNE

ACNE VULGARIS   Usually a self-limited disorder of teenagers and young adults. Comedo (small cyst formed in hair follicle) is clinical hallmark; become inflamed; may scar in severe cases.

Treatment   Careful cleaning and removal of oils; oral tetracycline or erythromycin 250–1000 mg/d; topical or systemic retinoic acid.

ACNE ROSACEA   Inflammatory disorder affecting predominantly the central face. Tendency toward exaggerated flushing, with eventual superimposition of papules, pustules, and telangiectasias. May lead to rhinophyma and ocular problems.

Treatment   Oral tetracycline 250–1500 mg/d; topical metronidazole and topical nonfluorinated glucocorticoids may be useful.

For a more detailed discussion, see Lawley TJ, Swerlick RA: Eczema, Psoriasis, Cutaneous Infections, Acne, and Other Common Skin Disorders, Chap. 56, in HPIM-12, p. 307

BASAL CELL CARCINOMA Most common form of skin cancer; most frequently on sun-exposed skin, esp. face.

Predisposing factors Fair complexion, chronic UV exposure, exposure to inorganic arsenic (i.e., Fowler's solution or insecticides such as Paris green), or exposure to ionizing radiation.

Types Five general types: *noduloulcerative* (most common), *superficial* (mimics eczema), *pigmented* (may be mistaken for melanoma), *morpheaform* (plaque-like lesion with telangiectasia—with keratotic is most aggressive), *keratotic* (basosquamous carcinoma).

Clinical appearance Classically a pearly, translucent, smooth papule with rolled edges and surface telangiectasia.

Treatment Local removal; metastases rare but may spread locally.

SQUAMOUS CELL CARCINOMA Less common than basal cell but more likely to metastasize.

Predisposing factors Fair complexion, chronic UV exposure, previous burn or other scar (i.e., scar carcinoma), exposure to inorganic arsenic or ionizing radiation.

General types

1. Bowen's disease: Erythematous patch or plaque, often with scale; noninvasive; involvement limited to epidermis and epidermal appendages.

2. Scar carcinoma: Suggested by sudden change in previously stable scar, esp. if ulceration or nodules appear.

3. Verrucous carcinoma: Most commonly on plantar aspect of foot; low-grade malignancy but may be mistaken for a common wart.

Clinical appearance Hyperkeratotic papule or nodule; may be ulcerated.

Treatment Local excision; radiation therapy in selected cases.

Prognosis Favorable if secondary to UV exposure; less favorable if in sun-protected areas or associated with ionizing radiation.

MALIGNANT MELANOMA Most dangerous cutaneous malignancy; high metastatic potential; poor prognosis with metastatic spread.

Predisposing factors Fair complexion, sun exposure, family history of melanoma, dysplastic nevus syndrome (autosomal dominant disorder with multiple nevi of distinctive appearance and cutaneous melanoma), and presence of a congenital nevus (esp. if >10 cm in diameter).

Types

1. Superficial spreading melanoma: Most common; begins with initial radial growth phase prior to invasion.

2. Lentigo maligna melanoma: Very long radial growth phase prior to invasion, lentigo maligna (Hutchinson's melanotic freckle) is precursor lesion, most common in elderly and in sun-exposed areas (esp. face).

3. Acral lentiginous: Most common form in darkly pigmented pts; occurs on palms and soles, mucosal surfaces, in nail beds and mucocutaneous junctions; similar to lentigo maligna melanoma but with more aggressive biologic behavior.

4. Nodular: Generally poor prognosis because of invasive growth from onset.

Clinical appearance Generally pigmented (rarely amelanotic); color of lesions varies, but red, white, and/or blue are common, in addition to brown and/or black. Suspicion should be raised by a pigmented skin lesion that is >6 mm in diameter, asymmetric, has an irregular surface or border, or has variation in color.

Prognosis Best with thin lesions without evidence of metastatic spread; with increasing thickness or evidence of spread, prognosis worsens.

Treatment Early recognition and surgical excision best treatment; metastatic disease requires chemotherapy or immunotherapy.

For a more detailed discussion, see Swanson NA: Skin Cancer, Chap. 307, p. 1633; and Sober AJ, Koh HK: Melanoma and Other Pigmented Skin Lesions, Chap. 308, p. 1634, in HPIM-12

SECTION 14 NUTRITION

184 ASSESSMENT OF NUTRITIONAL STATUS

Obesity and severe malnutrition can be recognized by history and physical examination, but subtle forms of undernutrition are frequently overlooked, particularly in the presence of edema. Quantitative assessment of nutritional status (Table 184-1) can reveal life-threatening undernutrition and allow assessment of progress once repletion is begun. Objective indicators of nutritional status correlate with morbidity and mortality, but no single measurement is of predictive value in individual patients.

ESTIMATION OF ENERGY REQUIREMENT To formulate an overall plan for nutritional management one must consider the components of daily energy expenditure:

1. Basal metabolic rate (basal energy expenditure, BEE)
2. Activity-related expenditure
3. Diet-induced thermogenesis
4. Illness-related expenditure

Daily caloric requirements can be estimated with the Harris-Benedict equation:

$$BEE_{women} = 655 + (9.5 \times W) + (1.8 \times H - (4.7 \times A)$$
$$(kcal/d)$$
$$BEE_{men} = 66 + (13.7 \times W) + (5 \times H) - (6.8 \times A)$$
$$(kcal/d)$$

where W is actual or usual weight (kg), H is height (cm), and A is age (years).

The energy of physical activity accounts for about one-third of total energy expenditure and may vary from 1.5 to 85 (kcal/kg body wt)/h. Diet-induced thermogenesis is the heat or energy production in excess of BEE caused by the ingestion of food. A mixed diet causes a 6–10% increase above basal levels. The daily energy requirement in serious illness is only slightly increased from the well state:

- Mild illness, BEE + 10%
- Moderate illness, BEE + 25%
- Severe illness, BEE + 50%
- Malabsorption: BEE + 2.5 × fecal energy loss from fat [which equals fat excretion (g) × 38 kJ/g (9 kcal/g)]

Even during the most severe illness energy requirements rarely exceed 12,500 kJ/d (3000 kcal/d).

NITROGEN BALANCE   Estimation of nitrogen balance (nitrogen intake minus nitrogen excretion) provides assessment of adequacy of nutritional support (Table 184-1). After growth ceases, rates of anabolism and catabolism are normally in equilibrium (nitrogen balance of zero). In catabolic states (trauma, infection, burns), increased protein losses and negative nitrogen balance ensue. Nitrogen intake is protein intake divided by 6.25. Normally, 95% of nitrogen is excreted in urine as urea, the remainder (about 2.5 g) in stool and skin. Hence, total daily nitrogen excretion equals 24-h urine nitrogen + 2.5 g. Nitrogen balance assessments give insight into nutritional status during the periods of observation but not about energy or protein stores, e.g., duration of malnutrition or overnutrition.

LEAN BODY MASS (LBM)   In the absence of edema, body weight as percent of ideal is a useful indicator of adipose tissue plus LBM. Ideal body weight can be estimated from a standardized height/weight table (Table 184-2) or as follows: women, 45 kg for first 152 cm of height + 0.9 kg for each cm above 152; men, 48 kg for first 152 cm + 1.1 kg for each cm above 152. Reduction of body weight/ideal body weight ratio to ≤80% usually indicates protein-energy undernutrition.

Skeletal muscle comprises about 30% of LBM. Anthropometric measurement of LBM requires only calipers and tape measure. In the nondominant arm, triceps skinfold is pulled away from triceps muscle midway between the acromial and olecranon processes. Skinfold is then measured with calipers (mm). Midarm muscle circumference is estimated from midarm circumference and skinfold thickness by the formula in Table 184-1. Normal ranges for skin thickness and muscle circumference are so wide that measurements are most useful as baselines for individual pts.

Since creatinine excretion is a function of the amount of skeletal muscle, muscle mass can be estimated by comparing the ratio of urinary creatinine excretion (g/d) either to height (cm) or to ideal urinary creatinine excretion (23 mg/kg body weight/d for men and 18 mg/kg body weight/d for women).

THE VISCERAL COMPARTMENT   The visceral compartment comprises 20% of LBM. When nutrition is inadequate, protein

TABLE 184-1 Measures of nutritional status

| | Normal | Deficiency | | |
| | | Mild | Mod | Severe |
	0–3	–1	–2	–3
Nitrogen balance (g/24 h):				
$\dfrac{\text{Protein intake (g)}}{6.25 \text{ (g protein per g N)}} - $ 24-h urine urea nitrogen (g) + 2.5				
Body weight:				
$\dfrac{\text{Actual body weight}}{\text{Ideal body weight}} \times 100$	100	80	70–80	<70
Adipose tissue:				
Triceps skin fold (mm)	Men 8–23 Women 10–30			
Lean body mass:				
Arm muscle circumference (cm) Arm circumference − 0.314 × triceps skinfold	Men 25.3 Women 23.2			
24-h urinary creatinine/height index (mg/cm)	Men 10.5 Women 5.8	8.4–9.5 4.6–5.2	7.4–8.4 4.1–4.6	<7.4 <4.1
Visceral protein compartment:				
Serum transferrin	200–260	180–200	160–180	<160
Serum albumin (g/L)	40	35–39	25–30	<25
Immune function:				
Total lymphocyte count/μL	>1800	1500–1800	900–1500	<900
Skin test (mm induration) (Tuberculin/PPD, Candida, streptokinase/streptodornase, mumps)	>10	5–10	0–5	0

737

TABLE 184-2   Weights at ages 25 to 59 based on lowest mortality*

Height		Small Frame	Medium Frame	Large Frame
Feet	Inches			
Men				
5	2	128–134	131–141	138–150
5	3	130–136	133–143	140–153
5	4	132–138	135–145	142–156
5	5	134–140	137–148	144–160
5	6	136–142	139–151	146–164
5	7	138–145	142–154	149–168
5	8	140–148	145–157	152–172
5	9	142–151	148–160	155–176
5	10	144–154	151–163	158–180
5	11	146–157	154–166	161–184
6	0	149–160	157–170	164–188
6	1	152–164	160–174	168–192
6	2	155–168	164–178	172–197
6	3	158–172	167–182	176–202
6	4	162–176	171–187	181–207
Women				
4	10	102–111	109–121	118–131
4	11	103–113	111–123	120–134
5	0	104–115	113–126	122–137
5	1	106–118	115–129	125–140
5	2	108–121	118–132	128–143
5	3	111–124	121–135	131–147
5	4	114–127	124–138	134–151
5	5	117–130	127–141	137–155
5	6	120–133	130–144	140–159
5	7	123–136	133–147	143–163
5	8	126–139	136–150	146–167
5	9	129–142	139–153	149–170
5	10	132–145	142–156	152–173
5	11	135–148	145–159	155–176
6	0	138–151	148–162	158–179

*Assumes indoor clothing weighing 5 lb for men and 3 lb for women; shoes with 1-in heels.
Source: Metropolitan Life Insurance Co., 1983.

synthesis declines, and metabolic pathways are altered; severe malnutrition impairs the immune system. Serum albumin and transferrin are sensitive indicators of the visceral protein pool. Transferrin has an average half-life of 8 d and provides a sensitive indicator of protein repletion after refeeding.

Immune competence requires normal protein nutrition (Table 184-1). Lymphocyte depletion and anergy to skin antigens (*Candida albicans,* mumps, streptokinase/streptodornase, and tuberculin/PPD) are associated with increase in morbidity and mortality. These parameters may revert to normal within weeks of initiating protein-energy repletion.

Once refeeding is initiated in the malnourished pt, weekly monitoring of weight, albumin, creatinine excretion, midarm circumference, skin thickness, and immune function should be performed.

For a more detailed discussion, see Rosenberg IH, Nutrition and Nutritional Requirements, Chap. 70, p. 403, and Mason JB, Rosenberg IH: Protein Energy Malnutrition, Chap. 71, p. 406, in HPIM-12

Malnutrition is common among alcoholics and the poor, elderly, and chronically ill. In hospitalized pts, common deficiency states are protein-energy undernutrition, beriberi, and scurvy. Vitamin excess, in contrast, is a disorder of affluence, due either to misguided nutritional concepts held by subjects themselves or therapeutic errors of physicians.

PROTEIN AND ENERGY UNDERNUTRITION Insufficient consumption of protein and energy causes progressive loss of lean body mass (LBM) and adipose tissue. Overt clinical deficiency develops when hypermetabolism, catabolism, anorexia, infection, or other illness supervene. Two syndromes of protein-energy malnutrition are: (1) *marasmus* (calorie deficiency), evident as stunted growth (children), loss of adipose tissue, generalized wasting of LBM without edema; and (2) *kwashiorkor* (protein deficiency), manifested by hypoalbuminemia, generalized edema, "flaky paint" dermatosis, enlarged, fatty liver, and relative preservation of adipose tissue. These syndromes rarely present in pure form and generally overlap.

The manifestations are often apparent on examination. A history of inadequate energy and protein intake is elicited. Listlessness, easy fatigability, swollen ankles, and cracked, dry skin may be accompanied by temporal wasting, exaggerated intercostal spaces, and dyspigmentation of skin and hair. Reversible alterations occur in cardiac structure, function, and conduction. In advanced cases, decubitus ulcers, hypothermia, and terminal infection supervene. Midarm and midarm muscle area and the ratio of 24-h urinary creatinine/height are decreased. Serum albumin, transferrin, and Hct are low. Immune function is impaired, and T-lymphocyte function is decreased, as evidenced by cutaneous anergy and lymphopenia (absolute lymphocyte count < 1200 cells/μL). Hormonal abnormalities include low circulating levels of insulin, increased growth hormone and glucagon, decreased somatomedins, and increased glucocorticoids. Serum triiodothyronine (T_3) and thyroxine (T_4) are decreased, and reverse T_3 is increased. Gonadal dysfunction may be primary or secondary.

Mortality rates vary from 15–40%, and institution of nutritional replacement is a medical emergency. Stupor, jaundice, petechiae, hyponatremia, and hypovitaminosis A are ominous signs. Death may be due to electrolyte imbalance, infection, hypothermia, or circulatory failure.

VITAMIN DEFICIENCY Vitamins of clinical significance are listed in Table 185-1, and recommended dietary allowances for vitamins and trace elements are given in Table 185-2.

Thiamine deficiency (beriberi) Thiamine deficiency occurs in alcoholics and food faddists or after chronic peritoneal dialysis, refeeding (without adequate thiamine) after starvation, or administration of glucose to asymptomatic thiamine-depleted pts. Clinical manifestations develop in only a fraction of subjects at risk, and genetic factors may be involved in susceptibility. The recommended dietary allowance (RDA) is 1.2–1.5 mg. Major manifestations involve the cardiovascular (wet beriberi) and nervous systems (dry beriberi). The typical pt has mixed symptoms involving both systems.

Beriberi heart disease comprises three derangements: (1) peripheral vasodilation leading to increased AV shunting and increased cardiac output, (2) biventricular myocardial failure, and (3) edema. Acute fulminant (shoshin) beriberi is characterized by myocardial dysfunction resulting in severe dyspnea, extreme tachycardia, restlessness, anxiety, marked cardiomegaly, hepatomegaly, "stocking-glove" cyanosis, atrial bruits, neck vein distention, and minimal or absent edema. Acute cardiovascular collapse and death can occur within hours to days.

In dry beriberi, peripheral neuropathy may or may not be painful and is characterized by symmetric impairment of sensory, motor, and reflex function that is more severe in distal segments of limbs. *Wernicke's encephalopathy* develops in an orderly sequence and consists of vomiting, nystagmus, palsies of the rectus muscles leading to ophthalmoplegia, fever, ataxia, and mental deterioration, eventuating in a global confusional state and even coma or death. Improvement occurs after thiamine replacement, although *Korsakoff's syndrome* may supervene, consisting of retrograde amnesia, impaired learning ability, and (usually) confabulation. Diagnosis is based upon clinical response to thiamine replacement. A decrease in heart rate, and occurrence or worsening of hypertension may occur within 12 h. The most reliable laboratory test is documentation of decreased erythrocyte transketolase activity. An increase in enzyme activity of more than 15% upon addition of thiamine diphosphate suggests a deficiency state. Treatment initially is 50 mg/d thiamine IM for several days, after which 2.5–5 mg/d can be given PO. Pts should also receive a multivitamin daily.

Riboflavin deficiency Deficiency almost invariably occurs in combination with other vitamin deficiencies. The RDA is 1.4–1.8 mg. An inadequate diet, especially in the

TABLE 185-1 Vitamins of clinical significance

Vitamin	Source	Major cause of deficiency	Clinical manifestation
Thiamine (B_1)	Wide distribution; rapidly destroyed by cooking	Alcoholism, highly refined diet	Wet beriberi: high output CHF; dry beriberi: peripheral neuropathy, Wernicke's encephalopathy, Korsakoff syndrome
Riboflavin (B_2)	Milk, meat, fish, leafy vegetables; destroyed by cooking	Alcoholism, malignancy	Sore mouth and tongue, glossitis, angular stomatis, dermatitis, anemia
Niacin (B_5) (nicotinic acid)	Whole-grain cereals, nuts, fish, meat; 60 mg tryptophan is converted to 1 mg niacin	Alcoholism, inadequate diet of amino acids	Pellagra: diarrhea, dermatitis, dementia
Pyridoxine (B_6)	Meats, vegetables, whole-grain cereals	Alcoholism, pregnancy; drugs: isoniazid, dopamine, estrogens, penicillamine	Seborrheic dermatitis, cheilosis, glossitis, nausea, vomiting, weakness, dizziness, peripheral neuropathy
Cobalamin (B_{12})	Liver, kidney, eggs, milk; gastric intrinsic factor required for absorption	Impaired absorption: gastric abnormalities, intestinal abnormalities, pancreatic insufficiency	Megaloblastic anemia, irritability, confusion, glossitis, fever, orthostatic hypotension, peripheral neuropathy, diarrhea
Ascorbic acid (C)	Fresh vegetables, citrus fruit	Inadequate diet, urban poverty	Scurvy: purpura, hemorrhages into joints and muscles, bleeding gums, loose teeth

Folic acid (C)	Green leafy vegetables	Defective absorption; impaired utilization: alcoholism, vitamin B_{12} deficiency; Increased requirements: chronic hemodialysis, hyperthyroidism, pregnancy	Megaloblastic anemia, diarrhea, cheilosis, glossitis
Retinol (A)	Animal foods, β-carotene in plant sources	Developed countries: malabsorption, TPN;* developing countries: inadequate diet	Night blindness, xerophthalmia (dry cornea and conjunctiva), keratomalacia, dry hyperkeratotic skin
Vitamin D	Fortified milk and other foods (D_2), fish, egg yolk, butter (D_3); endogenous conversion	Inadequate sunlight, inadequate diet, TPN	Rickets (children), osteomalacia (adults), osteoporosis, muscle weakness, muscle cramps, tetany, seizures
Vitamin E	Oils, fruits, vegetables, whole-grain foods	Chronic biliary obstruction, cystic fibrosis, abetalipoproteinemia	Areflexia, gait disturbances, ophthalmoplegia, poor proprioception and vibratory sense, edema, hemolytic anemia
Vitamin K	Vegetables; synthesis by bacteria	Anticoagulants, malabsorption, antibiotics, TPN	Bleeding

*TPN = total parenteral nutrition.

TABLE 185-2   **Recommended dietary allowances for healthy adults**

	Range of allowance	
	Men	Women
Protein, g	45–63	44–50
Vitamin A, μg retinol equivalents	1000	800
Vitamin D, μg	5–10	5–10
Vitamin E, mg α-tocopherol equivalents	10	8
Vitamin K, μg	45–80	45–65
Vitamin C, mg	50–60	50–60
Thiamine, mg	1.2–1.5	1–1.1
Riboflavin, mg	1.4–1.8	1.2–1.3
Niacin, mg niacin equivalents	15–20	13–15
Vitamin B_6, mg	1.4–2.0	1.4–1.6
Folate, μg	150–200	150–180
Vitamin B_{12}, μg	2.0	2.0
Biotin, μg*	30–100	50–100
Pantothenic acid, mg*	4–10	4–7
Calcium, mg	800–1200	800–1200
Phosphorus, mg	800–1200	800–1200
Magnesium, mg	270–400	280–300
Iron, mg	10–12	10–15
Zinc, mg	15	12
Iodine, μg	150	150
Selenium, μg	40–70	45–55
Copper, mg*	1.5–3	1.5–3
Manganese, mg*	2–5	2–5
Fluoride, mg*	1.5–4	1.5–4
Chromium, μg*	50–200	50–200
Molybdenum, μg*	75–250	75–250

*Estimated safe and adequate daily dietary intakes. From the National Research Council: *Recommended Dietary Allowances,* 10th ed. Washington, D.C., National Academy of Sciences, 1989.

setting of alcoholism or malignancy, is the major cause. Manifestations include soreness or burning of the mouth, tongue, and throat; hyperemia and edema of mucous membranes; glossitis; angular stomatitis; seborrheic dermatitis; and normochromic normocytic anemia due to red cell hypoplasia of the bone marrow. Multivitamin supplementation is recommended.

Niacin deficiency (pellagra)   Niacin is not a true vitamin because it can be formed from the essential amino acid tryptophan; 1 mg of niacin is formed for every 60 mg of tryptophan. Deficiency is usually associated with high intake of maize or millet and can be a secondary manifestation of carcinoid syndrome and Hartnup disease. Pellagra is a chronic wasting disease associated with diarrhea, dermatitis, and dementia. The dermatitis is bilateral, symmetric, desquamative, hyperpigmented, and photosensitive. Mucosal abnormalities include achlorhydria, glossitis, stomatitis, and vaginitis. Fatigue, apathy, and insomnia may precede development of encephalopathy. Niacin (10 g/d) with adequate dietary tryptophan is sufficient to cure pellagra. Niacin 20–40 mg/d may be required in Hartnup disease and carcinoid syndrome.

Pyridoxine (B$_6$) deficiency The RDA is 1.4–2.0 mg. Deficiency occurs in alcoholism and pregnancy and with drugs that act as pyridoxine antagonists: isoniazid, cycloserine, penicillamine, and oral contraceptive agents. Appropriate management includes supplementation of diet with 30 mg/d PO. Doses ≤100 mg/d may be required in patients given penicillamine.

Cobalamin (B$_{12}$) deficiency The RDA is 2 μg. Once the mechanism of deficiency is established, replacement is initiated with 100 μg IM qd for the first week, and a total of 2000 μg is recommended during the first 6 weeks of therapy. Thereafter, treatment is 100 μg IM every month. Reticulocytosis should occur after 4–5 days of therapy (see also Chap. 130).

Ascorbic acid deficiency (scurvy) Scurvy now usually occurs in areas of urban poverty. Many manifestations result from defective collagen synthesis, including perifollicular hyperkeratotic papules in which hairs become fragmented and buried; purpura beginning on the backs of the lower extremities coalescing to ecchymoses; hemorrhage into muscles of the extremities with secondary phlebothromboses; hemorrhages into joints; splinter hemorrhages in nailbeds; swelling, friability, bleeding, and secondary infection of gums and loosening of the teeth. Terminally, icterus, edema, and fever are common, and convulsions, shock, and death may occur abruptly.

If diagnosis is suspected, blood should be obtained for measurement of platelet ascorbate levels (if available), and ascorbic acid should be administered promptly. The usual dose in adults is 100 mg three to five times a day PO until 4 g has been administered, then 100 mg/d. Spontaneous bleeding, muscle and bone pain, and gums begin to improve within 2–3 d, and large ecchymoses resolve in 10–12 d.

Folic acid deficiency The RDA is 150–200 μg. Pts with this deficiency are malnourished. Megaloblastic anemia, GI symptoms, diarrhea, cheilosis, and glossitis are seen, but no neurologic abnormalities are present. The usual treatment is 1 mg/d PO, and a brisk hematologic response occurs after 4–5 d of therapy. Folate replacement can correct the anemia of B$_{12}$ deficiency but will not alter or may worsen the

TABLE 185-3 Vitamin excess

	Major cause	Clinical manifestation
Vitamin A and carotenes: carotenemia	Excess ingestion of carrots	Yellowing of skin (sclera remain white)
Hypervitaminosis A	Accidental overingestion by hunters (polar bear liver), food faddism, inappropriate therapy	Acute toxicity: abdominal pain, nausea, vomiting, headache, dizziness, sluggishness, papilledema, bulging fontanel in infants, followed by generalized desquamation of skin and recovery
		Chronic toxicity ($\geq 25,000$ U/d): bone and joint pain, hyperostoses, hair loss, dryness and fissures of lips, anorexia, benign intracranial hypertension, low grade fever, pruritus, weight loss
Hypervitaminosis D	Excessive ingestion, inappropriate therapy	Hypercalcemia, hyperphosphatemia, nausea, vomiting, dehydration, pruritus, azotemia, ectopic calcification, CNS manifestation
Hypervitaminosis E	Excessive ingestion	True toxicity described in oral anticoagulant users and premature infants
Pyridoxine	Excessive ingestion	Peripheral neuropathy, ataxia, perioral numbness
Niacin	Excessive ingestion	Flushing, pruritus, GI disturbances, elevated uric acid, hyperglycemia

neurologic abnormalities. Vitamin B_{12} deficiency must be excluded by laboratory testing. To test for folate deficiency both a red-cell folate and a B_{12} level must be obtained. A serum folate measurement is less sensitive.

Vitamin A deficiency The RDA for retinol is 800 µg/d for women and 1000 µg/d for men. Night blindness is the earliest symptom of deficiency, followed by conjunctival changes. This responds well to 30,000 IU of vitamin A daily for a week. Corneal damage constitutes a therapeutic emergency; treatment is 20,000 IU/kg body weight for 5 d.

Vitamin D deficiency (see Chap. 150 "Hyper- and Hypocalcemic Disorders")

Vitamin E deficiency The RDA is 10–30 mg/d. The vitamin is widely distributed in food, so a pure dietary deficiency state has never been recognized in otherwise healthy adults and children. Intestinal fat malabsorption is the most common cause. Treatment (50–100 IU/d) is most effective when initiated early.

VITAMIN EXCESS (See Table 185-3)

DISORDERS OF MINERAL METABOLISM (See Table 185-4)

TABLE 185-4 Disorders of metal metabolism in humans

Element	Deficiency	Excess
Fe	Anemia	Hepatic failure, diabetes, testicular atrophy, arthritis, cardiomyopathy, peripheral neuropathy, hyperpigmentation
Zn	Growth retardation, alopecia, dermatitis, diarrhea, immunologic dysfunction, failure to thrive, psychological disturbances, gonadal atrophy, impaired spermatogenesis, congenital malformations.	Gastric ulcer, pancreatitis lethargy, anemia, fever, nausea, vomiting, respiratory distress, pulmonary fibrosis
Cu	Anemia, growth retardation, defective keratinization and pigmentation of hair, hypothermia, degenerative changes in aortic elastin, mental deterioration, scurvy-like changes in skeleton	Hepatitis, cirrhosis, tremor, mental deterioration, Kayser-Fleischer rings, hemolytic anemia, renal dysfunction (Fanconi-like syndrome)
Mn	Bleeding disorder (increased prothrombin time)	Encephalitis-like syndrome, Parkinson-like syndrome, psychosis, pneumoconiosis

TABLE 185-4   Disorders of metal metabolism in humans
(*Continued*)

Element	Deficiency	Excess
Co	Anemia (B_{12} deficiency)	Cardiomyopathy, goiter
Mo	? Esophageal cancer	? Hyperuricemia
Cr	? Impairment of glucose tolerance	Renal failure, dermatitis (occupational), pulmonary cancer
Se	Cardiomyopathy, CHF, striated muscle degeneration	Alopecia, abnormal nails, emotional lability, lassitude, garlic odor to breath
Ni	?	Dermatitis (occupational), lung and nasal carcinomas, liver necrosis, pulmonary inflammation
Si	? Impaired early bone development	Pulmonary inflammation, granuloma, fibrosis
F	? Impaired bone and dental structure	Mottled dental enamel, nausea, abdominal pain, vomiting, diarrhea, tetany, cardiovascular collapse

From Falchuk KH: HPIM-12, p. 444.

For a more detailed discussion, see Mason JB, Rosenberg IH: Protein-Energy Malnutrition, Chap. 71, p. 406; Falchuk KH: Disturbances in Trace Element Metabolism, Chap. 77, p. 443; and Wilson JD: Vitamin Deficiency and Excess, Chap. 76, p. 434 in HPIM-12

Anorexia nervosa and bulimia are eating disorders predominantly in young women who develop a paralyzing fear of becoming fat. In anorexia nervosa, this fear causes radical restriction of energy intake, the end result being emaciation. In bulimia, massive binge eating is followed by self-induced vomiting and laxative abuse. Separation of the two conditions is not always clearcut (Table 186-1).

ANOREXIA NERVOSA (Table 186-2) While hypothalamic dysfunction (impaired regulation of gonadotropins, partial diabetes insipidus, and abnormal thermoregulation) is common in anorexia, most investigators favor a psychiatric cause. Interpersonal communication among family members tends to be inadequate, and there is a pathologic focus within family on food and eating behavior. Anorexia nervosa usually becomes apparent before or shortly after puberty. Despite

TABLE 186-1 The eating disorders

	Anorexia nervosa	Bulimia
Predominant sex	Female	Female
Method of weight control	Restriction of intake	Vomiting
Binge eating	Uncommon	Invariant
Weight at diagnosis	Markedly decreased	Near normal
Ritualized exercise	Usual	Rare
Amenorrhea	~100%	~50%
Antisocial behavior	Rare	Frequent
Cardiovascular changes (bradycardia, hypotension)	Common	Uncommon
Skin changes (hirsutism, dryness, carotenemia)	Usual	Rare
Hypothermia	Usual	Rare
Edema	+/−	+/−
Medical complications	Hypokalemia, cardiac arrhythmias	Hypokalemia, cardiac arrhythmias, aspiration of gastric contents, esophageal or gastric rupture

NOTE: These features are characteristic of pure anorexia nervosa and pure bulimia. Overlap syndromes occur, and anorexia may evolve to bulimia (the bulimia→ anorexia transformation is rare).
From Foster DW: HPIM-12, p. 418.

TABLE 186-2 Criteria for the diagnosis of anorexia nervosa

1. Onset prior to age 25
2. Anorexia with weight loss of at least 25% of original body weight
3. Distorted attitude toward eating, food, or weight that overrides hunger, admonitions, reassurances, and threats
4. No known medical illness that could account for the weight loss
5. No other known psychiatric disorder
6. At least two of the following manifestations:
   a. Amenorrhea
   b. Lanugo hair
   c. Bradycardia (persistent resting pulse of 60 beats per min or less)
   d. Periods of overactivity
   e. Episodes of bulimia
   f. Vomiting (may be self-induced)

From Foster DW: HPIM-12, p. 420. After Feighner et al, Arch Gen Psychiatry 26:59, 1972.

emaciation, pts deny hunger, thinness, or fatigue. Amenorrhea is common and may precede anorexia. Body fat may be undetectable, but breast tissue is often preserved. Parotid gland enlargement and edema may be accompanied by anemia, leukopenia, hypokalemia, and hypoalbuminemia. Basal luteinizing hormone (LH) and follicle-stimulating hormone (FSH) are low, accounting for the amenorrhea. Menses usually return with weight gain.

BULIMIA In bulimia episodic ingestion of large amounts of food in uncontrollable fashion is associated with an awareness that the eating pattern is abnormal, a fear that the eating cannot be stopped voluntarily, and feelings of depression after the act. Eating episodes are followed by induced vomiting, with or without ingestion of laxatives. Secrecy about the eating/vomiting sequence is characteristic. Weight loss is not as profound as with anorexia, and half continue to menstruate. Hypokalemia and metabolic alkalosis may be present.

COURSE The course of anorexia and bulimia is variable. Mortality is about 5–6%, major causes of death being starvation and suicide. Poor prognostic signs include onset after age 20, longer duration of illness, prominent vomiting, extreme weight loss, and significant depression.

THERAPY No specific therapy exists. Supportive treatment involves a combination of psychotherapy, family counseling, and hospitalization for nutritional support if malnutrition is severe or if hypokalemia, hypotension, or prerenal azotemia is present. Antidepressants may be used with some success. Treatment is long-term, rife with failure, and requires perseverance by subject, family, and physician.

For a more detailed discussion, see Foster DW: Anorexia Nervosa and Bulimia, Chap. 73, in HPIM-12, p. 417

187 OBESITY

Obesity implies ≥20% excess above ideal body weight, and a fifth of men and a third of women are obese. Mild obesity may not impart significant risk, but men who weigh 150–300% of ideal body weight have mortality rates 12 times those of nonobese men.

Excess weight can be assessed by comparison with standard tables for height and weight (see Table 184-2) or by calculation of body mass index (body weight in kg/height in meters). More precise estimates of adiposity may be obtained by skinfold measurements with skin calipers (see Table 184-1).

Most obesity is due to overeating. Genetic, environmental, and social factors are involved, but ultimately regulation of eating depends on interaction between hunger and satiety centers of hypothalamus, modulated by input from cerebral cortex. When energy intake exceeds expenditure, excess energy is stored in adipose tissue; if net positive energy balance is prolonged, obesity results.

Secondary obesity can be due to a variety of disorders. *Hypothyroidism* can cause obesity secondary to diminished energy needs. *Cushing's disease* causes obesity involving centripetal fat stores, the face, and cervical or supraclavicular fat deposits. *Insulinoma* causes obesity from increased energy intake secondary to recurrent hypoglycemia. Laurence-Moon-Biedl and Prader-Willis syndromes are rare disorders, thought to be hypothalamic in origin, and feature obesity and hypogonadism.

Obesity causes morbidity and mortality primarily through cardiovascular complications and sudden death. Impaired glucose tolerance and fasting hyperlipidemia may occur. Morbid obesity also produces mechanical and physical stresses that predispose to or aggravate osteoarthritis, thromboembolism, cholelithiasis, hypertension, hypoventilation, and hypoxemia.

Energy restriction is the cornerstone of weight reduction. Hyperinsulinemia, insulin resistance, diabetes, hypertension, and hyperlipidemia are ameliorated following weight loss. By estimating daily energy needs [approximately 138 kJ/kg (33 kcal/kg)], one can calculate the daily deficit needed to achieve a given rate of weight loss, which should be targeted at 0.5–1 kg per week. Low-energy diets should be balanced in protein, carbohydrate, and fat and should provide minerals and vitamins. Pts should be monitored closely while on weight-loss regimens (Table 187-1). Drugs are both ineffective in promoting weight loss and produce serious side effects and hence have no role in treatment.

Surgical treatment should be reserved for pts who have failed standard weight-reduction regimens and maintain a weight 50–100% over ideal body weight. Small-bowel bypass is effective in achieving weight reduction in such pts, but complications are common. Gastroplasty establishes a small upper gastric remnant attached to a larger gastric pouch by a 1.0–1.5 cm channel and thus delays gastric emptying. Weight loss with this procedure is without severe metabolic consequences.

A major problem in treatment is maintenance of reduced weight following weight loss. Techniques of behavior modification are sometimes useful.

TABLE 187-1 Complications of therapy for obesity

Treatment	Complication
DIETARY	
Total starvation	Anemia, hyperuricemia, gout, ketosis, potassium depletion, cardiac arryhthmias, sudden death
Carbohydrate depletion	Excessive water excretion, acidosis, ketosis, bone demineralization, cardiac arrhythmias, hypokalemia, hyperlipidemia
High-protein diet	Hypokalemia, cardiac arrhythmias
DRUG	
Diuretics	Hypokalemia, volume depletion, metabolic alkalosis
Laxatives	Hypokalemia, metabolic acidosis
Anorexiants	Cardiac arrhythmias, anxiety
Thyroid supplements	Cardiac arrhythmias, anxiety
SURGERY	
Jejunoileal bypass	Diarrhea, electrolyte disturbances, hepatic cirrhosis, urinary calculi, arthritis, cholelithiasis
Gastroplasty	Gastric outlet obstruction

For a more detailed discussion, see Olefsky JM: Obesity, Chap. 72, in HPIM-12, p. 411

188 DIET THERAPY

Diet prescription is essential for all hospitalized pts (Table 188-1), recognizing that for most a regular hospital diet containing about 8400–9200 kJ (2000–2200 kcal) and fed in three meals of $\frac{1}{5}$, $\frac{2}{5}$, and $\frac{2}{5}$ proportion will suffice.

Average energy expenditure is $1.37 \times$ basal energy expenditure $- 312$. For usual pt, recommended intake should equal energy expenditure. To maintain a positive energy balance when energy expenditure is increased (burns, infection, trauma, surgery, hyperthyroidism), energy intake should be 1.5–$2 \times$ this value.

In healthy adults, recommended protein intake is 0.8 (g/kg body weight)/d, but under conditions of stress, requirement may increase to 2–4 (g/kg body weight)/d. Optimal ratio of kJ (kcal) to g protein intake in the healthy individual is 625:1 (150:1), and intermediate ratios may be appropriate in conditions of altered growth or repair needs.

Needs for special restrictions and/or additions to diet depend on diagnosis (Table 188-1). Administration can be *oral intake, tube feeding,* or *parenterally.* For oral intake, consistency can vary from clear liquid to pureed or soft to regular, and for tube feedings and parenteral formulas, concentration and osmolality must be specified.

TUBE FEEDING When oral intake is inadequate or the GI tract is incapable of absorbing sufficient nutrients, enteral feeding may be indicated (Table 188-2). Such situations include anorexia, neurologic disorders such as dysphagia or cerebrovascular accidents, and malignancy. Enteral routes include nasogastric and nasoduodenal tubes, jejunostomy tubes, and gastrostomy tubes placed by percutaneous endoscopy. Small-bore Silastic or polyurethane tubes are as-

TABLE 188-1 Principles of diet prescription

Assess energy and protein needs
Designate route of administration:
  oral intake, tube feeding, parenteral nutrition
Select texture and/or concentration
Specify frequency and/or rate of feeding
Designate special restrictions:
  Na, Ca, K, fluid, gastric irritants, fiber, residue, gluten, fat, carbohydrate, protein, purine, tyrosine, galactose, sucrose, oxalate, lactate
Designate special additions:
  fiber, medium chain triglycerides, vitamins, prepared nutritional supplements

TABLE 188-2 Examples of formulas for tube feeding

Example	Osmolality mosmol/kg	kcal/*mL or g	Volume for 100% RDA,† mL/day	Composition, g/1000 kcal*			Electrolytes, mg/1000 kcal*	
				Protein/ amino acids	Carbohydrate	Fat	Na	K
ELEMENTAL								
Vivonex HN	810	1	3000	46	210	1	529	1173
Vital	460	1	1500	42	188	11	383	1167
Travasorb HN	560	1	2000	45	175	13	920	1170
POLYMERIC								
Sustacal	625	1	1080	60	138	23	920	2060
Osmolite HN	300	1	1400	44	131	47	708	1179
Ensure	450	1.1	1900	35	135	35	500	1250
Isocal	300	1.1	1900	32	125	42	704	1267
Ensure Plus HN	600	1.5	1920	37	133	35		
Two Cal HN	750	2	960	40	200	90		
MODULAR								
Polycose‡	850	2	NA	0	250	0	290	100
Casec‡	NA	3.7	NA	230	0	5	408	0
MCT oil‡	NA	7.7	NA	0	0	120	0	0

* For kJ multiply kcal by 4.1186.
† Recommended dietary allowance.
‡ Does not contain vitamins.

sociated with low rates of nasopharyngitis, rhinitis, otitis media, and stricture formation.

Elemental formulas   Composed of di- and tripeptides and/or amino acids, glucose oligosaccharides, and vegetable oils or medium-chain triglycerides. Residue is minimal, and little digestion is required. Such formulas may be of use in pts with short bowel syndrome, partial small bowel obstruction, pancreatic insufficiency, inflammatory bowel disease, radiation enteritis, or bowel fistula.

Polymeric formulas   Contain complex nutrients and can be used in most pts with a functional GI tract.

To initiate bolus feeding, 50–100 mL of isotonic or slightly hypotonic liquid is given q 3 h. This may be increased by 50 mL increments, if tolerated, until the daily target is reached. Gastric residual should not exceed 100 mL 2 h after feeding. If this occurs, hold the next feeding and recheck residual in 1 h.

Continuous gastric infusion is initiated with half-strength diet at a rate of 25–50 mL/h. This can be advanced as tolerated to full strength and energy target. The head of the bed must be kept elevated.

Complications of enteral feeding include:

1. Diarrhea
2. Gastric distention/retention
3. Aspiration
4. Electrolyte imbalances
   hyponatremia
   hyperosmolarity
5. Volume overload
6. Warfarin resistance
7. Sinusitis
8. Esophagitis

SINGLE-NUTRIENT MODULES FOR PROTEIN, CARBOHYDRATE, AND FAT   Can be combined to create formulas for specialized requirements, e.g., a high-energy, low-protein, low-sodium formula for a cachetic cirrhotic pt with ascites and encephalopathy.

PARENTERAL NUTRITION   When pts cannot eat or deteriorate on oral feeding, partial or complete nourishment via the parenteral route is needed. Indications for total parenteral nutrition (TPN) include malnourished pts who cannot tolerate oral feedings; bowel rest in pts with regional enteritis; well-nourished pts who require 10–14 d of abstinence from oral intake; prolonged coma when tube feeding is not possible; nutritional support in pts with hypercatabolism such as sepsis, burns, or trauma; pts receiving chemotherapy that precludes oral intake; and prophylactic use in malnourished pts undergoing surgery.

TPN should generally provide 140–170 kJ (32–40 kcal) per kg body weight and basal water intake of 0.3 mL/kJ (1.2 mL/kcal) per day. To this should be added a volume equivalent to losses from diarrhea, stomal output, nasogastric suction, and fistula drainage (Table 188-3). In oliguric pts, a basal intake of 750–1000 mL fluid should be given, plus a volume equal to urine and other losses. In edematous pts, Na intake should be limited to 20–40 mmoL/d.

Positive nitrogen balance can usually be achieved by infusing 0.5–1.0 g amino acids per kg of body weight/d, together with nonprotein energy. The protein-sparing effect of carbohydrate and fat is maximal at around 230–250 kJ (55–60 kcal) per kg ideal body weight/d. Carbohydrates and lipids can be infused with amino acids to provide sufficient nonprotein calories using a Y connector. A mixture in which lipid provides half the energy simulates the normal diet, causes neither hyperinsulinemia nor hyperglycemia, and eliminates the need for exogenous insulin.

Complications related to catheter insertion include pneumothorax, thrombophlebitis, catheter embolism, and hyperglycemia (from hypertonic glucose infusions). Disseminated candidiasis may occur after prolonged nutritional support. Hypokalemia, hypomagnesemia, and hypophosphatemia may result in disorientation, convulsions, and coma. Hyperchloremic acidosis may occur with inadequate sodium acetate supplementation. Hypoglycemia may result from abrupt discontinuation of the TPN secondary to relative insulin excess. The infusion rate should be tapered over 12 h, or a 10% dextrose infusion should be substituted for several hours.

TABLE 188-3 Representative daily protocols for TPN

Components	Fat free	50% Lipid	85% Lipid
Amino acids, g	60	60	75
Glucose, g	750	375	187
Lipids, g	0	100	150
Electrolyte mix, mL	60	60	60
Trace element mix, mL	5	5	5
Vitamins, mL	10	10	10
Na$^+$, mg	125	125	132
K$^+$, mg	81	80	87
Total kcal	2550	2375	2286
Total volume, mL	3075	2775	3075

* For kJ multiply kcal by 4.186.

For a more detailed discussion, see Dwyer JT, Roy J: Diet Therapy, Chap. 74, p. 420; and Howard LJ: Parenteral and Enteral Nutrition Therapy, Chap. 75, p. 427 in HPIM-12

SECTION 15

189 ADVERSE DRUG REACTIONS

Adverse drug reactions are among the most frequent problems encountered clinically and represent a common cause for hospitalization. They are caused by

1. Errors in self-administration of prescribed drugs (quite common in the elderly).
2. Exaggeration of intended pharmacologic effect (e.g., hypotension in a pt given antihypertensive drugs).
3. Concomitant administration of drugs with synergistic effects (e.g., aspirin and warfarin).
4. Cytotoxic reactions (e.g., hepatic necrosis due to acetaminophen).
5. Immunologic mechanisms (e.g., quinidine-induced thrombocytopenia, hydralazine-induced SLE).
6. Genetically determined enzymatic defects (e.g., primaquine-induced hemolytic anemia in G6PD deficiency).
7. Idiosyncratic reactions (e.g., chloramphenicol-induced aplastic anemia).

Table 189-1 lists a number of clinical manifestations of adverse effects of drugs. It is not designed to be complete or exhaustive.

TABLE 189-1 Clinical manifestations of adverse reactions to drugs

I MULTISYSTEM MANIFESTATIONS

Anaphylaxis
  Cephalosporins
  Dextran
  Insulin
  Iodinated drugs or contrast
    media
  Lidocaine
  Penicillins
  Procaine
Angioedema
  ACE inhibitors

Drug-induced lupus
erythematosus
  Cephalosporins
  Hydralazine
  Iodides
  Isoniazid
  Methyldopa
  Phenytoin
  Procainamide

Continued

TABLE 189-1   Clinical manifestations of adverse reactions to drugs (*continued*)

I MULTISYSTEM MANIFESTATIONS (*Cont.*)

Drug-induced lupus (*Cont.*)
  Quinidine
  Sulfonamides
  Thiouracil
Fever
  Aminosalicylic acid
  Amphotericin B
  Antihistamines

  Penicillins
Hyperpyrexia
  Antipsychotics
Serum sickness
  Aspirin
  Penicillins
  Propylthiouracil
  Sulfonamides

II ENDOCRINE MANIFESTATIONS

Addisonian-like syndrome
  Busulfan
  Ketoconazole
Galactorrhea (may also cause
  amenorrhea)
  Methyldopa
  Phenothiazines
  Tricyclic antidepressants
Gynecomastia
  Calcium channel antagonists
  Digitalis
  Estrogens
  Griseofulvin
  Isoniazid
  Methyldopa
  Phenytoin
  Spironolactone
  Testosterone
Sexual dysfunction
  Beta blockers
  Clonidine
  Diuretics

  Guanethidine
  Lithium
  Major tranquilizers
  Methyldopa
  Oral contraceptives
  Sedatives
**Thyroid function tests,
disorders of**
  Acetazolamide
  Amiodarone
  Chlorpropamide
  Clofibrate
  Colestipol and nicotinic acid
  Gold salts
  Iodides
  Lithium
  Oral contraceptives
  Phenothiazines
  Phenylbutazone
  Phenytoin
  Sulfonamides
  Tolbutamide

III METABOLIC MANIFESTATIONS

Hyperbilirubinemia
  Rifampin
Hypercalcemia
  Antacids with absorbable alkali
  Thiazides
  Vitamin D
Hyperglycemia
  Chlorthalidone
  Diazoxide
  Encainide
  Ethacrynic acid
  Furosemide
  Glucocorticoids

  Growth hormone
  Oral contraceptives
  Thiazides
Hypoglycemia
  Insulin
  Oral hypoglycemics
  Quinine
Hyperkalemia
  ACE inhibitors
  Amiloride
  Cytotoxics
  Digitalis overdose
  Heparin

Continued

TABLE 189-1   Clinical manifestations of adverse reactions to drugs (*continued*)

III METABOLIC MANIFESTATIONS (*Cont.*)

Hyperkalemia (*Cont.*)
  Lithium
  Potassium preparations
    including salt substitute
  Potassium salts of drugs
  Spironolactone
  Succinylcholine
  Triamterene
Hypokalemia
  Alkali-induced alkalosis
  Amphotericin B
  Diuretics
  Gentamicin
  Insulin
  Laxative abuse
  Mineralocorticoids,
    some glucocorticoids
  Osmotic diuretics
  Sympathomimetics
  Tetracycline
  Theophylline
  Vitamin B_{12}

Hyperuricemia
  Aspirin
  Cytotoxics
  Ethacrynic acid
  Furosemide
  Hyperalimentation
  Thiazides
Hyponatremia
  1. Dilutional:
    Carbamazepine
    Chlorpropamide
    Cyclophosphamide
    Diuretics
    Vincristine
  2. Salt wasting:
    Diuretics
    Enemas
    Mannitol
Metabolic acidosis
  Acetazolamide
  Paraldehyde
  Salicylates
  Spironolactone

IV DERMATOLOGIC MANIFESTATIONS

Acne
  Anabolic and androgenic
    steroids
  Bromides
  Glucocorticoids
  Iodides
  Isoniazid
  Oral contraceptives
Alopecia
  Cytotoxics
  Ethionamide
  Heparin
  Oral contraceptives
    (withdrawal)
Eczema
  Captopril
  Cream and lotion
    preservatives
  Lanolin
  Topical antihistamines
  Topical antimicrobials
  Topical local anesthetics

Erythema multiforme or Steven-Johnson syndrome
  Barbiturates
  Chlorpropamide
  Codeine
  Penicillins
  Phenylbutazone
  Phenytoin
  Salicylates
  Sulfonamides
  Sulfones
  Tetracyclines
  Thiazides
Erythema nodosum
  Oral contraceptives
  Penicillins
  Sulfonamides
Exfoliative dermatitis
  Barbiturates
  Gold salts
  Penicillins
  Phenylbutazone
  Phenytoin
  Quinidine
  Sulfonamides

Continued

TABLE 189-1   Clinical manifestations of adverse reactions to drugs (*continued*)

IV DERMATOLOGIC MANIFESTATIONS (*Cont.*)

Fixed drug eruptions
  Barbiturates
  Captopril
  Phenylbutazone
  Quinine
  Salicylates
  Sulfonamides
Hyperpigmentation
  Bleomycin
  Busulfan
  Chloroquine and other
    antimalarials
  Corticotropin
  Cyclophosphamide
  Gold salts
  Hypervitaminosis A
  Oral contraceptives
  Phenothiazines
Lichenoid eruptions
  Aminosalicylic acid
  Antimalarials
  Chlorpropamide
  Gold salts
  Methyldopa
  Phenothiazines
Photodermatitis
  Captopril
  Chlordiazepoxide
  Furosemide
  Griseofulvin
  Nalidixic acid
  Oral contraceptives
  Phenothiazines
  Sulfonamides
  Sulfonylureas

  Tetracyclines, particulary
    demeclocycline
  Thiazides
Purpura (see also
  thrombocytopenia)
  Aspirin
  Glucocorticoids
Rashes (nonspecific)
  Allopurinol
  Ampicillin
  Barbiturates
  Indapamide
  Methyldopa
  Phenytoin
Skin necrosis
  Warfarin
Toxic epidermal necrolysis
(bullous)
  Allopurinol
  Barbiturates
  Bromides
  Iodides
  Nalidixic acid
  Penicillins
  Phenylbutazone
  Phenytoin
  Sulfonamides
Urticaria
  Aspirin
  Barbiturates
  Captopril
  Enalapril
  Penicillins
  Sulfonamides

V HEMATOLOGIC MANIFESTATIONS

Agranulocytosis (see also
  pancytopenia)
  Captopril
  Carbimazole
  Chloramphenicol
  Cytotoxics
  Gold salts
  Indomethacin
  Methimazole
  Oxyphenbutazone
  Phenothiazines

  Phenylbutazone
  Propylthiouracil
  Sulfonamides
  Tolbutamide
  Tricyclic antidepressants
Clotting abnormalities/
Hypothrombinemia
  Cefamandole
  Cefoperazone
  Moxalactam

Continued

TABLE 189-1 Clinical manifestations of adverse reactions to drugs (*continued*)

V HEMATOLOGIC MANIFESTATIONS (*Cont.*)

Eosinophilia
  Aminosalicylic acid
  Chlorpropamide
  Erythromycin estolate
  Imipramine
  Methotrexate
  Nitrofurantoin
  Procarbazine
  Sulfonamides
Hemolytic anemia
  Aminosalicylic acid
  Cephalosporins
  Chlorpromazine
  Dapsone
  Insulin
  Isoniazid
  Levodopa
  Mefenamic acid
  Melphalan
  Methyldopa
  Penicillins
  Phenacetin
  Procainamide
  Quinidine
  Rifampin
  Sulfonamides
Hemolytic anemias in G6PD deficiency
  see Table 130-3
Leukocytosis
  Glucocorticoids
  Lithium
Lymphadenopathy
  Phenytoin
  Primidone
Megaloblastic anemia
  Folate antagonists
  Nitrous oxide
  Oral contraceptives
  Phenobarbital
  Phenytoin
  Primidone

  Triamterene
  Trimethoprim
Pancytopenia (aplastic anemia)
  Carbamazepine
  Chloramphenicol
  Cytotoxics
  Gold salts
  Mephenytoin
  ✳ Phenylbutazone
  Phenytoin
  Quinacrine
  Sulfonamides
  Trimethadione
  Zidovudine (AZT)
Pure red cell aplasia
  Azathioprine
  Chlorpropamide
  Isoniazid
  Phenytoin
Thrombocytopenia
  (see also pancytopenia)
  Acetazolamine
  Aspirin
  Carbamazepine
  Carbenicillin
  Chlorpropamide
  Chlorthalidone
  Furosemide
  Gold salts
  Heparin
  Indomethacin
  Isoniazid
  Methyldopa
  Moxalactam
  Phenylbutazone
  Phenytoin and other hydantoins
  Quinidine
  Quinine
  Thiazides
  Ticarcillin

VI CARDIOVASCULAR MANIFESTATIONS

Angina exacerbation
  Alpha blockers
  Ergotamine
  Excessive thyroxine
  Hydralazine

  Methysergide
  Minoxidil
  Nifedipine
  Oxytocin
  Propranolol withdrawal

Continued

TABLE 189-1   Clinical manifestations of adverse reactions to drugs (*continued*)

VI CARDIOVASCULAR MANIFESTATIONS (*Cont.*)

Angina exacerbation (*Cont.*)
  Vasopressin
Arrhythmias
  Adriamycin
  Antiarrhythmic drugs
  Atropine
  Anticholinesterases
  Beta blockers
  Digitalis
  Emetine
  Lithium
  Papverine
  Phenothiazines
  Sympathomimetics
  Thyroid hormone
  Tricyclic antidepressants
  Verapamil
AV block
  Clonidine
  Methyldopa
  Verapamil
Cardiomyopathy
  Adriamycin
  Daunorubicin
  Emetine
  Lithium
  Penothiazines
  Sulfonamides
  Sympathomimetics
Fluid retention or congestive heart failure
  Diazoxide
  Estrogens
  Indomethacin
  Mannitol
  Minoxidil

  Phenylbutazone
  Propranolol
  Steroids
  Verapamil
Hypotension
  Calcium channel blockers
  Citrated blood
  Diuretics
  Levodopa
  Morphine
  Nitroglycerin
  Phenothiazines
  Protamine
  Quinidine
Hypertension
  Clonidine withdrawal
  Corticotropin
  Cyclosporine
  Glucocorticoids
  Monoamine oxidase
    inhibitors with
    sympathomimetics
  NSAIDs (some)
  Oral contraceptives
  Sympathomimetics
  Tricyclic antidepressants
    with sympathomimetics
Pericarditis
  Emetine
  Hydralazine
  Methysergide
  Procainamide
Thromboembolism
  Oral contraceptives

VII RESPIRATORY MANIFESTATIONS

Airway obstruction
  Beta blockers
  Cephalosporins
  Cholinergic drugs
  NSAIDs
  Penicillins
  Pentazocine
  Streptomycin
  Tartrazine (drugs with yellow
    dye)

Cough
  ACE inhibitors
Pulmonary edema
  Contrast media
  Heroin
  Methadone
  Propoxyphene
Pulmonary infiltrates
  Amiodarone
  Azothioprine

Continued

TABLE 189-1   Clinical manifestations of adverse reactions to drugs (*continued*)

VII RESPIRATORY MANIFESTATIONS (*Cont.*)

Pulmonary infiltrates (*Cont.*)
  Bleomycin
  Busulfan
  Carmustine (BCNU)
  Chlorambucil
  Cyclophosphamide
  Melphalan
  Methotrexate
  Methysergide
  Mitomycin C
  Nitrofurantoin
  Procarbazine
  Sulfonamides

VIII GASTROINTESTINAL MANIFESTATIONS

Cholestatic jaundice
  Anabolic steroids
  Androgens
  Chlorpropamide
  Erythromycin estolate
  Gold salts
  Methimazole
  Nitrofurantoin
  Oral contraceptives
  Phenothiazines
Constipation or ileus
  Aluminum hydroxide
  Barium sulfate
  Calcium carbonate
  Ferrous sulfate
  Ion exchange resins
  Opiates
  Phenothiazines
  Tricyclic antidepressants
  Verapamil
Diarrhea or colitis
  Antibiotics (broad-
    spectrum)
  Colchicine
  Digitalis
  Magnesium in antacids
  Methyldopa
Diffuse hepatocellular damage
  Acetaminophen
    (paracetamol)
  Allopurinol
  Aminosalicylic acid
  Dapsone
  Erythromycin estolate
  Ethionamide
  Glyburide
  Halothane
  Isoniazid
  Ketoconazole
  Methimazole
  Methotrexate
  Methoxyflurane
  Methyldopa
  Monoamine oxidase inhibitors
  Niacin
  Nifedipine
  Nitrofurantoin
  Phenytoin
  Propoxyphene
  Propylthiouracil
  Pyridium
  Rifampin
  Salicylates
  Sodium valproate
  Sulfonamides
  Tetracyclines
  Verapamil
  Zidovudine (AZT)
Intestinal ulceration
  Solid KCl preparations
Malabsorption
  Aminosalicylic acid
  Antibiotics (broad-
    spectrum)
  Cholestyramine
  Colchicine
  Colestipol
  Cytotoxics
  Neomycin
  Phenobarbital
  Phenytoin
Nausea or vomiting
  Digitalis
  Estrogens
  Ferrous sulfate
  Levodopa
  Opiates

Continued

TABLE 189-1 Clinical manifestations of adverse reactions to drugs (*continued*)

VIII GASTROINTESTINAL MANIFESTATIONS (*Cont.*)

Nausea or vomiting (*Cont.*)
  Potassium chloride
  Tetracyclines
  Theophylline
Oral conditions
1. Gingival hyperplasia:
  Calcium antagonists
  Cyclosporine
  Phenytoin
2. Salivary gland swelling:
  Bretylium
  Clonidine
  Guanethidine
  Iodides
  Phenylbutazone
3. Taste disturbances:
  Biguanides
  Captopril
  Griseofulvin
  Lithium
  Metronidazole
  Penicillamine
  Rifampin

4. Ulceration:
  Aspirin
  Cytotoxics
  Gentian violet
  Isoproterenol (sublingual)
  Pancreatin
Pancreatitis
  Azathioprine
  Ethacrynic acid
  Furosemide
  Glucocorticoids
  Opiates
  Oral contracaptives
  Sulfonamides
  Thiazides
Peptic ulceration or hemorrhage
  Aspirin
  Ethacrynic acid
  Glucocoricoids
  NSAIDs

IX RENAL/URINARY MANIFESTATIONS

Bladder dysfunction
  Anticholinergics
  Disopyramide
  Monoamine oxidase inhibitors
  Tricyclic antidepressants
Calculi
  Acetazolamide
  Vitamin D
Concentrating defect with polyuria (or nephrogenic diabetes insipidus)
  Demeclocycline
  Lithium
  Methoxyflurane
  Vitamin D
Hemorrhagic cystitis
  Cyclophosphamide
Interstitial nephritis
  Allopurinol
  Furosemide
  Penicillins, esp.
    methicillin
  Phenindione

Sulfonamides
Thiazides
Nephropathies
  Due to analgesics (e.g., phenacetin)
Nephrotic syndrome
  Captopril
  Gold salts
  Penicillamine
  Phenindione
  Probenecid
Obstructive uropathy
  Extrarenal: methysergide
  Intrarenal: cytotoxics
Renal dysfunction
  Cyclosporine
  NSAIDS
  Triamterene
Renal tubular acidosis
  Acetazolamide
  Amphotericin B
  Degraded tetracycline
Tubular necrosis
  Aminoglycosides

Continued

TABLE 189-1   Clinical manifestations of adverse reactions to drugs (*continued*)

IX RENAL/URINARY MANIFESTATIONS (*Cont.*)

Tubular necrosis (*Cont.*)
  Amphotericin B
  Colistin
  Cyclosporin
  Methoxyflurane

  Polymyxins
  Radioiodinated contrast
    medium
  Sulfonamides
  Tetracyclines

X NEUROLOGIC MANIFESTATIONS

Exacerbation of myasthenia
  Aminoglycosides
  Polymyxins
Extrapyramidal effects
  Butyrophenones,
    e.g., haloperidol
  Levodopa
  Methyldopa
  Metoclopramide
  Oral contraceptives
  Phenothiazines
  Tricyclic antidepressants
Headache
  Ergotamine (withdrawal)
  Glyceryl trinitrate
  Hydralazine
  Indomethacin
Peripheral neuropathy
  Amiodarone
  Chloramphenicol
  Chloroquine
  Chlorpropamide
  Clofibrate
  Demeclocycline
  Disopyramide
  Ethambutol
  Ethionamide
  Glutethimide
  Hydralazine
  Isoniazid
  Methysergide
  Metronidazole

  Nalidixic acid
  Nitrofurantoin
  Phenytoin
  Polymyxin, colistin
  Procarbazine
  Streptomycin
  Tolbutamide
  Tricyclic antidepressants
  Vincristine
**Pseudotumor cerebri (or
intracranial hypertension)**
  Amiodarone
  Glucocorticoids,
    mineralocorticoids
  Hypervitaminosis A
  Oral contraceptives
  Tetracyclines
Seizures
  Amphetamines
  Analeptics
  Isoniazid
  Lidocaine
  Lithium
  Nalidixic acid
  Penicillins
  Phenothiazines
  Physostigmine
  Theophylline
  Tricyclic antidepressants
  Vincristine
Stroke
  Oral contraceptives

XI OCULAR MANIFESTATIONS

Cataracts
  Busulfan
  Chlorambucil
  Glucocorticoids
  Phenothiazines
Color vision alteration
  Barbiturates

  Digitalis
  Methaqualone
  Streptomycin
  Thiazides
Corneal edema
  Oral contraceptives

Continued

TABLE 189-1   Clinical manifestations of adverse reactions to drugs (continued)

XI OCULAR MANIFESTATIONS (*Cont.*)

Corneal opacities
  Chloroquine
  Indomethacin
  Mepacrine
  Vitamin D
Glaucoma
  Mydriatics
  Sympathomimetics
Optic neuritis
  Aminosalicylic acid
  Chloramphenicol

  Ethambutol
  Isoniazid
  Penicillamine
  Phenothiazines
  Phenylbutazone
  Quinine
  Streptomycin
Retinopathy
  Chloroqine
  Phenothiazines

XII EAR MANIFESTATIONS

Deafness
  Aminoglycosides
  Aspirin
  Bleomycin
  Chloroquine
  Erythromycin
  Ethacrynic acid

  Furosemide
  Nortriptyline
  Quinine
Vestibular disorders
  Aminoglycosides
  Quinine

XIII MUSCULOSKELETAL MANIFESTATIONS

Bone disorders
1. Osteoporosis:
  Glucocorticoids
  Heparin
2. Osteomalacia:
  Aluminum hydroxide
  Anticonvulsants
  Glutethimide

Myopathy or myalgia
  Amphotericin B
  Chloroquine
  Clofibrate
  Glucocorticoids
  Oral contraceptives
Myositis
  Lovastatin

XIV PSYCHIATRIC MANIFESTATIONS

Delirious or confusional states
  Amantadine
  Aminophylline
  Anticholinergics
  Antidepressants
  Cimetidine
  Digitalis
  Glucocorticoids
  Isoniazid
  Levodopa
  Methyldopa
  Penicillins
  Phenothiazines
  Sedatives and hypnotics

Depression
  Amphetamine withdrawal
  Beta blockers
  Centrally acting
    antihypertensives
    (reserpine, methyldopa,
    clonidine)
  Glucocorticoids
  Levodopa
Drowsiness
  Antihistamines
  Anxiolytic drugs
  Clonidine
  Major tranquilizers

Continued

TABLE 189-1 Clinical manifestations of adverse reactions to drugs (continued)

XIV PSYCHIATRIC MANIFESTATIONS (*Cont.*)

Drowsiness (*Cont.*)
  Methyldopa
  Tricyclic antidepressants
Hallucinatory states
  Amantadine
  Beta blockers
  Levodopa
  Meperidine
  Narcotics
  Pentazocine
  Tricyclic antidepressants
Hypomania, mania, or excited reactions
  Glucocorticoids
  Levodopa
  Monoamine oxidase inhibitors
  Sympathomimetics

  Tricyclic antidepressants
Schizophrenic-like or paranoid reactions
  Amphetamines
  Bromides
  Glucocorticoids
  Levodopa
  Lysergic acid
  Monoamine oxidase inhibitors
  Tricyclic antidepressants
Sleep disturbances
  Anorexiants
  Levodopa
  Monoamine oxidase inhibitors
  Sympathomimetics

Adapted from Wood AJJ, Oates JA: HPIM-12, p. 375.

For a more detailed discussion, see Wood AJJ, Oates JA: Adverse Reactions to Drugs, Chap. 66, in HPIM-12, p. 373

SECTION 16

---

190 LABORATORY VALUES OF CLINICAL IMPORTANCE

The system of international units (SI, Système International d'Unités) is now used in most countries and in virtually all medical and scientific journals. However, many clinical laboratories report values in traditional units. Therefore, both systems are utilized for the Appendix and for the text itself. Values in SI units appear first, and *traditional units appear in parentheses* after the SI units. This dual system is also followed in large part in the text. In those instances in which the numbers remain the same but only the terminology is changed (mmol/L for meq/L or IU/L for mIU/mL) only the SI units are given. In all other instances in the text the SI unit is followed by the traditional unit in parentheses. For a more complete listing, consult the Appendix of HPIM-12, pp. A-1 to A-10.

$$mmol/L = \frac{mg/dL \times 10}{atomic\ weight};$$

$$mg/dL = \frac{mmol/L \times atomic\ weight}{10}$$

BODY FLUIDS AND OTHER MASS DATA

Body fluid, total volume: 50% (in obese) to 70% (lean) of body weight
 Intracellular: 30–40% of body weight
 Extracellular: 20–30% of body weight
Blood:
 Total volume:
  Males: 69 mL/kg body weight
  Females: 65 mL/kg body weight
 Plasma volume:
  Males: 39 mL/kg body weight
  Females: 40 mL/kg body weight

RBC volume:
  Males: 30 mL/kg body weight (1.15–1.21 L/m² body surface area)
  Females: 25 mL/kg body weight (0.95–1.00 L/m² body surface area)

$$\text{Body surface area (m}^2) = \frac{(\text{wt in kg})^{0.425} \times (\text{ht in cm})^{0.725}}{139.315}$$

CSF

Glucose 2.2–3.9 mmol/L (40–70 mg/dL)
Total protein 0.2–0.4 g/L (20–45 mg/dL)
CSF pressure 50–180 mmH₂O
Leukocytes:
  Total <4 per mm³
  Differential:
    Lymphocytes 60–70%
    Monocytes 30–50%
    Neutrophils 1–3%

CHEMICAL CONSTITUENTS OF BLOOD

Albumin, serum: 35–55 g/L (3.5–5.5 g/dL)
Aldolase: 0–100 nkat/L (0–6 U/L)
Aminotransferases, serum:
  Aspartate (AST, SGOT): 0–0.58 μkat/L (0–35 U/L)
  Alanine (ALT, SGPT): 0–0.58 μkat/L (0–35 U/L)
Ammonia, whole blood, venous: 47–65 μmol/L (80–110 μg/dL)
Amylase, serum: 0.8–3.2 μkat/L (60–80 U/L)
Arterial blood gases:
  [HCO₃⁻]: 21–28 mmol/L (21–28 meq/L)
  P_{CO_2}: 4.7–6.0 kPa (35–45 mmHg)
  pH: 7.38–7.44
  P_{O_2}: 11–13 kPa (80–100 mmHg)
Bilirubin, total, serum (Malloy-Evelyn): 5.1–17 μmol/L (0.3–1.0 mg/dL)
  Direct, serum: 1.7–5.1 μmol/L (0.1–0.3 mg/dL)
  Indirect, serum: 3.4–12 μmol/L (0.2–0.7 mg/dL)
Calcium, ionized: 1.1–1.4 mmol/L (2.3–2.8 meq/L; 4.5–5.6 mg/dL)
Calcium, plasma: 2.2–2.6 mmol/L (4.5–5.5 meq/L; 9–10.5 mg/dL)
Carbon dioxide content, plasma (sea level): 22–38 mmol/L (27–28 meq/L)
Carbon dioxide tension (P_{CO_2}), arterial blood (sea level): 4.7–6.0 kPa (35–45 mmHg)

Chloride, serum: 98–106 mmol/L (98–106 meq/L)
Cholesterol, plasma:
  <29 years: <5.20 mmol/L (<200 mg/dL)
  30–39 years: <5.85 mmol/L (<225 mg/dL)
  40–49 years: <6.35 mmol/L (<245 mg/dL)
  >50 years: <6.85 mmol/L (<265 mg/dL)
Complement, serum:
  C3: 0.55–1.20 g/L (55–120 mg/dL)
  C4: 0.20–0.50 g/L (20–50 mg/dL)
Creatinine, serum: <133 μmol/L (<1.5 mg/dL)
Creatine phosphokinase, serum (total):
  Females: 0.17–1.17 μkat/L (10–70 U/L)
  Males: 0.42–1.50 μkat/L (25–90 U/L)
  Isoenzymes, serum: fraction 2 (MB) <5% of total
Digoxin, serum:
  Therapeutic level: 0.6–2.8 mmol/L (0.5–2.2 ng/mL)
  Toxic level: >3.1 mmol/L (>2.4 ng/mL)
Ethanol, plasma:
  Moderate intoxication 17–43 mmol/L (80–200 mg/dL)
  Marked intoxication   54–87 mmol/L (250–400 mg/dL)
  Severe intoxication   >87 mmol/L (>400 mg/dL)
Ferritin, serum: 15–200 μg/L (15–200 ng/mL)
Glucose (fasting), plasma:
  Normal: 4.2–6.4 mmol/L (75–115 mg/dL)
  Diabetes mellitus: >7.8 mmol/L (>140 mg/dL) (on more than one occasion)
Glucose, 2-h postprandial, plasma:
  Normal: <7.8 mmol/L (<140 mg/dL)
  Impaired glucose tolerance: 7.8–11.1 mmol/L (140–200 mg/dL)
  Diabetes mellitus: >11.1 mmol/L (>200 mg/dL) (on more than one occasion)
Hemoglobin, blood (sea level):
  Males: 140–180 g/L (14–18 g/dL)
  Females: 120–160 g/L (12–16 g/dL)
  Hemoglobin A_{1c}: Up to 6% of total hemoglobin
Immunoglobulins, serum:
  IgA: 0.9–3.2 g/L (90–325 mg/dL)
  IgD: 0–0.08 g/L (0–8 mg/dL)
  IgE: <0.00025 g/L (<0.025 mg/dL)
  IgG: 8.0–15.0 g/L (800–1500 mg/dL)
  IgM: 0.45–1.5 g/L (45–150 mg/dL)
Iron, serum: 14–32 μmol/L (80–180 μg/dL)
Iron-binding capacity, serum: 45–82 μmol/L (250–460 μg/dL)
  Saturation: 20–45%
Lactate dehydrogenase, serum:
  200–450 U/mL (Wrobleski)
  60–100 U/mL (Wacker)
  0.4–1.7 μkat/L (25–100 U/L)

Lipoproteins, plasma:
  LDL cholesterol: 1.3–4.9 mmol/L (50–190 mg/dL)
  HDL cholesterol: 0.8–2.4 mmol/L (30–90 mg/dL)
Magnesium, serum: 0.8–1.2 mmol/L (2–3 mg/dL)
Osmolality, plasma: 285–295 mosmol/kg of serum water
Phenytoin, plasma:
  Therapeutic range: 40–80 μmol/L (10–20 mg/L)
  Toxic level: >120 μmol/L (>30 mg/L)
Phosphatase, acid, serum: 0.90 nkat/L (0–5.5 U/L)
Phosphatase, alkaline, serum: 0.5–2.0 μkat/L (30–120 U/L)
Phosphorus, inorg., serum: 1.0–1.4 mmol/L (3–4.5 mg/dL)
Potassium, serum: 3.5–5.0 mmol/L (3.5–5.0 meq/L)
Proteins, total, serum: 55–80 g/L (5.5–8.0 g/dL)
Protein fractions, serum:
  Albumin: 35–55 g/L (3.5–5.0 g/dL) (50–60%)
  Globulin: 20–35 g/L (2.0–3.5 g/dL) (40–50%)
  Alpha$_1$: 2–4 g/L (0.2–0.4 g/dL) (4.2–7.2%)
  Alpha$_2$: 5–9 g/L (0.5–0.9 g/dL) (6.8–12%)
  Beta: 6–11 g/L (0.6–1.1 g/dL) (9.3–15%)
  Gamma: 7–17 g/L (0.7–1.7 g/dL) (13–23%)
Sodium, serum: 136–145 mmol/L (136–145 meq/L)
Triglycerides, plasma: <1.8 mmol/L (<60 mg/dL)
Urea nitrogen, serum: 3.6–7.1 mmol/L (10–20 mg/dL)
Uric acid, serum:
  Men: 0.15–0.48 mmol/L (2.5–8.0 mg/dL)
  Women: 0.09–0.36 mmol/L (1.5–6.0 mg/dL)

FUNCTION TESTS

Circulation

Cardiac output (Fick): 2.5–3.6 L/m^2 body surface area per min
Ejection fraction, stroke volume/end-diastolic volume (SV/EDV): Normal range: 0.55–0.78, average 0.67
Pulmonary vascular resistance: 2–12 kPa·s/L [(20–120 (dyn·s)/cm^5]
Systemic vascular resistance: 770–1500 kPa·s/L [(770–1500 (dyn·s)/cm^5]

Gastrointestinal

D-Xylose absorption test: After an overnight fast, 25 g xylose is given PO in aqueous solution; urine collected for the following 5 h should contain 33–53 mmol (5–8 g) (or >20% of ingested dose); serum xylose should be 1.7–2.7 mmol/L (25–40 mg per 100 mL) 1 h after the oral dose.

Gastric juice:
Volume:
  24 h: 2–3 L
  Nocturnal: 600–700 mL
  Basal, fasting: 30–70 mL/h
pH: 1.6–1.8
Acid output:
  Basal:
    Females (mean ± 1 SD): 0.8 ± 0.5 μmol/s (2.0 ± 1.8 meq/h)
    Males (mean ± 1 SD): 0.8 ± 0.6 μmol/s (3.0 ± 2.0 meq/h)
  Maximal (after subcutaneous histamine acid phosphate 0.004 mg/kg and preceded by 50 mg promethazine; or after betazole 1.7 mg/kg or pentagastrin 6 μg/kg):
    Females: 4.4 ± 1.4 μmol/s (16 ± 5 meq/h)
    Males: 6.4 ± 1.4 μmol/s (23 ± 5 meq/h)
Secretin test (pancreatic exocrine function: 1 U/kg body weight, IV):
  Volume (pancreatic juice): >2.0 mL/kg in 80 min
  Bicarbonate concentration: >80 mmol/L (>80 meq/L)
  Bicarbonate output: >10 mmol in 30 min (>10 meq in 30 min)

Metabolic and endocrine

Cortisol:
  8 A.M. 140–690 nmol/L (5–25 μg/dL)
  4 P.M. 80–330 nmol/L (3–12 μg/dL)
Adrenal steroids, urinary excretion:
  Aldosterone: 14–53 nmol/d (5–19 μg/d)
  Cortisol, free: 54–275 nmol/d (20–100 μg/d)
  17-Hydroxycorticosteroids: 5.5–28 μmol/d (2–10 mg/d)
  17-Ketosteroids:
    Men: 24–88 μmol/d (7–25 mg/d)
    Women: 14–52 μmol/d (4–15 mg/d)
Estradiol:
  Women: 70–220 pmol/L (20–60 pg/mL), higher at ovulation
  Men: <180 pmol/L (<50 pg/mL)
Progesterone:
  Men, prepubertal girls, preovulatory women, and postmenopausal women: <6 nmol/L (2 ng/mL)
  Women, luteal, peak: >16 nmol/L (>5 ng/mL)
Testosterone:
  Women: <3.5 nmol/L (<1 ng/mL)
  Men: 10–35 nmol/L (3–10 ng/mL)
  Prepubertal boys and girls: 0.17–0.7 nmol/L (0.05–0.2 ng/mL)

Thyroid function tests:
  Radioactive iodine uptake, 24 h: 5–30% (range varies in different areas due to variations in iodine intake)
  Resin T_3 uptake: 25–35% (varies among laboratories)
  Thyroid-stimulating hormone (TSH): <5 mU/L (<5 µU/mL)
  Thyroxine (T_4), serum radioimmunoassay: 64–154 nmol/L (5–12 µg/dL)
  Triiodothyronine (T_3), plasma: 1.1–2.9 nmol/L (70–190 ng/dL)

Renal

Clearances (corrected to 1.72 m² body surface area):
  Inulin clearance (mean ± 1 SD):
    Males: 2.1 ± 0.4 mL/s (124 ± 25.8 mL/min)
    Females: 2.0 ± 0.2 mL/s (119 ± 12.8 mL/min)
  Endogenous creatinine clearance: 1.5–2.2 mL/5 (91–130 mL/min)
Concentration and dilution test:
  Specific gravity of urine:
    After 12-h fluid restriction: 1.025 or more
    After 12-h deliberate water intake: 1.003 or less

HEMATOLOGIC EXAMINATIONS
(See also "Chemical Constituents of Blood")

Carboxyhemoglobin:
  Nonsmoker: 0–2.3%
  Smoker: 2.1–4.2%
Hemoglobin, adults Female: 14 ± 2.0 g/dL
                      Male: 16.0 ± 2.0 g/dL
Haptoglobin, serum: 0.5–2.2 g/L (50–220 mg/dL)
Leukocytes, total, adults 4500–11,000 cells/µL

Differential count	Approx % of total
Segmented neutrophils	40–70
Bands	1–5
Lymphocytes	20–50
Monocytes	2–6
Eosinophils	0–5
Basophils	0–3

Sedimentation rate:
  Westergren, <50 years of age:
    Males: 0–15 mm/h
    Females: 0–20 mm/h
  Westergren, >50 years of age:
    Males: 0–20 mm/h
    Females: 0–30 mm/h

Fibrinogen: 2–4 g/L (200–400 mg/dL)
Fibrin split products: <10 mg/L (<10 μg/mL)
Platelets: 130,000–400,000/mm³

URINE

Creatinine: 8.8–14 mmol/d (1.0–1.6 g/d)
Protein: <0.15 g/d (<150 mg/d)
Potassium: 25–100 mmol/d (25–100 meq/d) (varies with intake)
Sodium: 100–260 mmol/d (100–260 meq/d) (varies with intake)

Note: Page numbers with the letters f or t indicate figures and tables, respectively.